International Textbook of Obesity

Dedicated to Jules Hirsch

International Textbook of Obesity

Edited by

Per Björntorp

Sahlgrenska Hospital, Göteborg, Sweden

JOHN WILEY & SONS, LTD

Chichester • New York • Weinheim • Brisbane • Singapore • Toronto

Cover illustration copyright ©
Sofia Karlsson and Lars Sjöström.
Reproduced by permission.

Other Wiley Editorial Offices

John Wiley & Sons, Inc., 605 Third Avenue,
New York, NY 10158-0012, USA

WILEY-VCH Verlag GmbH, Pappelallee 3,
D-69469 Weinheim, Germany

John Wiley & Sons Australia, Ltd., 33 Park Road, Milton,
Queensland 4064, Australia

John Wiley & Sons (Asia) Pte, Ltd., 2 Clementi Loop #02-01,
Jin Xing Distripark, Singapore 129809

John Wiley & Sons (Canada), Ltd., 22 Worcester Road,
Rexdale, Ontario M9W 1L1, Canada

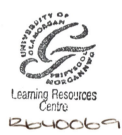

Library of Congress Cataloging-in-Publication Data

International textbook of obesity / edited by Per Björntorp,
     p.   cm.
  Includes bibliographical references and index.
  ISBN 0-471-98870-7 (cased)
  1. Obesity.   I. Björntorp, Per.

RC628.I58 2001
616.3′98—dc21   00-048591

British Library Cataloguing in Publication Data

A catalogue record for this book is available from the British Library

ISBN 0-471-98870-7

Typeset in 10/11.5pt Times from the author's disks by Vision Typesetting, Manchester
Printed and bound in Great Britain by Bookcraft (Bath) Ltd, Midsomer Norton, Somerset
This book is printed on acid-free paper responsibly manufactured from sustainable forestry,
in which at least two trees are planted for each one used for paper production.

Contents

Contributors

David B. Allison *Obesity Research Center, St Lukes/Roosevelt Hospital Center, 1090 Amsterdam Avenue, 14th Floor, New York, NY 10025, USA*
Email: dba8@columbia.edu

Björn Andersson *Department of Medicine, Sahlgrenska University Hospital, University of Göteborg, S-413 45 Göteborg, Sweden*
Email: bjorn.andersson@medfak.gu.se

Vicki J. Antipatis MSc *International Obesity Task Force, Rowett Research Institute, Greenburn Road, Bucksburn, Aberdeen AB21 9SB, UK*
Email: Vantipatis@aol.com

Angelo Avogaro *Department of Clinical and Experimental Medicine, University of Padova, Via Giustiniani 2, 35100 Padova, Italy*

Bengt-Åke Bengtsson *Research Center for Endocrinology and Metabolism, Sahlgrenska University Hospital, University of Göteborg, S-413 45 Göteborg, Sweden*

Per Björntorp MD PhD *Professor, Department of Heart and Lung Diseases, Sahlgrenska University Hospital, University of Göteborg, S-413 45 Göteborg, Sweden*
Email: Per.Bjorntorp@hjl.gu.se

George L. Blackburn MD PhD *Professor and Director of Nutritional Services, Department of Surgery, Beth Israel Deaconess Hospital, 330 Brookline Avenue, Boston MA 02215, USA*
Email: gblackbu@bidmc.harvard.edu

John E. Blundell *BioPsychology Group, University of Leeds, Leeds LS2 9JT, UK*
Email: J.E.Blundell@leeds.ac.uk

Leif Breum MD *Department of Medicine, Endocrine Unit, Køge Hospital, DK-4600 Køge, Denmark*
Email: leif.breum@dadlnet.dk

Maximilian P. de Courten MD MPH *International Diabetes Institute, 260 Kooyong Road, Caulfield Vic 3162, Australia*

Ivo H. De Leeuw *Department of Endocrinology, Metabolism and Clinical Nutrition, University Hospital Antwerp, Wilrijkstraat 10, 2650 Edegem, Antwerp, Belgium*

Jean-Pierre Després *Division of Kinesiology and Department of Food Sciences and Nutrition, Laval University, Ste-Foy, Quebec, Canada G1K 7P4*

Björn Ekblom *Department of Physiology and Pharmacology, Lidingövägen 2, Karolinska Institute, 11486 Stockholm, Sweden*

Madelyn H. Fernstrom PhD *Professor, Weight Management Center, University of Pittsburgh School of Medicine, Western Psychiatric Institute and Clinic, 3811 O'Hara Street, Pittsburgh PA 15213, USA*
Email: fernstrommh@msx.upmc.edu

Kevin R. Fontaine *Department of Medicine, Division of Gerontology, University of Maryland, VA Medical Center, Baltimore, Maryland, USA*

Tim P. Gill PhD RPHNutr *International Obesity TaskForce, Rowett Research Institute, Greenburn Road, Bucksburn, Aberdeen AB21 9SB, UK*
Email: tim.gill@iotf.org

Ronald R. Grunstein FRACP PhD MD *Centre for Respiratory Failure and Sleep Disorders, Level 9, E Block, Royal Prince Alfred Hospital, Camperdown, Sydney NSW 2050, Australia*
Email: rrg@mail.med.usyd.edu.au

T.S. Han PhD   *Wolfson College, University of Cambridge, Cambridge CB3 9BB, UK*
Email: tsh24@cam.ac.uk

Barbara C. Hansen PhD   *Professor and Director, Obesity and Diabetes Research Center, University of Maryland School of Medicine, 10 South Pine Street #6-00, Baltimore, Maryland 21201, USA*
Email: bchansen@aol.com

Helen H. Harris   *PHLS Communicable Disease Surveillance Centre, 61 Collindale Avenue, London NW9 5EQ, UK*
Email: HHarris@phls.org.uk

Berit Lilienthal Heitman   *Institute of Preventive Medicine, Copenhagen Health Services, Copenhagen Municipal Hospital, DK-1399 Copenhagen K, Denmark*
Email: Behe@glostruphosp.kbhamt.dk

Moonseong Heo   *Obesity Research Center, St Luke's/Roosevelt Center, 1090 Amsterdam Avenue, 14th Floor, New York, NY 10025, USA*

S. Heshka   *St Luke's/Roosevelt Hospital Center, 1111 Amsterdam Avenue, New York, NY 10025, USA*

Steven B. Heymsfield PhD   *Weight Control Unit, Obesity Research Center, St Luke's/Roosevelt Hospital Center, 1090 Amsterdam Avenue, 14th Floor, New York, NY 10025, USA*
Email: SBH2@Columbia.edu

Michael Hill DSc FRCPath   *Chairman, European Cancer Prevention Organisation; Professor, Nutrition Research Centre, South Bank University, 103 Borough Road, London SE1 0AA, UK*

Allison M. Hodge BAgSc BSc GradDipDiet   *International Diabetes Institute, 260 Kooyong Road, Caulfield, Victoria 3162, Australia*
Email: ahodge@accv.org.au

Daniel J. Hoffman PhD MPH   *Obesity Research Center, St Luke's/Roosevelt Medical Center, 1090 Amsterdam Avenue, 14th Floor, New York, NY 10025, USA*
Email: djh100@columbia.edu

Bernard Jeanrenaud   *Lilly Research Laboratories, Division of Endocrine Research and Clinical Investigation, Lilly Corporate Center, Indianapolis, Indiana 46285, USA*

Susan A. Jebb   *MRC Human Nutrition Research, Downhams Lane, Cambridge CB4 1XJ, UK*
Email: Susan.Jebb@mrc-hnr.cam.ac.uk

Gudmundur Johannsson   *Research Center for Endocrinology and Metabolism, Sahlgrenska University Hospital, University of Göteborg, S-413 45 Göteborg, Sweden*

Jan Karlsson   *Health Care Research Unit, Sahlgrenska University Hospital, University of Göteborg, S-413 45 Göteborg, Sweden*

Lalita Khaodhiar MD   *Fellow in Clinical Nutrition, Beth Israel Deaconess Medical Center, 1 Autumn Street, Harvard Medical School, Boston, Massachusetts 02215, USA*

Robert C. Klesges PhD   *University of Memphis Center for Community Health, 5350 Poplar Avenue, Memphis, TN 38119, USA*

John G. Kral MD PhD   *SUNY Downstate Medical Center, 450 Clarkson Avenue, Box 40, Brooklyn, New York 11203, USA*
Email: jgkral@hscbklyn.edu

M.E.J. Lean MA MD FRCP   *Department of Human Nutrition, University of Glasgow, Glasgow Royal Infirmary, Glasgow G31 2ER, UK*
Email: mej.lean@clinmed.gla.ac.uk

Bernt Lindahl MD   *Behavioural Medicine, Department of Public Health and Clinical Medicine, Umeå University, SE-901 87 Umeå, Sweden*
Email: bernt.lindahl@medicin.umu.se

Lauren Lissner   *Department of Medicine, Sahlgrenska University Hospital, University of Göteborg, S-413 45 Göteborg, Sweden*

Ilse L. Mertens   *Department of Endocrinology, Metabolism and Clinical Nutrition, University Hospital Antwerp, Wilrijkstraat 10, 2650 Edegem, Antwerp, Belgium*

Renato Pasquali MD   *Endocrinology Unit, Department of Internal Medicine and Gastroenterology, S. Orsola-Malphighi Hospital, Via Massarenti 9, 40138 Bologna, Italy*
Email: rpasqual@almadns.unibo.it

C.M. Pond   *Department of Biology, The Open University, Milton Keynes MK7 6AA, UK*
Email: C.M.Pond@open.ac.uk

Andrew M. Prentice   *MRC Human Nutrition Research, Elsie Widdarson Laboratory, Fulbourn Road, Cambridge CB1 9NL, UK*
Email: Andrew.Prentice@lshtm.ac.uk

Tracey D. Robinson MB BS FRACP   *Centre for Respiratory Failure and Sleep Disorders, Royal Prince Alfred Hospital, Camperdown, Sydney NSW 2050, Australia*
Email: traceyr@mail.med.usyd.edu.au

Françoise Rohner-Jeanrenaud   *Laboratoires de Recherches Metaboliques, Geneva University School of Medicine, Geneva, Switzerland*
Email: Jeanrenaud—Francoise@Lilly.com

Roland Rosmond   *Department of Heart and Lung Diseases, Sahlgrenska University Hospital, University of Göteborg, S-413 45 Göteborg, Sweden*

Stephan Rössner   *Professor, Obesity Unit, M73, Huddinge University Hospital, S-141 86 Stockholm, Sweden*
Email: Stephan.Rossner@medhs.ki.se

Jonathan R. Seckl   *University of Edinburgh, Endocrinology Unit, Department of Medical Sciences, Western General Hospital, Edinburgh EH4 2XU, UK*

Jacob C. Seidell PhD   *Department of Chronic Diseases Epidemiology, National Institute of Public Health and Environmental Protection, Institute for Research in Extramural Medicine, Free University Amsterdam, PO Box 1, 3720 BA Bilthoven, Amsterdam, The Netherlands*
Email: j.seidell@rivm.nl

Carol A. Shively PhD   *Department of Pathology (Comparative Medicine), Wake Forest University School of Medicine, Medical Center Boulevard, Winston-Salem, NC 27157-1040, USA*
Email: cschively@cpm.wfubmc.edu

Lars Sjöström   *Department of Internal Medicine, Sahlgrenska University Hospital, University of Göteborg, S-413 45 Göteborg, Sweden*
Email: lars.sjostrom@medfak.gu.se

Jeffery Sobal PhD MPH   *Division of Nutritional Sciences, Cornell University, 303 MVR Hall, Ithaca NY 14853, USA*
Email: js57@cornell.edu

Marianne Sullivan   *Professor, Health Care Research Unit, Sahlgrenska University Hospital, University of Göteborg, SE-413 45 Göteborg, Sweden*
Email: healthcare.research@medicine.gu.se

Charles Taft   *Health Care Research Unit, Sahlgrenska University Hospital, University of Göteborg, SE-413 45 Göteborg, Sweden*

Corrado Testolin   *Obesity Research Center, St Luke's/Roosevelt Hospital Medical Center, 1090 Amsterdam Avenue, 14th Floor, New York, NY 10025, USA*

Antonio Tiengo   *Department of Clinical and Experimental Medicine, University of Padova, Via Giustiniani 2, 35100 Padova, Italy*
Email: tiengo@ux1.unipd.it

Angelo Tremblay   *Division of Kinesiology and Department of Food Sciences and Nutrition, Physical Activity Sciences Laboratory, Laval University, Ste-Foy, Quebec, Canada G1K 7P4*
Email: angelo.tremblay@kin.msp.ulaval.ca

Luc F. van Gaal   *Professor, Department of Endocrinology, Metabolism and Clinical Nutrition, University Hospital Antwerp, Wilrijkstraat 10, 2650 Edegem, Antwerp, Belgium*

Mark W. Vander Weg PhD   *Professor, University of Memphis Center for Community Health, 5350 Poplar Avenue, Memphis, TN 38119, USA*

Valentina Vicennati   *Endocrinology Unit, Department of Internal Medicine and Gastroenterology, S. Orsola-Malpighi Hospital, Via Massarenti 9, 40138 Bologna, Italy*

Brian R. Walker   *University of Edinburgh, Endocrinology Unit, Department of Medical Sciences, Western General Hospital, Edinburgh EH4 2XU, UK*
Email: B.Walker@ed.ac.uk

Jeanne M. Wallace   *Department of Pathology (Comparative Medicine), Wake Forest University School of Medicine, Medical Center Boulevard, Winston-Salem, NC 27157-1040, USA*

ZiMian Wang   *Obesity Research Center, St Luke's/Roosevelt Hospital Center, 1090 Amsterdam Avenue, 14th Floor, New York, NY 10025, USA*

Kenneth D. Ward PhD   *Assistant Professor,*
University of Memphis Center for Community
Health, 5350 Poplar Avenue, Suite 675, Memphis,
TN 38119, USA
Email: kdward@memphis.edu

Paul Zimmet MD PhD FRACP   *Professor,*
International Diabetes Institute, 260 Kooyong
Road, Caulfield, Victoria 3162, Australia
Email: pzimmet@netscace.net.au

Preface

Why another book on obesity? Recently we have seen several similar books of which some are very comprehensive. The finalizing of this book has been delayed. It was originally meant to be presented at the Paris Congress as another armament in the current worldwide fight against obesity. This first planned book was rather limited in contents, but it was eventually decided to cover additional fields, and here is the result.

The field of modern obesity research is fairly young and has expanded considerably with time. The 'pioneers' who began this research are still to a large extent active, and several have contributed to this book with reviews in their respective sub-speciality of obesity research. One ambition with the present book was to invite several younger researchers to write chapters. In this way new angles of the problem have been presented. Rethinking and research should go hand in hand.

Although things appear to improve, I have the impression that at least in certain countries obesity is still not considered with sufficient seriousness. The economic arguments seem to have made some politicians and decision makers raise their eyebrows. The involvement of central, international organizations in making recommendations should have an effect. National problems of obesity are now also the subject of surveys in several countries and counteractions are planned.

A major problem is, however, that we still have difficulties impressing ourselves on adjacent areas of research. To take one example, during a recent major congress on diabetes mellitus I asked a handful of leading diabetes researchers the following questions: Which is the major problem in diabetes research? Unanimous answer: diabetes mellitus type 2. Which is the most frequent risk factor or precursor state to this type of diabetes? Unanimous

answer: obesity. I then suggested that we should join forces and see what can be done to prevent and treat obesity more successfully than is possible today. This was met with considerable enthusiasm.

The obesity and diabetes fields are largely overlapping. As a matter of fact obesity might be considered as the first step towards diabetes, where beta-cell insufficiency is eventually added. I think it would be extremely useful for both fields to collaborate more than is now the case. In a way the current situation is reminiscent of the clinical subspecialization where various organs are treated by different specialists, who have difficulties in seeing the world outside the fence, and thereby miss important information that might benefit the patient. What we could do, as an initial step, is to reserve large parts of obesity meetings for diabetes and vice versa. Several presidents for upcoming congresses in both obesity and diabetes have, as a response to a direct question, agreed that this is a good idea, and we will see if this is only lip-service or if the idea has been taken seriously.

The concept of the metabolic syndrome, a syndrome strongly associated with abdominal obesity, has been very helpful in facilitating the realization that we are to a large extent dealing with a common background to prevalent diseases. The awareness of this syndrome has had the consequence that the complex obesity–insulin resistance–dyslipidaemia–hypertension is often discussed as a cluster in congresses of diabetes, cardiology and hypertension. The realization of this clustering of symptoms has also had an impact on clinical activities, and has led to work-up outside one particular specialty. It is now more frequent that hypertensiologists determine circulating lipids and that cardiologists examine insulin resistance, and, most importantly, register height, weight and body circumferences.

This is clearly a large step forward.

Writing chapters for a book like this is a major task, interfering with the activities of an already busy day. I would like to thank the contributors who have taken on the task of writing chapters for this book, and also Wiley who asked me to organize it. The collaboration with Michael Osuch and Hannah Bradley has been very pleasant.

Per Björntorp
University of Göteborg, Sweden

Part I

Epidemiology

Obesity as a Global Problem

Vicki J. Antipatis and Tim P. Gill

Rowett Research Institute, Aberdeen, UK

INTRODUCTION

Obesity is a major public health and economic problem of global significance. Prevalence rates are increasing in all parts of the world, both in affluent Western countries and in poorer nations. Men, women and children are affected. Indeed, overweight, obesity and health problems associated with them are now so common that they are replacing the more traditional public health concerns such as undernutrition and infectious disease as the most significant contributors to global ill health (1). In 1995, the excess adult mortality attributable to overnutrition was estimated to be about 1 million deaths, double the 0.5 million attributable to undernution (2).

This chapter looks at obesity as a global problem. It begins with a brief overview of methods of classification, a critical issue for estimating the extent of obesity in populations. The serious impact of excess body weight on individuals and societies throughout the world in terms of associated health, social and economic costs is considered next. The body of the chapter concentrates on current prevalence and trends of adult obesity rates around the world, including projections for the year 2025. Comment is made on key features and patterns of the global epidemic followed by discussion of the major factors that are driving it. An overview of the emerging childhood obesity problem is given next. The chapter concludes with a call for global action to tackle the epidemic.

WHAT IS OBESITY AND HOW IS IT MEASURED?

At the physiological level, obesity can be defined as a condition of abnormal or excessive fat accumulation in adipose tissue to the extent that health may be impaired. However, it is difficult to measure body fat directly and so surrogate measures such as the body mass index (BMI) are commonly used to indicate overweight and obesity in adults. Additional tools are available for identification of individuals with increased health risks due to 'central' fat distribution, and for the more detailed characterization of excess fat in special clinical situations and research.

Measuring General Obesity

The BMI provides the most useful and practical population-level indicator of overweight and obesity in adults. It is calculated by dividing bodyweight in kilograms by height in metres squared $(BMI = kg/m^2)$. Both height and weight are routinely collected in clinical and population health surveys.

In the new graded classification system developed by the World Health Organization (WHO), a BMI of $30 \, kg/m^2$ or above denotes obesity (Table 1.1). There is a high likelihood that individuals with a BMI at or above this level will have excessive body fat. However, the health risks associated with overweight and obesity appear to rise progressively

International Textbook of Obesity. Edited by Per Björntorp.

Table 1.1 Classification of overweight and obesity in adults according to BMI

Classification	BMI (kg/m^2)
Underweight	<18.5
Normal range	18.5–24.9
Overweight	≥25
Pre-obese	25.0–29.9
Obese class I	30.0–34.9
Obese class II	35–39.9
Obese class III	≥40

Source: WHO (1).

Table 1.2 Sex-specific waist circumference measurements for identification of individuals at increased health risk due to intra-abdominal fat accumulation

	Risk of metabolic complications	Waist circumference (cm)	
		Men	Women
Alerting zone	Increased	94	80
Action zone	Substantially increased	102	88

Adapted from WHO (1).

with increasing BMI from a value below 25 kg/m^2, and it has been demonstrated that there are benefits to having a measurement nearer 20–22 kg/m^2, at least within industrialized countries. To highlight the health risks that can exist at BMI values below the level of obesity, and to raise awareness of the need to prevent further weight gain beyond this level, the first category of overweight included in the new WHO classification system is termed 'pre-obese' (BMI 25–29.9 kg/m^2).

Caution is required when interpreting BMI measurements in certain individuals and ethnic groups. The relationship between BMI and body fat content varies according to body build and body proportion, and a given BMI may not correspond to the same degree of fatness across all populations. Recently, a meta-analysis among different ethnic groups showed that for the same level of body fat, age and gender, American blacks have a 1.3 kg/m^2 higher BMI and Polynesians have a 4.5 kg/m^2 higher BMI compared to Caucasians. By contrast, BMIs in Chinese, Ethiopians, Indonesians and Thais were shown to be 1.9, 4.6, 3.2 and 2.9 kg/m^2 lower than in Caucasians (3). This suggests that population-specific BMI cut-off points for obesity need to be developed.

Measuring Central Obesity

For a comprehensive estimate of weight-related health risk it is also desirable to assess the extent of intra-abdominal or 'central' fat accumulation. This can be done by simple and convenient measures such as the waist circumference or waist-to-hip ratio. Changes in these measures tend to reflect changes in risk factors for cardiovascular disease and other forms of chronic illness. Some experts

believe that a health risk classification based on waist circumference alone is more suitable as a health promotion tool than either BMI or waist-to-hip ratio, alone or in combination (4). Recent work from the Netherlands has indicated that a waist circumference greater than 102 cm in men, and greater than 88 cm in women, is associated with a substantially increased risk of obesity-related metabolic complications (Table 1.2). The level of health risk associated with a particular waist circumference or waist-to-hip ratio may vary across populations.

THE HEALTH, SOCIAL AND ECONOMIC COSTS ASSOCIATED WITH OVERWEIGHT AND OBESITY

There is reason to be concerned about overweight and obesity as overwhelming evidence links both to substantial health, social and economic costs.

Overview of the Health Costs

US figures suggest that about 61% of non-insulin-dependent diabetes mellitus (NIDDM) and 17% of both coronary heart disease (CHD) and hypertension can be attributed to obesity. Indeed, as a person's BMI creeps up through overweight into the obese category and beyond, the risk of developing a number of chronic non-communicable diseases such as NIDDM, CHD, gallbladder disease, and certain types of cancer increases rapidly. There is also a graded increase in relative risk of premature death (Figure 1.1).

Before life-threatening chronic disease develops, however, many overweight and obese patients de-

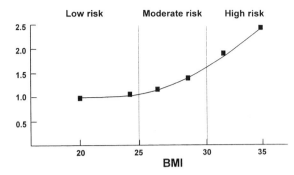

Figure 1.1 The relationship between risk of premature death and BMI. The figure is based on data from professional, white US women who have never smoked and illustrates the graded increase in relative risk of premature death as BMI increases. Adapted from WHO (1)

Table 1.3 Relative risk of health problems associated with obesity

Greatly increased (relative risk much greater than 3)	Moderately increased (relative risk 2–3)	Slightly increased (relative risk 1–2)
NIDDM	CDH	Certain cancers
Gallbladder disease	Hypertension	Reproductive hormone abnormalities
Dyslipidaemia	Osteoarthritis (knees)	Polycystic ovary syndrome
Insulin resistance	Hyperuricaemia and gout	Impaired fertility
Breathlessness		Low back pain due to obesity
Sleep apnoea		Increased anaesthetic risk
		Fetal defects arising from maternal obesity

Source: WHO (1).

velop at least one of a range of debilitating conditions which can drastically reduce quality of life. These include musculoskeletal disorders, respiratory difficulties, skin problems and infertility, which are often costly in terms of absence from work and use of health resources. Table 1.3 lists the health problems that are most commonly associated with overweight and obesity. In developed countries, excessive body weight is also frequently associated with psychosocial problems.

The risk of developing metabolic complications is exaggerated in people who have central obesity. This is related to a number of structural differences between intra-abdominal and subcutaneous adipose tissues which makes the former more susceptible to both hormonal stimulation and changes in lipid metabolism. People of Asian descent who live in urban societies are particularly susceptible to central obesity and tend to develop NIDDM and CHD at lower levels of overweight than other populations.

Overview of the Economic Costs

Conservative estimates clearly indicate that obesity represents one of the largest costs in national health care budgets, accounting for up to 6% of total expenditure in several developed countries (Table 1.4). In the USA in 1995, for example, the overall direct costs attributed to obesity (through hospitalizations, outpatients, medications and allied health professionals' costs) were approximately the same as those of diabetes, 1.25 times greater than those of coronary heart disease, and 2.7 times greater than those of hypertension (5). The costs associated with pre-obesity (BMI 25–30 kg/m^2) are also substantial because of the large proportion of individuals involved.

The economic impact of overweight and obesity does not only relate to the direct cost of treatment in the formal health care system. It is also important to consider the cost to the individual in terms of ill health and reduced quality of life (intangible costs), and the cost to the rest of society in terms of lost productivity due to sick leave and premature disability pensions (indirect costs). Overweight and obesity are responsible for a considerable proportion of both. Thus, the cost of lost productivity attributed to obesity in the USA in 1994 was $3.9 billion and reflected 39.2 million days of lost work. In addition, there were 239 million restricted-activity days, 89.5 million bed-days, and 62.6 million physician visits.

Estimates of the economic impact of overweight and obesity in less developed countries are not available. However, the relative costs of treatment if available are likely to exceed those in more affluent countries for a number of reasons. These include the accompanying rise in coronary heart disease and other non-communicable diseases, the need to import expensive technology with scarce foreign exchange, and the need to provide specialist training

Table 1.4   Conservative estimates of the direct economic costs of obesity

Country	Year	Obesity definition	Estimated direct costs	% National health care costs
USA	1995	BMI ≥ 30	US$52 billion	5.7
Australia	1989/90	BMI > 30	AUD$464 million	> 2
Netherlands	1981–89	BMI > 25	Guilders 1 billion	4
France	1992	BMI ≥ 27	FF 12 billion	2

Table 1.5   Estimated world prevalence of obesity

	Population aged ≥ 15 years (millions)	Prevalence of obesity (%)	Approximate estimate (mid-point) of number of obese individuals (millions)	
Established market economies	640	15–20	96–128	(112)
Former socialist economies	330	20–25	66–83	(75)
India	535	0.5–1.0	3–7	(5)
China	825	0.5–1.0	4–8	(6)
Other Asian countries and Islands	430	1–3	4–12	(8)
Sub-Saharan Africa	276	0.5–1.0	1–3	(2)
Latin America and Caribbean	280	5–10	14–28	(21)
Middle East	300	5–10	15–30	(22)
World	3616			(251)

Source: Seidell (4).

for health professionals. As many countries are still struggling with undernutrition and infectious disease, the escalation of obesity and related health problems creates a double economic burden.

THE GLOBAL OBESITY PROBLEM

The number of people worldwide with a BMI of 30 or above is currently thought to exceed 250 million, i.e. 7% of the world's adult population (Table 1.5) (4). When individual countries are considered, the range of obesity prevalence covers almost the full spectrum, from below 5% in China, Japan and certain African nations to more than 75% in urban Samoa. It is difficult to calculate an exact global figure because good quality and comparable data are not widely available. The assessment in Table 1.5 is a conservative estimate.

Important Issues Associated with Data Collation

Discussion and comparison of overweight and obesity rates throughout the world are complicated by a number of important issues associated with data collation. The first of these relates to the

limited availability of suitable data for an accurate assessment of obesity prevalence and trends in different countries. Although it is half a century since obesity was introduced into the International Classification of Diseases (ICD), overweight and obesity are rarely recognized by health professionals as a distinct disease or cause of death, and so are infrequently recorded on morbidity or mortality statistics. This means that we have to rely on BMI data collected as part of specific health screening surveys or scientific studies. Unfortunately, very few countries conduct national surveys on a regular basis, and even fewer report obesity prevalence. This reflects the fact that most national nutrition surveys, at least in developing countries, are still used to provide information about undernutrition in women and young children. The costs and resources required to conduct regular comprehensive national surveys are a major barrier to implementation.

The second issue relates to the need for caution when making comparisons of obesity rates between studies and countries. Comparison is complicated by a number of factors including differences in obesity classification systems, mismatched age groups, inconsistent age-standardization of study populations, discordant time periods and dates of data collection, and use of unreliable self-reported weight and height measurements for calculation of

BMI. In particular, the use of BMI cut-off points either above or below 30 kg/m^2 to denote obesity has a great impact on estimates of obesity prevalence in a given population. In the US, obesity has until very recently been routinely classified as a BMI at or above 27.8 kg/m^2 in men and 27.3 kg/m^2 in women. With these cut-off points, 31.7% of men and 34.9% of women were deemed obese in the period 1988–1994. These estimates fall to 19.9% of men and 24.9% of women when a BMI of 30 kg/m^2 is applied. Projects such as the WHO MONICA (MONItoring of trends and determinants in CArdiovascular diseases) study (see below), where data are collected from a large number of populations in the same time periods according to identical protocols, are particularly valuable for comparison purposes.

A third issue is the need to be aware that many countries such as Brazil and Mexico show great variation in wealth by region. Combining data from all areas into a single country figure, or from a number of countries into a regional figure, is likely to mask patterns of relationships between social variables and obesity.

Current Prevalence of Obesity

Despite the limited availability and fragmentary nature of suitable country-level data, it is clear that obesity rates are already high and increasing rapidly in all regions of the world. Table 1.6 shows the most current estimates of obesity prevalence, according to a BMI of 30 or greater, in a selection of countries from around the globe. Nationally representative data sets based on measured weight and height are presented where possible.

Examination of Table 1.6 reveals large variations in obesity prevalence between countries, both within and between regions. In Africa, for example, obesity rates are extremely high among women of the Cape Peninsula but very low among women in Tanzania.

Much of the developed world already has exceptionally high levels of overweight and obesity. In Europe, obesity prevalence now ranges from about 6 to 20% in men and from 6 to 30% in women. Rates are highest in the East (e.g. Russia, former East Germany and Czech Republic) and lowest in some of the Central European and Mediterranean countries. Recent data from the Russian Longitudinal Monitoring Survey indicate that Russia has a particularly serious obesity problem, especially among women where 28% of the population was obese in 1996. Results from the Italian National Health Survey indicate that Italy has one of the lowest levels of obesity in Europe. However, the Italian data may be underestimated due to self-reporting of weight and height measurements.

National figures for North America are similar to those of Europe, with approximately 20% of males and 25% of females currently obese in the USA, and 15% of all adults obese in Canada. Rates in the general populations of Australia and New Zealand are also in the range of 15–18%. Japan, at less than 3%, still has a very low level of obesity for an industrialized country.

In the oil-exporting countries of the Middle East, the adult populations appear to have a major obesity problem. Women in particular are affected, with prevalence several fold higher than that reported for many industrialized countries. Bahrain (urban), Kuwait, Jordan, Saudi Arabia (urban), and the United Arab Emirates all document female obesity rates well above 25%.

The highest obesity rates in the world are found in the Pacific Island populations of Melanesia, Polynesia and Micronesia. In urban Samoa, for example, approximately 75% of women and 60% of men were classified as obese in 1991. These figures correspond with some of the highest rates in the world of diabetes and other related chronic diseases. With regard to obesity, it should be noted that the prevalence figures may be slightly exaggerated because Polynesians are generally leaner than Caucasians at any given BMI.

From a nutrition perspective, research and policy in many Asian and lower-income countries have focused on undernutrition. However, there are clear indications that a number of these countries are now beginning, or are already experiencing, high levels of overweight and obesity. Urban China, urban Thailand, Malaysia and the Central Asian countries that were members of the Societ Union before 1992 (such as Kyrgyzstan) are all examples. Overweight is also becoming a serious problem in urban India, most notable in the upper-middle class. The situation in China and India is further complicated by the fact that chronic energy deficiency is still a major problem for large parts of the population.

Table 1.6 Prevalence of obesity (BMI $\geq 30\,\mathrm{kg/m^2}$) in a selection of countries

	Country	Year	Age	Prevalence of obesity (%)[a]	
				Men	Women
Europe	Finland	1991/93	20–75	14	11
	Netherlands	1995	20–59	8.4	8.3
	UK England	1997	16–64	17	20
	Scotland	1995	16–64	16	17
	[a]Italy	1994	15+	6.5	6.3
	France	1997?	15+	8.6	8.4
	Czech Republic	1995	20–65	22.6	25.6
	former East Germany	1992	25–69	21	27
	former West Germany	1990	25–69	17	19
	Russia	1996	Adults	10.8	27.9
North America	Canada	1991	18–74	15	15
	USA	1988–94	20–74	19.9	24.9
Central and South America	Mexico (urban)	1995	Adults	11	23
	Brazil	1989	25–64	5.9	13.3
	Curaçao	1993/94	18+	19	36
Middle East	Iran, Islamic Republic of (south)	1993/94	20–74	2.5	7.7
	Cyprus	1989/90	35–64	19	24
	Kuwait	1994	18+	32	44
	Jordan (urban)	1994–96	25+	32.7	59.8
	Bahrain (urban)	1991/92	20–65	9.5	30.3
	Saudi Arabia	1990/93	15+	16	24
Australasia and Oceania	Australia (urban)	1995	25–64	18.0	18.0
	New Zealand	1989	18–64	10	13
	Samoa (urban)	1991	25–69	58.4	76.8
	Papua New Guinea (urban)	1991	25–69	36.6	54.3
South and East Asia	Japan	1993	20+	1.7	2.7
	India (urban Delhi middle class)	1997	40–60	3.19	14.28
	China	1992	20–45	1.2	1.64
	Malaysia		18–60	4.7	7.9
	Singapore[b]	1992	Adults	4	6
	Kyrgyzstan	1993	18–59	4.2	10.7
Africa	Mauritius	1992	25–74	5.3	15.2
	Tanzania	1986/89	35–64	0.6	3.6
	Rodrigues (Creoles)	1992	25–69	10	31
	Cape Peninsula (Coloured)	1990	15–64	7.9	44.4

[a]Data are from the Italian National Health Survey and are self-reported.
[b]Obesity criterion: BMI $\geq 31\,\mathrm{kg/m^2}$.

A similar picture is emerging in Central and South America. Mexico and Brazil are already experiencing high levels of obesity, especially among low income and urban populations. Within the African region too, there are clear pockets where obesity is already a major problem. These include the coloured population of Cape Peninsula and the multiethnic island nation of Mauritius. Only the very underdeveloped countries of Africa appear to be avoiding the worldwide epidemic of obesity, although the lack of good quality data makes it difficult to judge their true weight status.

Recent Trends

Good quality data on trends in body composition are even harder to find than cross-sectional data on prevalence at one point in time, especially for countries outside Europe and the US. Fortunately, nationally representative or large nationwide data sets are now available for a small number of lower and middle income countries including Brazil, China, Mauritius, Western Samoa and Russia.

The countries of North America and Europe have seen startling increases in obesity rates over the last 10–20 years. In Europe, the most dramatic rise has been observed in England, where obesity prevalence more than doubled from 6% to 17% in men and from 8% to 20% in women after 1980. Prevalence has increased by about 10–40% over the last 10 years in the majority of other European countries.

Obesity rates in the USA have increased from 10.4% to 19.9% and from 15.1% to 24.9% in men and women, respectively, over the period 1960–1962 until 1988–1994. The largest increases, however, occurred from the period 1976–1980 onwards. In Japan, although overall rates of obesity remain below 3%, prevalence increased by a factor of 2.4 in the adult male population and by a factor of 1.8 in women aged 20–29 years.

Russia has seen a consistent increase in adult obesity from 8.4% to 10.8% in men and from 23.2% to 27.9% in women in only 4 years. This is despite marked shifts toward a lower fat diet in the post-reform period, during which price subsidies of meat and dairy products were removed. However, year-to-year fluctuations underscore the fact that the economy is in flux and that these changes cannot be used to predict trends. It is also worth noting that the prevalence of pre-obesity declined slightly between 1992 and 1994 in females but not in males.

Trend data from the western Pacific Islands indicate that obesity levels are not only high in these populations, but that the prevalence of obesity continues to increase considerably in each island (6).

Data from two comparable national surveys in Brazil conducted 15 years apart show that adult obesity has increased among all groups of men and women, especially families of lower income. National figures increased from 3 to 6% in men and from 8 to 13% in women. It is also of interest that the ratio between underweight and overweight—a measure of the relative importance of each problem in the population—changed dramatically between 1974 and 1989. This reversed from a ratio of 1.5:1 (underweight to overweight) in 1974 to a ratio of less than 0.5:1 in 1989 (7).

The level of obesity among Chinese adults remains low, but the marked shifts in diet, activity and overweight suggest that major increases in overweight and obesity will occur. During the most recent period of the national China Health and Nutrition Survey (CHNS), an ongoing longitudinal survey of eight provinces in China, data show a consistent increase in adult obesity in both urban and rural areas. Changes in diet and activity patterns are rapid in urban residents of all incomes but are even more rapid in middle and higher income rural residents.

Few countries seem to have escaped the rapid escalation in obesity rates in the last two decades. The Netherlands, Italy and Finland are rare exceptions where population height and weight data collected over this period indicate only small increases or even stabilization of the rates of obesity.

The MONICA Study

The WHO MONICA project provides a comprehensive set of obesity prevalence data from cities and regions. Information was collected in two risk surveys, conducted approximately 5 years apart from 38 populations. Most surveys were conducted in European cities but there were a few centres in North America, Asia and Australasia. Although they are not national data, they were collected from over 100 000 randomly selected participants aged 35 to 64 years, are age-standardized and are based on weights and heights measured with identical protocols. This provides a high level of confidence in the detailed analysis of the data, including comparisons between centres and observations over time. Such analysis is rarely possible with less rigorously collected data sets.

Analysis of the results from the first round of data collection between 1983 and 1986 showed that the average prevalence of obesity among European centres participating in the study was 15% in men and 22% in women, with the lowest in Sweden (Göteborg: 7% in men, 9% in women) and the highest in Lithuania (Kaunas: 22% in men, 45% in women).

The average age-standardized absolute changes in the prevalence of obesity over 5 years showed that rates increased in three-quarters of the populations for men and in half of the populations for women (8). The largest increases were observed in Catalonia, where there was a 9.4% rise in absolute prevalence in men and a 6.5% rise in women. A small number of populations actually saw a statistically significant decrease in obesity prevalence over the 5-year period. The most notable of these was in Ticino (Switzerland), where absolute rates fell by 11.7% in men and 9.6% in women. Charleroi in Belgium saw a 14.9% decrease in obesity prevalence in women but not in men.

Future Projections

Worldwide growth in the number of severely over-weight adults is expected to be double that of underweight adults between 1995 and 2025. Figure 1.2 presents some crude projections of the expected rise in obesity rates over the next 25 years for five of the countries included in Table 1.6. These estimates are based on a simple linear extrapolation of increases observed over the period 1975–1995 and indicate that by the year 2025, obesity rates could be as high as 40–45% in the USA, 30–40% in Australia, England and Mauritius, and over 20% in Brazil. It has even been suggested that, if current trends persist, the entire US population could be overweight within a few generations (9).

KEY FEATURES AND PATTERNS OF THE GLOBAL OBESITY EPIDEMIC

Closer analysis of obesity prevalence and trend data from around the world reveals a number of interesting patterns and features. These include an increase in population mean BMI with socioeconomic transition, a tendency for urban populations to have higher rates of obesity than rural populations, a tendency for peak rates of obesity to be reached at an earlier age in the less developed and newly industrialized countries, and a tendency for women to have higher rates of obesity than men. These and others are considered in some detail below.

Socioeconomic Status

Socioeconomic status (SES) is a complex variable that is commonly described by one or more simple indicators such as income, occupation, education and place of residence. Substantial evidence suggests that high SES is negatively correlated with obesity in developed countries, particularly among women, but positively correlated with obesity in populations of developing countries. As developing countries undergo economic growth, the positive relationship between SES and obesity is slowly replaced by the negative correlation seen in modern societies (see below, 'What is Driving the Global Obesity Epidemic?'

Modern Societies

In developed countries there is usually an inverse association between level of education and rates of obesity that is more pronounced among women. In the MONICA survey, a lower educational level was associated with higher BMI in almost all female populations (both surveys) and in about half of male populations. Between the two surveys, there was a strengthening of this inverse association and the differences in relative body weight by education increased. This suggests that socioeconomic inequality in health consequences associated with obesity may actually be widening in many countries (10). One analysis has shown that reproductive history, unhealthy dietary habits, and psychosocial stress may account for a large part of the association between low SES and obesity among middle-aged women (11).

There is some evidence to suggest that there are racial differences between BMI and SES in developed countries. Although women in the USA with low incomes or low education are more likely to be obese than those of higher SES overall, this association was not found in a large survey of Mexican American, Cuban American, and Puerto Rican adults (12). Similar findings have been reported for young girls where a lower prevalence of obesity was seen at higher levels of SES in white girls, but no clear relationship was detected in black girls (13), who tend to have much higher overall rates of obesity.

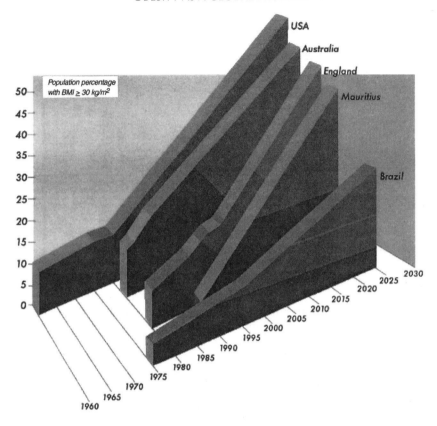

Figure 1.2   Projected increases in obesity prevalence. The figure illustrates the rate at which obesity prevalence is increasing in selected countries. It is based on crude projections from repeated national surveys. Source: IOTF unpublished

Developing and Transition Societies

New evidence from India illustrates the positive association between SES and obesity in developing countries. Nearly a third of males, and more than half of females, belonging to the 'upper middle class' in urban areas are currently overweight (BMI > 25). This is in stark contrast to the prevalence of overweight among slum dwellers (see Table 1.7) (14).

In Latin American and a number of Caribbean countries, a recent assessment of maternal and child obesity from national surveys since 1982 also found a tendency for higher obesity rates in poorly educated women throughout the region, except in Haiti and Guatemala where the reverse was true.

Urban Residence

Urban populations tend to have higher rates of obesity than rural populations, especially in less developed nations. Urbanization causes people to move away from their traditional way of living and is associated with a wide range of factors which adversely affect diet and physical activity levels. These include a shift to sedentary occupations, dependency on automated transport, reliance on processed convenience foods, and exposure to aggressive food marketing and advertising. Detrimental changes to family structures and value systems may also be an important contributor to reduced physical activity and poor diet associated with this shift.

In most countries, urbanization has led to populations consuming smaller proportions of complex carbohydrates, greater proportions of fats and animal products, more sugar, more processed foods, and more foods consumed away from home. Urbanization also has effects on physical activity levels. In Asian cities, bicycles are rapidly being displaced by motorbikes and cars with nearly

Table 1.7 Prevalence of overweight (BMI > 25) in urban adults by socioeconomic status in Delhi, India

	% Overweight	
Socioeconomic status	Males	Females
Middle class		
1. High	32	50
2. Middle	16	30
3. Low	7	28
Slum (poor)	1	4

Source: Gopalan (14).

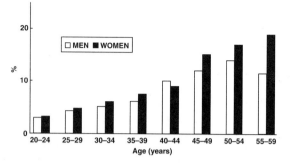

Figure 1.3 Obesity prevalence across the lifespan in the Netherlands. There is a consistent rise in the prevalence of obesity throughout all age groups in the Dutch population, reaching a peak in the seventh decade. Source: Seidell (15)

10 000 cars being added to the automobile fleet every month in Delhi. Meanwhile the rural populations are mainly engaged in agricultural occupations involving manual labour and a fairly high level of physical activity.

Steady urban migration has been an important feature of the ongoing developmental transition in all developing countries. Asia's urban population is expected to exceed 1242 million by the year 2000, a more than fivefold increase since 1950. This process is expected to continue in the decades to follow. By 2025, the world's urban population is expected to reach 5 billion (61% of the world's people), of whom 77% will live in less developed countries.

Age

Figure 1.3 shows the general pattern of overweight and obesity in the Netherlands, where a general rise in body weight and a modest increase in percentage body fat occur over the lifespan, at least until 60–65 years of age. This is reflected by an increase in obesity prevalence with age, reaching a maximum in the 60s, and then declining steadily thereafter. The decline is related in part to selective survival of people with a lower BMI. The issue is further complicated by the fact that BMI is not as reliable a measure of adiposity in old age because a decrease during this period often reflects a decrease in lean body mass rather than fat mass.

Peak rates of obesity and the associated health effects tend to be reached at a much earlier age in developing economies. In countries such as Western Somoa, the maximum rates of obesity tend to be reached at around 40 years of age (Figure 1.4).

Obesity rates tend to decline in age groups older than this in association with the high mortality that accompanies the rapidly developing diabetes and cardiovascular disease (CVD).

Gender Differences

More women than men tend to be obese whereas the reverse is true for overweight (BMI ≥ 25). This can be seen in countries as diverse as England, Mauritius, Japan and Saudi Arabia.

There are likely to be many social influences that differentially influence male and female food intake and energy expenditure patterns. However, it is clear that biological and evolutionary components are also important factors underlying the differences in rates of obesity between the sexes. In all populations, from contemporary hunting and gathering groups to those in complex industrial countries, women have more overall fat and much more peripheral body fat in the legs and hips than men. In addition, there appears to be a tendency for females to channel extra energy into fat storage in contrast to men who utilize a higher proportion of the energy to make protein and muscle. These gender differences are believed to be associated with the need for adequate fat deposits to ensure reproductive capacity in females. Men have, proportionally, much more central body fat. They also have a higher proportion of lean muscle mass which leads to a higher basal energy expenditure.

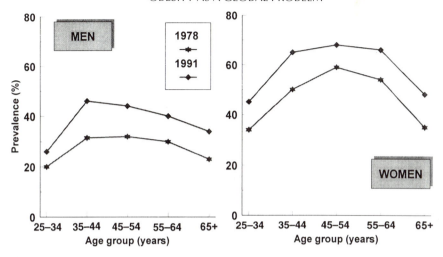

Figure 1.4 Obesity prevalence across the lifespan in Western Samoa. Peak rates of obesity are reached at around 40 years in communities of Western Samoa. Source: Hodge *et al.* (16)

High-risk Groups for Weight Gain

Minority Populations in Industrialized Countries

In many industrialized countries, minority ethnic groups are especially liable to obesity and its complications. Some researchers believe that this is the result of a genetic predisposition to store fat which only becomes apparent when the individuals are exposed to a positive energy balance promoted by modern lifestyles. Central obesity, hypertension and NIDDM are very common in urban Australian Aborigines, but can be reduced or even eliminated within a very short time by simply reverting to a more traditional diet.

It is likely that other factors, especially those associated with poverty, may also have a role to play in the far higher levels of obesity and its complications observed in minority populations. In native American and African American populations, for instance, where poverty is common, low levels of activity stem from unemployment and poor diets reflect dependence on cheap high-fat processed foods. Rates of hypertension among African American females below the poverty level are 40% compared with 30% of those at or above the poverty level. The particularly high levels of obesity among minority groups living in the USA are illustrated clearly in Figure 1.5.

Vulnerable Periods of Life

As outlined above, a general rise in body weight and a modest increase in percent body fat can be expected with age. However, there are certain periods of life when an individual may be particularly vulnerable to weight gain (Table 1.8).

Other Factors Promoting Weight Gain

A number of other groups have been identified as being at risk of weight gain and obesity for genetic, biological, lifestyle and other reasons. These include family history of obesity, smoking cessation, excessive alcohol intake, drug treatment for a wide range of medical conditions, certain disease states, changes in social circumstance, and recent successful weight loss. Major reductions in activity as a result of, for example, sports injury can also lead to substantial weight gain when there is not a compensatory decrease in habitual food intake.

WHAT IS DRIVING THE GLOBAL OBESITY EPIDEMIC?

The Changing Environment

Although research advances have highlighted the importance of leptin and other molecular genetic

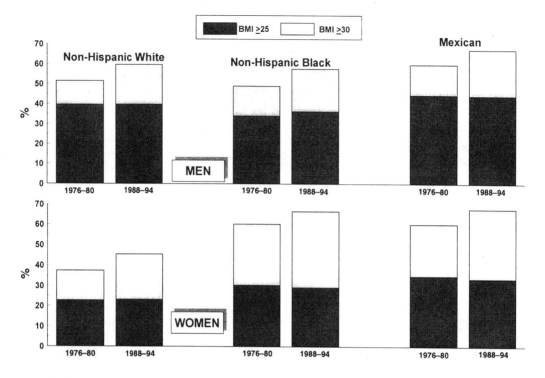

Figure 1.5   Obesity prevalence among ethnic groups in the USA, illustrating the disparity that exists between different ethnic groups, particularly amongst women, in the level of overweight and obesity in the USA. Source: Flegal *et al.* (17)

factors in determining individual susceptibility to obesity, these cannot explain the current obesity epidemic. The rapid rise in global obesity rates has occurred in too short a time for there to have been any significant genetic modifications within populations. This suggests that changes to the environment—physical, socio-cultural, economic and political—are primarily responsible for the epidemic and that genetics, age, sex, hormonal effects and other such factors influence the susceptibility of individuals to weight gain who are living in that environment.

There are a number of societal forces which underlie the environmental changes implicated in the obesity epidemic. These include modernization, economic restructuring and transition to market economies, increasing urbanization, changing occupational structures, technical and scientific developments, political change, and globalization of food markets. Many of these factors are associated with improved standards of living and other societal advances but urban crowding, increasing unemployment, family and community breakdown, and dis-

placement of traditional foodstuffs by Westernized high-fat products and other negative changes have also been a product of this process. The end result is often a move to weight-gain-promoting dietary habits and physical activity patterns.

Economic Growth and Modernization

A key factor in the global coverage of the obesity epidemic, particularly with respect to developing and transition countries, is economic growth. Rapid urbanization, changing occupational structures and shifts in dietary structure related to socioeconomic transition all affect population mean BMI. Demographic shifts associated with higher life expectancy and reduced fertility rates, as well as shifts in patterns of disease away from infection and nutrient deficiency towards higher rates of non-communicable diseases, are other components of this so-called 'transition'.

Table 1.8 Vulnerable periods of life for weight gain and the development of future obesity

Prenatal	Poor growth and development of the unborn baby can increase the risk of abdominal fatness, obesity and related illness in later life.
Adiposity rebound (5–7 years)	'Adiposity rebound' describes a period, usually between the ages of 5 and 7, when BMI begins to increase rapidly. This period coincides with increased autonomy and socialization and so may represent a stage when the child is particularly vulnerable to the adoption of behaviours that both influence and predispose to the development of obesity. Early adiposity rebound may be associated with an increased risk of obesity later in life.
Adolescence	This is a period of increased autonomy which is often associated with irregular meals, changed food habits and periods of inactivity during leisure combined with physiological changes. These promote increased fat deposition, particularly in females.
Early adulthood	Early adulthood is often associated with a marked reduction in physical activity. This usually occurs between the ages of 15 and 19 years in women but as late as the early 30s in men.
Pregnancy	The average weight gain after pregnancy is less than 1 kg although the range is wide. In many developing countries, consecutive pregnancies with short spacing often result in weight loss rather than weight gain.
Menopause	Menopausal women are particularly prone to rapid weight gain. This is primarily due to reductions in activity although loss of the menstrual cycle also affects food intake and reduces metabolic rate slightly.

Source: Gill (18).

Effect on BMI Distribution

Improvement in the socioeconomic conditions of a country tends to be accompanied by a population-wide shift in BMI so that problems of overweight eventually replace those of underweight (Figure 1.6). In the early stages of transition, undernutrition remains the principal concern in the poor whilst the more affluent tend to show an increase in the proportion of people with a high BMI. This often leads to a situation where overweight coexists with underweight in the same country. As transition proceeds, overweight and obesity also begin to increase among the poor.

Even in affluent countries, the distribution of body fatness within a population ranges from underweight through normal to obese. When the mean population BMI is 23 or below, there are very few individuals with a value of $30 \, kg/m^2$ or greater. However, when mean BMI rises above $23 \, kg/m^2$, there is a corresponding increase in the prevalence of obesity. An analysis by Rose (20) of 52 communities in the large multi-country INTERSALT Study found that there is a 4.66% increase in the prevalence of obesity for every single unit increase in population BMI above $23 \, kg/m^2$ (Figure 1.7).

The 'Nutrition Transition'

Generally, as incomes rise and populations become more urban, diets high in complex carbohydrates and fibre give way to varied diets with a higher proportion of fats, saturated fats and sugars. Recent analyses of economic and food availability data, however, reveal a major shift in the structure of the global diet over the last 30 years. Innate preferences for palatable diets coupled with the greater availability of cheap vegetable oils in the global economic have resulted in greatly increased fat consumption and greater dietary diversity among low income nations. As a result, the classic relationship between incomes and fat intakes has been lost, with the so-called 'nutrition transition' now occurring in nations with much lower levels of gross national product than previously. The process is accelerated by rapid urbanization (21).

The Relationship Between Undernutrition and Later Obesity

In countries undergoing transition where overnutrition coexists with undernutrition, the shift in population weight status has been linked to exaggerated problems of obesity and associated non-communicable diseases in adults.

Recent studies have shown that infants who were undernourished *in utero* and then born small have a greater risk of becoming obese adults (22,23). In particular, poor intrauterine nutrition appears to predispose some groups to abdominal obesity and results in an earlier and more severe development of comorbid conditions such as hypertension, CHD and diabetes (24–26). The apparent impact of intrauterine nutrition on the later structure and functioning of the body has become known as 'programming' and is often referred to as the 'Barker hypothesis', after one of the key researchers involved in developing this concept.

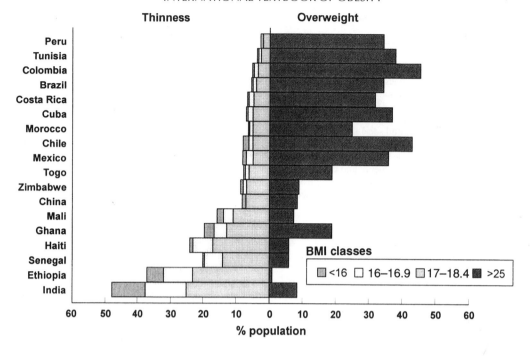

Figure 1.6 BMI distribution for various adult populations worldwide (both sexes). As the proportion of the population with a low BMI decreases there is a consequent increase in the proportion of the population with an abnormally high BMI. Many countries have a situation of unacceptably high proportions of both under- and overweight. Source: WHO (19)

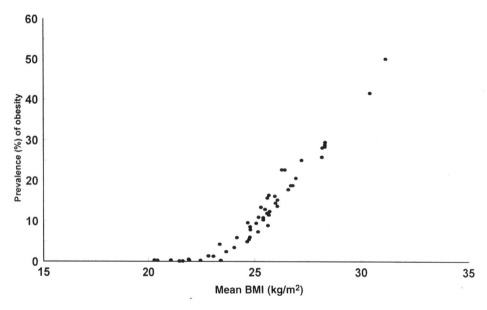

Figure 1.7 The relationship between population mean BMI and the prevalence of obesity, illustrating the direct association between population mean BMI and the prevalence of deviant (high) BMI values across 52 population samples from 32 countries (men and women aged 20–59 years). $r = 0.94$; $b = 4.66\%$ per unit BMI. Source: Rose (20)

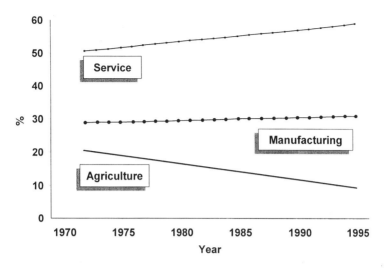

Figure 1.8 Shifts in distribution of occupations for lower income countries, 1972–1993. There has been a steady decline in employment in labour intensive agricultural occupations and a concomitant increase in employment within the less physical demanding service sector. Source: Popkin and Doak (7)

The ramifications of programming are immense for countries such as India and China where a large proportion of infants are still born undernourished. If these children are later exposed to high-fat diets and sedentary lifestyles associated with economic transition, and develop into obese adults, then it is likely that they will suffer severe consequences in the form of early heart disease, hypertension and diabetes.

Central obesity is already emerging as a serious problem in India, even at low relative weight; among non-overweight urban middle-class residents with BMI less than $25 \, kg/m^2$, nearly 20% of males and 22% of females had a high waist-to-hip ratio. In overweight subjects with a BMI over $25 \, kg/m^2$, abdominal obesity was found in a striking 68% of males and 58% of females.

In many populations undergoing rapid modernization and economic growth, high levels of obesity are associated with high rates of NIDDM, hypertension, dyslipidaemia and CVD as well as alcohol abuse and cigarette smoking. This has been descibed as the 'New World syndrome' and is responsible for the disproportionately high rates of mortality in developing nations and among the disadvantaged ethnic minority groups in developed countries.

Occupational Structure

Figure 1.8 shows the shift in the distribution of occupations that has been occurring in lower income countries during the past several decades. There has been a move towards more capital intensive and knowledge based employment that relies far less on physical activity. In China, the rapid decline in physical activity at work in urban areas has been associated with increased levels of adult obesity (27). Large shifts towards less physically demanding work have also been observed on a worldwide basis, both in the proportion of people working in agriculture, industry and services, and in the type of work within most occupations.

Other Possible Explanations

Changing Demographic Structure of Populations

Obesity, like many other non-communicable diseases, is age dependent and the highest rates are generally found in older age groups. The recent decline in fertility rates and increase in proportion of the population surviving into adulthood has led to a shift in the age structure of most populations with the result that they are generally older than a few decades ago. This is particularly evident in developing countries. It has been suggested that such changes in the demographics of societies could make a significant contribution to inflating the measured increase over time in a number of chronic diseases such as obesity (28). However, the finding that the greatest increases over the last few decades in mean body weight and rates of obesity have occurred in younger age groups does not support this explanation for the recent obesity epidemic.

Smoking Cessation and Increasing Obesity Rates

It has been suggested that the fall in smoking rates observed over recent years in many industrialized countries has made a significant contribution to the rises in mean body weight and rates of obesity. Studies have shown that smokers have significantly lower mean BMI than those who have never smoked and that male ex-smokers tend to have the highest level of BMI (29). Mean weight gain attributable to smoking cessation in a nationally representative cohort of smokers and non-smokers in the USA was 2.8 kg in men and 3.8 kg in women, with heavy smokers (> 15 cigarettes per day) and younger people at higher risk of weight gain (> 13 kg) on cessation (30). However, analyses of the contribution of smoking cessation to population weight gain have been equivocal. One study suggested that smoking cessation may account for up to 20% of the increase in overweight adults in the USA but other studies have indicated that the contribution may be much lower. Declines in self-reported cigarette smoking accounted for only 7% of change in BMI among males and 10% in females in a New Zealand Study (31). Studies from Australia (32) and Finland (33) did not find significant differences in the rates of weight increase over time between smokers, non-smokers and ex-smokers.

Cultural Body Shape Ideals

Culturally defined standards of a beautiful body vary between societies and across historical periods of time. 'Fatness' is still viewed as a sign of health and prosperity in many developing countries, especially where conditions make it easy to remain lean. 'Bigness' (large structure and muscularity but not necessarily fatness) also tends to be viewed as the male body ideal in most developed countries. Such views can inhibit patients from seeking treatment and support the continuing upwards trend in obesity rates.

OBESITY IN CHILDREN AND ADOLESCENTS

Obesity is also emerging as a serious global health problem among children and adolescents. Although good quality nationally representative data are still lacking, studies have generally reported a substantial rise in prevalence in both industrialized and developing countries.

Defining Obesity in Children and Adolescents

The major factor limiting our understanding of the true extent of the childhood obesity problem is the lack of a standard population-level methodology for measuring overweight and obesity in children and adolescents. Presently a number of different methods or indices are in use with a variety of cut-off points for designating a child as obese. The US National Center for Health Statistics (NCHS) growth reference charts have been recommended by the WHO for international use since the late 1970s but a number of serious technical and biological problems have been identified with their development and application.

An expert working group of the International Obesity Task Force investigated this issue and concluded that BMI-for-age, based on a redefined international reference population from 5 to 18 years, was a reasonable index of adiposity and could be used for population studies. They identified a novel approach to determine cut-off values that classify children as overweight or obese using percentiles that correlate to the standard cut-off points for BMI in adults (34). WHO is also in the process of developing a new growth reference for infants and children from birth to 5 years.

The Scale of the Childhood Obesity Problem

Despite the lack of agreement over childhood obesity classification, there is ample evidence to illustrate the scale of the problem across the world.

Using the existing WHO standards, the 1998 World Health Report indicated that about 22 mil-

Table 1.9 Prevalence of overweight[a] in 6- to 8-year-old children

	USA (1988–1991)	China (1993)	Russia (1994–1995)	South Africa (1994)	Brazil (1989)
Girls	24.2	12.2	17.8	20.3	10.5
Boys	21.3	14.1	25.6	25.0	12.8

[a]Defined as BMI higher than the US reference NHES 85th percentile.
Source: Popkin et al. (35).

lion children under 5 years are overweight across the world (2). This was based on weight-for-height data from 79 developing countries and a number of industrialized countries. Once the new growth reference is available a more realistic estimate should be possible.

Another comparison performed using the US NHES criteria also revealed the alarmingly high levels of overweight that exist in older children in both developed and developing countries. In some countries, up to a quarter of the school age child population is already overweight (Table 1.9).

Trend data suggest that the childhood obesity problem is increasing rapidly in many parts of the world. In the US, the percentage of young people aged 5–14 who are overweight has more than doubled in the past 30 years. Prevalence has risen from 15% in 1973–1974 to 32% in 1992–1994. Meanwhile, in England, triceps skinfold measurement increased by almost 8% in 7-year-old English boys and by 7% in 7-year-old girls between 1972 and 1994. In Scotland over the same period, triceps skinfold measurement increased by nearly 10% in 7-year-old boys and by 11% in 7-year-old girls. Weight for height index followed a similar pattern.

Childhood obesity is also increasing in Asia. In Thailand, the prevalence of obesity in 6- to 12-year-old children rose from 12.2% in 1991 to 15.6% in 1993. In Izumiohtsu city in Japan, the percentage of obese children aged 6–14 years doubled from 5 to 10% between 1974 and 1993.

Data from developing countries in Latin America show that urban residency, high SES and higher maternal education are associated with greater risk of overweight in children and that obesity is more common in girls than in boys. In developed countries an opposite association between SES and obesity is often found, with children from poorer educated parents with lower occupations more likely to be overweight.

Health Impact of Obesity in Childhood

Obese children and adolescents are at increased risk of developing a number of health problems. The most significant long-term consequence is the persistence of obesity and its associated health risks into adulthood. Some 30% of obese children become obese adults. This is more likely when the onset of obesity is in late childhood or adolescence and when the obesity is severe. Other obesity-related symptoms include psychosocial problems, raised blood pressure and serum triglycerides, abnormal glucose metabolism, hepatic gastrointestinal disturbances, sleep apnoea and orthopaedic complications.

Stunting and Obesity

A number of studies have indicated that there is an important association between stunting and overweight or obesity in a variety of ethnic, environmental and social backgrounds. Popkin et al. (35), for example, found that the income-adjusted risk ratios of being overweight for a stunted child in four nations undergoing transition ranged from 1.7 to 7.8. Obesity associated with stunting was also more common than obesity without stunting in a shanty-town population in the city of Sao Paulo, in both younger children and adolescents (36).

The association between stunting and obesity has serious public health implications, particularly for lower income countries, but the underlying mechanisms remain relatively unexplored. Recently, Sawaya et al. (37) suggested that stunting may increase the susceptibility to excess body fat gain in children who consume a high fat diet. A significant association was found between the baseline percentage of dietary energy supplied by fat and the gain in weight-for-height during follow-up in girls with mild stunting ($P = 0.048$), but not in the non-stunted control girls ($P = 0.245$). Despite clear indications that catch-up growth cannot be achieved outside critical growth windows, many countries continue with poorly targeted nutrition supplementation programmes based on energy-dense foods.

Key Factors Underlying the Increase in Childhood Obesity Rates

The fact that obesity is emerging as the most prevalent nutritional disease among children and adolescents in the developed world is hardly surprising. As outlined earlier, the highly technological societies of today have created an environment where it is increasingly convenient to remain sedentary whilst all forms of physical activity and active recreation are discouraged. Children are particularly susceptible to such changes as many of the decisions about diet and physical activity patterns are beyond their personal control. Parents are becoming increasingly concerned about the safety of their children and are preventing them from walking or cycling to school or playing in public spaces. In addition, lack of resources, space and staff for supervision has led to a reduction in the time spent in active play or sports when children are at school. As a result, the physical activity levels of children are dropping drastically and more sedentary pursuits such as television watching are replacing time once spent in active play. This is a trend that is spreading throughout many newly industrialized and developing countries as safety becomes a serious issue in overcrowded urban areas and consumer goods such as televisions become more accessible.

Television advertising and the rapid spread of ready-prepared foods directly marketed at children appear to have greatly influenced children's food preferences. There is a great deal of concern that the majority of food and drink advertisements screened during children's television programmes are for products high in fat and/or sugar, which clearly undermine messages for healthy eating. Only a very few countries such as Norway and Sweden have sought to restrict the level of television advertising directed towards children under 12 and during children's programmes. The globalization of world food markets has meant that traditional eating patterns of children are changing particularly rapidly in developing countries where high energy-dense, manufactured food is replacing less energy-dense traditional food and snacks based on cereals, fruits and vegetables.

THE NEED FOR GLOBAL ACTION

Obesity is a serious international public health problem which urgently needs action on a global scale. Governments, international agencies, industry/trade, the media, health professionals and consumers, among others, all have important roles to play in arresting this epidemic.

Strategies aimed at preventing weight gain and obesity are likely to be more cost effective, and to have a greater positive impact on long-term control of body weight, than treating obesity once it has developed. The majority of treatment therapies fail to keep weight off in the long-term and health care resources are no longer sufficient to offer treatment to all. In countries still struggling with high levels of undernutrition, tackling the problem of overweight and obesity poses even more of a challenge as many are not prepared institutionally to deal with problems of diet and chronic disease.

In the face of the current environment characterized by sedentary occupations and persistent temptation of high fat/energy-dense food, action to prevent obesity must include measures to reduce the obesity-promoting aspects of the environment. Previous attempts to improve community diet and physical activity habits have shown that efforts cannot rely solely on health education strategies aimed at changing individual behaviour. Living environments need to be improved so that they both promote and support healthy eating and physical activity habits throughout the life cycle for the entire population. Strategies are needed which address the underlying societal causes of obesity through action in sectors such as transport, environment, employment conditions, education, health and food policies, social and economic policies (Table 1.10).

For those individuals and subgroups of the population who have already developed, or are at increased risk of developing, obesity and the associated health complications, obesity management programmes within health care and community ser-

Table 1.10 Potential public health interventions to prevent obesity

Predominantly food related

1. Increase food industry development, production, distribution and promotion of products low in dietary fat and energy
2. Use pricing strategies to promote purchase of healthy foods
3. Improve quality of food labelling
4. Increase mass media promotion of healthy foods
5. Promote water as the main daily drink
6. Promote development and implementation of appropriate nutrition standards and guidelines for catering establishments (public and private)
7. Regulate food advertising and marketing practices aimed at children
8. Provide land in towns and cities for 'family' growing of vegetables, legumes and other healthy produce

Predominantly activity related

1. Improve public transport to reduce dependence on the motor car
2. Implement measures to promote walking and cycling as means of transport
3. Change building codes to promote use of stairs instead of elevators and escalators
4. Increase provision of affordable local exercise/recreational facilities and programmes
5. Provide flexible working arrangements to allow time for exercise (and to decrease reliance on convenience processed foods)
6. Provide exercise and changing facilities at work
7. Promote learning and practice of healthy physical activity (and nutrition) habits through schools

Health sector related

1. Mass media public awareness campaign on the need to maintain a healthy weight throughout life
2. Build economic incentives into health insurance plans
3. Provide adequate training in obesity prevention and management for physicians and other health care workers

Source: IOTF unpublished.

vices are essential. The effectiveness of such programmes is likely to be enhanced if improved and extended training of all relevant health care workers is provided. Obesity needs to be viewed as a disease in its own right and one which warrants intervention even when comorbidities are not present. Negative attitudes of health care professionals towards the condition are not helpful.

Finally, in all interventions aimed at preventing and managing overweight and obesity, systematic assessment and evaluation should be a routine element. Together with research into the development, consequences and scale of the global obesity epidemic, this has a key role in developing, improving and refining strategies to deal with it.

REFERENCES

1. World Health Organization. *Obesity: Preventing and Managing the Global Epidemic. Report of a WHO Consultation on Obesity. Geneva, 3–5 June 1997.* Geneva: World Health Organization, 1998 WHO/NUT/NCD/98.1.
2. World Health Organization. *The World Health Report 1998—Life in the 21st century: a vision for all.* Geneva: World Health Organization, 1998.
3. Deurenberg P, Yap M, van Staveren WA. Body mass index and percent body fat: a meta analysis among different ethnic groups. *Int J Obes* 1998; **22**: 1164–1171.
4. Seidell JC. Effects of obesity. *Medicine* 1998; 4–8.
5. Wolf AM, Colditz GA. Current estimates of the economic cost of obesity in the United States. *Obes Res* 1998; **6**: 97–106.
6. Hodge AM, Dowse GK, Zimmet PZ, Collins VR. Prevalence and secular trends in obesity in Pacific and Indian Ocean island populations. *Obes Res* 1995; **3** (Suppl 2): 77s–87s.
7. Popkin BM, Doak CM. The obesity epidemic is a worldwide phenomenon. *Nutr Rev* 1998; **56**: 106–114.
8. Dobson AJ, Evans A, Ferrario M, Kuulasmaa KA, Moltchanov VA, Sans S, Tunstall-Pedoe H, Tuomilehto JO, Wedel H, Yarnell J. Changes in estimated coronary risk in the 1980s: data from 38 populations in the WHO MONICA Project. World Health Organization. Monitoring trends and determinants in cardiovascular diseases. *Ann Med* 1998; **30**: 199–205.
9. Foreyt J, Goodrick K. The ultimate triumph of obesity. *Lancet* 1995; **346**: 134–135.
10. Molarius A, Seidell JC, Sans S, Tuomilehto J, Kuulasmaa K. Educational level and relative body weight, and changes in the association over 10 years—an international perspective from the WHO Monica project. *Int J Obes* 1998; **22**: S43.
11. Wamala SP, Wolk A, Orth-Gomer K. Determinants of obesity in relation to socioeconomic status among middle-aged Swedish women. *Prev Med* 1997; **26**: 734–744.
12. Khan LK, Sobal J, Martorell R. Acculturation, socioeconomic status, and obesity in Mexican Americans, Cuban Americans, and Puerto Ricans. *Int J Obes* 1997; **21**: 91–96.
13. Kimm SY, Obarzanek E, Barton BA, Aston CE, Similo SL, Morrison JA, Sabry ZI, Schreiber GB, McMahon RP. Race, socioeconomic status, and obesity in 9- to 10-year-old girls: the NHLBI Growth and Health Study. *Ann Epidemiol* 1996; **6**: 266–275.
14. Gopalan C. Obesity in the Indian urban 'Middle Class'. *Nutrition Foundation of India Bulletin* 1998; **19**: 1–5.
15. Seidell JC. Obesity in Europe. *Obes Res* 1995; **3** (Suppl 2): 89s–93s.
16. Hodge AM, Dowse GK, Toelupe P, Collins VR, Imo T, Zimmet PZ. Dramatic increase in the prevalence of obesity in Western Samoa over the 13-year period 1978–1991. *Int J Obes* 1994; **18**: 419–428.
17. Flegal KM, Carroll MD, Kuczmarski RJ, Johnson CL. Overweight and obesity in the United States: prevalence

and trends, 1960–1994. *Int J Obes* 1998; **22**: 39–47.

18. Gill TP. Key issues in the prevention of obesity. *Br Med Bull* 1997; **53**: 359–388.

19. World Health Organization. *Physical Status: the use and interpretation of anthropometry. Report of a WHO Expert Committee.* Geneva: World Health Organization, 1995 (WHO Technical Report Series, No. 854).

20. Rose G. Population distributions of risk and disease. *Nutr Metab Cardiovasc Dis* 1991; **1**: 37–40.

21. Drewnowski A, Popkin BM. The nutrition transition: new trends in the global diet. *Nutr Rev* 1997; **55**: 31–43.

22. Ravelli GP, Stein ZA, Susser M. Obesity in young men after famine exposure in utero and early infancy. *N Eng J Med* 1976; **295**: 349–353.

23. Jackson AA, Langley-Evans SC. McCarthy HD. Nutritional influences on early life upon obesity and body proportions. In: Chadwick DJ, Cardew GC (eds) *The Origins and Consequences of Obesity.* Chichester: Wiley, 1996: 118–137 (Ciba Foundation Symposium 201).

24. Law CM, Barker DJ, Osmond C, Fall CH, Simmonds SJ. Early growth and abdominal fatness in adult life. *J Epidemiol Community Health* 1992; **46**: 184–186.

25. Schroeder DG, Martorell R, Flores R. Infant and child growth and fatness and fat distribution in Guatemalan adults. *Am J Epidemiol* 1999; **149**: 177–185.

26. Barker DJ. Maternal nutrition, fetal nutrition, and disease in later life. *Nutrition* 1997; **13**: 807–813.

27. Popkin BM, Paeratakul S, Zhai F, Ge K. Dietary and environmental correlates of obesity in a population study in China. *Obes Res* 1995; **3** (Suppl 2): 135s–143s.

28. Pellitier DL, Rahn, M. Trends in body mass index in developing countries. *Food Nutr Bull* 1998; **19**: 223–239.

29. Molarius A, Seidell JC, Kuulasmaa K, Dobson AJ, Sans S. Smoking and relative body weight: an international perspective from the WHO MONICA Project. *J Epidemiol Community Health* 1997; **51**: 252–260.

30. Williamson DF. Smoking cessation and severity of weight gain in a national cohort. *N Eng J Med* 1991; **324**: 729–745.

31. Simmons G, Jackson R, Swinburn B, Yee RL. The increasing prevalence of obesity in New Zealand: is it related to recent trends in smoking and physical activity. *NZ Med J* 1996; **109**: 90–92.

32. Boyle CA, Dobson AJ, Egger G, Magnus P. Can the increasing weight of Australians be explained by the decreasing prevalence of smoking? *Int J Obes* 1994; **18**: 55–60.

33. Laaksonen M, Rahkonen O, Prattala R. Smoking status and relative weight by educational level in Finland, 1978–1995. *Prev Med* 1998; **27**: 431–437.

34. Dietz WH, Robinson TN. Use of the body mass index (BMI) as a measure of overweight in children and adolescents. *J Pediatr* 1998; **132**: 191–193.

35. Popkin BM, Richards MK, Montiero CA. Stunting is associated with overweight in children of four nations that are undergoing the nutrition transition. *J Nutr* 1996; **126**: 3009–3016.

36. Sawaya AL, Dallal G, Solymos G, de Sousa MH, Ventura ML, Roberts SB, Sigulem DM. Obesity and malnutrition in a Shantytown population in the city of Sao Paulo, Brazil. *Obes Res* 1995; **3** (Suppl 2): 107s–115s.

37. Sawaya AL, Grillo LP, Verreschi I, da Silva AC, Roberts SB. Mild stunting is associated with higher susceptibility to the effects of high fat diets: studies in a shantytown population in Sao Paulo, Brazil. *J Nutr* 1998; **128** (2 Suppl): 415S–420S.

2

The Epidemiology of Obesity

Jacob C. Seidell

National Institute of Public Health and the Environment, Bilthoven, The Netherlands

CLASSIFICATION OF OBESITY AND FAT DISTRIBUTION

The epidemiology of obesity has for many years been difficult to study because many countries had their own specific criteria for the classification of different degrees of overweight. Gradually during the 1990s, however, the body mass index (BMI; weight/height^2) became a universally accepted measure of the degree of overweight and now identical cut-points are recommended. This most recent classification of overweight in adults by the World Health Organization is shown in Table 2.1 (1).

In many community studies in affluent societies this scheme has been simplified and cut-off points of 25 and 30 kg/m^2 are used for descriptive purposes. The prevalence of very low BMI (< 18.5 kg/m^2) and very high BMI (40 kg/m^2 or higher) is usually low, in the order of 1–2% or less. Already researchers in Asian countries have criticized these cut-points. The absolute health risks seem to be higher at any level of the BMI in Chinese and South Asian people, which is probably also true for Asians living elsewhere. There are some developments that indicate that the cut-points to designate obesity or overweight may be lowered by several units of BMI. This would of course greatly affect the estimates of the prevalence of obesity in these populations. For instance, the prevalence of overweight measured as BMI > 27 kg/m^2 in the 1989 China Health and Nutrition Survey (2) was 6% in the North, 3% in Central China and 1% in the South. If the cut-off point was lowered to 25 kg/m^2 the prevalence

would be increased to, respectively, 15%, 9% and 6%. In countries such as China and India, each with over a billion inhabitants, small changes in the criteria for overweight or obesity potentially increase the world estimate of obesity by several hundred million (currently estimates are about 250 million worldwide).

Much research over the last decade has suggested that for an accurate classification of overweight and obesity with respect to the health risks one needs to factor in abdominal fat distribution. Traditionally this has been indicated by a relatively high waist-to-hip circumference ratio. Recently it has been accepted that the waist circumference alone may be a better and simpler measure of abdominal fatness (3,4). Table 2.2 gives some tentative cut-points for the waist circumference. These are again based on data in white populations.

In June 1998 the National Institutes of Health (National Heart, Lung and Blood Institute) adopted the BMI classification and combined this with waist cut-off points (6). In this classification the combination of overweight (BMI between 25 and 30 kg/m^2) and moderate obesity (BMI between 30 and 35 kg/m^2) with a large waist circumference (> 102 cm in men or 88 cm in women) is proposed to carry additional risk.

GLOBAL PREVALENCE OF OBESITY AND TIME TRENDS

In many reviews it has been shown that obesity (defined as a BMI of 30 kg/m^2 or higher) is a

International Textbook of Obesity. Edited by Per Björntorp.
© 2001 John Wiley & Sons, Ltd.

Table 2.1 WHO classification of overweight and obesity (1)

Classification	BMI (kg/m^2)	Associated health risks
Underweight	< 18.5	Low (but risk of other clinical problems increased)
Normal range	18.5–24.9	Average
Overweight	25.0 or higher	
Pre-obese	25.0–29.9	Increased
Obese class I	30.0–34.9	Moderately increased
Obese class II	35.0–39.9	Severely increased
Obese class III	40 or higher	Very severely increased

prevalent condition in most countries with established market economies (7). There is a wide variation in prevalence of obesity between and within these countries. It is quite easy to find instances of at least a twofold difference in the prevalence of obesity within one country (e.g. Toulouse in France with a prevalence of obesity of 9% in men and 11% in women and Strasbourg in France with 22% of men and 23% of women being obese). Usually, obesity is more frequent among those with relatively low socioeconomic status and the prevalence increases with age until about 60–70 years of age, after which the prevalence declines (8). In most of these established market economies it has been shown that the prevalence is increasing over time (8). Tables 2.3 and 2.4 show the increases in the prevalence of obesity in men and women aged 35–64 years in several centres participating in the WHO MONICA project (9). It is clear that there is a rapid increase in the prevalence of obesity in most centres from countries in the European Union, particularly in men. In centres in countries from Central and Eastern Europe the prevalences of obesity in women may have stabil-

Table 2.2 Sex-specific cut-off points for waist circumference. Level 1 was established to replace the classification of overweight (BMI ≥ 25 kg/m^2) but not combined with a high waist-to-hip ratio (WHR ≥ 0.95 in men and ≥ 0.80 in women). Level 2 was based on classification of obesity BMI ≥ 30 kg/m^2 and BMI between 25 and 30 kg/m^2 in combination with high waist-to-hip ratio (5)

	Level 1 ('alerting zone')	Prevalence	Level 2 ('action level')	Prevalence
Men	≥ 94 cm (~ 37 inches)	24.1%	≥ 102 cm (~ 40 inches)	18.0%
Women	≥ 80 cm (~ 32 inches)	24.4%	≥ 88 cm (~ 35 inches)	23.9%

Table 2.3 Prevalence of obesity (age standardized % with BMI > 30 kg/m^2) of centres in EU countries participating in the first round of the MONICA study (May 1979 to February 1989) and the third round (June 1989 to November 1996)

	Men		Women	
EU country (Centre)	First round	Third round	First round	Third round
Belgium (Ghent)	9	10	11	11
Denmark (Glostrup)	11	13	10	12
Finland (north Karelia)	17	22	23	24
Finland (Kuopio)	18	24	20	25
Finland (Turku/Loimaa)	19	22	17	19
France (Toulouse)	9	13	11	10
France (Lille)	13	17	17	22
Germany (Augsburg, urban)	18	18	15	21
Germany (Augsburg, rural)	20	24	22	23
Italy (area Brianza)	11	14	15	18
Italy (Friuli)	15	17	18	19
Spain (Catalonia)	10	16	23	25
Sweden (North)	11	14	14	14
United Kingdom (Belfast)	11	13	14	16
United Kingdom (Glasgow)	11	23	16	23
Mean	*13.5*	*17.3*	*16.4*	*18.8*

Table 2.4   Prevalence of obesity (age standardized % with BMI $> 30\,kg/m^2$) of centres in countries outside the European Union participating in the first round of the MONICA study (May 1979 to February 1989) and the third round (June 1989 to November 1996)

Country (centre)	Men		Women	
	First round	Third round	First round	Third round
Other European countries				
Iceland (Iceland)	12	17	14	18
Switzerland (Vaud/Fribourg)	12	16	12	9
Switzerland (Ticino)	19	13	14	16
Poland (Warsaw)	18	22	26	28
Poland (Tarnobrzeg)	13	15	32	37
Russia (Moscow)	14	8	33	21
Russia (Novosibirsk)	13	15	43	43
Czech Republic (rural CZE)	22	22	32	29
Yugoslavia (Novi Sad)	18	17	30	27
Mean	*15.6*	*16.1*	*26.2*	*25.3*
Outside Europe				
China (Beijing)	3	4	10	8
USA (Stanford)	10	22	14	23

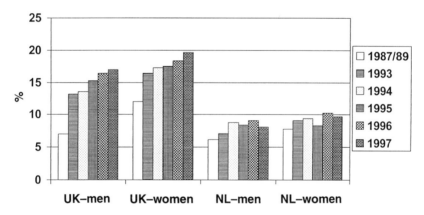

Figure 2.1   Time-trends of the prevalence of obesity in adults in the Health Survey for England (ages 16+), 1987–1997 and in the Netherlands (MORGEN project, ages 20–65 years), 1987–1997

ized or even slightly decreased but still those prevalences remain among the highest in Europe. The study by Molarius *et al.* (9) showed that the social class differences in the prevalence of obesity are increasing with time. Obesity is increasingly becoming an almost exclusively lower class problem in Europe.

Figure 2.1 shows the extraordinary increase in the prevalence of obesity in England. In the mid 1980s the prevalence of obesity in men from the Netherlands and England was about the same but in 1997 it was at least twice as high in england. The most recent (1988–1994) estimates of obesity in

adults in the USA are about 20% in men and 25% in women (8). In other parts of the world obesity is also frequent. Martorell *et al.* recently described the prevalence of obesity in young adult women aged 15–49 years (10). The estimated prevalence of obesity was on average 10% in Latin American countries and 17% in countries in North Africa and the Middle East.

Obesity is uncommon in sub-Saharan Africa, China and India, although in all regions the prevalence seems to be increasing, particularly among the affluent parts of the population in the larger cities (11). In these countries we quite often see the paradoxical condition of both increasing undernutrition and overnutrition. This is clearly related to growing inequalities in income and access to food in these regions. In addition, it has already been mentioned that classification criteria based on Europid populations (i.e. those of European ancestry) might not be appropriate for Asian populations.

There is some uncertainty around most national estimates of obesity prevalence because of the lack of solid data, and the large differences between countries within the same region and secular trends. The numbers corresponding to the midpoint of the estimates add up to about 250 million obese adults, which is about 7% of the total adult world population. It does not seem unreasonable that the true prevalence of obesity is likely to be in the order of 5–10%. In most countries the prevalence of overweight (BMI between 25 and 30 kg/m^2) is about two to three times the prevalence of obesity, which would mean that there may be as many as one billion people who are overweight or obese.

EXPLANATIONS FOR THE GROWING EPIDEMIC OF OBESITY

On an ecological or population level these time trends are not too difficult to explain although exact quantification of different factors is almost impossible. On the one hand, the average energy supply per capita is increasing. The World Health Report (12) has estimated that the average energy supply per capita in the world was 2300 kcal in 1963, 2440 kcal in 1971, and 2720 kcal in 1992; and it is estimated that in 2010 this will be 2900 kcal. These increases are obviously not evenly distributed across the world's population and, sadly, many remain undernourished although in Asia (particularly China and India) and most of Latin America these numbers are declining. The number of people with access to at least 2700 kcal has increased from 0.145 billion in 1969–1971 to 1.8 billion in 1990–1992 and is estimated to grow to 2.7 billion in 2010. Even when corrected for the increase in the world's population this implies a more than 10-fold increase in the number of people having access to high caloric diets. The globalization of agricultural production and food processing has not only affected the quantity of energy available per capita but also the energy density.

At the same time, there are continuing changes in the physical demands of work and leisure time. Increasingly we are at leisure during working hours and we work out during leisure time. Mechanization of many types of work and changes in transportation are causing ever-increasing numbers of people to be sedentary for most of the time.

Increasing sedentary behaviour has been proposed as one of the principal reasons for a further increase in the prevalence of obesity in countries with established market economies. Sedentary behaviour is poorly measured by the number of hours engaged in sports only. Large and important differences can be seen in the number of hours spent at sedentary jobs and behind television or computer screens during leisure time. Transportation is almost certainly a factor as well. For example, of short trips in the Netherlands 30% are done by bicycle and 18% by walking. In the UK these percentages are 8% by cycling and 12% by walking and in the USA 1% by bicycle and 9% by walking (13). These daily activities accumulated over a year can easily explain the small but persistent changes in energy balance needed to increase the prevalence of obesity.

Given the changes in lifestyles over the last decades in many parts of the world it is not surprising that people gain weight on the average although for many individuals this seems to remain a mystery. With small changes in average body weight the prevalence of obesity increases rapidly. For every unit increase in BMI there is an increase in the prevalence of obesity of around five percentage points (14).

PREVALENCE OF A LARGE WAIST CIRCUMFERENCE

The data of the WHO MONICA population (second survey carried out between 1987 and 1992) have recently been analysed with respect to waist cut-off points (15). From this analysis it is clear that the use of these single cut-off points of the waist circumference to replace classification by BMI and waist-to-hip ratio varies greatly from country to country. The prevalence of a large waist circumference (≥ 102 cm in men and ≥ 88 cm in women) and of obesity (BMI ≥ 30 kg/m^2) is shown in Table 2.5.

Table 2.5 Prevalence of a large waist circumference (102 cm or more in men or 88 cm or more in women) and of obesity (BMI 30 or more) in 19 centres participating in the WHO MONICA study (second round, 1987–1992). Adapted from reference 16

Population (countries by alphabetical order)	Men		Women	
	Large waist (%)	Obesity (%)	Large waist (%)	Obesity (%)
Australia (Newcastle)	24	20	31	19
Australia (Perth)	15	14	17	14
China (Beijing)	4	4	21	8
Czech Republic (Rural)	32	25	48	30
Denmark (Glostrup)	18	11	17	8
Finland (Kuopio Province)	16	16	23	20
Finland (North Karelia)	19	19	23	21
Finland (Turku/Loimaa)	18	16	21	19
France (Toulouse)	19	12	—	—
Germany (Augsburg Rural)	21	18	26	21
Germany (Augsburg Urban)	19	15	25	15
Germany (Halle County)	29	18	40	26
Italy (Area Brianza)	11	12	23	17
Italy (Friuli)	15	15	26	15
Spain (Catalonia)	23	17	33	22
Sweden (Göteborg)	12	9	14	10
Sweden (Northern Sweden)	13	11	18	11
United Kingdom (Glasgow)	22	14	27	19
Yugoslavia (Novi Sad)	17	15	32	26

In general, the prevalence of a large waist is higher than the prevalence of obesity and this is because it also includes overweight subjects with abdominal obesity.

OBESITY IN CHILDREN AND ADOLESCENTS

Comparison of prevalence data of obesity in children and adolescents around the world remains difficult because of the lack of standardization and interpretation of indicators of overweight and obesity in these age groups. Usually local or national percentile distributions for weight-for-age, weight-for-height, or BMI-for-age are used. Not only do these differ between regions and nations but they are also subject to change over time. In addition, different percentile cut-off points are used for the definition of overweight or obesity (e.g. 85th, 90th, 95th and 97th percentiles are used in different countries).

Another difficulty with these criteria is that when they are applied to older adolescents they do not correspond to the criteria for classification of overweight based on BMI for adults. Recently Cole *et al.* (17) used data from six large nationally representative cross-sectional growth studies from various parts of the world. They established centiles of the distribution of BMI by age. Those centile curves that, at age 18 years, passed through the widely used cut-points of 25 and 30 kg/m² for adult overweight and obesity were then used to define BMI cut-points by age. These proposed cut-points are less arbitrary and more internationally based than current alternatives.

With respect to the interpretation of criteria of overweight in different age groups it is also important to know whether or not they are predictive of later obesity. It is now generally accepted that body weight before the age of 6 years has very limited predictive power for the chances of becoming an overweight or obese adult irrespective of the family history of obesity (18). Data at this age may, however, be predictive in another way, as has been suggested by Rolland-Cachera and others (19). The BMI-for-age from infancy until adulthood has the form of a J-shape. The nadir of this curve usually is in the age range of 5 to 7 years of age. It has been

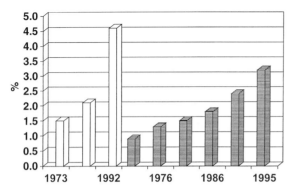

Figure 2.2 Time-trend in the prevalence of obesity (BMI $\geq 30\,kg/m^2$) among Danish (open bars) and Swedish (striped bars) male conscripts (adapted from references 2, 28)

suggested that when this nadir occurs at a relatively early age ('early-adiposity-rebound') the chances of adult obesity are higher than when there is a relatively late adiposity rebound (19,20). In addition, time trends in overweight may be sensitive indicators of secular changes in energy balance.

The World Health Organization has now tentatively recommended the use of BMI-for-age as an indicator of overweight or obesity (14). In the Netherlands, the French reference curves (> 97th percentile of BMI-for-age) have been used to evaluate some recent trends and a slight increase in the prevalence of obesity during the early 1990s was observed (21). Similar trends have also been observed in other countries, particularly the USA (22–24) and the United Kingdom (25). Military conscript data have been shown to be particularly useful in giving an unbiased view of long-term national time trends. Such data have been reported from Denmark (26) and in Sweden (27).

Figure 2.2 shows these time trends in overweight and obesity among young Danish and Swedish men and they illustrate a persistent increase in both countries.

Currently, a subgroup of the WHO International Obesity Task Force (IOTF) is trying to develop international BMI-by-age standards that can be used universally and which are preferably based on longitudinal tracking data of BMI for children and adolescents and which match around age 20 with the adult classification of BMI. Body mass index may not be a very precise indicator of body fatness on an individual level but there are many studies that support the use of BMI as an indicator of fatness on a population level (5,28).

The interpretation of these increases in childhood and adolescent obesity rates is difficult. Explanations require unbiased and precise estimates of energy intake and energy expenditure and these are often unavailable. Small secular changes in obesity may be the result of minute shifts in energy balance which are all well within the margin of error of all available methods. This is further complicated by the likelihood that reported energy intake in children is considerably underestimated (29). However, the USA is among those countries in which, despite a dramatic recent increase in the prevalence of obesity, there is no good evidence for any appreciable change in energy intake over the last decades and there may even have been some improvement (30). Some crude evidence suggests that the reduction in energy expenditure in children and adults is the most important determinant and it is not difficult to see that quite major changes in lifestyle have occurred in youngsters over the last few decades (16). Several studies report low physical activity in obese children compared to their lean counterparts (31,32). This may be the cause or the consequence of their obesity. Prospective studies, however, have also linked sedentary behavior such as television viewing to the development of obesity (33,34).

CONCLUSIONS

The increase in the prevalence of obesity among children, adolescents and adults in many countries around the world is alarming. Prevention of obesity should be among the high priorities in public health. This should be particularly aimed at encouraging healthy lifestyles in all age groups including children and adolescents. This cannot be achieved by efforts aimed at the individual level. Communities, governments, the media and the food industry need to work together to modify the environment so that it is less conducive to weight gain (1).

REFERENCES

1. WHO. *Obesity: Preventing and Managing the Global Epidemic.* Geneva: WHO, 1998. WHO/NUT/NCD/98.1.
2. Popkin BM, Leyou G, Fengying Z, Guo X, Haijiang M, Zohoori N. The nutrition transition in China: a cross-

sectional analysis. *Eur J Clin Nutr* 1993; **47**: 333–346.

3. Lean MEJ, Han TS, Seidell JC. Impairment of health and quality of life in men and women with a large waist. *Lancet* 1998; **351**: 853–856.

4. Han TS, Van Leer EM, Seidell JC, Lean MEJ. Waist circumference action levels in the identification of cardiovascular risk factors: prevalence study in a random sample. *Br Med J* 1995; **311**: 1401–1405.

5. Deurenberg P, Weststrate JA, Seidell JC. Body mass index as a measure of body fatness: age- and sex-specific prediction formulas. *Br J Nutr* 1991; **65**: 105–114.

6. National Institutes of Health. 1998. *Clinical Guidelines on the Identification, evaluation, and treatment of overweight and obesity in adults. The Evidence Report.* NIH, NHLBI, June 1998.

7. Seidell JC. Time trends in obesity: an epidemiological perspective. *Horm Metab Res* 1997; **29**: 155–158.

8. Seidell JC, Flegal KM. Assessing obesity: classification and epidemiology. *Br Med Bull* 1997; **53**; 238–252.

9. Molarius A, Seidell JC, Sans S, Tuomilehto J, Kuulasmaa K. Educational level and relative body weight and changes in their associations over ten years—an international perspective from the WHO MONICA project. *Am J Public Health* 2000; **90**: 1260–1268.

10. Martorell R, Kahn LK, Hughes ML, Grummer-Strawn LM. Obesity in women from developing countries. *Eur J Clin Nutr* 2000; **54**: 247–252.

11. Seidell JC, Rissanen A. World-wide prevalence of obesity and time-trends. In: Bray GA, Bouchard C, James WPT (eds). *Handbook of Obesity*, New York: M. Dekker, 1997: 79–91.

12. WHO *The World Health Report 1998. Life in the 21st Century—a Vision for All.* Geneva; WHO, 1998.

13. Pucher J. Bicycling boom in Germany: a revival engineered by public policy. *Transportation Quarterly* 1997; **51**: 31–46.

14. WHO. Physical status: the use and interpretation of anthropometry. *WHO Technical Report Series #854.* Geneva: WHO, 1995.

15. Molarius A, Seidell JC, Sans S, Tuomilehto J, Kuulasma K. Varying sensitivity of waist action levels to identify subjects with overweight or obesity in 19 populations of the WHO MONICA project. *J Clin Epidemiol* 1999; **52**: 1213–1224.

16. Jebb SA. Aetiology of obesity. *Br Med Bull* 1997; **53**: 264–285.

17. Cole TJ, Bellizzi MC, Flegal KM, Dietz WH. Establishing a standard definition for child overweight and obesity worldwide: international survey. *BMJ* 2000; **320**: 1240–1243.

18. Whitaker R, Wright J, Pepe M *et al.* Predicting adult obesity from childhood and parent obesity. *N Engl J Med* 1997; **337**: 869–873.

19. Rolland-Cachera MF, Deheeger M, Guilloud-Bataille M, Avons P, Sempe M. Tracking the development of adiposity from one month of age to adulthood. *Ann Hum Biol* 1987; **14**:
219–229.

20. Dietz WH. Critical periods in childhood for the development of obesity. *Am J Clin Nut* 1994: **59**: 955–959.

21. Seidell JC. Obesity, a growing problem. *Acta Paediatr* 1999; (Suppl 428): 46–51.

22. Troiano RP, Flegal KM, Kuczmarski RJ, Campbell SM, Johnson CL. Overweight prevalence and trends for children and adolescents. *Arch Pediatr Adolesc Med* 1995; **149**: 1085–1091.

23. Mei Z, Scanlon KS, Grummer-Strawn LM, Freedman DS, Yip R, Trowbridge FL. Increasing prevalence of overweight among US low-income preschool children: the CDC Pediatric Nutrition Surveillance 1983 to 1995. *Pediatrics* 1997; **101**(1). URL: http//www.pediatrics.org/cgi/content/full/101/1/e12.

24. Ogden CL, Troiano RP, Briefel RR, Kuczmarski RJ, Flegal KM, Johnson CL. Prevalence of overweight among preschool children in the United States, 1971 through 1994. *Pediatrics* 1997; **99**(4). URL: http//www.pediatrics.org/cgi/content/full/99/4/e1.

25. Hughes JM, Li L, Chinn S, Rona RJ. Trends in growth in England and Scotland, 1972 to 1994. *Arch Dis Child* 1994; **76**: 182–189.

26. Sörensen HT, Sabroe S, Gillman M, Rothman KJ, Madsen KM, Fischer P, Sörensen TIA. Continued increase in prevalence of obesity in Danish young men. *Int J Obes* 1997; **21**: 712–714.

27. Rasmussen F, Johansson M, Hansen HO, Trends in overweight and obesity among 18-year old males in Sweden between 1971 and 1995. *Acta Paediatr* 1999; **88**: 431–437.

28. Pietrobelli A, Faith MS, Allison DB, Gallagher D, Ciumello G, Heymsfield SB. Body mass index as a measure of adiposity among children and adolescents: a validation study. *J Pediatr* 1998; **132**: 204–210.

29. Champagne CM, Baker NB, Delany JP, Harsha DW, Bray GA. Assessment of energy intake underreporting by doubly labelled water and observations on reported nutrient intakes in children. *J Am Diet Assoc* 1998; **98**: 426–433.

30. Kennedy E, Powell R. Changing eating patterns of American children: a view from 1996. 1997. *J Am Coll Nutr* **16**: 524–529.

31. Harrell JS, Gansky SA, Bradley CB, McMurray RG. Leisure time activities of elementary school children. *Nut Res* 1997; **46**: 246–253.

32. Maffeis C, Zaffanello M, Schutz Y. Relationship between physical inactivity and adiposity in prepubertal boys. *J Pediatr* 1997; **131**: 288–292.

33. Gortmaker S, Must A, Sobel A, Peterson K, Colditz GA, Dietz WH. Television viewing as a cause of increasing obesity among children in the United States. *Arch Pediatr Adolesc Med* 1996; **150**: 356–362.

34. Robinson TN. Does television cause childhood obesity? *JAMA* 1998; **279**: 959–960.

3

Body Weight, Body Composition and Longevity

David B. Allison[1], Moonseong Heo[1], Kevin R. Fontaine[2]
and Daniel J. Hoffman[1]

[1]*St Luke's/Roosevelt Hospital Center, New York and* [2]*University of Maryland, Baltimore, USA*

INTRODUCTION

The question of the effect of variations in body weight on longevity is of enormous importance. Due in large part to the industrial and agricultural revolutions, relative body weight has been steadily increasing in the United States and most of the Western world (1). Consequently, rates of obesity have risen dramatically (2). As agricultural and industrial technology spreads into much of the non-Western world, evidence suggests that the relative body weights and rates of obesity are increasing in those populations as well (1). Given this background and the fact that weight is something that is possessed by all humans and therefore of potential interest to all humans, it is not surprising that enormous attention has been focused on relative body weight. Relative body weight is the subject of government policies and guidelines (1), employment policies and guidelines, public education campaigns, insurance policies, a target of the food and pharmaceutical industries, and substantial scientific investigation.

Despite all of this effort and attention, the effect of variations in relative body weight on longevity remains the subject of considerable debate (3–6). At one extreme, some authors suggest that the relationship between relative body weight and longevity is monotonic decreasing (7). In other words, one can never be too thin. At the other extreme, some authors have suggested that relative body weight has little important impact on longevity (8). In the middle, several authors have suggested that the relationship between relative body weight and mortality within a given period of time is U-shaped or J-shaped (9), that the relationships may vary as a function of individuals' demographic characteristics such as age, sex, and race (10,11), or that the relationships are simply not fully understood at this time (12,13).

We divide this chapter in two broad sections. First, because methodological issues have been and continue to be so prominent in this area, we begin with a review of a few methodological points. We then follow this with a discussion focusing on current findings and needs for future research.

METHODOLOGICAL ISSUES

Beginning in approximately 1987, a number of methodologically oriented reviews have appeared addressing this topic (4,5,14,15). Collectively, these reviews often imply that the effect of relative body weight on mortality depends critically on how the data from prospective cohort studies are analyzed. It has been suggested that the relationship between

International Textbook of Obesity. Edited by Per Björntorp.

relative body weight and mortality within a defined period of time is monotonic increasing (at least above a body mass index of $19 \, kg/m^2$) when the following conditions hold: (1) the sample is large; (2) the follow-up is long; (3) subjects dying during the first few years are excluded from the analysis to eliminate the confounding effects of pre-existing disease; (4) smoking is properly controlled for to eliminate its confounding effects; and (5) one does not mistakenly control for variables that are on the causal path from increased relative body weight to mortality (e.g. hypertension, dyslipidemias, glucose intolerance). It is our perception that until recently these statements had been largely accepted as statements of fact.

In addition, though less explicitly advocated, it appears that standard practice has come to favor certain analytic approaches to prospective cohort studies assessing the effect of relative body weight on mortality. Specifically, it appears to have become the standard that: (1) a continuous measure of relative body weight such as body mass index (BMI; kg/m^2) is accepted as a valid proxy for the conceptually desired variable of adiposity; (2) a continuous measure of relative body weight such as BMI should be categorized (usually on the basis of quintiles) prior to conducting an analysis; (3) the range of relative body weight associated with minimal mortality is best determined by examining the quintile-defined category in which mortality is at a minimum as opposed to fitting some statistical model to the data and finding the minimum via this model; and (4) individuals with weight fluctuation should be eliminated from the data set.

In this chapter, we question these assumptions. In many cases, these statements and/or practices seem to be based primarily on tradition or assertion. That is, these statements and practices have not been based on mathematical proofs, statistical simulations, or clear empirical demonstrations. In the remainder of this chapter, we critically evaluate these assumptions and practices. We follow this with a discussion of the implications of this work in terms of proposed methodological approaches to the study of relative body weight and mortality, a description of what currently available data seem to show, and finally a speculative discussion on what the currently available data may mean and suggestions for future research.

Measures of Relative Body Weight as Proxies for Adiposity

The use of BMI (and other measures of relative body weight) as a measure of relative adiposity has been documented in a number of studies and is generally reported to be highly correlated (~ 0.70–0.80) to the percentage of body weight as fat (16). However, an inherent difficulty in using BMI as a proxy for adiposity is that BMI is composed of two components, fat mass (FM) and fat-free mass (FFM). That is: $BMI = mass/stature^2 = (fat \, mass + fat\text{-}free \, mass)/stature^2 = fat \, mass/stature^2 + fat\text{-}free \, mass/stature^2$. The index $FM/stature^2$ has been referred to as the body fat mass index (BFMI) and fat-free mass/$stature^2$ has been used as an indicator of relative FFM (17). Thus, it may be that the use of BMI as a proxy for adiposity actually masks differential health consequences associated with both FM and FFM.

The rate of mortality associated with BMI is generally higher for lower and higher BMI values and lower for moderate levels of BMI. This curve, generally termed a U-shape curve, may be a function of any number of influences. (The term 'U-shaped' is used colloquially and does not imply the symmetry of a perfect U. Rather, it is intended to convey that the relation is convex and non-monotonic with regions at the extremes of the curve in which the mortality rate exceeds the rate at points between those regions.) The most common explanation is that persons with low BMI may suffer from pre-existing diseases that increase their risk for mortality, independent from BMI. Another hypothesis is that BMI, as a reflection of both adiposity and leanness, is not capturing the true relationship between body composition and mortality. Several studies have reported a positive health outcome for increased FFM and negative for increased FM (18). Thus, persons with low BMI may suffer from early mortality not because of BMI per se, but rather because inadequate levels of FFM increase their mortality rate. Stated another way, it may be that the risk of death increases with increasing FM and decreases with increasing FFM.

Recently we explored *possible* relationships between body composition and mortality using body composition measurements obtained on 1136 healthy subjects. We sought to evaluate the plausible effects of using BMI when FM and FFM had differential effects on mortality (6). Hypothetical models of mortality were generated (using the real BMI data) in which mortality rate increased monotonically with FM and decreased monotonically with FFM. Using this model we showed that a U-shaped association between BMI and mortality could occur even when: (a) mortality rate increased monotonically with FM; (b) mortality rate decreased monotonically with FFM; and (c) percent body fat increased monotonically (indeed almost linearly) with BMI. Thus, BMI does not necessarily adequately capture the effect of adiposity on mortality rate despite its high correlation with adiposity. Therefore, the need exists for longitudinal studies using precise body composition techniques to study more accurately the relationship between mortality rate and FM and FFM. That is, our analyses suggest that BMI alone may be insufficient to elucidate the relations between body fatness and mortality rate.

There are several studies that are consistent with this hypothesis, but are based on weak body composition measurements. First, although fatness per se and body fat distribution are clearly not synonymous, examining the differential patterns of mortality that have been found as function of fat distribution versus BMI may be illuminating. Folsom et al. (19) followed 41 837 women from the Iowa Women's Health Study Cohort for 5 years, testing the independent effects of BMI and waist-to-hip circumference ratio (WHR) on mortality rate. Cox regression revealed a U-shaped association between BMI and mortality rate. In contrast, the 'waist/hip circumference ratio was strongly and positively associated with mortality in a dose-dependent manner' (p. 483). These conclusions were not substantially changed after controlling for a number of covariates including smoking level, marital status, estrogen use, and alcohol use, such that a 0.15 unit increase in WHR was associated with a 60% greater hazard ratio.

In a small but rigorous study, Keys et al. (20) examined 20-year coronary heart disease (CHD) incidence among 279 middle-aged Minnesota men. Measures were taken of subjects' BMI, another index of relative body weight (RBW), skinfolds, and body density by under-water weighing at baseline. Twenty-year incidence rates were then evaluated as a function of these variables. It is noteworthy that results tended to be slightly stronger for measures of adiposity than the weight indices. However, due to its very small sample size, this study cannot support firm conclusions.

In a 10-year prospective study in Italy, Menotti et al. (21) examined the association of BMI with mortality rate and skinfold measurements among 8341 men and 1199 women. Among both men and women, results showed a consistent and clear U-shaped association between BMI and mortality. In contrast, the analysis of skinfold data among men showed 'similar but definitely less clear-cut findings' (p. 296) and an 'irregular trend' after excluding certain subjects. Among women, analyses of skinfold data were less clear and suggested 'a tendency toward a positive trend with increasing levels of [adiposity]' (p. 296). Notably, among women, the greatest relative risk (RR) was observed among those with low BMI and high skinfolds, a pattern suggestive of low lean body mass. Unfortunately, BMI and skinfolds were not simultaneously entered into a model to estimate independent effects. A recent analysis by Lee and Jackson (22) also presented mortality data involving measurements of body composition but did not estimate the independent effects of FM and FFM. This is problematic because, given the high correlation between FFM and FM, confounding will occur if each has independent effects on mortality rate and each is evaluated only in separate models.

In summary, very limited data regarding fatness (as opposed to just weight) and its effects on mortality exist. However, those data that do exist suggest the possibility that the elevated risks associated with excessively high BMIs will be seen to be worse when proper body fat rather than body measurements are used.

Categorizing the BMI/Adiposity Measure: Advantages and Disadvantages

The majority of studies of the BMI–mortality relation have transformed the continuously measured variable (BMI) into a polytomous variable. The most common approach seems to be to break the distribution up into five ordered categories with equal numbers of subjects per group based on sample quintiles. There seems to be a perception in some circles that this is the optimal way to analyze the data and, perhaps, even the only way. In contrast, we suggest that is certainly not the only way and may not be the best way.

With respect to alternatives, it is well known that survival/mortality outcomes can be modeled as a function of continuous predictor variables through techniques including logistic regression and Cox regression (23). Given that there are alternatives to categorization available, we wish to address some limitations of analyzing the continuous variables as categorical variables and point out a few nuances. The first nuance we wish to address is simply terminological. Many authors refer to the 'bins' containing the categories of subjects as the quintiles. For example, they may state that subjects in the fifth quintile are at a relative risk of such-and-such compared to subjects in the first quintile. It should be noted that this is an incorrect use of terminology. There are not five quintiles in a distribution, rather there are four quintiles which cut the distribution into five segments or bins of equal density. The term *quintile* refers to the cut-points and not the bins created by the cut-points.

Moving beyond terminological trivia, there are some substantive reasons to avoid the use of a categorized measure. First, it is well established that, all other things being equal, categorization can markedly reduce power (24). Second, if the variable being categorized is also being used as a covariate in the analysis, this categorization may result in incomplete control for the variable and therefore residual confounding (25). Third, and perhaps most importantly, the use of a categorized measure can create interpretive difficulties.

Suppose, for example, one investigator studies the relation between BMI and mortality among Pima Indians and another investigator studies the relation between BMI and mortality among Swedes. Because these two groups have such markedly different distributions of BMI, the BMI values represented by subjects with scores above the fifth quintile will be dramatically different in the two studies. If one investigator reports that the RR among subjects in the highest category is much different between the two studies, it is difficult to determine whether this is due to a true difference in the association of BMI with mortality across the two populations or whether this is simply due to the different BMI distributions in the two populations.

Another interpretive difficulty arises when one wishes to make a specific statement about the risk or hazard associated with a given BMI value. Suppose, for example, an investigator wishes to answer the question 'what is the absolute (or relative) risk of mortality in some defined period of time for an individual with a BMI of 34?' If a continuous risk function is presented using BMI as a continuous variable, this is a simple question to answer. In contrast, if one only has the absolute risk or RR available for subjects put into various categories, one can only answer questions about the risks for the 'average' individual in that category. So, for example, if the only information the investigator has available is the absolute risks or RRs among people with BMI of 32 or greater, then that investigator can say nothing about the risk among individuals with BMI of 32, 34, 36, or any other value. They can only say 'for the *average* individual with a BMI of 32 or greater, the risk is...' One can immediately see the limitation this places on interpreting data in a fine grained way. Among other things, this precludes use of the results of such studies for making predictions about individuals for future research or even in clinical work.

Finally, because the distribution of BMI tends to decrease in density as one moves away from the center of the distribution for virtually every population ever examined, this implies that distributions in the highest and lowest categories are likely to be markedly skewed. This further implies that the means of the 'bins' of BMI will be more disbursed than are the medians. This will be especially true in the first and last bins. This will result in the following visual anomaly. If some function of mortality rate (e.g. probabilities of death within some defined period of time) increases linearly with BMI, the plot of that same function of mortality rate as a function of ordinal BMI categories will appear to accelerate. The appearance of acceleration can even occur if the true relation between BMI and the function of mortality is monotonic increasing but decelerating. Thus, the frequently observed graphs in the BMI mortality literature which imply, at least visually, that functions of mortality rate accelerate (i.e. have positive second derivatives) with BMI above a certain level may exaggerate the degree of acceleration. Thus, the use of a categorical BMI measure may create a 'visual illusion' that causes us to overestimate the true effect of BMI on mortality.

Given the above, it is our opinion that analyzing mortality as a function of categories of BMI is not optimal and should not be the primary analysis. Some investigators prefer the use of the categorical data because it allows for marked non-linearity in the association between BMI mortality. However, as has been pointed out elsewhere (26), after an initial exploration with categorized variables, this can be easily accommodated through techniques such as polynomials of BMI.

Estimating the Range of BMI Associated with Minimal Mortality

Estimating the point of BMI associated with minimal mortality rate (i.e. the 'optimal' BMI) and the range around the point that still represents 'reasonable' BMIs for people is a challenging task involving empirical, statistical and conceptual issues. The empirical issue concerns the fact that the BMIs associated with minimal mortality seem to vary with subject characteristics such as age, sex, and race as described elsewhere in this chapter and may also vary as a function of other factors such as genotype. However, beyond the factors of age and sex, knowledge is very limited. Therefore, just as separate standards for BMI ranges associated with greater longevity are sometimes produced for men and women and people of different ages, perhaps the future will bring separate standards for people depending on other factors including ethnicity or genotype. Until greater information is available about genetic modifiers of the BMI–mortality relation, family history may be a useful proxy. For example, the optimal BMI for a person with a strong family history of osteoporosis and no family history of cardiovascular disease (CVD) may be substantially higher than the optimal BMI for a similar person with no family history of osteoporosis and a strong family history of CVD. This remains to be evaluated and is likely to be a fruitful area for future research.

The statistical issues are fairly straightforward. Although the most common approach is again to categorize BMI on the basis of sample quantiles and declare the category with the lowest sample risk or rate as the region of optimal BMI, this may not be an ideal approach. This is because, as stated above, the risk or hazard estimate for each bin is an estimate of the *average* risk or hazard for people in that bin. Therefore, there is no guarantee that the BMI bin with the lowest risk or hazard contains the BMI point with the lowest risk or hazard. Similarly,

it is entirely possible that, if the bins are wide and the curvature of the BMI–mortality curve acute, then the range of the bin may be far greater than the range of BMI associated with reasonably low mortality rate. Of course, the converse is also true.

The alternative is to treat BMI as a continuous variable and estimate the minimum of a polynomial curve fitted to the data. It had been suggested that this would cause a systematic underestimation of the nadir of the curve (27). However, Allison and Faith (28) showed that, though either over- or underestimation could occur, there was no a priori reason to expect a particular bias. Thus, the calculus can be used to determine the BMI associated with minimum mortality rate and confidence intervals can be placed around such estimates using methods described elsewhere (29). In addition, Durazo-Arvizu *et al.* (30) demonstrated how change-point models can also be used to estimate the BMI associated with minimal mortality rate when the data may not be well characterized by a polynomial.

With respect to the conceptual issues, things are perhaps a bit trickier. Thus far, we have described methods for obtaining a point-estimate of the BMI associated with minimum mortality rate and, possibly, a confidence interval around that estimate. However, of equal importance is developing a *range* around that point-estimate. Without such a range, one would be left in the absurd position of stating, for example, that the optimal BMI for such-and-such a person is 24.65 and anything above (e.g. 24.7) or below (e.g. 24.6) is not good. So how does one declare such a range? One possibility would be to use the 95% (or other) confidence interval. However, this would conflate statistical precision of estimation with biological 'tolerability' of variation in BMI. That is, a wide interval could occur because nature truly tolerates a wide interval of BMIs for the class of individuals under study or because the sample size is small, or both. Conversely, a narrow interval could occur because nature only tolerates a narrow interval of BMIs for the class of individuals under study or because the sample size is large, or both. Alternatively, one might scale the relative risk, odds ratios, or hazard ratios to the average risk, odds, or hazard over the entire sample, find the points where the curve crosses a value of 1.0, and treat those points as the limits of the range. However, this essentially reifies the average and says 'your hazard of death is OK as long as it's not above average'. Who wants to be average when it comes to longevity?

The above methods of determining a range of BMIs associated with minimum mortality rate are flawed because they essentially try to take a judgement that is inherently a subjective value-based judgement and make it objective. Assuming the BMI–mortality curve is convex and differentiable (which seems likely), then the risk is always elevated once one moves off the nadir in either direction. Trying to find points where it is not elevated therefore seems unwise. In contrast, we suggest a simple two-stage approach where the first step is explicitly subjective and the second step involves objective quantification. The first step is to decide how big an increase in risk (either absolute or relative) one is willing to accept. Then, define the limits of the acceptable BMI range as the points on either side of the estimated nadir associated with that degree of elevation.

Eliminating Early Deaths

Rationale

In prospective studies of the BMI–mortality relationship it has become standard to analyze data without those cohort members who have died early (e.g. within the first 5 years of follow-up) as a means of controlling for confounding from pre-existing diseases. The rationale originates from the observation that many serious illnesses lead to both weight loss and an increased risk of death. Therefore, pre-existing occult disease could confound the BMI–mortality relation and lead spuriously to an apparent increase in the rate of mortality among persons with low BMIs. Thus, many reports have asserted the need to eliminate these confounding deaths by simply disregarding those persons who die early in the follow-up and analyze only those deaths that are less likely to have resulted from pre-existing morbidities. The practice of excluding early deaths in the study of longevity and obesity requires that cohort members who have died in the first 'k years' of follow-up be completely excluded from the data analysis. This technique became standard practice in the absence of analytic proof, Monte Carlo simulations, or even detailed statistical discussions of its properties and effectiveness in reducing confounding due to pre-existing disease.

In order to evaluate the effectiveness of such exclusions we conducted three separate studies using analytic methods, Monte Carlo simulations, and meta-analysis. Our analytic proofs (31) showed that the use of 'k-years exclusion', that is excluding subjects who die during the first k years of follow-up, does not necessarily lead to a reduction in bias in the estimated effect of a risk factor on mortality when this relation is confounded by the presence of occult disease. In fact, it was shown that such exclusion can actually exacerbate the bias in some situations. The analytic studies tell us what can happen but not necessarily what is likely to happen. To provide information on what is likely to happen, we conducted an extensive set of computer simulations (32). These simulations used an actual BMI distribution and overall death rates from large databases representative of the US civilian non-institutionalized population. A hypothetical occult disease was assigned to small proportions of the population and the effects of such occult disease on mortality was set to be strong to exaggerate any effects of excluding early deaths. The results of the simulation were consistent with those of the above analytical study such that removal of persons dying early in the study did not necessarily reduce bias in the estimated BMI–mortality curve due to confounding. In fact, elimination of early deaths usually had little discernable effect on the outcome. Moreover, as the analytic results showed, in some cases elimination of early deaths could even exacerbate the effects of such confounding. While this simulation provides no evidence that the true relationship between BMI and mortality is or is not U-shaped, it does indicate that exclusion of subjects who die early is not as effective as once proposed. Therefore, as stated earlier, it is essential that alternative methods to control for the influence of occult diseases on the relationship between BMI and mortality be explored.

To further examine the effect of k-year exclusions on changes in study outcomes, a meta-analysis was conducted on the effect of early death exclusion on the relationship between BMI and mortality. Studies were selected from a MEDLINE search for the years 1966 to 1996, other meta-analyses, reviews of obesity and mortality, and ancestry analyses. The analysis was conducted on 29 studies with almost 2 million subjects and used a strict set of inclusion criteria for study selection. It was found that the difference in results when early deaths were included and excluded was statistically significant, but extremely small and the shape of the curve did not change appreciably. From these results, it was concluded that exclusion of early deaths from the analysis of the BMI–mortality relationship has only a very small and not clinically significant effect (33).

Thus, it is evident from this discussion that the practice of excluding early deaths from analyses of mortality and weight is not statistically sound. The simulation study and meta-analysis both demonstrate that the shape of the mortality risk curve remains U-shaped with or without the exclusion of early deaths. This suggests that *either* the higher rates of mortality at lower BMIs are not simply artifacts from persons suffering from occult diseases which may precipitate weight loss, or such confounding does exist and early death elimination is incapable of reducing the bias thereby induced. Therefore, more emphasis needs to be placed on acquiring 'clean' data rather than on ad hoc statistical fix-ups.

Dealing with Weight Fluctuation

Recently, excluding subjects who have lost more than some minimal amount of weight and/or have had more than some minimal degree of weight fluctuation has become popular (7,34,35). Like excluding early deaths (see above), this practice has been introduced in the absence, to our knowledge, of mathematical proofs, computer simulations, or even detailed statistical discussions of its merits. Though it is beyond the scope of this review to undertake a detailed exploration of this technique, we point out that, like early death exclusion, this elimination of subjects reduces power. Moreover, the degree of weight loss or fluctuation is a continuous variable and it is not necessary to make it categorical and eliminate subjects in one category. Rather, one can simply include the degree of loss or fluctuation in a model as a covariate and also model interactions between it and baseline BMI. Thus, before the practice of eliminating subjects with weight loss or fluctuation becomes *de rigueur* or is used as a primary analytic approach for BMI mortality studies, proponents of this technique should publish careful analyses of its merits.

RESEARCH FINDINGS

Overall Findings

Having stressed the methodological issues above and their impact on the results of studies, the obvious question is 'What conclusions can the currently available data support?' Describing what the currently available data show is relatively simple. When the overall body of literature available is reviewed, the data clearly show that the association between BMI and mortality is U- or J-shaped. Among non-elderly white males and females the nadirs of the curve tend to be around the mid to high 20s. The nadir of the curve can vary substantially as a function of age, sex, race, and possibly other variables. However, the shape of the curve and its nadir does not vary substantially regardless of whether or how one adjusts for smoking, whether or how one adjusts for variables that are likely to be on the causal path from obesity to mortality, and whether or not one eliminates subjects dying during the first few years of analysis or makes other attempts to control for pre-existing disease. Though isolated studies may occasionally show other results, the aforementioned conclusions are those that are clearly supported by the overall body of data (9).

The Effect of Smoking

Smoking is thought typically to be a major confounder of the BMI–mortality relation and to contribute artifactually to the elevated mortality rate at the low end of the BMI continuum. This is hypothesized because smoking strongly increases mortality rate and also has an inverse association with adiposity (4). If this is so, then failure to control for the effects of smoking might help account for the overall J- or U-shaped association typically observed. If it were established that smoking consistently confounds the BMI–mortality association, it would suggest that studies that have not controlled for the effects of smoking would have systematically underestimated the deleterious effect of high BMIs and overestimated the deleterious effect of low BMIs on longevity. Table 3.1 summarizes recent studies that investigated whether smoking confounds the BMI–mortality association. As can be

Table 3.1 Does smoking confound the BMI–mortality association?

Authors	Data source	Sample	Years follow-up	Deaths	Covariates	Results
Fontaine et al. (38)	Panel Study of Income Dynamics	1355 American women ≥ 50	4.5 years	110	Age, BMI², smoking, education, 4 health status variables	U-shaped relation with and without smoking in the model
Sempos et al. (39)	Framingham Heart Study	5209 men and women (28–62 years at baseline)	30 years	>1900	Age, illness, education, smoking	J-shaped relation; similar BMI at minimum risk of death for smokers and non-smokers
Brenner et al. (40)	Cohort of German construction workers	7812 men (age 25–64 at baseline)	Mean 4.5 years	167	Age, nationality, alcohol, occupation, smoking	Excess mortality in lowest BMI category reduced but not eliminated by control of smoking
Dorn et al. (41)	Buffalo Health Study	1308 men and women (age 20–96 at baseline)	29 years	576	Age, education, smoking	U-shaped quadratic relation
Chyou et al. (42)	Cohort of Japanese-Americans in Hawaii	8006 men (age 45–68 at baseline)	22 years	2667	Age, alcohol consumption, smoking	J-shaped relation
Seidell et al. (43)	Consultation Bureau Project of Cardiovascular Diseases	48 287 men and women (age 30–54 at baseline)	Mean 12 years	818	Age, cholesterol, hypertension, diabetes, smoking	In men, excess mortality in lowest BMI category reduced but not eliminated by control of smoking; no relation for women
Manson et al. (1995)	Nurses' Health Study	115 195 women (age 30–55 at baseline)	16 years	4726	Age, contraception, hormone use, family history of myocardial infarction, menopausal status, smoking	Apparent excess risk associated with leanness eliminated when smoking and many other factors were accounted for
Wienpahl et al. (44)	Members of Kaiser Foundation Health Plan	5184 black men and women (age 40–79 at baseline)	15 years	676	Age, antecedent illness, education, alcohol use, smoking	J-shaped curve for men after controlling for smoking; flat association for women
Rissanen et al. (45)	Cohort of Finnish men	22 995 (age > 25 years)	Median 12 years		Age, smoking, cholesterol, blood pressure	U-shaped high mortality in lean men 'not entirely attributable to smoking'
Wannamethee and Shaper (46)	Cohort of British men	7735 (age 40–59 at baseline)	Mean 9 years	660	Age, pre-existing disease, smoking	Increased mortality in lean men seen only in current smokers
Garrison et al. (36)	Framingham Heart Study	5209 (age 28–62 at baseline)	26 years	679	Age, smoking	BMI–mortality relation in lean subjects confounded by smoking

seen, although at least three studies (7,36,37) suggest that smoking is an important confounder in that the left-most elevation in the J-shaped curve diminished substantially when controlling for smoking (statistically or by restricting the analysis to never smokers), the overwhelming majority of studies have found that the increased mortality among thin subjects (i.e. the J- or U-shaped association) persisted, though often slightly attenuated somewhat, after controlling for smoking.

The minimal power of smoking to account for the excess mortality among thin individuals is further supported by recent comprehensive analyses. In the first, Troiano and colleagues (9) performed a quantitative synthesis of 19 prospective cohort studies and found a U-shaped relation between BMI and mortality regardless of whether or not smoking was controlled for statistically or smokers were eliminated. In a second analysis, The BMI in Diverse Populations Collaborative Group (47) analyzed pooled data from 15 separate epidemiologic studies involving over 200 000 subjects and found that the BMI–mortality association remained essentially unchanged and quadratic (i.e. U-shaped) irrespective of whether or not and how smoking was controlled for or treated in their analyses. Collectively the quantitative syntheses suggest that smoking does not appear to be a major cause of the elevated mortality among the thin.

Nevertheless, when smoking information is available, as it is in most epidemiologic studies, there is no reason not to adjust for it and a possible (though apparently small) benefit in doing so. One question that arises is *how* one should adjust for smoking. Some investigators prefer to keep the entire data set intact and statistically adjust for smoking. Others seem to believe that the only valid approach is to eliminate any subject who has ever smoked from the data set. The answer to this questions sees to depend, in part, on what one is prepared to believe and see as paramount in the BMI–smoking–mortality relationship. Two non-exhaustive possibilities seem to predominate current thinking: (1) Smoking confounds the BMI–mortality relation, smoking is poorly measured in epidemiologic studies, people can accurately report if they have *ever* smoked, and the true causal relation (not the observed association) between BMI and mortality rate is unaffected by smoking status; and (2) the true causal relation (not the observed association) between BMI and

mortality rate may be affected by smoking status and measurements of smoking status in epidemiologic studies perfectly capture all of the variance in exposure to any of the deleterious aspects of smoking (e.g. tar exposure). If the first possibility were true, then any attempt to control for smoking statistically would fail as a result of measurement error induced residual confounding (25), whereas studies of *never*-smokers only would yield unbiased estimates of the effects of BMI on mortality for both never-smokers and ever-smokers. In contrast, were the second possibility true, then statistical adjustment will fully control for any confounding by smoking and including all subjects in the analysis will provide the best estimate of the *average* effect of BMI on mortality rate across the whole population of smokers and non-smokers. Of course, in this second case, one would probably wish to estimate effects of BMI on mortality rate that varied as a function of smoking status and this could be accomplished by use of interaction terms (23). In reality, neither of the two possibilities listed above is likely to be strictly true and the best approach may be to fit the model involving interactions with smoking status where a category is explicitly coded for never-smokers. This allows simultaneous estimation of the effects among never-smokers and among smokers. Both can then be viewed and readers can determine for themselves what the most plausible estimate is for the overall population and different smoking subgroups.

Aging and the Elderly

A number of studies have investigated whether age modifies the relation between body weight and mortality. Certainly several studies of BMI and mortality among older adults have reported weak effects of obesity on mortality rate and/or very high nadirs for the BMI–mortality curves (38,41,48–50). The Build Study (51) found that the relation between BMI and mortality was U-shaped, and that the BMI associated with minimal mortality increased with age. In a Norwegian study (27), plots of the log of the mortality rate against BMI categories also revealed a U-shaped association. Although it was less clear whether the BMI associated with minimal mortality increased with age, the overall curves did flatten substantially with age. However, it should be noted that Waaler (27) did not control for the effects of smoking.

More recent studies that examined the effect of age on the BMI–mortality association have controlled for smoking. In a Finnish cohort of 17 000 women followed for 12 years, there was a U-shaped BMI-all-cause mortality relation among non-smokers 25 to 64 years of age. Among women aged 65 or greater, mortality varied little according to BMI (52). Among white women from the Seventh Day Adventist cohort who never smoked, the RR of death associated with elevated BMI was lower among 55- to 74-year-olds than for 30- to 54-year-olds. For these older women, the minimal mortality was in the group with BMIs from 23 to 24.8 (53). Although the nadirs of the curves were much higher, a recent study by Seccareccia et al. (54) of over 60 000 Italian subjects again shows the increase in the nadir with age.

In one of the largest studies, Stevens et al. (34) investigated mortality over 12 years as a function of BMI across six age groups (30–44, 45–54, 55–64, 65–74, 75–84, and ≥ 85) among 324 135 never-smokers with no apparent pre-existing disease from the American Cancer Society's Cancer Prevention Study I. Results indicated that, although greater BMI was associated with higher all-cause and CVD mortality, the RR associated with greater BMI declined somewhat with age (e.g. for men the RR of CVD mortality with an increment of 1.0 BMI units was 1.10 for 30–44-year-olds and 1.03 for 65–74-year-olds).

Bender and colleagues (55) recently examined the effect of age on excess mortality associated with obesity among 6193 obese persons enrolled in the Duseldorf Obesity Mortality Study (DOMS). When grouped into four groups based on approximate quartiles of age and BMI, it was found that the overall risk of death increased with increased body weight, but that obesity-related excess mortality declined with age at all levels of BMI.

On the whole, these studies suggest that the relative increase in rate of death associated with increased BMI is somewhat lower for older adults than for younger adults and the BMI associated with minimum mortality rate increases with age. However, as Stevens et al. (56) point out, the *absolute* increase in rate of death can be higher in an older than younger person even when the *relative* increase is lower.

Ethnicity

The majority of research on the effects of body weight, body composition and longevity has been conducted on samples of European Americans (57). While it is clear that obesity in African Americans, most notably women, is associated with a number of risk factors (58,59), the relation between obesity and mortality/longevity among African Americans is not as clear as it is in white individuals.

On the basis of a 14-year mortality study with X-ray-determined adiposity, Comstock et al. (60) concluded that the excess mortality of overweight/ obese persons was more marked for European Americans than for African Americans. By the same token, in a cohort of 2731 African American women members of the Kaiser Foundation Health Plan who were followed for 15 years, Wienpahl et al. (44) found an essentially flat BMI–mortality association across the entire range of BMI. However, although the U-shaped relation between BMI and all-cause mortality was not significant, Stevens et al. (61) found that, among African American men, obesity was associated with increased risk of mortality from ischemic heart disease (IHD). More recently, Stevens et al. (11) examined the association of BMI to all-cause and CVD mortality among 100 000 White and 8142 African American women from the American Cancer society Prevention Study I. At the 12-year follow-up, they found a significant interaction between ethnicity and BMI for both all-cause and CVD mortality. That is, among white women BMI was associated with all-cause mortality in all four groups (defined by smoking status and educational attainment). In African American women with less than a high school education there was no significant association between BMI and all-cause mortality. However, there was a significant association among high school-educated African American women. Models using the lowest BMI as the reference group among never smoking women with at least a high school education indicated a 40% higher risk of all-cause mortality at a BMI of 35.9 in the African American women versus 27.3 in the white women. Stevens et al. concluded that, although educational attainment modifies the impact of BMI on mortality, BMI was a less potent risk factor in the African American women than in the white women.

Similar results have been obtained by others (35,62–65). That is, the bulk of the studies conducted suggest that the effect of given BMI increase on mortality rate may be less deleterious among African Americans. Two more recent studies have emerged with relatively large and high quality samples of African Americans (66,67). These studies show that there clearly is a deleterious effect of obesity on mortality rate among African Americans, though the BMIs associated with minimum mortality rate may be slightly higher among African Americans.

With regard to the BMI–mortality association among persons of other ethnic origins, the data are relatively sparse. In a sample of Micronesian Nauruans and Melanesian and Indian Fijians, obesity was not significantly associated with an elevated mortality rate (68). Among a sample of 8006 Japanese American men living in Hawaii who were followed for 22 years, a significant quadratic (J-shaped) relation was found between BMI and mortality independent of the effects of smoking and alcohol consumption (42). Similarly, among a cohort of over 2000 Japanese adults over age 40, there was a U-shaped relation between BMI and mortality rate with a nadir in the range of 23–25. However, among a cohort of 2546 East Indian and Melanesian Fijians followed for 11 years, the association of BMI to all-cause and CVD mortality was generally inconsistent (69). Despite the known associations between body weight and diabetes and other obesity-related diseases found among Mexican Americans, data have revealed lower than expected rates of mortality, based on known body weights (70). To date, the data available on the BMI–mortality association among other ethnic groups (e.g. Native Americans, Alaska Natives) are limited. Hanson *et al.* (71) found that, among a cohort of 814 diabetic and 1814 non-diabetic Pima Indians, a U-shaped relationship between BMI and mortality was found in men, but not women. It was reported that excess mortality among lighter individuals was present in those persons who were gaining weight. Thus, they concluded that pre-existing illness may only partially explain the high mortality among lighter persons.

Could the Elevated Mortality Rate Among the Thin Be Causal?

As we have pointed out, most studies find that thin people (e.g. $18 < BMI < 24$) tend to have higher mortality rates than more 'mid-BMI' people (e.g. $24 < BMI < 28$). There are several non-exclusive possible explanations for this. The most commonly mentioned is that this is due to confounding by smoking or pre-existing disease. A second is that this has to do with using BMI as a proxy for adiposity. These two possibilities were discussed elsewhere in this chapter. A possibility that seems to receive less consideration is that being in the mid-BMI range may *cause* one to be at lower risk of death from certain causes. Consider a few examples that range from well-supported to plausible-but-highly-speculative. It is clear that relative to thinness, being in the mid-BMI range is protective against osteoporosis (72,73). There is a clear biological mechanism because thinness is a clear risk factor for hip fracture (74) which is in turn a risk for mortality (72,75). Thus, it is plausible that thinness (at least among the elderly) causes increased mortality rate through an osteoporosis/fracture pathway.

Though more speculative, it is possible that, relative to being in the mid-BMI range, people in the thin range are more potently affected by or more susceptible to certain forms of infection and injury. Finally, given that most modern Americans (as well as the members of many other countries) have inadequate intake of fruit, vegetables, fiber, and many micronutrients (76,77), it may be that thin people, simply by virtue of eating less total food, are at increased risk of nutrient deficiencies despite adequate caloric intake. That is, just as laboratory animals live longer when calorically restricted only when one insures adequate micronutrient intakes (78,79), thinness in humans may be deleterious only because it is, among many people, associated with inadequate intake of certain nutrients.

Though many of the potential explanations above are speculative, they are plausible. We believe the possibility that thinness *causes* increased mortality rate deserves to be taken seriously and that further research to *understand* rather than dismiss the observed elevated mortality rate among the thin is warranted.

Putting the Results in Perspective

Statements about RRs, hazard ratios, and odds ratios are interpretable to many scientists but often do not have an intuitive appeal to clinicians, policy makers, and the lay public. Therefore, it is useful to consider the effect of varying levels of BMI on mortality rate with different metrics. Two metrics that may be useful are the number of annual deaths due to obesity and the years of life an individual can expect to lose from being a given degree above the optimal BMI. The former may be especially useful for policy makers whereas the latter may be more useful for clinicians and individual patients.

Attributable Deaths

At a societal level, one can estimate the number of deaths each year that are attributable to obesity and overweight. Recently, Allison et al. (32) estimated that of adults who were alive in the United States at the beginning of 1991, somewhere between 280 000 and 325 000 fewer would have died during that year, if they had never been overweight or obese. More than 80% of these deaths occurred among individuals with BMIs over 30.

Estimated Years of Life Lost

The individual patient may be less concerned with numbers for the whole population than with answers to questions like 'How many years less am I expected to live given that my BMI is such-and-such?' This question calls for an analysis of years of life lost (YLL). Stevens et al. (56) recently published such an analysis. However, they restricted this analysis to a 12-year period rather than estimating YLL across the remaining life. We believe that this will markedly underestimate YLL and is likely to create spurious positive correlations between baseline age and YLL. Therefore, we believe additional studies estimating YLL across the entire life are necessary to provide meaningful values in this metric.

Change in Weight

Dramatic effects of obesity on mortality rate have been demonstrated in studies of laboratory rodents (80). When obese animals are compared to nonobese, the lean outlive the obese regardless of the type of obesity (e.g. polygenic factors or dietary induction). These findings are buttressed by the life-prolonging effects shown to be achieved by caloric restriction (CR). CR should not be conflicted with lower body weight or lower body fat. However, CR clearly results in lower body weight and is the most common method by which humans achieve lower body weight. Therefore, it is worth noting that CR achieved by various means and resulting weight loss has been demonstrated to result in increased longevity in a variety of animal species, such as spiders, water fleas, fish, and laboratory rodents (81).

Obesity (at least when severe) is clearly associated with an increased mortality rate. Moreover, weight loss is clearly associated with reductions in many risk factors. Therefore, one might wish to conclude that weight loss among the obese will increase lifespan. However, to date, data to support this conjecture are sparse at best. Indeed, after a review 13 papers from 11 samples of adults in the United States and Europe, Andres et al. (10) wrote:

Despite the diversity of the populations studied, the degree of 'clinical clean-up' at entry, the techniques used to assess weight change, and the differences in analytic techniques (including consideration of potentially confounding variables), certain conclusions may be drawn. Evidence suggests that the highest mortality rates occur in adults who either have lost weight or have gained excessive weight. The lowest mortality rates are generally associated with modest weight gain. (p. 737).

However, the puzzling finding that weight loss is predictive of increased mortality rate is still subject to considerable inquiry. In an insightful review of the literature, Williamson (82) noted that analyses should be restricted to those for whom weight loss is generally recommended, i.e. obese individuals. Furthermore, as in the study of BMI per se, in the study of the effects of changes in BMI the possibility of confounding by occult disease remains a substantial issue. This is illustrated by Williamson (82) who show that unintentional weight loss is at least as common as is intentional weight loss. Williamson describes a study (83) of intentional weight loss among 203 adults with recent myocardial infarction who had been instructed to lose weight. The results of this study indicated that subjects losing at least 5 kg had a 54% lower mortality rate during the subsequent year. In an observational study, Lean et al. (84) found that weight loss was associated with greater longevity among identified and treated diabetics. These results suggest possible benefits to weight loss among obese individuals suffering from comorbidities.

Recently, a series of large epidemiological studies

Table 3.2 Two by two table weight loss by intention

	No intention to lose weight	Intention to lose weight
Did not lose weight	0.187	0.414
Lost weight	0.045	0.354

Based on Meltzer and Everhart (88).

have been conducted to address this issue. Williamson and colleagues observed that when analyses are restricted to weight loss among never-smoking, overweight individuals who reported that their weight loss was intentional, weight loss was associated with either a beneficial effect or no effect. For further discussion of these studies, see French *et al.* (85), Kuller (86), and Williamson *et al.* (87).

However, it is important to realize that the so-called intentional weight loss studied by these investigators may often by unintentional. Consider the following. Meltzer and Everhart (88) studied participant attributions of weight loss intention in a large population-based survey. Among women, they found the following:

- 76.8% of overweight women reported attempting to lose weight.
- Of those women attempting to lose weight, 46.1% did lose weight.
- The adjusted odds ratio for weight loss given that one intends to lose weight is reported to be 3.52.

Similar results were obtained for men. Using these three numbers and some algebra, one can derive the 2×2 table shown in Table 3.2 expressed in proportions. Applying the standard attributable risk approach, this implies that 46% of overweight women who intend to lose weight do lose weight, but that 19% would have lost weight even if they had not intended to do so. Therefore, the fraction of weight loss among overweight women who intend to lose weight that is due to factors other than their intention is about 41% (i.e. 19/46). These calculations suggest that some large sub-portion of those who have been designated as intentional weight losers in past studies may have actually lost weight through some other mechanism such as occult illness. If this were true, the currently observed equivocally beneficial effects of what we currently label intentional weight loss may markedly underestimate true benefits due to residual confounding by occult disease. This points out the severe limitations of observational (non-experimental) studies in this area.

Moreover, perhaps we are misguided by focusing on 'intentionality' at all. In many of the observational studies of so-called intentional weight loss, subjects were initially measured decades ago (82, 87). By what methods did they achieve weight loss decades ago? Among others, by drugs and surgical procedures that are far less safe than those currently available. Even as late as 1997 some widely prescribed drugs were removed from the market because of dangerous effects (89). Still today, methods for intentionally inducing weight loss include fad diets (90), herbal supplements of untested safety, bulimia and other methods of highly questionable safety. Hence, it appears ill advised to estimate the effects weight loss achieved by medically recommended methods by studying weight loss that is merely reported to be 'intentional.' What is needed is studies of weight loss that is produced among obese humans by modern methods that are accepted by mainstream medicine.

Presently, a well-controlled *non-randomized*, study of weight loss produced by surgery among morbidly obese adults is underway (91). Mortality results are not yet available. A randomized clinical trial (RCT) testing whether producing weight loss through medically accepted methods among obese people can reduce mortality rate could settle these issues (92). Presently, the National Institute of Diabetes, Digestive and Kidney Diseases is designing a large multi-center study termed *SHOW*. Although this RCT will examine mortality as a secondary outcome, it is not necessarily powered to detect differences in mortality rates.

Our perspective of the admittedly incomplete evidence regarding the effect of weight loss on mortality rate is portrayed in Figure 3.1—an iconic representation of the currently available literature and a conjecture of what the future might bring. This figure is intended to convey that as studies of weight loss and mortality rate have become methodologically more sound, what initially appeared to be a harmful effect has progressively shifted to be neutral

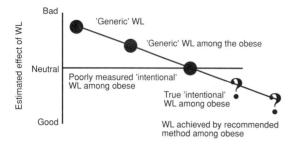

Figure 3.1 Iconic presentation of the estimated effects of weight loss (WL) on mortality with varying study designs

at worst and possibly even somewhat positive. When studies of weight loss that is intentionally induced among obese individuals through accepted medical interventions are included, it is plausible to conjecture that the effect may become strongly positive. Still, there is a great gap between conjecture and demonstration and we must continue to look for stronger studies that can provide this demonstration (or lack thereof).

Change in Body Composition

Finally, as discussed above, studies of body composition at a single point in time, as opposed to just body weight at a single point in time, may tell different stories. The same may hold true for studies of *change* in body composition versus *change* in weight. To examine this possibility, Allison *et al.* (32) analyzed mortality rate in two epidemiologic studies, the Tecumseh Community Health Study and the Framingham Heart Study. In both, change in weight and fat (via skinfolds) across two points in time were available. In both studies, weight loss and fat loss were, respectively, associated with an elevated and reduced mortality rate. Each standard deviation (SD) of weight loss (approximately 5.5 kg across both studies) was estimated to increase the hazard of mortality by about 35%. In contrast, each SD of fat loss (10.0 mm in Tecumseh and 4.8 mm in Framingham) reduced the hazard of mortality by about 16%. Thus, among individuals that are not severely obese, weight loss (conditional upon fat loss) is associated with increased mortality rate and fat loss (conditional upon weight loss) with decreased mortality rate. These results, if confirmed in future studies, have important implications for clinical and public health recommendations regarding

weight loss. They suggest that weight loss should only be recommended under conditions where a sufficient proportion of the weight lost can be expected to be fat. Unfortunately, what those conditions are and what the minimum proportion is remains unknown at his time.

DISCUSSION

In this discussion section, we begin by reiterating key methodological conclusions. We follow this with a discussion of what we believe the currently available data on relative body weight and mortality show and what the currently available data on body weight and mortality mean. We can point out that these are not necessarily the same thing.

Based on the information reviewed above, we reach the following conclusions:

1. While controlling for smoking either by stratification or statistical adjustment is a sound process and smoking is a plausible confounder of the BMI–mortality relationship, in actual data sets, adjusting for smoking has very little impact on the results of the analysis. This does not imply that one should not control for smoking. It only implies that smoking appears to be an unlikely explanation for the U- and J-shaped relationships frequently observed between BMI and mortality.

2. Excluding subjects who die during the first few years of follow-up is not a reliable way of controlling for confounding due to occult disease. In the presence of confounding due to occult disease such exclusions can either increase or decrease the bias, although in practice such exclusions appear to make little difference. Because such exclusions can actually increase the bias under some circumstances and result in an overall reduction of sample size, we do not recommend that subjects dying during the first few years be excluded from the analyses.

3. There is no a priori reason to assume, if a quadratic model is fitted to describe the relationship between BMI and mortality and the minimum of this quadratic equation solved for the resulting estimated BMI associated with minimum mortality, that the estimate will systematically overestimate the true BMI associated with minimum mortality. However, other methods for es-

timating the BMI associated with minimum mortality are available and may be superior. These methods do not require that BMI be categorized into quantiles but can be applied to BMI treated as a continuous variable.

4. BMI is a continuous variable and, as with other continuous variables, there is little advantage to categorizing BMI in the final analysis. It is certainly useful to treat BMI categorically in an exploratory manner. However, it is possible to treat BMI continuously in the final analysis and there are a number of advantages to doing so.

5. Though highly correlated with body fatness, BMI is not a true measure of body fatness and it cannot be assumed that BMI will have the same relationship with mortality in either direction or form as will a valid measure of body composition. Therefore, it is strongly suggested that future research consider including measures of body composition rather than just BMI.

6. There is substantial variation in results from study to study, some of which is probably due solely to random sampling variations. Because of this, selective review of the data can be used to support virtually any conclusion. Therefore, it is essential that reviews of the literature, if they are intended to be objective, evaluate the entire body of the literature to the greatest extent possible. This approach is exemplified in the recent papers by Allison *et al.* (32), Troiano *et al.* (9), and The BMI in Diverse Populations Collaborative Group (47).

7. The relationship between BMI and mortality appears to vary substantially by age, sex, and race. Other variables yet to be fully explored may also moderate this relationship. Therefore, it is ill advised to generalize from studies in the one population (e.g. white middle-aged females) to other populations (e.g. young black males or elderly Asian females). Moreover, investigators who wish to make broad statements about the overall 'average' relationship between BMI and mortality for the US population will need to rely on samples that are representative of the US population. Finally, this implies that it is wise for investigators to attempt to stratify by or fit interaction terms with their demographic variables and other possible moderators when analyzing the relationship between BMI and mortality.

What the Available Data Show

The above conclusions can be used to guide future research investigating the effect of variations in relative body weight on longevity. Collectively, they suggest that measures of body composition should be used over measures of body weight whenever possible, that subjects dying during the first several years not be excluded from the analysis, that measures of either body composition or relative body weight can be treated as continuous variables, that statistical methods can be used to estimate the BMI (or degree of adiposity) associated with minimum mortality, and, finally, that alternative methods be pursued to reduce the possibility of confounding due to occult disease (e.g. more careful clinical evaluation at baseline).

However, what the data show and what the data mean are not necessarily the same thing. Because the association between BMI and mortality is U-shaped does not mean that the causal relationship between BMI and mortality is U-shaped. As we have shown, the fact that relationship persists even after eliminating subjects who die during the first several years of follow-up cannot be taken as evidence that this relationship is not due to confounding for pre-existing disease. Moreover, as we have shown, the fact that the relationship between BMI and mortality may be U-shaped does not necessarily imply that the relationship between adiposity and mortality is U-shaped. Thus, it is difficult to know exactly what to conclude from the currently available data. Certainly, the currently available data do demonstrate that unusually high levels of BMI (e.g. BMIs greater than the high 20s) are associated with increased mortality and this is entirely consistent with a great deal of clinical and basic laboratory research. However, over the range of BMI from about 28 down, the picture is not clear. The human epidemiological data suggest that lower BMIs are associated with increased mortality but, as we have argued, there are limits to the strength of the conclusions one can draw from here. Moreover, these data are not easily reconcilable with the results of animal work which show that caloric restriction is capable of producing substantial increases in longevity (81). Finally, such work is not consistent with the clinical evidence that suggests that intentional weight loss is almost always associated with a reduction in morbidities even among those who are only mildly overweight (93).

It appears that, to date, the approaches that investigators have taken for evaluating the association between variations in relative body adiposity and mortality have been to rely on weak epidemiologic data. By 'weak' we mean data in which the measured independent variable (e.g. BMI) is only a proxy for the conceptual independent variable (i.e. adiposity) and the most plausible confounding factor (i.e. occult disease) is not measured but only inferred. In the face of such weak data, the approach that some authors seem to believe will yield valid conclusions is a strong statistical analysis. In our opinion, this is an example of what has been called 'under-design and over-analysis'. Though we are as appreciative of the power and beauty of good statistical models as anyone, we believe that no amount of statistical analysis will make weak data strong. If stronger conclusions are to be drawn from future studies we believe that stronger measurements and designs will have to be employed. Such designs should clearly include measures of adiposity, detailed and thorough clinical evaluations of health status at study onset, and possibly even the use of large-scale randomized trials (92).

ACKNOWLEDGEMENTS

This work was supported in part by National Institutes of Health grants R01DK51716, P30DK26687.

REFERENCES

1. WHO. *Obesity. Preventing and Managing the Global Epidemic*. Geneva: World Health Organization, 1998.
2. Kuczmarski RJ, Flegal KM, Campbell SM, Johnson CL. Increasing prevalence of overweight among US adults. The National Health and Nutrition Examination Surveys, 1960 to 1991. *JAMA* 1994; **272**(3): 205–211.
3. Simopoulos AP, Van Itallie TB. Body weight, health, and longevity. *Ann Intern Med* 1984; **100**: 285–295.
4. Manson JE, Stampfer MJ, Hennekens CH, Willett WC. Body weight and longevity: A reassessment. *JAMA* 1987; **257**: 353–358.
5. Samaras TT, Storms LH. Impact of height and weight on life span. *Bull WHO* 1992; **70**: 259–267.
6. Allison DB, Faith MS, Heo M, Kotler DP. Hypothesis concerning the U-shaped relation between body mass index and mortality. *Am J Epidemiol*; 1997; **146**: 339–349.
7. Manson JE, Willett WC, Stampfer MJ, Colditz GA, Hunter DJ, Hankinson SE, Hennekens CH, Speizer FE. Body weight and mortality among women. *N Eng J Medi* 1995; **333**: 677–685.
8. Ernsberger P, Haskew P. Rethinking obesity. An alternative view of its health implications. *J Obes Weight Regulation* 1987; **6**.
9. Troiano RP, Frongillo EA Jr, Sobal J, Levitsky DA. The relationship of body weight and mortality: a quantitative analysis of combined information from existing studies. *Int J Obes Relat Metab Disord* 1996; **20**: 63–75.
10. Andres R, Muller DC, Sorkin JD. Long-term effects of change in body weight on all-cause mortality. A review. *Ann Intern Med* 1993; **110** (7 Pt 2): 737–743.
11. Stevens J, Plankey MW, Willaimson DF, Thun MJ, Rust PF, Palesch Y, O'Neil PM. The body mass index–mortality relationship in White and African American women. *Obes Res* 1998; **6**: 268–277.
12. Lee CD, Jackson AS, Blair SN. US weight guidelines: is it also important to consider cardiorespiratory fitness? *Int J Obes Relat Metab Disord* 1998; **22**: S2–7.
13. Blair SN, Brodney S. Effects of physical inactivity and obesity on morbidity and mortality: current evidence and research issues. *Med Sci Sports Exerc* 1999; **31**: S646–662.
14. Kushner RF. Body weight and mortality. *Nutr Rev* 1993; **51**(5): 127–136.
15. Michels KB, Greenland S, Rosner BA. Does body mass index adequately capture the relation of body composition and body size to health outcomes? *Am J Epidemiol* 1998; **147**: 167–172.
16. Roche AF, Siervogel RM, Chumlea WC, Webb P. Grading body fatness from limited anthropometric data. *Am J Clin Nutr* 1981; **34**: 2831–2838.
17. Van Itallie TB, Yang MU, Boileau RA, *et al*. Applications of body composition technology in clinical medicine: Some issues and problems. In: Kral JG, Van Itallie TB (eds) *Recent Developments in Body Composition Analysis*: Methods and Applications. London: Smith-Gordon, 1993; 87–97.
18. Segal KR, Dunaif A, Gutin B, Albu J, Nyman A, Pi-Sunyer FX. Body composition, not body weight, is related to cardiovascular disease risk factors and sex hormone levels in men. *J Clin Invest* 1987; **80**: 1050–1055.
19. Folsom AR, Kaye SA, Sellers TA *et al*. Body fat distribution and 5-year risk of death in older women. *JAMA* 1993; **142**: 483–487.
20. Keys A, Taylor HL, Blackburn H, Brozek J, Anserson JT, Simonson E. Mortality and coronary heart disease among men studied for 23 years. *Arch Intern Med* 1971; **128**: 201–214.
21. Menotti A, Descovich GC, Lanti M. Indexes of obesity and all-causes mortality in Italian epidemiological data. *Prev Med* 1993; **22**: 293–303.
22. Lee CD, Jackson AS. Cardiorespiratory fitness, body composition, and all-cause and cardiovascular disease mortality in men. *Am J Clin Nutr* 1999; **69**: 373–380.
23. Collett D. *Modeling Survival Data in Medical Research*. New York: Chapman & Hall, 1994.
24. Selvin S. Two issues concerning the analysis of grouped data. *Eur J Epidemiol* 1987; **3**: 284–287.
25. Becher H. The concept of residual confounding in regression models and some applications. *Stat Med* 1992; **11**: 1747–1758.
26. Zhao LP, Kolonel LN. Efficiency loss from categorizing

quantitative exposures into qualitative exposures in case-control studies. *Am J Epidemiol* 1992; **136**(4): 464–474.

27. Waaler HT. Height, weight, and mortality: the Norwegian experience. *Acta Med Scand Suppl* 1984; **679**: 1–56.

28. Allison DB, Faith MS. On estimating the minima of BMI-mortality curves. *Int J Obes* 1995; **20**: 496–498.

29. Graybill FA, Iyer HK. *Regression Analysis. Concepts and Applications*. Belmont, CA: Wadsworth Publishing, 1994.

30. Durazo-Arvizu R, McGee D, Li Z, Cooper R. Establishing the nadir of the body mass index–mortality relationship: A case study. *J Am Stat Assoc* 1997; **92**: 1312–1319.

31. Allison DB, Heo M, Flanders DW, Faith MS, Williamson DF Examination of 'early mortality exclusion' as an approach to control for confounding by occult disease in epidemiologic studies of mortality risk factors. *Am J Epidemiol* 1997; **146**: 672–680.

32. Allison DB, Fontain KR, Manson JE, Stevens J, VanItallie TB. Annual deaths attributable to obesity in the United States. *JAMA* 1999; **282**: 1530–1538.

33. Andres R. Beautiful hypotheses and ugly facts: the BMI–mortality association. *Obes Res* 1999; **7**: 417–419.

34. Stevens J, Cai J, Pamuk ER, Williamson DF, Thun MJ, Wood JL. The effect of age on the association between body-mass index and mortality. *N Eng J Medicine* 1998; **338**: 1–7.

35. Calle EE, Thun MJ, Petreli JM, Rodriguez C, Heath CW. Body-mass index and mortality in a prospective cohort of US adults. *N Engl J Med* 1999; **341**: 1097–1105.

36. Garrison RJ, Feinleib M, Castelli WP *et al.* Cigarette smoking as a contributor of the relationship between relative weight and long-term mortality: The Framingham Heart Study. *JAMA* 1983; **249**: 2199–2203.

37. Lew EA, Garfinkel L. Variations in mortality by weight among 750,000 men and women. *J Chronic Dis* 1979; **32**: 563–576.

38. Fontaine KR, Heo M, Cheskin LJ, Allison DB. Body mass index, smoking, and mortality among older American women. *J Women's Health* 1998; **7**: 1257–1261.

39. Sempos CT, Durazo-Arvizu R, McGee DL, Cooper RS, Prewitt TE. The influence of cigarette smoking on the association between body weight and mortality: The Framingham Heart Study revisited. *Ann Epidemiol* 1998; **8**: 289–300.

40. Brenner H, Arndt V, Rothenbacher D, Schuberth S, Fraisse E, Fliedner TM. Body weight, pre-existing disease, and all-cause mortality in a cohort of male employees in the German construction industry. *J Clin Epidemiol* 1997; **50**: 1099–1106.

41. Dorn JM, Schisterman EF, Winkelstein W Jr, Trevisan M. Body mass index and mortality in a general population sample of men and women. The Buffalo Health Study. *Am J Epidemiol* 1997; **146**: 919–931.

42. Chyou PH, Burchfiel CM, Yano K, Sharp DS, Rodriguez BL, Curb JD, Nomura AM. Obesity, alcohol consumption, smoking, and mortality. *Ann Epidemiol* 1997; **7**: 311–317.

43. Seidell JC, Verschuren WM, van Leer EM, Kromhout D. Overweight, underweight, and mortality: A prospective study of 48,287 men and women. *Arch Intern Medi* 1996; **156**: 958–963.

44. Wienpahl J, Ragland DR, Sidney S. Body mass index and 15-year mortality in a cohort of black men and women. *J Clin Epidemiol* 1990; **43**: 949–960.

45. Rissanen A, Heliovaara M, Knekt P, Aromaa A, Reunanen A, Maatela J. Weight and mortality in Finnish men. *J Clin Epidemiol* 1989; **42**: 781–789.

46. Wannamethee G, Shaper AG. Body weight and mortality in middle aged British men: Impact of smoking. *Lancet* 1989; **299**: 1497–1502.

47. The BMI in Diverse Populations Collaborative Group. Effect of smoking on the body mass index–mortality relation: Empirical evidence from 15 studies. *Am J Epidemiol* 1999; **150**: 1297–1308.

48. Allison DB, Gallagher D, Heo M, Pi-Sunyer FX, Heymsfield SB. Body mass index and all-cause mortality among people age 70 and over: the Longitudinal Study of Aging. *Int J Obes Relat Metab Disord* 1997; **21**: 424–431.

49. Brill PA, Giles WH, Keenan NL, Croft JB, Davis DR, Jackson KL, Macera CA. Effect of body mass index on activity limitation and mortality among older women. The National Health Interview Survery, 1986–1990. *J Women's Health* 1997; **6**: 435–440.

50. Diehr P, Bild DE, Harris TB, Duxbury A, Siscovick D, Rossi M. Body mass index and mortality in nonsmoking older adults: the Cardiovascular Health Study. *Am J Public Health* 1998; **88**: 623–629.

51. *Build Study 1979*. Chicago: Society of Actuaries and Association of Life Insurance Medical Directors of America, 1980.

52. Rissanen A, Knekt P, Heliovaara M, Aromaa A, Reunanen A, Maatela J. Weight and mortality in Finnish women. *J Clin Epidemiol* 1991; **44**: 787–795.

53. Lindsted KD, Singh PN. Body mass and 26-year risk of mortality among women who never smoked: Findings for the Adventist Mortality Study. *Am J Epidemiol* 1997; **146**: 1–11.

54. Seccareccia F, Lanti M, Menotti A, Scanga M. Role of body mass index in the prediction of all cause mortality in over 62,000 men and women. The Italian RIFLE Pooling Project. Risk Factor and Life Expectancy. *J Epidemiol Community Health* 1998; **52**: 20–26.

55. Bender R, Jockel KH, Trautner C, Spraul M, Berger M. Effect of age on excess mortality in obesity. *JAMA* 1999; **281**: 1498–1504.

56. Stevens J, Cai J, Juhaeri, Thun MJ, Williamson DF, Wood JL. Consequences of the use of different measures of effect to determine the impact of age on the association between obesity and mortality. *Am J Epidemiol* 1999; **150**: 399–407.

57. Van Itallie TB, Lew EA. In search of optimal weights for US men and women. In: Pi-Sunyer FX, Allison DB (eds) *Obesity Treatment*: Establishing Goals, Improving Outcomes, and Reviewing the Research Agenda. New York: Plenum, 1995; 1–20.

58. Allison, DB, Edlen-Nezin, L, Clay-Williams, G. Obesity among African American women: Prevalence, consequences, causes, and developing research. *Women's Health*: Research on Gender, Behavior, and Policy 1997; **3**: 243–274.

59. Nabulsi AA, Folsom AR, Heiss G, Weir SS, Chambless LE, Watson RL, Eckfeldt HH. Fasting hyperinsulinemia and cardiovascular disease risk factors in nondiabetic adults: Stronger associations in lean versus obese subjects. *Metabolism* 1995; **44**: 914–922.

60. Comstock GW, Kendrick MA, & Livesay VT. Subcutaneous fatness and mortality. *Am J Epidemiol* 1966; **83**: 548–563.

61. Stevens J, Keil JF, Rust PF *et al.* Body mass index and body

girths as predictors of mortality in black and white men. *Am J Epidemiol* 1992; **135**: 1137–1146.

62. Cornoni-Huntley JC, Harris TB, Everett DF, Albanes D, Micozzi MS, Miles TP, Feldman JJ. An overview of body weight of older persons, including the impact on morality. *J Clin Epidemiol* 1991; **44**: 743–753.

63. Johnson JL, Heineman EF, Heiss G, Hames CG, Tyroler HA. Cardiovascular disease risk factors and mortality among Black women and White women aged 40–64 years in Evans County, Georgia. *Am J Epidemiol* 1986; **123**: 209–220.

64. Sorkin JD, Zonderman AB, Costa PT, Jr, Andres RA. Twenty-year follow-up of the NHANES I cohort: Test of methodological hypotheses. *Obes Res* 1996; **4**: S12.

65. Stevens J, Keil JE, Rus PF, Tyroler HA, Davis CE, Gazes PC. Body mass index and body girths as predictors of mortality in Black and White women. *Arch Intern Med* 1992; **152**: 1257–1262.

66. Durazo-Arvizu R, Cooper RS, Luke A, Prewitt TE, Liao Y, McGee DL. Relative weight and mortality in U.S. blacks and whites: findings from representative national population samples. *Ann Epidemiol* 1997; **7**: 383–395.

67. Durazo-Arvizu RA, McGee DL, Cooper RS, Liao Y, Luke A. Mortality and optimal body mass index in a sample of the US population. *Am J Epidemiol* 1998; **14**: 739–749.

68. Hodge AM, Dowse GK, Collins VR, Zimmet PZ. Mortality in Micronesian Nauruans and Melanesian and Indian Fijians is not associated with obesity. *Am J Epidemiol* 1997; **143**: 442–455.

69. Collins VR, Dowse GK, Cabealawa S, Ram P, Zimmet PZ. High mortality from cardiovascular disease and analysis of risk factors in Indian and Melanesian Fijians. *Int J Epidemiol* (1996). **25**: 59–69.

70. Stern MP, Patterson JK, Mitchell BD, Haffner SM, Hazuda HP. Overweight and mortality in Mexican Americans. *Int J Obes* 1990; **14**: 623–629.

71. Hanson RL, McCance DR, Jacobsson LT, Narayan KM, Nelosn RG, Pettitt DJ, Bennett PH, Knowler WC. The U-shaped association between body-mass index and mortality-relationship with weight-gain in a Native-American population. *J Clin Epidemiol* 1995; **48**: 903–915.

72. Cummings SR, Nevitt MC, Browner WS, Stone K, Fox KM, Ensrud KE, Cauley J, Black D, Vogt TM. Risk factors for hip fracture in white women. *N Eng J Medi* 1995; **332**: 767–773.

73. Ensrud KE, Cauley J, Lipschutz R, Cummings SR. Weight change and fractures in older women. Study of Osteoporotic Fractures Research Group. *Arch Intern Medi* 1997; **157**: 857–863.

74. Slemenda C. Protection of hip fractures: risk factor modification. *Am J Med* 1997; **103**: 65S–71S.

75. Huuskonen J, Kroger H, Arnala I, Alhava E. Characteristics of male hip fracture patients. *Ann Chir Gynaecol* 1999; **88**: 48–53.

76. Norris J, Harnack L, Carmichael S, Pouane T, Wakimoto P, Block G. US trends in nutrient intake: the 1987 and 1992 National Health Interview surveys. *Am J Public Health* 1997; **87**: 740–746.

77. Peterson S, Sigman-Grant M, Eissenstat B, Kris-Etherton P. Impact of adopting lower-fat food choices on energy and nutrient intakes of American adults. *J Am Diet Assoc* 1999; **99**: 177–183.

78. Frame LT, Hart RW, Leakey JE. Caloric restriction as a mechanism mediating resistance to environmental disease. *Environ Health Perspect* 1998; **106** (Suppl 1): 313–324.

79. McCarter RJ. Role of caloric restriction in the prolongation of life. *Clin Geriatr Med* 1995; **11**: 553–565.

80. Weindruch R. The retardation of aging by caloric restriction: studies in rodents and primates. *Toxicol Pathol* 1996; **24**: 742–745.

81. Walford RL, Harris SB, Weindruch R. Dietary restriction and aging: historical phases, mechanisms and current discussion. *J Nutr* 1987; **117**: 1650–1654.

82. Williamson DF. Intentional weight loass: Patterns in the general populations and its association with morbidity and mortality. *Int J Obes Relat Metab Disord* 1997; **21** (Suppl 1): S14–S19.

83. Singh R, Rastogi SS, Verma R *et al*. Randomized controlled trial of cardioprotective diet in patients with recent acute myocardial infarction: results of one year follow up. *BMJ* 1992; **304**: 1015–1019.

84. Lean ME, Powrie JK, Anderson AS, Garthwaite PH. Obesity, weight loss and prognosis in type 2 diabetes. *Diabet Med* 1990; **7**: 228–233.

85. French SA, Folsom AR, Jeffery RW *et al*. Prospective study of intentionaly of weight loss and mortality in older women: The Iowa Women's Health Study. *Am J Epidemiol* 1999; **149**: 504–514.

86. Kuller L. Invited commentary on 'Prospective study of intentionaity of weight loss and mortality in older women: The Iowa Women's Health Study' and 'Prospective study of intentional weight loss and mortality in overweight white men aged 40–64 years'. *Am J Epidemiol* 1999 **149**: 515–516.

87. Williamson DF, Pamuk E, Thun M *et al*. Prospective study of intentional weight loss and mortality in overweight white men aged 40–64 years. *Am J Epidemiol* 1999; **149**: 491–503.

88. Meltzer A, Everhart J. Correlations with self-reported weight loss in overweight US adults. *Obes Res* 1996; **4**: 479–486.

89. Wadden TA, Berkowitz RI, Silvestry F *et al*. The Fen-phen finale: A study of weight loss and valvular heart disease. Obes Res 1998; **6**: 278–284.

90. Anomyous. The fallacy of fad diets. *Harvard Women's Health Watch* 1998; **6**(3): 1.

91. Sjostrom L, Larsson B, Backman L, Bengtsson C, Bouchard C, Dahlgren S, Hallgren P, Jonsson E, Karlsson J, Lapidus L *et al*. Swedish obese subjects (SOS). Recruitment for an intervention study and a selected description of the obese state. *Int J Obes Relat Metab Disord* 1992; **16**(6): 465–479.

92. Stern MP. The case for randomized clinical trials on the treatment of obesity. *Obes Res* 1995; **3** (Suppl 2): 299s–306s.

93. Goldstein DJ. Beneficial health effects of modest weight loss. *Int J Obes Metab Disord* 1992; **16**: 397–415.

Part II

Diagnosis

4

Anthropometric Indices of Obesity and Regional Distribution of Fat Depots

T.S. Han[1,2] and M.E.J. Lean[2]

[1]*Wolfson College, Cambridge and* [2]*Glasgow Royal Infirmary, Glasgow*

INTRODUCTION AND BACKGROUND

Body fatness and body shapes have been topics of interest to people over the ages because of health considerations, but scientific assessment and presentation have been complicated by changing fashions and a range of myths. Many methods of measuring body fatness have been developed for epidemiological field studies or clinical use, based on laboratory methods such as underwater weighing as a conventional 'gold standard'. This two-compartment model estimates body composition with the assumption that the densities of lean (1.1 kg/L) and adipose (0.9 kg/L) tissues are constant (1). Indices of obesity have been derived to assess body composition and health at the present, and to predict future health. Rarely a method has been developed specifically for self-monitoring by lay people. One of the tantalizing features of research in body composition is the lack of any true gold standard from which to calibrate other methods. Direct measurement by chemical analysis, either by macroscopic dissection or by lipid extraction, is of limited value as it cannot be related to measurements *in vivo*.

PURPOSES AND APPLICATIONS OF ANTHROPOMETRY

Simple and cheap anthropometric methods are useful for epidemiological surveys of large numbers of subjects across the population. For clinical use, anthropometric methods are useful tools for diagnosis and monitoring patients. The most appropriate methods may vary depending on whether the need is for cross-sectional or longitudinal assessment. In research studies, physiological characterization of individuals is assessed by a range of anthropometric measurements. One of the most fundamental issues in employing anthropometric measurements to assess body fat is that the prediction equations must be validated in a similar population to that to which the equations are being applied.

METHODS COMMONLY USED TO MEASURE BODY FATNESS

Laboratory Standard Methods

For small studies, total body fat is estimated by standard methods (Table 4.1) such as underwater

International Textbook of Obesity. Edited by Per Björntorp.

Table 4.1 Methods of measuring body fat and fat distribution

Methods	Accuracy	Practicality	Sensitivity to change	Cheapness	Fat distribution detection
Laboratory: 'standard' methods					
Underwater weighing	+ + + +	+ +	+ + +	+ + +	−
Potassium-40 counting	+ + +	+ + +	+	+ + +	−
Dual-energy X-ray absorptiometry	+ + +	+ +	+ +	+ +	+ +
Computerized tomography	+ + + + +	+ + +	+ + +	+	+ + + + +
Magnetic resonance imaging	+ + + + +	+ + + +	+ + +	+	+ + + + +
Multi-compartment models	+ + +	+	+	+	−
Air displacement (BOD POD)	?	+ + + +	?	+ +	−
Field: anthropometric methods					
Skinfold thickness	+ + +	+ + + +	+ + +	+ + + + +	−
Circumference	+ + +	+ + + +	+ + +	+ + + + +	+ + + + +
Body mass index	+ + +	+ + + +	+ + + + +	+ + + + +	−

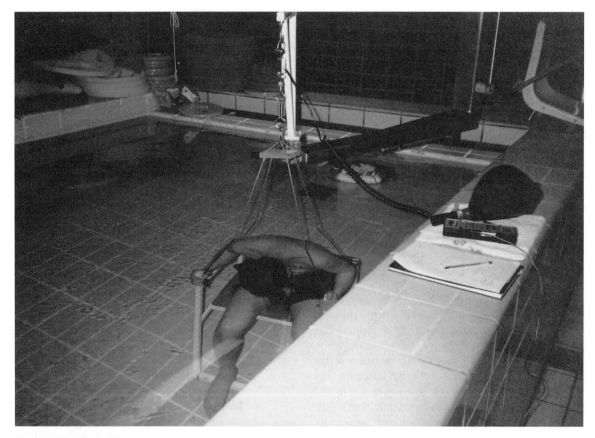

Figure 4.1 Measuring total body fat by underwater weighing

weighing (Figure 4.1), potassium-40 (^{40}K) counting, or more recently by imaging techniques such as dual-energy X-ray absorptiometry (DEXA) (which was itself calibrated against underwater weighing), computerized tomography (CT) scan and magnetic resonance imaging (MRI) (Figure 4.2). All these methods make assumptions about composition of 'average' tissues, e.g. density of fat, constant ^{40}K of

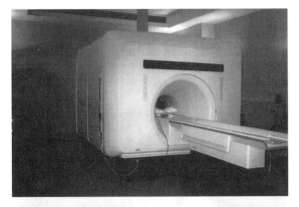

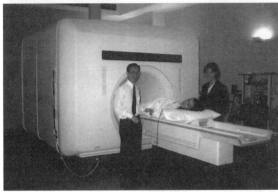

Figure 4.2 Magnetic resonance imaging scanner used to image body tissues

muscles, or attenuation to X-rays from fat and lean tissues, and thus all the methods have inherent error. Overhydration and dehydration also affect the estimation of body composition. In attempts to overcome these problems, three- and four-compartment models to predict body composition have been developed, which employ separate measurements of body fat, muscle mass, body water and bones. These multi-compartment methods may improve accuracy of measurement but patients are subjected to many tests. Time and costs will limit the number of subjects that can be studied, and accumulated errors from these methods also make this model unattractive. A recently invented technique based on air displacement (BOD POD; Life Measurements Instruments, Concord, CA) has been introduced. This method measures rapidly and is less intimidating; thus it is useful for measuring body composition of children and the elderly.

It is important to recognize that there is in fact no true gold standard or reference method for body composition analysis. Thus scanning methods de-pend on the resolution of imaging, and they also fail to detect fat within organs such as liver, muscles and bones. Cadaver dissection, coupled with chemical analysis, should theoretically overcome this problem, but there is a very real practical limitation through the time required for dissection and alteration in tissue hydration.

Field Anthropometric Methods

Using an underwater weighing method to predict body fat is impractical for large field studies, requiring facilities and the cooperation of subjects and expertise of the investigators. Proxy anthropometric methods (Table 4.1) have been employed including skinfolds (2), body mass index (BMI) (3), and skinfolds combined with various body circumferences (4–6) to predict body fat estimated by underwater weighing. Body fat predicted from these equations shows high correlations with body fat measured by underwater weighing and relatively small errors of prediction. However, there have been few major validations of these equations in independent populations to test their generalizability or applicability in special population subgroups. The most widely used field method for total fat has been the four-skinfold methods (Figure 4.3), derived from underwater weighing (2). Recognizing possible errors of predicting body fat in subpopulations with altered fat distribution, regression equations including waist circumference (Figure 4.4) appear to have advantages in predicting total body fat by taking some account of this variation in fat distribution (6). Waist circumference, alone, predicts health (7) as well as body composition and is recommended for public health promotion (8,9).

Previously, little attention has been paid to developing an index of adiposity that could be used by lay people. The BMI has been the traditional index of obesity, but its concept and calculations are not readily understood by many. Criteria for classification of overweight and obesity have been inconsistent. Conventional classification of BMI, using the same criteria for both men and women, is based on life insurance and epidemiological data. Waaler (10) has shown a U-shaped relationship between BMI and mortality rates, with exponential increases of mortality in adult subjects with high BMI ($> 30 \, \text{kg/m}^2$) or low BMI ($< 20 \, \text{kg/m}^2$). These cri-

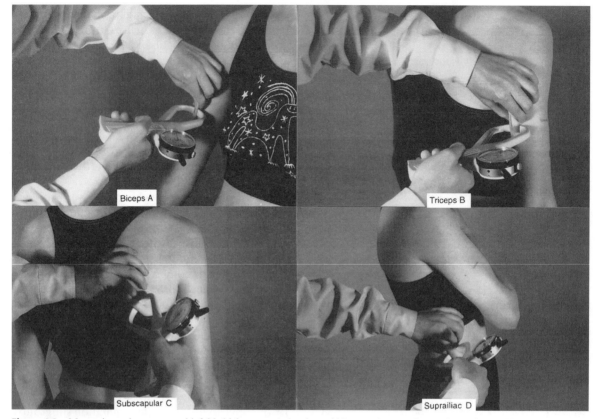

Figure 4.3 Measuring subcutaneous skinfold thicknesses at the sites of biceps, triceps, subscapular and suprailiac using skinfold calipers

teria for interpreting BMI do not apply to children, whose BMI is normally much lower than that of adults. The arbitrary cut-offs for overweight at BMI 25 and for obesity at BMI 30 kg/m² have now been adopted by the National Institutes of Health (8) in America and World Health Organization (11). These cut-offs have been used widely in Europe for many years.

MEASURING BODY COMPOSITION IN SPECIAL GROUPS

There are major effects of age on body composition which mean that anthropometric methods may not always be valid. A major pitfall is the unquestioning use of equations to predict body fat derived from one population group, without subsequent validation in another specific population group.

Infants and Children

For infants, the 'reference' methods used to determine body composition in infants include ¹⁸O isotope dilution (12) and DEXA (13). The ponderal index (weight divided by height cubed) has been used as an anthropometric method to assess body fatness. Measuring children's body composition is problematic, as their tissue composition varies with growth, the rate and timing of growth vary widely, and physical activity influences the composition of fat free mass (14). Several studies have used doubly labelled water to monitor children's growth and estimate their total body water, and thus body composition. Reference values for body weight and triceps skinfold thickness of British children have been provided by Tanner and co-workers (15–17), although the Tanner reference values for weight are no longer appropriate in the UK. In a validation study, Reilly et al. (18) have shown that the skinfold method produces large errors in predicting body fat

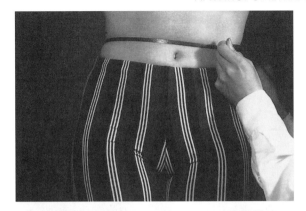

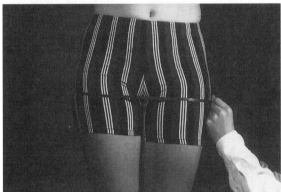

Figure 4.4 Measuring waist circumference midway between iliac crest and lowest rib margin, and hip circumference at the level of the greater trochanters

of 9-year-old children. These workers used underwater weighing as the reference method and found it acceptable even to very young children. As a generalization, anthropometric methods to estimate body fat are not reliable in children. BMI can be used, but with caution in its interpretation because of variable stages of development at the same age. There are standard BMI reference curves (Figure 4.5) developed by Cole *et al.* (19) for the Child Growth Foundation.

Ageing and Elderly

Intra-abdominal fat increases with age and immobility, and thereby tends to invalidate the subcutaneous skinfold methods. In postmenopausal women, body fat may accumulate intra-abdominally as a result of hormonal changes. Consequently, subcutaneous skinfold methods may underestimate their total body fat.

Athletes

In athletes, BMI does not reflect body fat very well, particularly in power athletes who have large muscle mass. Inaccuracies in anthropometric prediction equations stem from the reference methods, such as underwater weighing, from which they are derived since the density of these subjects' lean tissues is considerably higher than the 1.1 kg/L value (1) used for estimating body composition in the 'normal' population. Muscle varies considerably as a proportion of total lean body mass.

Illness

Conventional anthropometric prediction equations break down with altered relative body composition. For example, patients with advanced tuberculosis and cancer or with benign oesophageal stenosis may have similar BMIs as a result of weight loss, but muscle loss is likely to be greater in a cachectic inflammatory condition. Errors will therefore result from using the same body composition prediction equations. Illnesses that result in considerable loss of minerals or specific tissues, e.g. muscle wasting in patients with acquired immune deficiency syndrome (AIDS), may result in an overestimation of body fat using conventional prediction equations. In contrast, in patients with non-insulin-dependent diabetes mellitus (NIDDM) (Type 2 diabetes) who have increased intra-abdominal fat, there is underestimation of body fat using skinfold methods, which increases with the amount of central fat deposition (20). There is a problem in measuring body composition of amputees whose substantial absence of muscle mass gives unrealistic BMI values. In bed- or chair-bound patients, height measurement is not available for calculation of BMI. Alternative methods including arm span and lower leg length can be used to predict height with an accuracy within 4 cm (21).

ANTHROPOMETRIC ASSESSMENT OF OBESITY

Predicting Total Body Fat from Skinfold Thicknesses

Four skinfold thicknesses are conventionally meas-

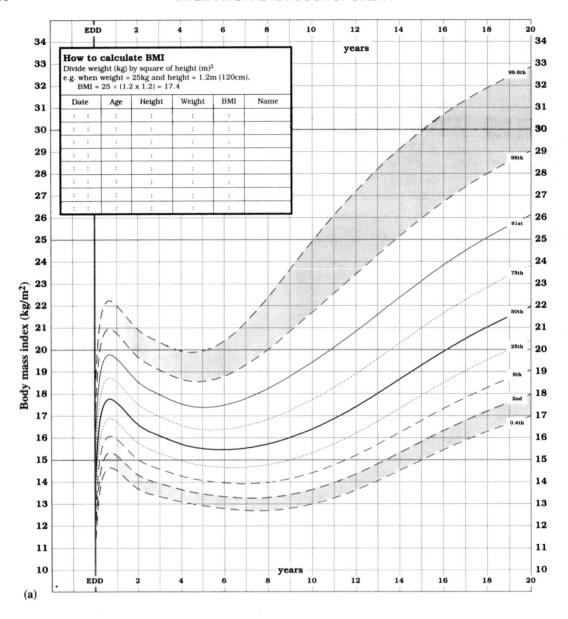

Figure 4.5   Standard body mass index curves from birth to 20 years for boys (a, *above*) and girls (b, *opposite*). Copyright © Child Growth Foundation. Reproduced by permission. Copies of the CGF BMI charts are available from Harlow Printing, Maxwell Street, South Shileds NE33 4PU, UK

ured (Figure 4.3), using calipers at biceps, triceps, subscapular and suprailiac, and the sum of all four skinfolds (equation 1), or just the triceps skinfold (equation 2), with subjects' age, are used in linear multiple regression to predict total body fat. The original equations for use in adults (2) have been cross-validated in a separate sample and found to be robust in adults aged 20–60 years (6), but tend to

underestimate substantially the total fat in the elderly, particularly women (6,22) (Figure 4.6).

$$\text{Body fat \% (men)} = [30.9 \times \log_{10} \textstyle\sum_4 \text{skinfolds (mm)}] + [0.271 \times \text{Age (years)}] - 39.9 \quad (1)$$

$$\text{Body fat \% (women)} = [30.8 \times \log_{10} \textstyle\sum_4 \text{skinfolds (mm)}] + [0.274 \times \text{Age (years)}] - 31.7$$

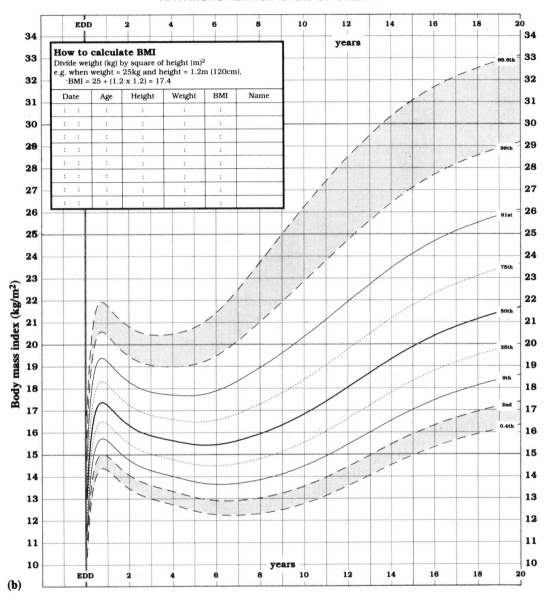

(b)

$$\text{Body fat \% (men)} = (1.31 \times \text{Triceps}) + (0.430 \times \text{Age}) - 9.2 \qquad (2)$$

$$\text{Body fat \% (women)} = (0.944 \times \text{Triceps}) + (0.279 \times \text{Age}) + 4.6$$

Predicting Total Body Fat from Waist Circumference and Triceps Skinfold

Han and Lean (20) have observed a systematic underestimation of body fat by equations using subcutaneous skinfold thicknesses (2) in subjects with increased intra-abdominal fat mass, reflected by a high waist circumference or waist-to-hip ratio, including the elderly and those with type 2 diabetes. Waist circumference (Figure 4.4) has been found to correlate highly with both intra-abdominal and total fat masses (6,23), and was used on its own and with skinfold thicknesses to develop new regression equations to correct for the intra-abdominal fat mass (6). These equations were validated in a large Dutch sample from previous study of body fat distribution (3).

Equations using waist circumference alone, adjusted for age (equation 3), showed good prediction of body fat in the independent Dutch sample ($r^2 = 78\%$) with similar error of prediction as other equations. These equations are particularly good for estimating body fat in the elderly without the systematic underestimation of body fat that occurs in the subcutaneous skinfold method (Figure 4.6).

Body fat % (men) = [0.567 × Waist circumference (cm)] + [0.101 × Age (years)] − 31.8   (3)
Body fat % (women) = [0.439 × Waist circumference (cm)] + [0.221 × Age (years)] − 9.4

Equations combining waist circumference and triceps skinfold, adjusted for age (equation 4), have been shown to improve predictive power of body fat estimation without systematic errors over equations employing subcutaneous skinfolds alone in subjects with type 2 diabetes who had increased intra-abdominal fat mass (20).

Body fat % (men) = [0.353 × Waist (cm)] + [0.756 × Triceps (mm)] + 0.235 × Age (years)] − 26.4   (4)
Body fat % (women) = [0.232 × Waist (cm)] + [0.657 × Triceps (mm)] + [0.215 × Age (years)] − 5.5

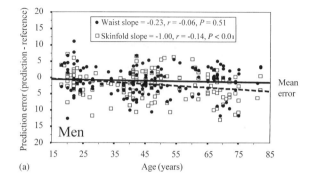

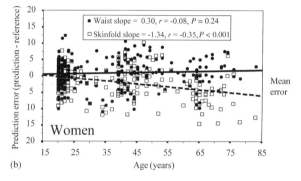

Figure 4.6 Plots of errors of predicting body fat by underwater weighing from equations using waist circumference (—●—, Lean *et al.* (6) and subcutaneous skinfolds (---□---, Durnin and Womersley (2) against age in men (a) and women (b) aged 18 to 83 years

Calculations of Body Mass Index (Quetelet Index), and its Use to Predict Body Fat

Bigger people—both taller and fatter—are heavier than small people. Body weight includes fat, muscle and all other organs. For people of the same height, most of the variation in weight is accounted for by different amounts of body fat. BMI aims to describe weight for height in a way which will relate maximally to body weight (or body fat) with minimal relation to height (24). BMI is calculated as the ratio of weight in kilograms divided by height squared (m²). Since BMI uses height, the height measurement needs to be very accurate. Classification of BMI (Table 4.2) uses the same criteria for both men and women is now adopted by both the NIH (8) and WHO (25). A BMI of 18.5 to 24.9 kg/m² is considered as in the normal range, above 25 kg/m² as overweight and above 30 kg/m² as obese. For some purposes, the obese category is subclassified by the

WHO (25) as 30–34.9 (moderately obese), 35–39.9 (severely obese), and greater than 40 (very severely obese) kg/m².

BMI can be used to predict body fat from underwater weight ($r^2 = 79\%$) with age and sex corrections (3). Our derived equations using BMI to predict body fat were validated in the independent sample provided by Deurenberg *et al.* (3) and showed similarly good prediction of body fat as other equations currently in use (equation 5).

Body fat % (men) = [1.33 × BMI (kg/m²)] + [0.236 × Age (years)] − 20.2   (5)
Body fat % (women) = [1.21 × BMI (kg/m²)] + [0.262 × Age (years)] − 6.7

ANTHROPOMETRIC ASSESSMENT OF BODY FAT DISTRIBUTION

People with central fat distribution in both sexes

tend to have a distinct body shape, said to resemble that of an apple (Figure 4.7), a physical characteristic of men (termed 'android' by Vague) which tends to be associated with metabolic abnormalities and chronic diseases (26–31).

Body circumferences and their ratios are used to indicate the distribution of body fat. The most important variations, in terms of health associations, are between the amounts of fat in internal, mainly intra-abdominal sites, as distinct from subcutaneous sites (Figure 4.8). The 'gold standard' for measuring fat depots in these sites is scanning by MRI (Figure 4.2). CT gives almost equal information but the small radiation exposure limits its acceptability.

Waist-to-hip Ratio

The ratio of waist-to-hip circumferences (Figure 4.4) was the first anthropometric method developed from epidemiological research as an indicator of fat distribution in relation to metabolic diseases. Waist-to-hip ratio is related more closely to the ratio of intra-abdominal fat/extra-abdominal fat mass than the absolute amount of intra-abdominal fat mass (32), and has been shown to relate to mortality from coronary heart disease and type 2 diabetes independent of BMI (28,29). Most of the value in indicating body fat is derived from waist circumference, the hip circumference probably reflecting several other body tissues such as bones and muscles. The waist-to-hip ratio may have some particular value in reflecting diseases which involve muscle reduction as well as fat deposition, e.g. type 2 diabetes (33).

Waist-to-thigh Ratio

In some studies waist-to-thigh ratio has been used as an index for fat distribution to relate to metabolic risk factors (34). This ratio is also influenced by abdominal fat as well as fat mass, muscle mass and bone structures of the thigh, which may be a strong indicator of certain health conditions involving both abdominal fat accumulation and skeletal muscle wasting such as NIDDM.

Table 4.2 Classification of body mass index for body fatness adopted by the World Health Organization (25) and US National Institutes of Health (8)

BMI (kg/m^2)	Classification
18.5–24.9	Acceptable
25–29.9	Overweight—increased health risks
≥ 30	Obesity—high health risks

Conicity Index

The conicity index was formulated by Valdez (35) to estimate abdominal fat, based on the theory that leaner subjects have a body shape similar to a cylinder, but as fat is accumulated around the abdomen, the body shape changes towards that of a double cone (two cones with a common base at the waist). With the assumption that the average human body density is 1.05 kg/m^3, the equation was derived as:

$$\text{Conicity index} = \frac{\text{Waist}}{(0.109 \times \sqrt{\text{weight/height}})} \quad (6)$$

The conicity index is theorized to have a built-in adjustment for height and weight so that abdominal adiposity can be compared across different populations of varying heights and weights (36). The index is related to the ratio of intra-abdominal fat/extra-abdominal fat mass similarly to waist-to-hip ratio, and may be useful when hip measurement is not available. Valdez et al. (36) found the conicity index to be correlated to cardiovascular risk factors similarly to that of waist-to-hip ratio in different countries. A drawback is that the index has not been cross-validated to ensure applicability.

Sagittal Abdominal Diameter

The use of sagittal diameter of the waist has been proposed as an index of abdominal fatness based on a theory that fat deposition in the anteroposterior axis is more 'dangerous' than lateral fat deposition. This index has not been validated in an independent population. Sagittal diameter can be measured using a pelviometer in the standing position, or a more sophisticated instrument that is modified from a sliding stadiometer in the supine position (37). Gadgets are on sale with a back plate which is

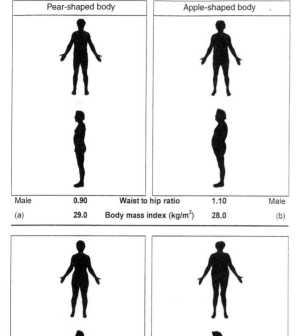

| Male | 0.90 | Waist to hip ratio | 1.10 | Male |
| (a) | 29.0 | Body mass index (kg/m²) | 28.0 | (b) |

| Female | 0.70 | Waist to hip ratio | 1.20 | Female |
| (c) | 30.0 | Body mass index (kg/m²) | 30.5 | (d) |

Figure 4.7 Silhouette photographs showing variation in human body fat distribution

flexible, thereby introducing enormous errors. The measurement of sagittal diameter of the waist has not been used very widely. This method has recently been validated by CT scanning and found to have high reproducible results.

Abdominal Cross-sectional Area

Abdominal cross-sectional area (CSA$_A$) has also been proposed by van der Kooy et al. (38) as an index of abdominal fat and is calculated from waist sagittal (WSD) and waist transverse diameters (WTD) as: CSA$_A$ = $(4 \times WSD \times WTD)/\pi$, but this

more complicated method is not likely to be much different from a circumference or a single measurement of waist diameter.

Waist Circumference

Recent proposals for the use of waist circumference as a single measurement of body fat and fat distribution have now been adopted by several major public health promotion agencies and organizations (8,9,21).

Waist circumference has been suggested as a simple measurement to identify individuals with high BMI or high waist-to-hip ratio. Waist circumference correlates significantly with BMI (both men and women: $r = 0.89$; $P < 0.001$). Lean et al. (39) have derived the 'action levels' for weight management based on the waist circumference of over 2000 men and women (Table 4.3). Action level 1: Waist circumference of ≥ 94 cm in men or ≥ 80 cm in women identifies as overweight with increased health risks, those with BMI ≥ 25 kg/m² and high waist-to-hip ratio (≥ 0.95 for men; ≥ 0.80 for women). These subjects are advised not to gain further body weight and to increase physical activity. Action level 2: Waist circumference of ≥ 102 cm in men or ≥ 80 cm in women identifies as overweight with high health risks, those with BMI ≥ 30 kg/m² and high waist-to-hip ratio (≥ 0.95 in men and ≥ 0.80 in women). Weight loss and consultation of health professionals are recommended for these individuals. These action levels for weight management have a sensitivity (correctly identifies individuals who need weight management by waist circumference above action levels) and a specificity (correctly identifies individuals who do not need weight management by waist circumference below action levels) of more than 96% for identifying overweight and obese subjects with high waist-to-hip ratio. Waist circumference is not importantly influenced by height (40) (Figure 4.9), thus it is not necessary to divide waist by height when using waist circumference as an index of adiposity. To avoid problems with over-tightening during waist measurement, a specially designed 'Waist Watcher' spring-loaded tape measure has been produced with three colour bands based on cut-offs of the waist circumference action levels (Figure 4.10).

Table 4.3 Action levels to identify overweight and obese men and women with increased abdominal fat

Action level	cm	Body mass index	Waist-to-hip ratio	Classification of health risks	Weight management
Waist circumference		Approximate equivalents			
Men					
Action level 1	≥ 94	≥ 25	≥ 0.95	Increased health risks	Prevent further weight gain, try to get down to below action level 1 (94 cm)
Action level 2	≥ 102	≥ 30	≥ 0.95	High health risks	Seek advice to lose weight, aim for 5–10% weight loss permanently
Women					
Action level 1	≥ 80	≥ 25	≥ 0.80	Increased health risks	Prevent further weight gain, try to get down to below action level 1 (80 cm)
Action level 2	≥ 88	≥ 30	≥ 0.80	High health risks	Seek advice to lose weight, aim for 5–10% weight loss permanently

METHODS FOR ANTHROPOMETRIC MEASUREMENTS

Body Weight

Weight is measured by digital scales or beam balance to the nearest 100 g. For those unable to stand, electronic chair scales (Weighcare C, Marsden Ltd, London) are available. For field work, portable scales are used. Equipment is calibrated regularly by standard weights (4 × 10 kg and 8 × 10 kg), and the results of test weighing recorded in a book. Subjects are weighed in light clothing, fasting and with an empty bladder, preferably at the same time of day.

Height

Height is measured by stadiometer to the nearest millimetre, which is calibrated by meter rule before use. When possible, a wall mounted stadiometer is preferred. For field work, a portable stadiometer (Leicester Height Measure, Child Growth Foundation, London, UK; Holtain, Crymych, UK) is available. Subjects stand in bare feet which are kept together and pointing forward. The head is level with horizontal Frankfurt plane (line from lower border of the eye orbit to the auditory meatus). Subjects are encouraged to stretch upwards by applying gentle pressure at the mastoid processes and height is recorded with subjects taking in a deep breath for maximum measurement.

Limb Lengths

When height measurement is not available in bed- and chair-bound patients. Height can be predicted from arm span or lower leg length (21). Arm span is measured between finger tips with subjects standing against the wall, and both arms fully stretch horizontally. Demi-arm span is measured as the horizontal distance from the web space between middle and fourth fingers to the midpoint of the sternal notch to the nearest millimetre, in the sitting position. Lower leg length is measured with subjects sitting in a chair adjusted to about their knee height, and the lower legs and bare feet flexed at 90°. The lower legs, 25–30 cm apart, are adjusted to vertical position both side and front views. A ruler standing on its edge is placed on top of the patellae. Lower leg length is taken to the nearest millimetre from the midpoint of the ruler to the floor with a wooden metre rule.

Waist Circumference

Waist circumference is measured midway between the lower rib margin and iliac crest, with a horizontal tape at the end of gentle expiration (Figure 4.4), with feet kept 20–30 cm apart. Subjects should be asked not to hold in their stomach, and a constant tension spring-loaded tape device reduces errors from over-enthusiastic tightening during measurement. Waist circumference measurement reflects body fat and does not include most of the bone

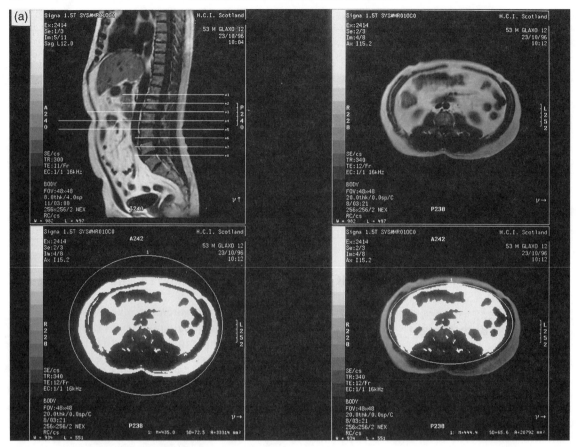

Figure 4.8 Subcutaneous and intra-abdominal fat images obtained from magnetic resonance imaging. (a, *above*) Male; (b, *opposite*) female. Light areas indicate fat

structure (only the spine) or large muscle masses, whose variations between subjects might otherwise introduce errors.

Hip Circumference

Maximum hip circumference is measured with a horizontal steel tape at the widest part of the trochanters at horizontal position (Figure 4.4) with feet kept 20–30 cm apart. It is related more closely to subcutaneous fat than to intra-abdominal fat mass. Hip circumference has limited value on its own in body composition estimation. The circumference of the hip is influenced by gluteal muscle mass and pelvic size, which vary between subjects, as well as by fat.

Thigh Circumference

Thigh circumference is measured at the level of gluteal fold with the leg being measured relaxed by placing it forward and slightly bent, with body weight transferred to the other leg. It estimates fat on the thigh but will also be altered by muscle mass.

Waist Diameter

Abdominal fat deposition is further classified into medial (fat is accumulated at the middle of the abdomen) and lateral (fat is accumulated at the sides of the abdomen). Waist diameters are measured using a pelviometer or a more expensive device that measures the supine sagittal abdominal diameter (37). The pelviometer is a cheaper instrument

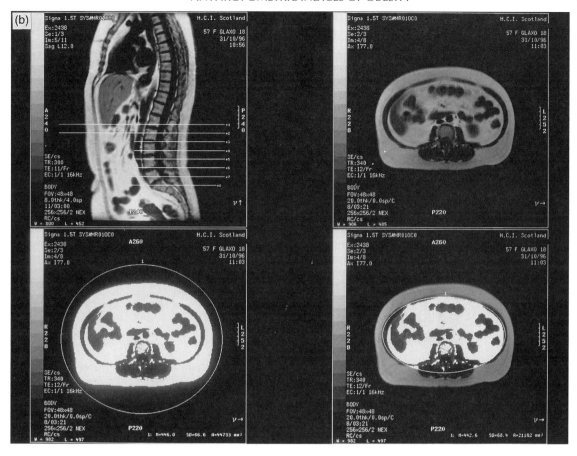

that looks like a pair of large calipers and measures the waist diameter at the level between the lower rib margin and iliac crest. Waist sagittal diameter is taken as the distance from the back to the front of the abdomen measured with the subject standing. Waist transverse diameter is taken as the distance from the sides of the abdomen.

Skinfold Thickness

Skinfold thicknesses are measured on the left side of the body with calipers (Holtain Ltd, Crymych, UK) in triplicate, to the nearest 0.2 mm. All the sites intended for measurements should be marked clearly on the skin after making measurements from bony landmarks (Figure 4.3). When the subjects relax their mucles, the subcutaneous fat layer (commonly referred to as skinfold thickness) covering the muscles is relatively loose and can usually be pinched easily by two fingers (thumb and index finger) which hold the skinfold firmly throughout the measurement (11). The pinch is made at about 1 to 2 cm above the ink mark so that the jaw of the calipers can be applied at the mark. The thickness of the skinfold is read about 2 seconds after closing the jaw of the calipers.

Biceps and triceps skinfold thicknesses are made at the midpoint of the upper arm, between the acromion process and the tip of the bent elbow. Subscapular skinfold thickness is picked up at the natural fold about 2–3 cm below the shoulder blade in an oblique angle. Suprailiac skinfold is pinched at about 2–3 cm above the iliac crest, in either a vertical or oblique angle on the lateral side and mid-axillary line. The upper limit of skinfold calipers is 50 mm, which is exceeded for the subscapular site when BMI is greater than $40 \, \text{kg/m}^2$. Thus for very overweight people, other methods are required.

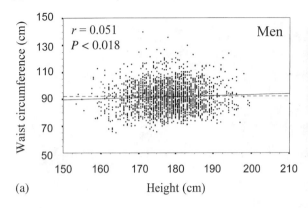

(a)

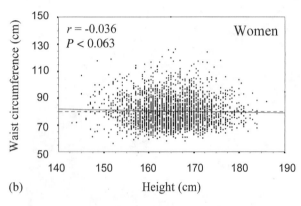

(b)

Figure 4.9 The relationship between waist circumference and height in 2183 men (a) and 2698 women (b) showing regression line (solid) and the line of zero correlation (dashed)

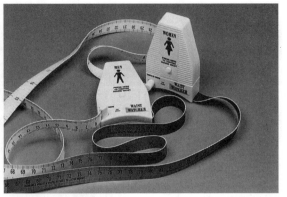

Figure 4.10 "Waist Watcher" tape measures with three colour bands (green, orange and red) based on cut-off waist circumference action levels. (BGA, The Spire, Egypt Road, Nottingham NG7 7GD, UK)

REFERENCES

1. Siri. WE. Body composition from fluid spaces and density analysis of methods. IN: Brozek J, Henschel A (eds) *Technique for Measuring Body Composition.* Washington DC: Natural Academy of Sciences, 1961: 223–244.
2. Durnin JVGA, Womersley J. Body fat assessed from total body density and its estimation from skinfold thickness: measurements on 481 men and women aged from 16 to 72. *Br J Nutr* 1974; **32**: 77–97.
3. Deurenberg P, Weststrate J, Seidell JC. Body mass index as a measure of body fatness: age- and sex-specific prediction formulas. *Br J Nutr* 1991; **65**: 105–114.
4. Jackson AS, Pollock ML. Genealised equations for predicting body density of men. *Br J Nutr* 1978; **40**: 497–504.
5. Jackson AS, Pollock ML, Ward A. Generalised equations for predicting body density of women. *Med Sci Sports Exerc* 1980; **12**: 175–182.
6. Lean MEJ, Han TS, Deurenberg P. Predicting body composition by body density from simple anthropometric measurements. *Am J Clin Nutr* 1996; **63**: 4–14.
7. Lean MEJ, Han TS, Seidell JC. Impairment of health and quality of life in people with large waist circumference. *Lancet* 1998; **351**: 853–856.
8. National Institutes of Health, National Heart, Lung and Blood Institute. *Clinical guidelines on the identification, evaluation, and treatment of overweight and obesity in adults—the evidence report.* Bethesda, MD: NIH, 1998 (June).
9. Scottish Intercollegiate Guidelines Network. *Obesity in Scotland. Integrating Prevention with Weight Management.* Edinburgh: Scottish Intercollegiate Guidelines Network, 1996.
10. Waaler HT. Height, weight and mortality. The Norwegian experience. *Acta Med Scand Supplement* 1984; **679**: 1–56.
11. World Health Organization. *Physical status; the use and interpretation of anthropometry. Report of a WHO Expert Committee.* Geneva: World Health Organization Technical Report Series, 1995.
12. De Bruin NC, Westerterp KR, Degenhart HK, Visser HK. Measurement of fat-free mass in infants. *Pediatr Res* 1995; **38**: 411–417.
13. Rigo J, Nyamugabo K, Picaud JC, Gerard P, Pieltain C, Curtis MD. Reference values of body composition obtained by dual X-ray absorptiometry in preterm and term neonates. *J Pediatr Gastroenterol Nutr* 1998; **27**: 184–190.
14. Lohman TG. Applicability of body composition techniques and constants for children and youths. *Exerc Sport Sci Rev* 1986; **14**: 325–357.
15. Tanner JM, Whitehouse RH, Takaishi M. Standards from birth to maturity for height, weight, height velocity, weight velocity: British children, 1965, Part I. *Arch Dis Child* 1966; **41**: 454–471.
16. Tanner JM, Whitehouse RH, Takaishi M. Standards from birth to maturity for height, weight, height velocity, weight velocity: British children, 1965. Part II. *Arch Dis Child* 1966; **41**: 613–643.
17. Tanner JM, Whitehouse RH. Revised standards for triceps and subscapular skinfolds in British children. *Arch Dis Child* 1975; **50**: 142–145.
18. Reilly JJ, Wilson J, Durnin JV. Determination of body composition from skinfold thickness: a validation study. *Arch Dis Child* 1995; **73**: 305–310.

19. Cole TJ, Freeman JV, Preece MA. Body mass index reference curves for the UK, 1990. *Arch Dis Child* 1995; **73**: 25–29.

20. Han TS, Lean MEJ. Body composition in patients with non-insulin-dependent diabetes and central fat distribution. *Diabet Med* 1994; **11**(Suppl 1): S39.

21. Han TS, Lean MEJ. Lower leg length as an index of stature in adults. *Int J Obes* 1996; **20**: 21–27.

22. Reilly JJ, Murray LA, Durnin JVGA. Measuring the body composition of elderly subjects: a comparison of methods. *Br J Nutr* 1994; **72**: 33–44.

23. Han TS, McNeill G, Seidell JC, Lean MEJ. Predicting intra-abdominal fatness from anthropometric measures: the influence of stature. *Int J Obes* 1997; **21**: 587–593.

24. Khosla T, Lowe CR. Indices of obesity derived from body weight and height. *Br J Prev Med* 1967; **1**: 122–128.

25. World Health Organization. *Obesity: Preventing and Managing the Global Epidemic*. Geneva: World Health Organization, WHO/NUT/NCD/98.1, 1998.

26. Vague J. The degree of masculine differentiation of obesity—factors determining predisposition to diabetes, atherosclerosis, gout and uric calculus. *Am J Clin Nutr* 1956; **4**: 20–34.

27. Kissebah AH, Vydeligum N, Murray R, Eveans DJ, Hartz J, Kalkhoff RK, Adams PW. Relation of body fat distribution to metabolic complications of obesity. *J Clin Endo-crinol Metab* 1982; **54**: 254–260.

28. Lapidus L, Bengtsson C, Larsson B, Pennert K, Rybo E, Sjöström L. Distribution of adipose tissue and risk of cardiovascular disease and death. 12 year follow-up of participants in the population study of women in Gothenburg, Sweden. *BMJ* 1984; **289**: 1261–1263.

29. Larsson B, Svardsudd K, Welin L. Wilhelmsen L, Björntorp P, Tiblin G. Abdominal adipose tissue distribution, obesity, and risk of cardiovascular disease and death: 13 year follow-up of participants in the study of men born in 1913. *BMJ* 1984; **228**: 1401–1404.

30. Ohlson LO, Larsson DC, Svärdsudd K, Wellin L, Erikson H, Wilhelmsen L *et al.* The influence of body fat distribution on the incidence of diabetes mellitus—13.5 years of follow-up of the participants in the study of men born in 1913. *Diabetes* 1985; **34**: 1055–1058.

31. Björntorp P. Metabolic implications of body fat distribution. *Diabetes Care* 1991; **12**: 1132–1143.

32. Ashwell M, Cole TJ, Dixon AK. Obesity: new insight into the anthropometric classification of fat distribution shown by computed tomography. *BMJ* 1985; **250**: 1692–1694.

33. Seidell JC, Han TS, Feskens EJM, Lean MEJ. Narrow hips and broad waist circumferences independently contribute to increased risk of NIDDM. *J Intern Med* 1997; **242**: 401–406.

34. Seidell JC, Bakx E, de Boer E, Deurenburg P, Hautvast JGAJ. Fat distribution of overweight persons in relation to morbidity and subjective health. *Int J Obes* 1985; **9**: 363–374.

35. Valdez R. A simple model-based index of abdominal adiposity. *J Clin Epidemiol* 1991; **44**: 955–956.

36. Valdez R, Seidell JC, Ahn YI, Weiss KM. A new index of abdominal adiposity as an indicator of risk factor for cardiovascular disease. A cross-population study. *Int J Obes* 1993; **17**: 77–82.

37. Kahn HS, Williamson DF. Sagittal abdominal diameter. *Int J Obes* 1993; **17**: 187–196.

38. Van der Kooy K, Leenen R, Seidell JC, Deurenberg P, Visser M. Abdominal diameters as indicators of visceral fat: comparison between magnetic resonance imaging and anthropometry. *Br J Nutr* 1993; **70**: 47–58.

39. Lean MEJ, Han TS, Morrison CE. Waist circumference as a measure for indicating need for weight management. *BMJ* 1995; **311**: 158–161.

40. Han TS, Seidell JC, Currall JEP, Morrison CE, Deurenberg P, Lean MEJ. The influences of height and age on waist circumference as an index of adiposity in adults. *Int J Obes* 1997; **21**: 83–89.

5

Screening the Population

Bernt Lindahl

Umeå University, Umeå, Sweden

An epidemic of obesity and type 2 (non-insulin-dependent) diabetes is in progress across the world. The global burden of diabetes has been projected to rise, with an increase in the total number of people with type 2 diabetes from about 120 million in 1997 to about 215 million in 2010 (1). The obvious remedy for this development is to combat overweight and obesity, and to counteract the sedentary lifestyle of modern society. The basis for these actions must be a population strategy of prevention. However, an equally important mission, not least from an ethical standpoint, is to find and engage those individuals that are in most need of help (high-risk strategy). The screening procedure is used to identify these high-risk individuals. Screening in this chapter refers to prescriptive screening, whose aim is to use early detection and early treatment to control the outcome of the disease. In epidemiological surveys, the principal aim of the screening is to explore the prevalence and natural history of the variable in question and not to bring patients to treatment.

PRINCIPLES OF SCREENING

Screening may be defined as the examination of apparently well or asymptomatic people in order to find out if they are likely or unlikely to suffer from disease. They can then, if they are likely to have the disease, be placed under treatment early in the natural course of the disease. The goal of screening is to detect and treat the disease as early as possible and

thereby reverse or retard the disease process. Sometimes the object of the screening procedure is to find people at high risk of getting a disease. By identifying precursors of disease and correcting these, the disease may be postponed or at best prevented. There is no sharp line between a risk factor and a disease (2).

The screening procedure must always be followed by a treatment programme offering treatment to those found to have a disease or an increased risk of getting the disease. A screening programme can thus be divided into a diagnostic and a therapeutic component. In 1968, an increased interest in screening inspired the WHO to publish a Public Health Paper with the title 'Principles and practice of screening for disease' (3). This presented basic principles of screening together with practical and ethical considerations (Table 5.1). Launching a screening programme is a complex task, which if not done appropriately may lead to serious consequences. Several questions of an ethical and practical nature must be considered. By using certain screening principles, the chance of success will increase and the risk of serious adverse consequences will diminish.

The Importance of the Problem

The importance of the health problem needs to be regarded from the point of view of the individual as well as of the community. An uncommon condition with serious consequences for the individual, such

International Textbook of Obesity. Edited by Per Björntorp.
© 2001 John Wiley & Sons, Ltd.

Table 5.1   Principles of screening

1. The condition sought should be an important health problem
2. There should be an accepted treatment for patients with recognized disease (condition)
3. Facilities for diagnosis and treatment should be available
4. There should be a recognizable latent or early symptomatic stage
5. There should be a suitable test
6. The natural history of the condition, including development from latent to manifest disease, should be adequately understood

Modified from Wilson and Jungner (3).

as phenylketonuria, may warrant screening measures just as much as a more common but individually less serious condition.

The Necessity of an Accepted Treatment and Resources for its Implementation

Perhaps the most important criterion for a screening programme is to have an accepted treatment for those screened positive. It must be admitted that there are many difficulties in evaluating the outcome of a screening programme. Often, months or years must pass before the gains may be measurable. It is vitally important to determine whether earlier treatment really does give a better prognosis. If this is not the case, then there is no advantage in alerting the patient of the risk condition by early detection. No screening programme should be implemented without first having ensured that there are adequate resources in personnel and equipment for all individuals in need of treatment to get it. The responsibility is clearly on the health care organization that has initiated the screening examination and urged the individual to respond.

A Latent or Early Symptomatic Stage of the Disease

The disease must have a recognizable latent or early stage that can be detected by the screening test. The interval from this detection to the time when diagnosis ordinarily would have been made due to symptoms, which would make the person seek medical attention, is known as the lead time. In other words, lead time is the amount of time by which treatment may be begun earlier due to the screening programme. To summarize, if early treatment is not especially helpful, then there is no point in early detection.

Characteristics of the Screening Test

The validity of a screening test is measured by its sensitivity and specificity. 'Sensitivity' is the ability of the test to classify people as positive when they have the disease or the risk factor under study. 'Specificity' is defined as the ability of the test to classify people as negative when they do not have the disease or the risk factor under study. Having or not having the disease or risk factor in question should ideally be determined by a test that is a part of the diagnostic procedure. A diagnostic test may take more time and be more expensive to perform, and may have a lower degree of safety, but it is essential that it has the highest degree of accuracy. Consequently, an estimate of sensitivity should be regarded as the sensitivity of one test (the screening test) relative to another (the diagnostic test). The same kind of argument may be applied to the use of specificity. In reality, it is often impossible to use the diagnostic test on all screenees to verify the result of the screening test. For instance, the diagnostic test in cancer screening might be extensive surgery.

False positives are people who tested positive but do not have the disease or risk factor under study and false negatives are people who tested negative but do show the disease or risk factor under study. The 'positive predictive value' is the ability of the screening test to predict that there is a state of early disease or a high risk. The positive predictive value will depend in part on the screening test characteristics (sensitivity and specificity) and in part on the prevalence of the disease or risk situation. The reliability of the test is its capacity to give the same result on repeated measurements. Ideally, a screening test should be valid, safe, simple to perform, acceptable to the subject and inexpensive. The sensitivity of the test may be increased or decreased by changing the level at which the test is considered positive. An increase in the sensitivity will decrease the specificity and vice versa (Figure 5.1).

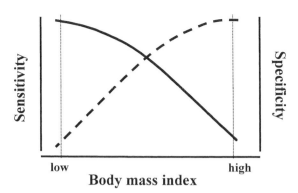

Figure 5.1 Schematic illustration of the relationship between different cut-off points and sensitivity and specificity of defining high-risk individuals and normals. Sensitivity is represented by the solid line and specificity by the dotted line

Adequate Understanding of the Natural History of the Target Disease

Whether a screening programme will be useful to a given population or not depends to a large extent on the natural history of the target disease. A main question is: Does early detection and treatment affect the course and prognosis of the disease? In order to answer that question well-planned and preferably randomized experimental studies must be conducted. In many cases, these clinical trials must be started as soon as possible. If not carried out speedily enough, the time trend may change the practice of treatment and treating the latent stage of the disease may be regarded as normal practice. In such a situation, it would no longer be considered ethical to perform a randomized clinical trial. As a result of this, scientific evidence, showing that the early detection and treatment really changes the natural course of the disease and improves its prognosis, may be lacking.

SCREENING FOR A RISK FACTOR INSTEAD OF A DISEASE

When it comes to the use of screening for a risk factor instead of a disease, two additional points may be formulated (4). The first of these defines the purpose of the screening. The intention must be to find *reversible risk*—not risk factors. The object of the screening procedure must be to find those persons who will benefit from an ensuing intervention.

It is the effect of the intervention that may increase the individual's health and not the risk classification per se. The second point states that *selected screening* is more cost effective than mass screening. Simple and easily attainable information, such as age and sex, may help to select a segment of the population with a heightened risk. The screening procedure may then be done within that segment. In a situation where there is a lack of resources for advice and long-term support, it is better to concentrate the resources on those who need it most.

Obesity is a predisposing factor for type 2 diabetes and cardiovascular disease (CVD). In a screening programme focused on obesity with the aim of preventing or postponing diabetes and CVD, obesity may be regarded as a detectable but asymptomatic phase of these outcomes, i.e. a preclinical phase of CVD or type 2 diabetes. The distinction between screening for a risk factor and screening for a disease is that when a disease is the object of the screening, as in the case of breast cancer, then eventually most screen-detected cases will develop symptomatic disease. When a risk factor is the object of the screening, often only a minority will develop symptomatic disease. This has been the case in screening for hypertension, where only a minority of those screened as mild hypertensives will develop stroke or myocardial infarction.

MASS SCREENING, OPPORTUNISTIC SCREENING OR SELF-REFERRAL

A screening programme uses a screening test to detect early disease or a risk factor for future disease. This detection part of a screening programme need not to be that costly. At least, this is what is to be expected in screening for obesity irrespective whether body mass index or other anthropometric measures are used as screening tools. However, to treat those screened to be high-risk individuals, in a long-term weight management programme, will need considerable resources.

The decision to launch a mass screening programme (the whole population) for overweight and obesity must incorporate a commitment to allocating enough resources to give all high-risk individuals the opportunity to participate in a treatment programme. Otherwise such a decision would be unethical.

An alternative could be to use an opportunistic screening procedure, using all visits made by individuals to the health care centre for whatever reasons to screen for overweight and obesity. In Sweden, more than three-quarters of the population would be reached in this way within a 5-year period (5). Some minor resources would be saved by using a programme based on opportunistic instead of mass screening. However, the greater part of the costs for screening of overweight and obesity would come from the treatment programme and these costs must be the same irrespective of the screening procedure used.

In recent years, many magazines have been offering their readers a chance to calculate their own body mass index (BMI) and along with that a table is presented, prescribing treatment alternatives for different ranges of BMI. This form of magazine-initiated screening puts the responsibility for initiating a suitable treatment on the subjects themselves and not on the health care system. Some may, by self-referral, seek professional help for their weight problem. However, many individuals will appraise the situation of an increased risk, but will not have the strength or the social support to initiate a treatment on their own. Furthermore, most health care systems are not able to cope with a situation where large groups of people seek help for problems with overweight and obesity. A clear disadvantage of this magazine-related screening for obesity is that it alerts people of a risk without offering enough help, and this may create a feeling of helplessness. Probably, such a situation will enlarge the inequity in health already present in contemporary society. Another problem is the impact magazine-related screening may have on eating disorders, especially among young women.

SELECTIVE AND MULTIPLE SCREENING

The term selective screening is used when the screening procedure is concentrated on a special high-risk sector within a population. By using health indicators, information that is already at hand or at least is easy to obtain such as age, sex and race, costs for a screening programme can be reduced. We know that the prevalences of disease and pre-clinical disease often increase with age. One

way of cutting costs in a screening programme could be to select only individuals above a certain age. In this way a larger percentage of those screened will be classified as high-risk individuals. The positive predictive value will be higher since the prevalence of pre-clinical disease is higher and this will reduce costs for the screening procedure. However, as stated above, the main costs in screening for obesity will come from the treatment programme.

The term multiple (or multiphasic) screening has been defined as the application of two or more screening tests in combination to a large group of people. From an economic standpoint it seems logical to offer more than one screening test at the same time, at least if much energy has been spent on getting a high participation rate in the screening programme. Many different pre-clinical diseases may then be examined at the same time. However, multiple screening tests may also be used to specify the high-risk group more precisely. In such a situation only screenees with a positive result in all screening tests are classified as high-risk individuals. The advantage would be that individuals in a smaller and more refined high-risk group would be able to get a more specified treatment programme, in which also more resources could be spent on each individual in the programme. A screening programme targeted to the primary prevention of type 2 diabetes might combine one screening test for obesity and one test for glucose tolerance. In that way, only participants having the combination of obesity and impaired glucose tolerance are classified as high-risk individuals. A further refinement of the programme, at least if the object is to reduce numbers-needed-to-screen to detect a high-risk individual, would be to choose a high-risk sector of the population and offer the programme only to certain age groups.

EVALUATION OF SCREENING

How do we know that our screening is doing more good than harm? Most screening programmes must be continuously evaluated and the evaluation of screening is often complex. Mass screening for breast cancer in women provides a good illustration of this. Despite more than a decade of screening results, the scientists still disagree on the value of these mass screening programmes for breast cancer and whether they should be continued or not (6). Most of the discussion is concerned with how to interpret mortality and survival rates.

There are many difficulties in the evaluation of the outcome of screening (2). Often, the gains are several months or years in the future. It is not acceptable simply to compare survival of screen-detected cases with that of cases detected by symptoms. There are two main reasons for this. A higher survival rate among screen-detected cases could be explained by the fact that the diagnosis was made earlier (lead time). Another explanation could be that a screening programme tends to detect more benign cases (prognostic selection bias). We know that the clinical course of a disease may vary substantially, even if two patients are diagnosed at the same time. A long clinical course, a sign of a more benign disease, is often preceded by a long pre-clinical phase. The probability of detecting a given case in a screening procedure increases as the length of the pre-clinical phase increases.

Comparing overall mortality rate or disease-specific mortality rate would be unbiased in this respect. A lower mortality rate in the screened group would suggest a beneficial effect of early treatment. In general, it is appropriate to compare the rate of development of advanced symptomatic disease between screened and unscreened groups (2).

What is more, even if a reliable evaluation does establish that we are doing more good than harm with our screening programme, we still have to reflect on the alternative use of the resources spent on the screening programme. What would the result be if the resources instead were to be allocated to another sector of the health care system or perhaps to a sector outside the health care system? What would that mean in terms of public health? The strategy of prevention and the balance between preventive and curative work to improve health are two additional issues that have to be included in answering whether screening is worthwhile or not.

BENEFICIAL AND ADVERSE EFFECTS OF SCREENING

Who will gain and who will lose on participating in a screening programme? Since the evaluation of screening programmes is often complex, especially when screening for risk factors, no simple and clear-cut answers can be given. In part, it will depend on the ability of the chosen screening test to correctly separate those that will become ill from those that will continue to be healthy. In part, it will depend on whether the instituted early treatment on those classified to be at high risk is effective or not. In other words, whether the early treatment really prevents or postpones the target disease of the screening programme.

As mentioned earlier, screening for early disease has some advantages compared to screening for a risk factor. In screening for disease, e.g. breast cancer in women, most of the true positives and perhaps some of the false negatives will develop symptomatic disease. This makes it possible, even though not easy, to evaluate on an individual level the gains and losses that are at stake.

In screening for a risk factor, as in screening for hypertension or obesity, most of those screened to be at high risk will not, during a foreseeable time period, develop the target disease of the screening programme whether myocardial infarction, stroke or type 2 diabetes. In such a situation our ability to predict the outcome on an individual level is very limited.

Those who benefit most from participating in a screening programme are individuals in whom the serious consequences of the target disease have been prevented or postponed by the early treatment. This is also the reason why we do the screening in the first place. What about those screened to be at high risk, where serious consequences of the target disease do not develop, even if followed for a very long time. Psychologically, they may be in a lose situation. They have been alerted of a serious risk, without having cause to be alarmed, and may react with anxiety and depression. How much unjustified anxiety and depression is evoked in individuals participating in different screening programmes? The question is impossible to answer in any precise manner and has not received much attention in the evaluation of screening programmes.

A study examining potential adverse psychological effects of screening for cardiovascular risk factors showed that a minority (about 20%) of those screened to be at high risk reacted with some degree of anxiety and confusion (7). Another study, also examining adverse psychological effects of screening, found a mild degree of worry in people labelled as having high cholesterol levels when compared to those labelled as normals. However, the level of anxiety did not influence mood, participation in social activities or life satisfaction. The conclusion was that the screening did not create any adverse psychosocial consequences (8). A similar result was found in a study of screening for hypertension. Individuals with mild to moderate hypertension were compared to individuals with normal blood pressure. Assessment for psychological effects was made repeatedly during a 12-month follow-up. A self-administered questionnaire comprising general health issues was used. A diagnostic psychiatric interview was conducted if the questionnaire indicated a high risk of developing psychiatric manifestations. In the study, no support was given for the belief that the screening programme evoked psychiatric symptoms among the participants. In fact, the reverse was suggested. Based on the interviews, individuals treated for hypertension showed less anxiety than individuals not in the treatment programme. There may, of course, be several explanations for this effect. Regularly attending a clinic could be one explanation. There could also be anxiolytic side effects in the antihypertensive medications that were used (9).

What about those found to be healthy in a screening programme? As stated above, our ability to predict the outcome for an individual is very limited. On that account, there is reason to assume that some individuals classified by the screening test as normal may in fact have an increased risk of becoming ill (false negatives). A harmful effect of screening may also arise in a situation where an individual on testing is found to be without risk factors. A negative screening test may be regarded by the individual as a proof of being healthy and living a healthy life. Ideas of not overdoing things starts to rankle. The next step in the chain might be a worsening in the lifestyle of that individual. This justification for an unhealthy behaviour has sometimes been called the 'certificate of health' effect and must be considered an adverse effect of the screening programme (7).

THE ROLE OF SCREENING IN THE STRATEGY OF PREVENTION

Whether to approach high-risk individuals or the whole population in order to improve health and to prevent disease is often a matter of opinion. Both strategies have their strong and weak points (4). Many of our most important cardiovascular risk factors, e.g. blood pressure, serum cholesterol and body weight, are measured on a continuous scale. They are often normally distributed in the population. The implication of this in risk assessment is that relatively few people have a substantially increased risk, whereas many more people have different degrees of slightly increased risk situations. A specific pattern often emerges when the relative risk of getting a disease for an individual is compared with the total distribution of the disease in the population. Most cases of the disease are derived from the large majority of the population having a slight increase in risk and relatively few cases are derived from the high-risk group. Rose called this phenomenon 'the prevention paradox' and stated 'a preventive measure that brings large benefits to the community offers little to each participating individual' (10). From this it follows that we cannot successfully control modern disease, mainly cardiovascular disease and cancer, solely by detecting and intervening on high-risk individuals. Prevention must embrace both the population and the high-risk approach. The two strategies are complementary and have their respective strengths and limitations.

The screening procedure is a means to identify individuals at high risk of developing disease. Screening is thus a part of a high-risk strategy of prevention. The basic idea behind high-risk strategy is to concentrate the resources for advice and support on those who need it most. The high-risk approach offers a more cost-effective use of available resources and this is especially important when the needed treatment both has to be intense and must continue for a long time. This is clearly the case in the treatment of obesity. The rationale of this high-risk strategy is easy to understand and accept in the medical care system. Giving most resources to those who need it most is a principle that feels familiar to health professionals and is considered more as an extension of the ongoing curative work. This strategy also seems natural to most high-risk individuals. They have been examined and classified as being at risk for future disease. A person who appraises such a situation rationally also realizes that there is a lot to be gained from a treatment programme, and this is likely to increase motivation. Unfortunately, even if we can accurately estimate the average risk for a group, our ability to predict what will happen to an individual is much more uncertain. This uncertainty often has a hampering effect on the individual's motivation.

SCREENING FOR OBESITY

Although obesity should be regarded as a disease entity of its own, many of its more serious consequences are due to the strong relations that exist between obesity and some common chronic diseases. Obesity is an important risk factor for type 2 diabetes, cardiovascular disease, sleep apnoea, gallbladder disease and certain types of cancer.

Why Screen for Obesity?

The association between obesity and type 2 diabetes is perhaps the strongest of all reasons why a crusade against overweight and obesity must be initiated in the near future. The ongoing secular trends in Westernized societies are alarming. It is a healthy sign that the medical profession is showing an increasing interest in and awareness of the impact lifestyle has on health. However, many health professionals express a pessimistic view over the future with regard to many of our chronic diseases, if the 'Westernized' way of living continues to expand over the world. Headlines such as, 'obesity—a time bomb to be defused' (11) and 'non-insulin dependent diabetes mellitus—an epidemic in progress' (12), have been used. The global burden of diabetes has, as stated above, been projected to rise from about 120 million type 2 diabetic individuals in 1997 to about 215 million in 2010 (1).

The 1980s and the 1990s research in cell and molecular biology has presented a body of evidence that supports many years of past clinical experience. Sustained high levels of free fatty acids (FFAs) seem to affect both insulin secretion and insulin action in susceptible individuals by interfering with the glucose transporter mechanism in the pancreatic islet cells and in the muscle and fat cells. Caloric restriction and exercise training have, in animal experiments, been shown to counteract the suppression of glucose transporters, verifying on a cellular level over forty years of experience from observational and experimental studies in humans on the relationships between body weight, physical activity and glucose tolerance. The amount of body fat mass and the metabolic activity in different fat cells seem to regulate the production of FFAs and the consumption of FFAs is largely dependent on the level of physical activity. High levels of stress (cortisol and catecholamines) seem to be implicated both in the enlargement of the visceral fat depots and in boosting their activity. A long-term lifestyle change therefore seems to be the obvious remedy.

The Screening Test—Measuring Body Mass Index or Waist Circumference or Both

The purpose of screening for obesity must be to find individuals at high risk of developing future disease that is caused by a long-standing effect of obesity. Since 'obesity' is associated with a certain level of BMI (more than or equal to 30), the term obesity in this passage will be replaced by the term 'excess storage of body fat'. Excess storage of body fat may be measured in many different ways. Some methods measure the amount of body fat very precisely, but are not suitable for screening purposes. They are often laborious and expensive. Ideally, a screening test should be safe, valid, rapid and inexpensive. The identification of high-risk individuals based on measuring body weight seems, at least compared to many other screening tests, relatively simple and straightforward. The measurements are easy to obtain, safe to use, and reliable. What about validity? Some studies imply that BMI correlates well with percentage of body fat (13). Other studies, using modern imaging techniques, have found significant variations in the percentage of body fat across the whole range of BMI (14). Yet, it is reasonable to believe that measuring BMI would for most subjects capture the increased risk for comorbities that is linked to an excess storage of body fat. Furthermore, BMI is much more stable as a measurement than blood pressure or serum cholesterol, and consequently more suitable as a screening tool. Stress or anxiety can, within seconds, change the level of blood pressure but will have no effect on an individual's BMI.

If measuring BMI is simple and strightforward, the issue of where to draw the line between a high-risk situation and a normal situation is more complex. Body mass index, like many other risk factors, is measured on a continuous scale. However, when used as a screening test, the purpose is to divide the screened population into a minority assessed as having a high risk of developing future disease and a majority assessed as normal. A cut-off point at a low level of BMI will define our high-risk group more broadly, ensuring that practically all individuals with excess storage of body fat are classified as high-risk individuals (true positives). This is easily understood if we hypothetically choose a BMI of $20 \, \text{kg/m}^2$ as a cut-off point. The sensitivity would be high in such a situation (Figure 5.1). However, a broadly defined high-risk group would also include many individuals not having excess storage of body fat. These would be falsely regarded as high-risk individuals (false positives). Another way of expressing this is to say that the screening test does not correctly classify as negative those individuals without excess storage of body fat. The specificity of such a test would be low (Figure 5.1). Similarly, if a high level of BMI was chosen as the cut-off point, the high-risk group would be defined narrowly. This is most easily understood if we hypothetically choose a BMI of $35 \, \text{kg/m}^2$ as a cut-off point. In such a situation, many individuals having excess storage of body fat would by the screening test be classified as negatives, i.e. belonging to a normal risk situation (false negatives). The sensitivity of the test would be low. However, the specificity would be high, since practically all those without excess storage of body fat would be classified as normals (true negatives).

Many different considerations have to be taken into account when deciding which cut-off point to use in a screening test. All individuals found to have a high risk are entitled to a treatment programme. If obesity is to be treated successfully on a long-term basis, a lot of professional support is needed. In this way, the amount of resources allocated to the treatment component of the screening programme will have a major impact on how broadly or narrowly the high-risk group is to be defined. Of course, a cut-off point that is already generally accepted by the medical profession, and represents a level of BMI above which the risk curve for comorbidities rises more steeply, would seem natural. A BMI of more than or equal to $30 \, \text{kg/m}^2$ would define between 10 and 25% of most Western populations as high-risk individuals (15).

As mentioned earlier, intensive research in cardiovascular disease and type 2 diabetes, over more than two decades, has pointed to visceral fat accumulation and free fatty acids as key factors in the aetiology of these diseases. This clearer understanding of the mechanisms by which obesity contributes to cardiovascular disease and type 2 diabetes may also imply that waist circumference, abdominal sagittal diameter or waist-to-hip ratio are more accurate measures of the risk of future disease than BMI and should therefore be preferred as screening tests. Abdominal obesity has in prospective studies independently, after controlling for BMI, been associated with the incidence of cardiovascular disease (16) and type 2 diabetes (17). However, the picture is not entirely clear-cut. In the Health Professionals' Follow-up Study, although waist circumference was shown to be a good predictor, a high BMI was the dominant risk factor for type 2 diabetes (18).

The new techniques for measuring body fat introduced during the 1980s and the 1990s, such as computed tomography and magnetic resonance imaging (MRI), have the ability to determine accurately not only total body fat but also the body fat content in different compartments. This makes it possible to measure the amount of visceral fat in a more precise manner (14). Several studies have already been performed using these new techniques to measure the amount of visceral fat. The visceral fat content has been linked to different anthropometric indices and to the presence of cardiovascular and metabolic risk factors. Pouliot and colleagues showed, by using computed tomography, that waist circumference and abdominal sagittal diameter correlated better than the more commonly used waist-to-hip ratio with both the amount of visceral fat accumulation and the different metabolic risk factors (19). From the data in this study it was suggested that a waist circumference of above 100 cm, or an abdominal sagittal diameter of above 25 cm, would indicate an increased risk situation for the development of cardiovascular disease and/or type 2 diabetes. However, since the sagittal diameter in the study was measured indirectly using an abdominal scan obtained with computed tomography, further studies need to be performed where the abdominal sagittal diameter is measured clinically, before the method can be recommended for clinical purposes.

The use of waist circumference has also been advocated. In this context, it should be pointed out that the relationship between waist circumference (or waist-to-hip ratio) and abdominal visceral fat accumulation may be age-specific. Older subjects seem to have more visceral fat for each given value of waist circumference (or waist-to-hip ratio) than younger adults (20). From a public health point of view, it might be argued that measuring waist circumference on large subgroups of a population, and then using age-specific threshold values to identify individuals at risk, would present no major problems. In a study from Glasgow, the waist circumference was found to relate closely to both BMI and waist-to-hip ratio. By using a combination of these two measures of adiposity as a 'gold standard' and calculating sensitivity and specificity with respect to waist circumference, two action levels for waist circumference were suggested. A waist circumference of more than or equal to 94 cm in men and 80 cm in women (lower action level) identified' with a sensitivity of 96% and a specificity of 97.5%, subjects having either a BMI more than or equal to 25 kg/m^2, or a waist-to-hip ratio that was high (≥ 0.95 for men and ≥ 0.80 for women). The higher action level was defined as a waist circumference of more than or equal to 102 cm for men and 88 cm for women. These levels identified, with the same degree of sensitivity and specificity, subjects with either a BMI of more than or equal to 30 kg/m^2, or a high waist-to-hip ratio. The conclusion was that waist circumference is a suitable tool to use in health promotion programmes to identify, i.e. screen for, individuals who might benefit from weight management programmes (21). It was also suggested that individuals identified to be above the lower action level should acknowledge being in an increased risk situation and take action to avoid weight gain, and that individuals above the higher action level should seek professional help to lose weight and maintain a lowered body weight.

From samples within the Nurses' Health Study and the Health Professionals' Follow-up Study, the validity of self-reported body weights and waist and hip circumferences has been explored. The self-reported measurement was compared to a measurement conducted by a specially trained technician in the study. An especially high degree of correlation was found for body weight (0.97) and waist circumference (0.95 in men and 0.89 in women) (22). Recently, national guidelines for the management of obesity in Scotland were presented by the Scottish Intercollegiate Guidelines Network (23). Their report recommended the use of BMI and waist circumference as screening tests for obesity.

A point of caution is warranted if using these new action levels of waist circumference on populations other than Caucasian. A study comparing the prevalence of glucose intolerance in Chinese and Europid men and women showed similar age-adjusted prevalences in men (13%) but higher prevalence of glucose intolerance in Chinese women (20%) compared to Europid women (13%), despite the fact that the study found mean BMI and waist circumference to be lower in Chinese men and women than in Europids. Furthermore, the mean waist-to-hip ratio in Chinese women was higher than in Europid women (24).

Taken together, total body fat measured as body mass index and body fat distribution measured as waist circumference seem to supplement each other in indicating a cardiovascular or metabolic risk situation for an individual. They seem both to be suitable as screening tests and should preferably be used together in health promotion programmes. The action levels that have been suggested are based on our present knowledge of using simple proxy measures to assess total and visceral fat accumulation. However, as stated earlier, the choice of cut-off point in screening programmes must be determined by the level of resources allocated to take care of those identified to be at high risk. Alerting without offering advice and support is harmful. It goes without saying that different degrees of risk may need different levels of treatment programmes. It is crucial that every high-risk individual feels that the screening programme offers something they experience as beneficial.

SCREENING FOR OBESITY TO PREVENT TYPE 2 DIABETES

The primary prevention of type 2 diabetes is an urgent issue and weight control in the population seems to be the most important part of the preventive process. The drastic predictions concerning the time trends of obesity and type 2 diabetes call urgently for research aimed at finding a solution or more probably several solutions to the problem. One approach could be a mass screening programme examining the whole population for body weight and offering obese individuals the opportunity to participate in a weight management programme. Another approach could be a selective screening procedure where only some especially high-risk segments of the population are examined.

Type 2 Diabetes and its Complications—a Serious Health Problem

People with diabetes have a substantially reduced life expectancy. Atherosclerosis is the most common long-term complication of diabetes, at least in Caucasian populations. People with diabetes are two to three times more likely to die from coronary heart and cerebrovascular disease than are people without diabetes. The relationship is even more accentuated in peripheral artery disease, which is four times more common among diabetes patients. Retinopathy develops in about 60% of those with type 2 diabetes (25) and seems to be present prior to the clinical onset of the disease in 10–30% of individuals (26). In the USA, kidney disease was 17 times more common in diabetic than in non-diabetic individuals, and diabetic kidney disease is considered the leading cause of renal disease requiring dialysis or transplantation. More than 50% of all non-traumatic lower-limb amputations conducted in the USA are associated with diabetes and the overall risk of amputation is 15 times greater in diabetic than in non-diabetic individuals (25).

Impaired Glucose Tolerance—an Intermediate Stage in the Development of Type 2 Diabetes

Both insulin resistance and beta cell dysfunction seem necessary for an individual to develop type 2 diabetes mellitus. Controversy exists about which of the two pathogenic mechanisms is the primary one. Genetic as well as environmental factors participate in the process. Using the two-step model for diabetes proposed by Saad, the diabetic process can be divided into a first step, which includes the transition from the normal to impaired glucose tolerance (IGT) and where insulin resistance seems to be the main determinant. The second step is the worsening from IGT to type 2 diabetes, where beta cell dysfunction seems to play a major role (27). In six prospectives studies the worsening of IGT to diabetes varied from 3.6% to 8.7% per year (28). In

the combined analysis of all six studies, but not in all of the separate studies BMI was associated with the diabetes incidence independently of fasting and post-load glucose levels. Family history of diabetes was not associated with the progression of IGT to diabetes. It has been estimated that by the time the diagnosis of diabetes is determined according to a criterion of a fasting plasma glucose level of above 7.7 mmol/L (compare the new threshold of 7.0 mmol/L), 75% of the beta cell function has been lost (29).

A few long-term intervention studies, with the intention to prevent diabetes by treating IGT subjects, have been conducted. In the Malmö study, a combination of diet and exercise reduced the progression from IGT to diabetes during a 6-year period from 29% in the control group to 11% in the treatment group (30). The Chinese Da Qing IGT and Diabetes study showed similar results with a decrease in the incidence of diabetes in the diet and exercise treatment group of 42% compared to the control group at follow-up after 6 years (31). These two studies show that long-term lifestyle intervention may prevent or at least postpone the worsening of IGT to type 2 diabetes.

Taken together, many indications suggest that once the diagnosis of the diabetes is made, the reversibility of the diabetic state is lost, a state which probably has been present as a glucose–insulin feedback disturbance for 5–10 years (32), and what remains is to use all efforts possible to diminish further deterioration in beta cell function and diabetes disease. In contrast, lifestyle interventions have been shown to prevent the progression of IGT to diabetes. Furthermore, the effect on future macrovascular disease, due to a state of insulin resistance and hyperinsulinaemia for several years before the diagnosis of diabetes is made, must also be included in the discussion of primary prevention.

An important point that must be considered in a screening programme aimed at preventing type 2 diabetes is how the distribution of BMI in the population affects the screening procedure. In the population a majority of people will be of normal weight or have a slight excess of body fat (overweight). A few will be seriously obese. Since the number of diabetic cases that will develop is dependent on both the relative risk and the number of people sharing that risk, one may argue from a population perspective that most diabetic cases will develop among the many having a slight increase in risk and

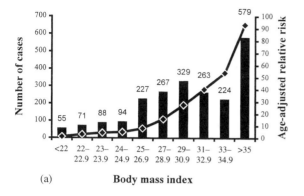

(a)

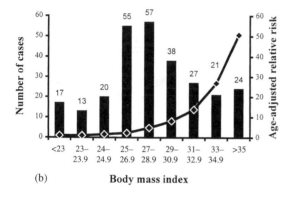

(b)

Figure 5.2 (a) The age-adjusted relative risk for developing diabetes during 14 years of observation (curve) among women in different classes of body weight and the distribution of incident diabetic cases in the study (bars). Based on data from Colditz *et al.* (33) (b) The age-adjusted relative risk for developing diabetes during 5 years of observation (curve) among men in different classes of body weight and the distribution of incident diabetic cases in the study (bars). Based on data from Chan *et al.* (18)

not among the few having the large increase in risk. In other words, most high-risk individuals will not develop diabetes at least during a foreseeable time period and many low-risk individuals will develop diabetes (the prevention paradox).

Above Which Level of Body Mass Index is the Risk Considered as High—Results from two Prospective Studies

Figure 5.2 and Table 5.2 are based on data from two well-cited prospective studies that have explored the association between BMI and the development of type 2 diabetes in the population. In the Nurses'

Table 5.2 Comparing the distribution of new diabetes cases at three different levels of body mass index in two populations

Reference	Body mass index	Diabetes cases (% of total)	Person-years of follow-up (% of total)
Colditz (33)[a]	≥ 27	76	22.1
	≥ 31	49	8.3
	≥ 35	26	3.1
Chan (18)[b]	≥ 27	61	23.5
	≥ 31	27	4.2
	≥ 35	9	0.7

[a]The Nurses' Health Study.
[b]The Health Professionals' Follow-up Study.

Health Study more than 100 000 nurses participated and were followed with respect to diabetes incidence over 14 years. More than 2000 cases of diabetes were diagnosed during 1.49 million person-years of follow-up (33). In the Health Professionals' Follow-up Study, more than 50 000 male health professionals participated. During 5 years of observation, 272 cases of diabetes were diagnosed (18). Both studies show a progressively increased relative risk of getting type 2 diabetes when groups with successively higher BMIs were compared to a group with the lowest BMI.

In the Nurses' Health Study, the age-adjusted relative risk of getting diabetes during a 14-year follow-up was found to be more than 90 times higher if BMI was more than $35 \, kg/m^2$ compared to less than $22 \, kg/m^2$ (33). Correspondingly, the age-adjusted relative risk for diabetes after 5 years of follow-up in men was 50 times higher if BMI was $35 \, kg/m^2$ or more compared to less than $23 \, kg/m^2$ (18). It was also shown that the relative risk for diabetes already started to increase in the upper range of normal weight and became ever more pronounced as body weight increased. Nevertheless, looking at the problem from another angle, more than 85% of the subjects in the highest weight class (BMI $\geq 35 \, kg/m^2$) did not develop diabetes during the observational period (14 and 5 years, respectively).

If instead of relative risk we concentrate on the distribution of new diabetes cases during the follow-up, a pattern of increasing incidence along with higher BMI emerges. However, at a point where BMI reaches $31 \, kg/m^2$ in the female study and $29 \, kg/m^2$ in the male study, the number of diabetic cases starts to fall in spite of a still increasing relative risk for the disease. As stated earlier, at more extreme levels of BMI fewer individuals are to be found, in accordance with the normal distribution curve of BMI in the population. In the Nurses' Health Study, there is one large exception to this pattern. Individuals having a BMI of 35 or more presented such a large risk increase that even though they were relatively few, they generated more than 25% of all the diabetic cases. This indicates that the relation between body weight and type 2 diabetes does not strictly follow the pattern of the preventive paradox.

By choosing different cut-off points in BMI, the proportion of a population that will be designated as high-risk individuals will vary and this in turn means that the number of potential diabetes cases that could be prevented or postponed will vary (Table 5.2). A cut-off value of $27 \, kg/m^2$ would designate more than 20% of the population as high-risk individuals, to whom a treatment programme should be offered. According to these two prospective studies, between 60 and 70% of future type 2 diabetic cases would be involved and at best prevented or postponed. A less resourceful screening programme using a cut-off of $35 \, kg/m^2$ would designate 3% of the population in the Nurses' Health Study and 0.7% of the population in the Health Professionals' Study as high-risk individuals (Table 5.2). As much as 26% of future type 2 diabetic cases would be involved in such a programme according to the Nurses' Health Study. This should be compared to 9% in the male study, which also had a shorter period of observation. A screening programme where extensive treatment is to be offered to less than 3% of the population is certainly feasible. The impact of such a programme on public health would not be large but would not be insignificant either. However, the main objective of the screening programme is to provide treatment for those found to be at high risk and the impact on these high-risk individuals may be substantial (high-risk strategy).

To sum up, to achieve a large impact on public health our preventive efforts need to be concentrated on changing attitudes and behaviour in the whole population (population approach). However, it is also evident, especially from the Nurses' Health Study, that a high-risk approach is warranted in the prevention of type 2 diabetes.

The Gain of the Game—What are the Potential Benefits?

As stated above, most would agree that a high-risk strategy certainly would be beneficial to many high-risk individuals. But the question is, may such a strategy also be justified from a public health point of view? Earlier in this chapter the prevention paradox was discussed, with its emphasis on the importance of having the whole population making small changes in lifestyle. When scrutinizing the results from the Nurses' Health Study, looking at the association between BMI and the incidence of type 2 diabetes, a surprisingly large percentage (26%) of the incident cases was found in the highest BMI group ($\geq 35 \, kg/m^2$).

What would the gain be, at best, using a screening programme to detect all individuals in the population with a BMI of $35 \, kg/m^2$ or more, and offering these high-risk individuals a long-term weight management programme? Hypothetically, a crude calculation on the data from the Nurses' Health Study can be made. Assuming that the whole population participates in the screening procedure and that the treatment programme is 100% effective in bringing down the body weight to a BMI between 29 and $30.9 \, kg/m^2$. As shown in Table 5.3, the incidence of diabetes in the highest BMI group would be reduced by more than 70%. Converting this figure into its effect on the whole population in the study, there would be a decrease in incident diabetic cases in the population of 19% (414/2197 fewer cases). In this example 3% of the population (i.e. 3% of observed person-years in the study) would be classified as high-risk individuals. Enlarging the screening programme to all individuals having a BMI $\geq 31 \, kg/m^2$, and achieving the same result concerning weight management, would reduce the incidence of type 2 diabetes on a population level by 29% (628/2197 fewer cases), but in this alternative 8% of the population had to be offered the treatment programme. Of course, there are many good arguments questioning the basis for this calculation. The two most obvious would perhaps be the participation rate in the screening and the effectiveness of the treatment programme. However, the point to illustrate in this calculation is that in the case of obesity and type 2 diabetes a high-risk strategy really seems worthwhile.

Table 5.3 Hypothetical calculation of reduction in number of incident diabetic cases in women during 14 years of follow-up. The assumption is that an intervention successfully achieved a weight decline to a body mass index range of 29.0–30.9 kg/m² in all individuals. The calculations are performed on data from the Nurses' Health Study (33)

Body mass index	Diabetic cases	Person-years of follow-up	Age-standardized incidence rate[a]	Hypothetical number of diabetic cases[b]
29.0–30.9	329	84 880	354.5	329
31.0–32.9	263	47 119	521.2	167
33.0–34.9	224	29 885	703.6	106
≥ 35	579	46 636	1190.5	165

[a]Age-standardized rate per 100 000 persons.
[b]Hypothetical number of cases has been calculated by using the incidence rate among individuals in the BMI range of 29.0–30.9.

THREE SELECTIVE SCREENING PROGRAMMES FOR OBESITY—A PROPOSITION

As stated earlier, the screening procedure for obesity, whether using BMI or waist circumference or both as screening tools, will not be the expensive part of the screening programme. These measurements of obesity are easy to obtain and the measurements could be performed with a high accuracy at many different locations such as work sites, schools and primary health care centres. The expensive part of the screening programme arises when all screenees classified as high-risk individuals are to be treated. Considerable resources must then be allocated if success is to be expected in performing weight management programmes on a large scale.

Recently, the Scottish Intercollegiate Guidelines Network (SIGN) released a report on the management of obesity in Scotland (23). The report pointed out the need for earlier identification of children and adults that are gaining weight, especially if they come from overweight families. To solve this problem, the recommendation was to institute regular screening of the whole population at 3-year intervals with recording of BMI and waist circumference. Furthermore, weight management programmes were to be introduced in primary health care centres and evaluated regularly in a strict manner.

There are many reasons to involve the primary health care system in the early detection and treatment of obesity. There is one obvious question, concerning these interventions, that must be

answered: 'Do those who really need the intervention most participate in the screening programme?' In 1985, a community intervention programme on cardiovascular disease and diabetes prevention was launched in the province of Västerbotten in northern Sweden. The programme combined a population strategy and an individually oriented strategy. The latter was mainly carried out within the primary health care system. Evaluation by comparing participants and non-participants in the intervention programme showed the social selection bias to be quite modest. The result was explained by the close involvement of the primary health care organization in the programme. The primary health care centres in Sweden seem to attract and interact with all groups in the local society, independent of social position, education, employment and income level (34).

Another observation derives from a small community in Sweden, where opportunistic screening was used to find undiagnosed diabetes. In this community, primary care was provided through a single health care centre. It was shown that as much as 75–85% of the whole population participated in the screening programme during a 5-year period of observation (5). It is important to emphasize that all screening for obesity must be evaluated on a regular basis, whether we choose to use a mass screening approach or opportunistic screening, and whether we select some sector of the population to participate or the whole population. There is a need to conduct different kinds of screening programmes for obesity and in different populations. The results from these studies may then form the basis for future planning of screening programmes for obesity.

In the light of these facts, three potentially interesting areas of screening for obesity will be highlighted, namely screening for obesity in children, for severe obesity and for the combination of obesity and impaired glucose tolerance.

The Prevention of Obesity in Children

About 30% of obese children become obese adults (35). Furthermore, obese adults whose obesity started to develop at a young age seem to suffer more serious consequences because of their excess body fat resulting in higher morbidity and mortality rates (36). It often takes years for obesity to develop, but once there it is hard to treat. A promising approach worth exploring would be to prevent childhood obesity becoming adulthood obesity. In a randomized study, obese children treated in a family-based weight reduction programme were found to have a decrease in percentage overweight (− 7.5%) at follow-up after 10 years. The non-specific control group in the study had an increase at follow-up of more than 14% (37). However, two points must be emphasized when working with weight management programmes in children. First, in order to promote healthy growth and to avoid future eating disorders, a child must be fed properly, i.e. the child must receive an adequate nutrition and the meal frequency should be regular. Second, every effort must be made to counteract potential negative effects that may appear as a consequence of classifying some children as high-risk individuals and others as normals. All signs of these obese children being frozen out by their peers should be taken seriously (38).

Intensive Treatment in Severely Obese

A number of indications suggest that the treatment of severely obese people, i.e. a BMI more than or equal to $35 \, \text{kg/m}^2$, should be intensified. Perhaps the most important reason is the marked increase in risk for developing diabetes that exists among the severely obese. As mentioned earlier when discussing the Nurses' Health Study, those defined as severely obese (BMI $\geq 35 \, \text{kg/m}^2$) consituted 3% of the observed person-years but 26% of the incidence in diabetes. In the Swedish Obese Subjects (SOS)

Study, it was shown that a large weight loss (about 20 kg) was associated with a 14-fold risk reduction for type 2 diabetes (39). A non-randomized study, where excess body weight in the severely obese was reduced by 50%, prevented progression from impaired glucose tolerance to type 2 diabetes more than 30-fold compared to a control group (40). The large weight loss in these studies was achieved by surgical treatment. In general surgery is today considered the most effective way of reducing weight in the severely obese. Due to the gravity of the health situation for the severely obese, immediate steps to identify and treat this group of people ought to be taken. One possibility could be to institute an opportunistic screening programme within the primary health care system. In other words, whenever an obese person makes an appointment at the primary health care centre, the routine is to measure BMI and waist circumference. Of course, different treatment alternatives, and not only surgery, must be offered to those classified as high-risk individuals in such a large-scale operation. Not everyone will or should accept surgery as the only, or as the first, treatment alternative.

Screening for the Combination of Obesity and Impaired Glucose Tolerance

Impaired glucose tolerance (IGT) implies an increased risk for CVD and for type 2 diabetes mellitus. In fact, some consider IGT as the strongest measurable risk factor for future type 2 diabetes. However, not all individuals with IGT seem to develop diabetes and the conversion rate varies considerably between different ethnic populations. The thrifty genotype syndrome, originally described by Neel, has been suggested as a possible explanation for this phenomenon (41). In the Västerbotten Intervention Programme in north Sweden, a strong association was found between obesity and IGT. As shown in Figure 5.3, BMI was divided into seven subgroups from underweight ($< 20 \, \text{kg/m}^2$) to severe obesity ($\geq 35 \, \text{kg/m}^2$). The relative frequency of IGT among obese subjects (BMI $\geq 30 \, \text{kg/m}^2$) was four times that of subjects with normal body weight (BMI $20–24.9 \, \text{kg/m}^2$). Subjects with overweight (BMI $25–29.9 \, \text{kg/m}^2$) had a frequency of IGT twice that of subjects with normal weight. However, com-

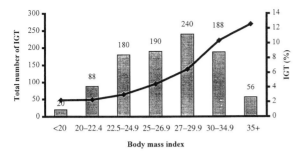

Figure 5.3 The age-adjusted prevalence of impaired glucose tolerance (curve) and the total numbers of subjects with impaired glucose tolerance (bars) in relation to body weight in the Väster-botten Intervention Programme ($n = 21\,057$). From Lindahl *et al.* (42). Reproduced by permission from *Diabetes Care*

paring absolute numbers of individuals with IGT in the different body weight classes, as indicated by the bars in the figure, did show that the majority of individuals with IGT were found among those with a modestly increased body weight (45%) or with a normal body weight (27%). Only 25% of the subjects with IGT were classified as obese (42). In the study, the impact of selecting certain age groups to be screened was examined by calculating the numbers-needed-to-screen to find one individual with abnormal glucose tolerance. It was shown that three to six times as many 40-year-old men and women were needed to be screened when compared to 60-year-old subjects, after adjustments were made for body weight and heredity for diabetes.

Although the relative risk of having IGT increased with increased body weight and with reported heredity for diabetes, the study also clearly demonstrated that the majority of IGT subjects were non-obese and had no heredity for diabetes. The implication of this in screening programmes aimed at preventing type 2 diabetes must be that the screening procedure for IGT should not be targeted solely towards obesity, at least, if we assume that IGT is the predominant risk variable for progression to diabetes. On the other hand, if the screening was to target only 60-year-old individuals with overweight, it ought to be effective from a cost–benefit point of view, even if the chosen subgroup represents only a small portion of IGT in the population. Another way of reasoning could be that our screening strategy should be adjusted to our ability in preventing diabetes by lifestyle and/or pharmacological interventions. Logically, then, it feels as though there is more to offer to obese subjects.

CONCLUSIONS

The prevention of type 2 diabetes by combating obesity and counteracting a sedentary lifestyle is one of the most important health issues of today, and based on projections of future development the issue will be even more important tomorrow. There is much to indicate that our preventive efforts must be based on a population strategy, engaging different sectors of the society. Having health-promoting legislation and agreements with the food industry go hand in hand with health professionals' ambition to change people's attitudes and lifestyles. However, at the same time, not least for ethical reasons, there must be a concentration of resources within the health care system to treat as effectively as possible those identified to be at highest risk of suffering serious health consequences by their choice of lifestyle (high-risk strategy).

Looking at the association between obesity and type 2 diabetes, many indications suggest that a high-risk strategy may be worthwhile, not only from an individual standpoint, but also from a population perspective. The role of screening programmes is to identify and treat these high-risk individuals. The question from a cost-effective point of view, when screening for obesity, is not how to find these high-risk individuals, whether by using mass screening, opportunistic screening or screening by educating people to seek advice and support from the health care system when BMI or waist circumference is above a certain level. The costs for the detection of obesity in screening programmes will be within reasonable limits, irrespective of screening methods used. A potential danger is that many high-risk individuals from low socioeconomic groups will abandon the screening activities. We must remember that the central issue, with respect to obesity, is to find an acceptble treatment open to all defined as high-risk individuals. In other words to allocate enough resources for the treatment programme.

Selective rather than mass screening programmes have been advocated and exemplified in the second part of this chapter. These screening proposals may be regarded as the first line of screening programmes for obesity, especially in view of the present level of resources for prevention within most health care systems.

REFERENCES

1. Amos, AF, McCarty DJ, Zimmet P. The rising global burden of diabetes and its complications: Estimates and projections to the year 2010. *Diabet Med* 1997; **14**: S7–S85.
2. Morrison AS. *Screening in Chronic Disease*. New York: Oxford University Press, 1992.
3. Wilson JMG, Jungner G. Principles and practice of screening for disease. Public Health Papers No. 34. Geneva: World Health Organization, 1968.
4. Rose G. *The Strategy of Preventive Medicine*. New York: Oxford University Press, 1992.
5. Andersson DKG, Lundblad E, Svärdsudd K. A model for early diagnosis of type 2 diabetes mellitus in primary health care. *Diabet Med* 1993; **10**: 167–173.
6. Mayor S. Swedish study questions mammography screening programmes. *BMJ* 1999; **318**: 621.
7. Tymstra T, Bieleman B. The psychological impact of mass screening for cardiovascular risk factors. *Fam Pract* 1987; **4**: 287–290.
8. Irvine MJ, Logan AG. Is knowing your cholesterol number harmful? *J Clin Epidemiol* 1994; **47**: 131–145.
9. Mann AH. The psychological effect of a screening programme and clinical trial for hypertension upon the participants. *Psychol Med* 1977; **7**: 431–438.
10. Rose G. Strategy of prevention: lessons from cardiovascular disease. *BMJ* 1981; **282**: 1847–1851.
11. Bray GA. Obesity: a time bomb to be defused. *Lancet* 1998; **352**: 160–161.
12. Zimmet PZ, Alberti KGMM. The changing face of macrovascular disease in non-insulin-dependent diabetes mellitus: an epidemic in progress. *Lancet* 1997; **350**: 1–4.
13. Deurenberg P, Weststrate JA, Seidell JC. Body mass index as a measure of body fatness: age- and sex-specific prediction formulas. *Br J Nutr* 1991; **65**: 105–114.
14. Thomas EL, Saeed N, Hajnal JV, Brynes A, Goldstone AP, Frost G, Bell JD. Magnetic resonance imaging of total body fat. *J Apply Physiol* 1998; **85**: 1778–1785.
15. The WHO MONICA Project. Geographical variation in the risk factors of coronary heart disease in men and women aged 35–64 years. *World Health Stat Q* 1988; **41**: 115–140.
16. Larsson B, Svärdsudd K, Welin L, Wilhelmsen L, Björntorp P, Tibblin G. Abdominal adipose tissue distribution, obesity, and risk of cardiovascular disease and death: 13 year follow up of participants in the study of men born in 1913. *BMJ* 1984; **288**: 1401–1404.
17. Ohlsson L-O, Larsson B, Svärdsudd K, Welin L, Eriksson H, Wilhelmsen L, Björntorp P, Tibblin G. The influence of body fat distribution on the incidence of diabetes mellitus. 13.5 years of follow-up of the participants in the study of men born in 1913. *Diabetes* 1985; **34**: 1055–1058.
18. Chan JM, Rimm EB, Colditz GA, Stampfer MJ, Willett WC. Obesity, fat distribution, and weight gain as risk factors for clinical diabetes in men. *Diabetes Care* 1994; **17**: 961–969.
19. Pouliot M-C, Després J-P, Lemieux S, Moorjani S, Bouchard C, Tremblay A, Nadeau A, Lupien PJ. Waist circumference and abdominal sagittal diameter: Best simple anthropometric indexes of abdominal visceral adipose tissue accumulation and related cardiovascular risk in men and women. *Am J Cardiol* 1994; **73**: 460–468.
20. Lemieux S, Prud'homme D, Bouchard C, Tremblay A, Després J-P. A single threshold value of waist girth identifies normalweight and overweight subjects with excess visceral adipose tissue. *Am J Clin Nutr* 1996; **64**: 685–693.
21. Lean MEJ, Han TS, Morrison CE. Waist circumference as a measure for indicating need for weight management. *BMJ* 1995; **311**: 158–161.
22. Rimm EB, Stampfer MJ, Colditz GA, Chute CG, Litin LB, Willett WC. Validity of self-reported waist and hip circumferences in men and women. *Epidemiology* 1990; **1**: 466–473.
23. SIGN report. *Obesity in Scotland. Integrating Prevention with Weight Management*. Scottish Intercollegiate Guidelines Network, SIGN. 1996.
24. Unwin N, Harland J, White M, Bhopal R, Winocour P, Stephenson P, Watson W, Turner C, Alberti KGMM. Body mass index, waist circumference, waist–hip ratio, and glucose intolerance in Chinese and Europid adults in Newcastle, UK. *J Epidemiol Community Health* 1997; **51**: 160–166.
25. World Health Organization. Prevention of diabetes mellitus. *WHO Technical Report Series 844*. Geneva: WHO, 1994.
26. Harris MI, Klein R, Welborn TA, Knuiman MW. Onset of NIDDM occurs at least 4–7 yr before clinical diagnosis. *Diabetes Care* 1992; **15**: 815–819.
27. Saad MF, Knowler WC, Pettitt DJ, Nelson RG, Charles MA, Bennett PH. A two-step model for the development of non-insulin-dependent diabetes. *Am J Med* 1991; **90**: 229–235.
28. Edelstein SL, Knowler WC, Bain RP, Andres R, Barrett-Connor EL, Dowse GK, Haffner SM, Pettitt DJ, Sorkin JD, Muller DC, Collins VR, Haman RF. Predictors of progression from impaired glucose tolerance to NIDDM. An analysis of six prospective studies. *Diabetes* 1997; **46**: 701–710.
29. Porte Jr D. Banting lecture 1990. Beta cells in type II diabetes mellitus. *Diabetes* 1991; **40**: 166–180.
30. Eriksson K-F, Lindgärde F. Prevention of type 2 (non-insulin-dependent) diabetes mellitus by diet and physical exercise. The 6-year Malmö feasibility study. *Diabetologia* 1991; **34**: 891–898.
31. Pan X, Li G, Hu Y, Wang J, Yang W, An Z, Hu Z, Lin J, Xiao J, Cao H, Liu P, Jiang X, Jiang Y, Wang J, Zheng H, Zhang H, Bennett PH, Howard BV. Effects of diet and exercise in preventing NIDDM in people with impaired glucose tolerance. The Da Qing IGT and diabetes study. *Diabetes Care* 1997; **20**: 537–544.
32. DeFronzo RA, Bonadonna RC, Ferrannini E. Pathogenesis of NIDDM. *Diabetes Care* 1992; **15**: 318–368.
33. Colditz GA, Willett WC, Rotnitzky A, Manson JE. Weight gain as a risk factor for clinical diabetes mellitus in women. *Ann Intern Med* 1995; **122**: 481–486.
34. Weinehall L, Hallgren C-G, Westman G, Janlert U, Wall S. Reduction of selection bias in primary prevention of cardiovascular disease through involvement of primary health care. *Scand J Prim Health Care* 1998; **16**: 171–176.
35. Dietz WH. Therapeutic strategies in childhood obesity. *Horm Res* 1993; **39** (Suppl 3): 86–90.
36. Seidell JC, Verschuren WMM, van Leer EM, Kromhout D. Overweight, underweight, and mortality. A prospective study of 48 287 men and women. *Arch Intern Med* 1996; **156**: 958–963.

37. Epstein LH, Valoski A, Wing RR, McCurley J. Ten-year follow-up of behavioral, family-based treatment for obese children. *JAMA* 1990; **264**: 2519–2523.

38. Gill TP. Key issues in the prevention of obesity. *Br Med Bull* 1997; **53**: 359–388.

39. Sjöström L, Narbro K, Sjöström D. Costs and benefits when treating obesity. *Int J Obes* 1995; **19** (Suppl 6): S9–S12.

40. Long SD, O'Brien K, MacDonald Jr KG, Leggett-Frazier N, Swanson MS, Pories WJ, Caro JF. Weight loss in severely obese subjects prevents the progression of impaired glucose tolerance to type II diabetes. *Diabetes Care* 1994; **17**: 372–375.

41. Neel JV. Diabetes mellitus: A 'thrifty' genotype rendered detrimental by 'progress'? *Am J Hum Genet* 1962; **14**: 353–362.

42. Lindahl B, Weinehall L, Aslplund K, Hallmans G. Screening for impaired glucose tolerance. Results from a population-based study in 21,057 individuals. *Diabetes Care* 1999; **22**: 1988–1992.

6

Evaluation of Human Adiposity

Steven B. Heymsfield, Daniel J. Hoffman, Corrado Testolin
and ZiMian Wang

St. Luke's/Roosevelt Hospital Center, New York, USA

INTRODUCTION

Human body weight is normally precisely regulated to maintain a weight which reflects habitual energy intake and output. When a positive balance of energy exists there is a greater tendency for the body to store energy and become overweight or obese. Obesity reflects a long-term positive energy balance and excessive weight gain. Accordingly, body weight is a reflection of total body energy content and long-term weight change is a measure of energy balance.

Based upon this view the human body consists mainly of two related parts, one of energy-yielding fuels (i.e. fat, protein and glycogen; Figure 6.1) and the other water (1). Water is bound or closely associated with two of the fuels, glycogen and protein. The remaining energy-yielding compounds, lipids, consist primarily of triglycerides or 'fat'. This simple model ignores the contribution of bone and other minerals to body mass.

Although body weight consists mainly of water and energy-yielding substrates, the actual components of the human body are obviously far more complex. Thus, one can consider the body to be composed of any number of components, such as fat mass and fat-free mass, different molecules, and even different elements. Traditionally techniques to measure whole-body composition have proposed that the body can be organized into five levels consisting of over 40 distinct components (1).

Atomic Level

Body weight represents the lifetime accumulation of only six main elements, oxygen, carbon, hydrogen, nitrogen, calcium and phosphorus (Figure 6.2). Less than 2% of body weight is accounted for by sulfur, potassium, sodium, chlorine, magnesium, and ~ 40 other elements that normally occur in amounts of less than 10 g (2).

Molecular Level

Elements are distributed into molecular components which can be grouped into the five main categories of lipids, proteins, glycogen, water and minerals (Figure 6.3) (1). The main atomic level elements are organized into molecular level components.

The molecular level is often divided, for practical purposes, into two main components, fat and fat-free mass (FFM). Fat-free mass is usually considered to be the metabolically active portion of body mass at the molecular body composition level.

Another molecular level model is based on three components: fat, lean soft tissue and bone mineral (3) (Figure 6.3). This model is appropriate for use with the dual-energy X-ray absorptiometry methods described in later sections.

Three-, four-, and even six-component molecular

International Textbook of Obesity. Edited by Per Björntorp.
© 2001 John Wiley & Sons, Ltd.

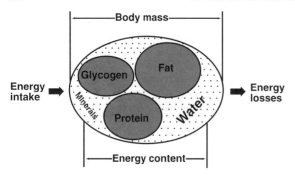

Figure 6.1 Interrelations between energy intake, output and stores

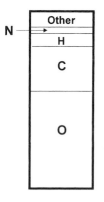

Figure 6.2 Atomic level of body composition. O, oxygen, C, carbon; H, hydrogen; N, nitrogen

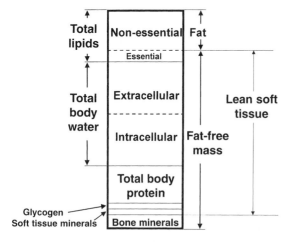

Figure 6.3 Molecular level of body composition

level models are applied with body volume measurements as a core and other additional measurements added for quantifying more components.

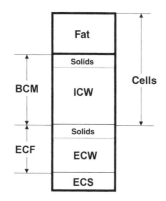

Figure 6.4 Cellular level of body composition. BCM, body cell mass; ECF, extracellular fluid; ECS, extracellular solids; and ECW, extracellular water

Cellular Level

Molecular level body composition components form the basis of functioning cells, and the cellular level of body composition is usually described as three components: cells, extracellular fluid and extracellular solids (Figure 6.4). Cell mass, for measurement purposes, is further divided into fat (a molecular level component) and a metabolically active portion referred to as body cell mass (1,4). The resulting four components are fat, body cell mass, extracellular fluid and extracellular solids.

Tissue–Organ Level

The cellular level components form the tissues and organs of the body such as adipose tissue, skeletal muscle, bone, skin, heart, and other visceral organs (Figure 6.5). These organs and tissues comprise the human body and ultimately complete the link in the five levels of body composition, atomic, molecular, cellular, tissue-system and whole-body.

Body weight, according to this model, represents a complex interplay of energy–nutrient exchange associated with ~ 40 components at the first four levels of body composition. Methods for evaluating adiposity are summarized in Table 6.1. The following section presents a summary of selected methods based on their clinical and research applicability.

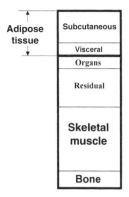

Figure 6.5 Tissue–organ level of body composition

MEASUREMENT OF ADIPOSITY

Whole-body Level

Body Mass Index

Body mass reflects energy content, although actual energy stores are also related to stature, age and gender (5). The usual approach today is to adjust body weight for stature as body mass index (BMI) calculated as body weight (kg)/height (m^2) or 705 × (pounds/inches^2).

BMI has a curvilinear relationship with the body's main energy store, fat, when fatness is expressed as a percentage. Cross-sectional studies suggest that percentage fat is also related to at least three additional factors after considering BMI, those of gender, age and ethnicity (5). BMI is thus a rough marker of adiposity across populations, although over the long term, body weight and BMI are reasonable markers of energy balance for individuals.

BMI has been related to fatness using various modeling strategies in a number of studies. A typical set of percent fat prediction formulas are presented in Table 6.2 (5). These formulas provide a rough estimate of body fat in healthy adults and they do not apply to subjects who are engaged in vigorous exercise training programs.

In practice, BMI is usually used to classify subjects as underweight (i.e. < 18.5), normal weight (≥ 18.5 < 25), overweight (≥ 25 < 30) or obese (≥ 30) (6). BMI may also be used in appropriate subjects as a means of estimating their expected percent fat using equations such as those presented in Table 6.2. The subject's actual measured values can then be compared to the predicted percent fat. For example, a muscular subject would likely have a lower actual body fat than predicted from BMI.

Skinfolds

Another approach at the whole-body level is to estimate fatness using various anthropometric methods that typically include body weight, stature, skinfold and circumference measurements. Various prediction formulas, based on reference body fat measurements, are then applied for predicting body fat.

Although many anthropmetric formulas are applied, the most widely used and cross-validated approach at present is that reported by Durnin and Womersley (7). The corresponding four skinfold

Table 6.1 Adiposity measurement methods

Level	Component	Measurement methods
Molecular	Fat[a]	Dual-energy X-ray absorptiometry (DEXA)
		Tracer dilution (D$_2$O, ^{3}H$_2$O)
		Hydrodensitometry
		Air plethysmography
		In vivo neutron activation (IVNA)
		Whole-body ^{40}K counting
		Multicompartment models
		Bioimpedance analysis (BIA)
		Anthropometry
Cellular	Adipocytes	None
Tissue-system	Adipose tissue	Computerized axial tomography (CT)
		Magnetic resonance imaging (MRI)
		Ultrasound

[a]Refers to lipids in general and specifically storage fats or tryglycerides.

Table 6.2 Prediction formulas for percent fat based upon Body Mass Index (5)

Ethnic group	Prediction formula
Caucasian and African American	% fat = 64.5 − 848 × (1/BMI) + 0.079 × Age − 16.4 × SEX + 0.05 × SEX × Age + 39.0 × SEX × (1/BMI) (SEX = 1 for male, = 0 for female)
Asian	Female: % fat = 64.8 − 752 × (1/BMI) + 0.016 × Age Male: % fat = 51.9 − 740 × (1/BMI) + 0.029 × Age

measurement sites and calculation equations are presented in Tables 6.3 and 6.4. Other equations and methods can be found in the reviews of Heymsfield *et al.* (8) and Roche (9).

In addition to predicting whole-body fatness, anthropometric measurements are also used to estimate regional fat either as absolute individual skinfold measurements or as mid-extremity fat areas using the following formula:

$$\text{limb fat area} = [(\text{mid limb circumference} \times \text{skinfold})/2] - [(\pi \times \text{skinfold}^2)/4] \qquad [1]$$

Mid-arm, calf, and thigh fat areas can be estimated using equation 1 along with corresponding circumferences and skinfolds (8).

Anthropometric methods based upon skinfold measurements are inexpensive, safe, and practical to apply in all settings. Technician training and periodic evaluation is required if measurements are to be reliable and precise. As with many body composition methods, available anthropometric prediction formulas are population specific and cross-validation is required when new populations are evaluated. Lastly, there are technical concerns when skinfold measurements are applied in elderly or very obese populations.

Adipose Tissue Distribution

Visceral adipose tissue is an independent predictor of obesity health-related risks (10). Measures of visceral adipose tissue and adipose tissue distribution are therefore often collected in clinical and research settings.

The most important whole-body level measure of visceral adipose tissue is waist circumference (6).

Table 6.3 Skinfold and circumference measurement methods and sites

Methods of measuring skinfolds
1. Arrive at the anatomic site as defined.
2. Lift the skin and fat layer from the underlying tissue by grasping the tissue with the thumb and forefinger.
3. Apply calipers about 1 cm distal from the thumb and forefinger, midway between the apex and base of the skinfold.
4. Continue to support the skinfold with the thumb and forefinger for the duration of the measurement.
5. After 2 to 3 seconds of caliper application, read skinfold to the nearest 0.5 mm.
6. Measurements are then made in triplicate until readings agree within 1.0 mm; results are then averaged.

Skinfold measurement sites
Biceps. Lift the skinfold on the anterior aspect of the upper arm, directly above the center of the cubital fossa, at the same level as the triceps skinfold and midarm circumference. The arm hangs relaxed at the patient's side, and the crest of the fold should run parallel to the long axis of the arm.
Triceps. Grasp the skin and subcutaneous tissue 1 cm above the midpoint between the tip of the acromial process of the scapula and the olecranon process of the ulna. The fold runs parallel to the long axis of the arm. Care should be taken to ensure that the measurement is made in the midline posteriorly and that the arm hangs relaxed and vertical.
Subscapular. The skin is lifted 1 cm under the inferior angle of the scapula with the patient's shoulder and arm relaxed. The fold should run parallel to the natural cleavage lines of the skin; this is usually a line about 45° from the horizontal extending medially upwards.
Suprailiac. Pick up this skinfold 2 cm above the iliac crest in the midaxillary line. The crest of this fold should run horizontally.

Methods of measuring circumferences
1. The tape should be maintained in a horizontal position touching the skin and following the contours of the limb, but not compressing underlying tissue.
2. Measurements should be made to the nearest millimeter, in triplicate, as previously described for skinfolds.

Circumference measurement sites
Waist. A flexible inelastic measuring tape is placed at the level of the narrowest part of the torso, as viewed anteriorly. Waist measurements are made at the end of normal expiration.
Hip. Circumference measured at the level of maximum extension of the buttocks as viewed from the side.

Methods for optimizing precision
1. Observers should be trained by skilled professionals.
2. One rather than multiple observers should be used if possible, particularly for the same subject followed over time.
3. The anatomic landmarks, how to grasp the skinfold, how long to compress the skinfold site, and how to read the caliper scale properly should be taught to all anthropometrists.
5. Periodically assess inter-observer and between-day measurement differences of the staff.

Table 6.4 Skinfold method of estimating total body fat (7)

1. Determine the patient's age and weight (kg).
2. Measure the following skinfolds in mm; biceps, triceps, subscapular, and suprailiac.
3. Compute $\sum$ by adding the four skinfolds.
4. Compute the logarithm of $\sum$.
5. Apply one of the following age- and sex-adjusted equations to compute body density (D, g/ml).
    Equations for men:
    Age range
    17–19 D = 1.1620 − 0.0630 × (log $\sum$)
    20–29 D = 1.1631 − 0.0632 × (log $\sum$)
    30–39 D = 1.1422 − 0.0544 × (log $\sum$)
    40–49 D = 1.1620 − 0.0700 × (log $\sum$)
    50 + D = 1.1715 − 0.0779 × (log $\sum$)
    Equations for women:
    Age range
    17–19 D = 1.1549 − 0.0678 × (log $\sum$)
    20–29 D = 1.1599 − 0.0717 × (log $\sum$)
    30–39 D = 1.1423 − 0.0632 × (log $\sum$)
    40–49 D = 1.1333 − 0.0612 × (log $\sum$)
    50 + D = 1.1339 − 0.0645 × (log $\sum$)
6. Fat mass is then calculated as fat mass (kg) = body weight (kg) $\times \left[\dfrac{4.95}{D} - 4.5 \right]$
7. Fat-free body mass is then calculated as FFM (kg) = body weight (kg) − fat mass (kg)

Reproduced with permission from Heymsfield SB, McManus III C, Seitz S, Nixon D, Smith J. Anthropometric assessment of adult protein-energy malnutrition. In: Wright RA and Heymsfield SB (eds). *Nutritional Assessment of the Hospitalized Patient*. Boston: Blackwell Scientific Publications, Inc, 1984: 27–82.

Additionally, the waist-to-hip circumference ratio is a useful, although less often used measured of adipose tissue distribution. The measurement sites for waist and hip circumferences are summarized in Table 6.3.

Various skinfold ratios are also reported in the literature as measures of adipose tissue distribution (9). The application of skinfold ratios to describe the differences in adipose tissue distribution is useful given the economical means of measuring the subcutaneous adipose tissue. In addition, skinfold measurements can be used to estimate the amount of deep adipose tissue in various parts of the body.

Tissue-system Level

All major tissues and organs can now be measured *in vivo* using either computerized axial tomography (CT) (11) or magnetic resonance imaging (MRI) (12). Cross-sectional images are prepared at one or more predefined anatomic locations and the amount of adipose tissue present is then quantified as a slice 'area' or across multiple slices into a 'volume' estimate. Volume estimates can then be converted to mass after adjusting for adipose tissue density (i.e. $0.92 \, \text{g/cm}^3$). Imaging methods are usually reserved for research studies and are not able to be applied in field settings since the required scanners are costly, require trained personnel for operation, and technical expertise is needed for scan analysis and adipose tissue quantification. Imaging methods often serve as the reference for quantifying whole-body and regional adiposity, particularly visceral adiposity (13).

Computerized axial tomography provides high resolution standardized images at preselected anatomic locations. Images may be produced as a single slice or by 'spiral' imaging of whole regions (11,12). Ideally whole-body adipose tissue is measured by head-to-toe contiguous imaging, but it is often more typical that slices several centimeters apart are collected and the evaluated adipose tissue areas integrated. Various studies have reported that from 20 to 40 cross-sectional images are required for accurate whole-body analysis (11).

Analysis of CT images is well developed and usually does not require special hardware or software beyond that of CT system components. Pixels, or picture elements, are expressed in Hounsfield units, and calibrations are the same from scanner to scanner. Water is arbitrarily defined as HU = 0, with adipose tissue ~ -90 HU and lean tissues ~ 120 HU (11,12). Segmentation of each image is accomplished using a combination of tracing and HU range setting procedures.

Although CT rapidly provides high resolution images, radiation exposure is a concern, particularly when multiple studies are planned or children and young women are the subject of study. Nevertheless, CT can be applied as the reference for tissue-system level components against which other methods are compared or calibrated (12). The CT number of evaluated pixels, expressed as Hounsfield units, can also be used not only as a means of separating one tissue from another, but also as a measure of tissue composition (12). For example, the lipid content of liver or skeletal muscle can be estimated from the CT number (12).

Magnetic resonance imaging also provides high

resolution cross-sectional images, although longer image development times lead to motion artifacts in peristaltic tissues, such as the gastrointestinal tract. A major advantage of MRI is the lack of radiation exposure and the capability of carrying out whole-body scans in less than 30 minutes (12,14). Male and female subjects of all ages can therefore be studied on a repeated basis and MRI is ideally suited for longitudinal studies. As with CT, imaging cost tends to be high and instrument access is often limited or erratic due to clinical exigencies. Unlike CT, MRI image pixels of the same tissue may vary within an image, between images on the same subject, and between scanners. This lack of pixel uniformity requires additional observer time and technical skill. While images can be read on the conventional MRI scanner console, most investigators now transfer images to their own computer system coupled with specialized analysis software (12,14). The usual approach to scan analysis is application of specialized software (e.g. Tomovision Inc., Montreal, Canada) by a trained technician.

Both CT and MRI represent major advances in the study of human body composition at the tissue-system body composition level. While they are best suited for use in research and/or hospital settings, the ease of measuring body composition with these techniques greatly improves the use of such data in cross-sectional or longitudinal studies.

Adipose Tissue Distribution

Both CT and MRI are capable of producing cross-sectional images of the abdomen, although CT has the advantage of shorter image production times and thus less peristaltic movement artifact. Imaging methods often serve as the reference against which other adipose tissue distribution methods are compared or calibrated (12). The usual approach is to collect and analyze one image, typically at the L4–L5 interspace (15). Occasionally, three or more images are collected by investigators with the aim of estimating total visceral adipose tissue volume.

Cellular Level

Adiposity at the cellular level is represented by fat cells or adipocytes. Unfortunately, it is not possible at present to quantify fat cell mass *in vivo*. One rough approach is to evaluate total body adipose tissue mass with CT or MRI and to combine this information with biopsy-derived adipose tissue cell mass concentration. This method, which assumes representative biopsy sampling of adipose tissue, can provide approximations of total fat cell mass.

Most investigators model the cellular level as shown in Figure 6.4. Included in this model is the molecular level component fat, rather than fat cell mass, which can be estimated as reviewed in the next section.

Body cell mass is the 'metabolically active' compartment at the cell level and several measurement strategies are recognized. The classical approach is to assume stable intracellular potassium concentrations (150 mmol/kg H_2O) and then to measure total body or exchangeable potassium using whole-body counting or multiple isotopic methods (16). An alternative is to measure intracellular water, a compartment similar to BCM, as the difference between total body water and extracellular water. A number of isotope dilution methods can be used to evaluate total body water and extracellular water (17).

Molecular Level

Fat, or triglyceride, is the major relevant component at the molecular body composition level. Three of the methods used to measure body composition at this level are often used either alone or in combination with each other. These methods are body volume analysis, labeled water dilution, and dual-energy X-ray absorptiometry (DEXA).

Body Volume Analysis

Body volume is a measurable physical property of the human body that can be used in the classic two-compartment model originally proposed by Behnke (18). Behnke, and those who followed his lead, proposed that two components comprise body mass, fat and fat-free mass (FFM). Fat has a relatively stable density of $0.900 \, g/cm^3$ at body temperature while FFM, assuming stable proportions of water, protein and minerals, has a density of $1.100 \, g/cm^3$ (19). These two assumed constants can be used to develop a two-component model (Table 6.5). Body volume is measured in a temperature-controlled underwater weighing tank with correc-

Table 6.5 Models for estimating total body fat mass (kg) based on measured body weight and volume

Two-compartment model
Fat = (4.95 × BV) − (4.50 × BW)
Multi-compartment models
Fat = (2.118 × BV) − (0.78 × TBW) − (1.351 × BW)
Fat = (6.386 × BV) + (3.961 × mineral) − (6.09 × BW)
Fat = (2.75 × BV) − (0.714 × TBW) + (1.129 × Mo) − (2.037 × BW)
Fat = (2.513 × BV) − (0.739 × TBW) + (0.947 × Mo) − (1.79 × BW)
Fat = (2.75 × BV) − (0.714 × TBW) + (1.148 × mineral) − (2.05 × BW)

BV, body volume (L); BW, body weight (kg); Mo, bone mineral; TBW, total body water (kg).

tion for residual lung volume (20). The underwater weighing apparatus is relatively simple to construct, the method is safe, and measurements are inexpensive. However, some patients find water submersion difficult and the apparatus cannot be easily moved from one location to another.

The recent introduction of an operational air plethysmograph (BOD POD®; Life Measurements Instruments, Concord, CA) offers an alternative to underwater weighing as a means of measuring body volume (21). The measurement of body volume is carried out by application of classical gas laws within a two-chambered air plethysmograph. Small changes in chamber volume are produced and the corresponding changes in pressure are then measured. The subject's whole-body volume is determined by subtraction of the chamber's volume while empty. Additional corrections are applied for body volume based on body surface area and thoracic gas volume. Body volume is measured while the subject sits quietly inside the system chamber for 60 seconds. An average of several trials is used in estimating body volume. Lung air volume or thoracic gas volume are estimated during normal tidal breathing using a tube connected to the system breathing circuit. The subject puffs gently into the tube while the tube is mechanically obstructed. The two-compartment equation in Table 6.5 or a similar counterpart is used to derive an estimate of adiposity.

The BOD POD system compares favorably with underwater weighing as a means of estimating body volume in adults (21). Simplicity, safety, and lack of need for active subject participation are all favorable characteristics of this new body volume measurement system. The system costs more than a typical underwater weighing apparatus and the current model is not optimally designed for pediatric use.

Hydrometry

The total body water (TBW) compartment can be quantified using three water isotopes, two of which are stable (i.e., ^2H_2O and $H_2{}^{18}O$) and one of which is radioactive (^3H_2O) (17). Isotopes are administered either orally or intravenously and saliva, blood or urine samples are collected several hours later after equilibration. Isotope dilution volume is then estimated, usually after correction for urinary losses. Dilution volumes tend to marginally overestimate TBW, making appropriate adjustments necessary along with volume to mass conversion in order to arrive at a measure of water mass (17). The average fat-free mass hydration of mammals is 0.73 and this stable coefficient also applies to adult humans. Therefore, fat-free mass can be calculated as TBW/0.73 or 1.37 × TBW (17,22,23). Fat mass is calculated as the difference between body weight and FFM.

The total body water method of quantifying adiposity is widely applied in adults as it is simple, portable and practical. Specimen analysis is also simple and inexpensive for tritiated water, although isotope radioactivity may limit use in children and young women, particularly women who are pregnant. Deuterium overcomes the radioactivity concerns of tritium, although analysis is more complex and costly. Oxygen-18 labeled water is costly and analysis is complex and may be expensive owing to the requirement for a mass spectroscopy measurement system.

Dual-energy X-ray Absorptiometry (DEXA)

Dual-energy X-ray absorptiometry allows for evaluation of both regional and total body adiposity (24). Systems vary in design, speed, and cost, although operating principles are all similar. An X-ray source and filter produce two main photon energies and the emitted photons pass through the subject (3). Emerging photon intensity is then measured by system detectors. Relative photon attenuation of the two energies depends upon the elemental make-up of traversed tissues. Fat, lean soft tissue, and bone mineral have high proportions of carbon, oxygen, and calcium, respectively (3). These differing tissue properties influence relative attenuation in a manner that allows separation of pixel mass into two components: soft tissue + bone mineral in pixels with bone, and fat + lean soft tissue in pixels without bone. Mathematical algorithms are then used to solve for whole-body and regional fat, lean soft tissue and bone mineral mass (Figure 6.3). Animal and human cadaver and *in vivo* studies support DEXA accuracy in most circumstances; results may not be accurate using conventional systems in very small animals (e.g. $< 300\,g$) and severely obese subjects (i.e. BMI $> 35\,kg/m^2$).

An important feature of DEXA is software capable of providing both regional and whole-body measurements (24). Whole-body scans usually include a default setting with manual adjustment for separating the body into several appendicular and truncal segments. Manual analysis of specific regions is also possible with newer DXA systems.

DEXA is an important innovation in the body composition field as three clinically relevant components can be accurately quantified in specific regions or the whole body with low radiation exposure, good accuracy, and high reproducibility. Systems are widely available, although whole-body measurements are moderately expensive.

Multicomponent Models

Molecular level methods are available for estimating total body fat using between two and six components (Table 6.5) (19). One important group of multicomponent models presented in Table 6.5 is formulated around body volume measurement and the two-component model originated by Behnke (18). Multicomponent models include three or more components, and measurements in addition to body volume are required. The classic three-component model of Siri is formulated upon measured body volume, body mass and TBW (25). This model has an advantage over the two-component model in subjects or groups who have hydration levels that differ from the assumed ~ 0.73. Four- and six-component models include measured bone mineral (i.e. by DEXA) in addition to the three-component model measurements. These more complex models improve over the two- and three-component models by accounting for individual differences in relative bone mineral mass.

The body-volume-based group of multicompo-

nent models is widely used as a reference for comparison or calibration of other available methods. Adding more measured properties and components reduces model error, which is useful when evaluating subjects varying widely in age, gender, ethnicity and health. Measurement error also increases when multicomponent models are applied and care should be taken that additional error does not offset the accuracy gained (26,27). Multicomponent models are usually applied only in research settings.

Bioimpedance Analysis (BIA)

An alternating electrical current passing across tissues experiences a voltage drop in relation to tissue specific resistivity (28). High specific resistivity components, such as bone and adipose tissue, impede electrical current passage whereas low resistivity components, such as skeletal muscle and visceral organs, readily pass an electrical current. This phenomenon gives rise to the BIA method: between-individual variation in whole-body or regional impedance is associated with corresponding tissue composition (28). Accordingly, prediction formulas have been developed linking measured impedance with tissue water, fluid, and related lean soft tissue (29).

Impedance, usually measured at 50 kHz, is adjusted for stature as a surrogate for electrical path length (28). Reactance and resistance together determine impedance, and some systems are designed for separate measurement of these electrical properties of tissue (30).

Although systems designed for analysis of total body fat are often designed for use at 50 kHz, multiple frequencies can be measured. Multiple frequency BIA systems are typically designed for analysis of fluid distribution in addition to body fat (28).

Electrical skin contacts also vary from applied gel electrodes to stainless steel contact electrodes (31). Varying positioning and number of electrodes allows analysis of 'half-body' (i.e. arm to leg), 'whole-body' (i.e. both arms to both legs), and regional (e.g. limb or limb portion) impedance, resistance and reactance (32). Lean tissue prediction formulas can be developed that correspond to the various measured regions, although fat analysis is only available for the whole body.

Prediction formulas are developed by first calibrating the BIA system against measured adipose-tissue free mass, FFM or TBW using a reference method such as MRI or DEXA (29). Total body water can be used to estimate FFM as noted earlier. Subjects are then evaluated under carefully controlled pre-specified conditions using the reference method and BIA (33). Impedance, resistance, reactance and other potential predictor variables are then entered into multiple linear regression statistical analyses and appropriate models are developed and used for final model development (34). Developed equations are then cross-validated before they are applied in commercial systems or in the research setting. Fat mass is usually calculated as the difference between body weight and FFM, although some BIA systems are calibrated directly to body fat or percent fat.

Prediction formulas are, by their nature, population specific and care should be taken to confirm that evaluated subjects are similar to those on whom the system formula was developed. Subjects should also be studied under the specified conditions such as room temperature, time of day, length of time standing or recumbent, and so on (33).

As there are so many variations in BIA technology, it is difficult to provide a global statement surrounding measurement accuracy and reproducibility. Highly developed and well-calibrated systems, when used appropriately, are now often used in large-scale research studies of obesity and weight loss. The advantages of BIA are that it is relatively cheap, safe and simple to use, practical, and has excellent reproducibility when measurement conditions are carefully controlled. An additional advantage of BIA is the potential for estimation of components other than fat, such as TBW, intracellular and extracellular fluid, FFM, and skeletal muscle mass. Poorly designed and calibrated systems or lack of attention to protocol when carrying out subject evaluations can lead to unreliable body fat analyses.

Fat Distribution

Adipose tissue, or more specifically fat, distribution can be estimated from regional DEXA measurements (34). First, various regional ratios, such as the trunk-to-extremity fat ratio, can be used as simple measures of adipose tissue distribution. Second, fat at specific anatomic sites, such as at the umbilical and mid-thigh levels, can be measured using investigator-guided software. Third, regional DEXA

measurements can be combined with other techniques such as skinfold measurement of subcutaneous adipose tissue, as a means of deriving visceral fat estimates (35).

While all of these approaches show some merit, none fully replace either MRI or CT as accurate predictors of visceral and regional subcutaneous adipose tissue.

Atomic Level

Total Body Potassium (TBK)

A small but constant proportion of TBK is radioactive ^{40}K. The characteristic ^{40}K gamma ray can be measured in a heavily shielded whole-body counter (16). As the proportion of TBK as ^{40}K is constant, whole-body counting can be used as a means of quantifying total body potassium content *in vivo*. There are now approximately 40 operational whole-body counters worldwide.

As potassium is distributed primarily in the intracellular compartment, TBK can be used as a measure of body cell mass (BCM) (4) and related FFM (16). Classical two-compartment models link TBK with FFM by assuming a stable and known ratio of TBK to FFM. This method requires that one first measures the amount of ^{40}K and from this value calculates TBK. Developed models are then used to link TBK with FFM; fat mass is derived as the difference between body mass and FFM.

While the TBK method is important from a historical perspective, very few investigators now use whole-body counting as a means of quantifying total body fat. This is primarily a result of the fact that access to systems is limited and construction costs are high. Some concern also exists regarding the accuracy of TBK conversion via developed models to fat-free mass and fat (36). On the other hand, some advantages of the method are the lack of radiation exposure and children can be safely evaluated.

Total Body Nitrogen and Carbon (TBN and TBC)

A group of methods referred to collectively as *in vivo* neutron activation analysis (IVNA), when combined with whole-body counting, are capable of measuring all major elements found in humans

(Figure 6.2). Two important multicomponent models, used for research purposes, can be developed from measured elements.

The first approach is formulated around measured total body nitrogen (TBN). Nitrogen is found almost entirely in protein and TBN can be measured using prompt gamma neutron activation analysis (37). Total body calcium (TBCa), found almost entirely in bone and measured with delayed gamma neutron activation analysis, can be used to estimate total body bone minerals (38). Other neutron activation methods, along with whole-body counting, can be used to quantify soft tissue minerals (e.g. K, Na, Cl). Total body water, measured using isotope dilution methods, combined with protein, mineral and an estimate of glycogen, can be summed to provide FFM (39). Fat is then calculated as the difference between body mass and FFM.

The second and more recent approach is based upon total body carbon (TBC) (40). A large proportion of carbon is found in fat, and non-fat carbon is found in protein, glycogen, and bone minerals. A multicomponent model proposed by Kehayias *et al.* (40) derives total body fat from TBC, measured using inelastic neutron scattering, corrected for protein (i.e. TBN), glycogen and bone minerals (i.e. TBCa).

Neutron activation methods of estimating total body fat have made major contributions to our understanding of human body composition. The measured atomic level components provide a means of deriving chemical components independently from most other body composition methods. Access to systems, however, is limited and radiation exposure limits studies in children and potentially child-bearing women. Measuring body fat using IVNA is therefore limited primarily to selected research applications at centers specializing in body composition research.

REFERENCE VALUES

The National Institutes of Health and the World Health Organization have both adopted the same BMI ranges as follows: underweight < 18.5; normal weight $\geq 18.5 < 25$; overweight $\geq 25 < 30$; obese, ≥ 30 (6). The corresponding adipose tissue distribution levels for high risk are, for waist circumference, 94 cm (37 in) for men and 80 cm (32 in) for women.

A number of studies report national distributions for skinfolds and percent fat (8). However, nations that have a high prevalence of obesity do not serve as a reference source for healthy percent fat ranges. Thus it is possible to establish a subject's fatness relative to the population as a whole but there are no experimentally developed ranges set for optimum health. As a working alternative, our group and two others derived percent fat ranges in accord with the three BMI thresholds (6). Two methods for estimating fatness were applied as the reference, DEXA and four-compartment (4C). There were three groups of subjects, Caucasian, African American, and Japanese-Asian. Regression models were developed linking percent fat with BMI and other predictor variables. Two prediction models were developed, one for African Americans and Caucasians and the other for Japanese-Asians. The developed percent fat ranges are presented in Tables 6.6 and 6.7. A subject's measured percent fat can be classified according to sex, age, and race as consistent with underweight, normal weight, or obese. Hence, a bodybuilder according to this approach might be overweight but not over-fat. Although these percent fat ranges are tied to 'healthy' BMI ranges, the need remains over the long term to prospectively establish optimum body fatness levels.

METHOD SELECTION

The selection of a particular method for evaluating body composition is determined primarily by the intended use of the data and the need for varying degrees of accuracy. In addition, cost and convenience play significant roles in determining which particular method should be utilized.

Clinical evaluation of body composition requires methods which range from easy and inexpensive to moderately difficult and expensive. The primary objective in determining the method best suited for clinical evaluations is that the method be both reproducible for within-subject measurements and simple to use in either an office or hospital setting. The use of anthropometric measurements to estimate body composition is suitable for such evaluations since it is reliable for the same subject when

Table 6.6 Predicted % fat ranges for African Americans and Caucasians[a]

BMI	% fat		
	20–39 years	40–59 years	60–79 years
Females			
Normal			
≥ 18.5 < 25	≥ 21 < 33	≥ 23 < 34	≥ 24 < 36
Obese			
≥ 30	≥ 39	≥ 40	≥ 42
Males			
Normal			
≥ 18.5 < 25	≥ 8 < 20	≥ 11 < 22	≥ 13 < 25
Obese			
≥ 30	≥ 25	≥ 28	≥ 30

[a]Calculated using a 4C-based prediction formula for estimating % fat and centering on ages 30, 50, and 70 (5).

Table 6.7 Predicted % fat ranges for Asians[a]

BMI	% fat		
	20–39 years	40–59 years	60–79 years
Females			
Normal			
≥ 18.5 < 25	≥ 25 < 35	≥ 25 < 35	≥ 25 < 36
Obese			
≥ 30	≥ 40	≥ 41	≥ 41
Males			
Normal			
≥ 18.5 < 25	≥ 13 < 23	≥ 13 < 24	≥ 14 < 24
Obese			
≥ 30	≥ 28	≥ 29	≥ 29

[a]Asians are Japanese. Calculated using a 4C-based prediction formula for estimating % fat and centering on ages 30, 50, and 70 (5).

the same investigator conducts the measurements and it may be used in almost any setting. On the other hand, the accuracy of anthropometric measurements is not as high as other methods and significant training is required for accurate measurements, but they are able to determine differences in truncal versus peripheral adiposity.

Another method for clinical use is BIA. As noted earlier, BIA has been validated against more precise methods and is excellent for clinical settings since it is relatively cheap and the amount of training required is minimal. A disadvantage to using BIA is that the accuracy may vary depending on the hydration status and degree of fatness of the subject.

DEXA is also well suited to both clinical and hospital settings and for longitudinal research studies. The fact that DEXA is accurate both between and within subjects, coupled with its non-invasive technique, adds to its advantages. Two disadvantages are that it is expensive to purchase and operate and training for both operation and evaluation is extensive.

Finally, the BOD POD is proving to be a new option for many clinical studies. It is much less invasive and provides more reliable between-subject estimates of body fat than hydrodensitometry. In addition, once the initial cost of purchasing the equipment is incurred there is minimal maintenance cost and technician training is also minimal. The two disadvantages to the BOD POD are the initial cost and that it has not been validated for use in young children or extremely obese subjects.

Research settings outside of a hospital or clinic have significantly different needs and capabilities and the appropriate method of choice varies greatly. For example, given the variability in facilities in field or remote settings, such as lack of energy sources, limited personnel and/or training, cultural concerns, and so on, methods which are cheap, require minimal training, and are non-invasive will prove to be best. Anthropometric measurements are by far one of the most inexpensive means to measure body composition and are well suited for field work since they require only a flexible measuring tape and skinfold calipers. Two disadvantages are that they require a fair amount of training and most measurements (e.g. subscapular and suprailiac) require the patient to partially disrobe.

The next logical method for field work would be BIA since minimal training is required and the method is relatively inexpensive. A disadvantage of BIA is the need for a power source, which makes it impractical for use over several days or weeks at some remote sites.

Finally, measuring body composition by isotope dilution is an option for some studies. Isotope dilution is neither invasive nor time-consuming and can be used in almost any site where samples can be stored and shipped for storage. The major disadvantage to using isotope dilution is the cost of buying the isotope and analyzing the fluid sample for dilution content.

CONCLUSION

Methods of evaluating adiposity and adipose tissue distribution have advanced substantially in the past decade. Stimulated by the rising worldwide prevalence of obesity, new methods are under development that promise to advance the field. The point has now been reached, however, at which excellent methods of quantifying fatness are available for application in field, clinical, and research settings.

REFERENCES

1. Wang ZM, Pierson RN Jr, Heymsfield SB. The five level model: a new approach to organizing body composition research. *Am J Clin Nutr* 1992; **56**: 19–28.
2. Snyder WM, Cook MJ, Nasset ES, Karhausen LR, Howells GP, Tipton IH. *Report of the Task Group on Reference Man.* Oxford: Pergamon Press, 1975.
3. Pietrobelli A, Formica C, Wang ZM, Heymsfield SB. Dual-energy x-ray absorptiometry body composition model: review of physical concepts. *Am J Physiol* 1997; **271**: E941–E951.
4. Moore FD, Oleson, KH, McMurray, JD, Parker HV, Ball MR, Boyden CM. *The Body Cell Mass and its Supporting Environment.* Philadelphia: WB Saunders, 1963.
5. Gallagher D, Heymsfield SB, Heo M, Jebb SA, Murgatroyd PR, Sakamoto Y. Healthy percent body fat ranges: an approach for developing guidelines based upon body mass index. *Am J Clin Nutr* 200; **72**: 694–701.
6. NIH. Clinical guidelines on the identification, evaluation, and treatment of overweight and obesity in adults-the evidence report. *Obes Res* 1998; **6**: 54S.
7. Durnin JVGA, Womersley J. Body fat assessed from total body density and its estimation from skinfold thickness: measurements on 481 men and women aged from 16 to 72 years. *Br J Nutr* 1974; **32**: 77–97.
8. Heymsfield SB, Baumgartner RN, Pan SF. Nutrition assessment of malnutrition by anthropometric methods. In: Shils ME *et al. Modern Nutrition in Health and Disease.* Baltimore, MD: Williams & Wilkins, 1999: 903–922.
9. Roche AF. Anthropometry and ultrasound. In: Roche AF, Heymsfield SB, Lohman TG (eds), *Human Body Composition*, Champaign, IL: Human Kinetics, 1996: 167–190.
10. Albu JB, Murphy L, Frager DH, Johnson JA, Pi-Sunyer FX. Visceral fat and race-dependent health risks in obese non-diabetic premenopausal women. *Diabetes* 1997; **46**: 456–462.
11. Sjöström L. A computer-tomography based multicomponent body composition technique and anthropometric predictions of lean body mass, total and subcutaneous adipose tissue. *Int J Obes* 1991; **15**: 19–30.
12. Heymsfield SB, Ross R, Wang ZM, Frager D. Imaging techniques of body composition: advantages of measurement and new uses. In: *Emerging Technologies for Nutrition Research.* Washington, DC: National Academy Press, 1997: 127–150.
13. Seidell JC, Oosterlee A, Thijssen M, Burema J, Deurenberg P, Hautvast J, Josephus J. Assessment of intra-abdominal and subcutaneous abdominal fat: relation between anthropometry and computed tomography. *Am J Clin Nutr* 1987; **45**: 7–13.
14. Heymsfield SB, Wang ZM, Baumgartner RN, Ross R. Human body composition: advances in models and methods. *Ann Rev Nutr* 1997; **17**: 527–528.
15. Depres JP, Ross R, Lemieux S. Imaging techniques applied to the measurement of human body composition. In: Roche AF, Heymsfield SB, Lohman TG (eds), *Human Body Composition.* Champaign, IL: Human Kinetics, 1996: 149–166.
16. Forbes GB. *Human Body Composition.* New York: Springer-Verlag, 1987.
17. Schoeller DA. Hydrometry. In: Roche AF, Heymsfield SB, Lohman TG (eds) *Human Body Composition*, Champaign, IL: Human Kinetics, 1996: 25–44.
18. Behnke AR, Feen BG, Welham WC. The specific gravity of healthy men. *JAMA* 1942; **118**: 495–498.
19. Heymsfield SB, Wang ZM, Withers R. Multicomponent molecular-level models of body composition analysis. In: Roche AF, Heymsfield SB, Lohman TG (eds) *Human Body Composition.* Champaign, IL: Human Kinetics, 1996: 129–148.
20. Going SB. Densitometry. In: Roche AF, Heymsfield SB, Lohman TG (eds) *Human Body Composition.* Champaign IL: Human Kinetics, 1996: 3–24.
21. McCrory MA, Gomez TD, Bernauer EM, Mole PA. Evaluation of a new air displacement plethysmograph for measuring human body composition. *Med Sci Sports Exerc* 1995; **27**: 1686–1691.
22. Wang ZM, Deurenberg P, Wang W, Pietrobelli A, Baumgartner RN, Heymsfield SB. Hydration of fat-free body mass: review and critique of a classic body composition content. *Am J Clin Nutr* 1999. **69**: 833–841.
23. Wang ZM, Deurenberg P, Wang W, Pietrobelli A, Baumgartner RN, Heymsfield SB. Hydration of fat-free body mass: new physiological modeling approach. 1999. *Am J Physiol* 1999; **276**: E995–E1003.
24. Mazess, RB, Barden H, Bisek J, Hanson J, Dual energy X-ray absorptiometry for total-body and regional bone-mineral and soft-tissue composition. *Am J Clin Nutr* 1990; **51**: 1106–1112.
25. Siri WE. Body composition from fluid spaces and density: analysis of methods. In: Brozek J, Henschel A (eds). *Techniques for Measuring Body Composition.* Washington, DC: National Academy of Sciences–National Research Council, 1961: 223–244.
26. Friedl KE, DeLuca JP, Marchitelli LJ, Vogel JA. Reliability of body-fat estimations from a four-component model by using density, body water, and bone mineral measurements. *Am J Clin Nutr* 1992; **55**: 764–770.
27. Roche AF, Guo S. Development, testing and use of predictive equations for body composition measures. In: Kral JG, VanItallie TB (eds) *Recent Developments in Body Composition Analysis: Methods and Applications.* London: Smith-Gordon, 1993: 1–16.
28. Baumgartner RN, Chumlea WC, Roche AF. Impedance for body composition. *Exerc Sport Sci Rev* 1990; **18**: 193–224.
29. Houtkooper LB, Lohman TG, Going SB, Howell WH. Why bioelectrical impedance analysis should be used for estimating adiposity. NIH Technology Assessment Conference. *Am J Clin Nutr* 1996; **64**: 436S–448S.

30. Chumlea WC, Guo SS. Bioelectrical impedance and body composition: present status and future directions. *Nutr Rev* 1994; **52**: 123–131.

31. Nunez C, Gallagher D, Visser M, Pi-Sunyer FX, Wang ZM, Heymsfield SB. Bioimpedance analysis: evaluation of leg-to-leg system based on pressure contact foot-pad electrodes. *Med Sci Sports Exerc* 1997; **29**: 524–531.

32. Tan YX, Nunez C, Sun YG, Zhang K, Wang ZM, Heymsfield SB. New electrode system for rapid whole-body and segmental bioimpedance assessment. *Med Sci Sports Exerc* 1997; **29**: 1269–1273.

33. Kushner RF, Gudivaka R, Scholler DA. Clinical characteristics influencing bioelectrical impedance analysis measurements. *Am J Clin Nutr* 1996; **64**: 423S–427S.

34. Guo SS, Chumlea WC, Coockram DB. Use of statistical methods to estimate body composition. *Am J Clin Nutr* 1996; **64**: 428S–435S.

35. Jensen MD, Kanaley JA, Reed JE, Sheedy PF. Measurement of abdominal and visceral fat with computed tomography and dual-energy x-ray absorptiometry. *Am J Clin Nutr* 1995; **61**: 274–278.

36. Heymsfield SB, Waki M. Body composition in humans: advances in the development of multicompartment chemical models. *Nutr Rev* 1991; **49**: 97–108.

37. Chettle DR, Fremlin JH. Techniques of in vivo neutron activation analysis. *Phys Med Biol* 1984; **29**: 1011–1043.

38. Dilmanian FA, Weber DA, Yasumura S, Kamen Y, Lidofsky L. Performance of the neutron activation systems at Brookhaven National Laboratory. In: Yasumura S, McNeill KG, Woodhead AD, Dilmanian FA. *Advances in in Vivo Body Composition Studies.* New York: Plenum Press, 1990.

39. Cohn SH. In vivo neutron activation analysis: state of the art and future prospects. *Med Phys* 1981; **8**: 145–153.

40. Kehayias JJ, Heymsfield SB, LoMonte AF, Wang J, Pierson RN Jr. In vivo determination of body fat by measuring total body carbon. *Am J Clin Nutr* 1991; **53**: 1339–1344.

Part III

Appetite Regulation and Obesity Prevention

7

Role of Neuropeptides and Leptin in Food Intake and Obesity

Bernard Jeanrenaud[1] and Françoise Rohner-Jeanrenaud[2]

[1]*Lilly Corporate Center, Indianapolis, Indiana, USA and* [2]*Geneva University School of Medicine, Geneva, Switzerland*

Interrelationships Between Hypothalamic Neuropeptides and Leptin in the Maintenance of Body Weight Homeostasis, or Evolution to Obesity

It is now accepted that body weight homeostasis is maintained via a series of complex interactions that occur between the brain, the hypothalamus in particular, and the periphery (1–3), notably via a hormone, leptin, synthesized in and secreted from adipose tissue (4). Secreted leptin, although it may have direct peripheral effects, exerts its action principally within the brain. Following its transport through the blood–brain barrier, possibly via the short leptin receptor isoform (ObRa), leptin reaches the hypothalamic area where it binds to its long receptor isoform (ObRb). Following a specific signaling cascade, leptin inhibits many of the orexigenic neuropeptides, while favoring many of the anorexigenic ones, as discussed below. By doing so, leptin exerts its effects of decreasing food intake and body weight, increasing fat oxidation and energy expenditure, thus favoring leanness (5–11).

In the present review, the characteristics of the main orexigenic and anorexigenic neuropeptides will be summarized (Figure 7.1) and putative effects of leptin thereon described or, when such effects of leptin are defective, the main reasons for the estab-

lishment of a state of obesity will be outlined (Figure 7.2).

OREXIGENIC NEUROPEPTIDES

Effects of Neuropeptide Y (NPY)

NPY is a 36 amino acid neuropeptide that is widely distributed in the brain. In the hypothalamus, it is synthesized in the arcuate nucleus and released in the paraventricular nucleus. It stimulates food intake by binding to Y1 and/or Y5 receptor subtypes (12–14). This increase in feeding can be observed upon infusing the peptide intracerebroventricularly (i.c.v.) in normal rats and is accompanied by a rapid, sustained and marked increase in body weight (15,16). Central NPY infusion also stimulates insulin secretion via an activation of the parasympathetic nervous system reaching the endocrine pancreas (17). Concomitantly, central NPY administration increases the activity of the hypothalamo-pituitary-adrenal axis, with resulting hypercorticosteronemia and increased susceptibility to stressful situations (15,17). Finally, central NPY reduces the activity of the efferent sympathetic nerves reaching brown adipose tissue, with resulting decrease in energy dissipation as heat (18,19).

The metabolic consequences of the hormonal

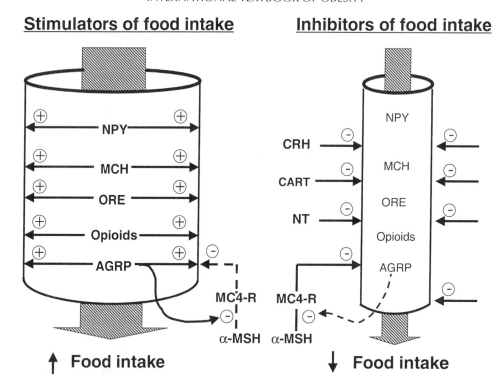

Figure 7.1 Diagram of food intake regulation by orexigenic and anorexigenic neuropeptides. Stimulators of food intake are depicted as increasing the diameter of a tube by exerting a pressure (+) from inside, with agouti-related peptide (AGRP) mainly exerting its action by inhibiting the melanocortin system (α-MSH and MC4 receptor), the effect of which is to reduce this diameter. Inhibitors of food intake are depicted as reducing (−) the diameter of the tube, with AGRP having little effect on the melanocortin system, allowing the latter to largely contribute to reducing this diameter. NPY, neuropeptide Y; MCH, melanin concentrating hormone; ORE, orexins; α-MSH, α-melanocyte-stimulating hormone and the melanocortin-4 (MC4-R) receptor; CRH, corticotropin-releasing hormone, CART, cocaine- and amphetamine-regulated transcript; NT, neurotensin. Not all neuropeptides are represented. Solid lines indicate marked effects, dotted ones weak effects

changes produced by central NPY infusion (increased plasma insulin and corticosterone levels) are increased adipose tissue and liver lipogenic activity, changes mainly due to hyperinsulinemia (15,16), together with decreased insulin-stimulated glucose utilization by muscles (15,16). This muscle insulin resistance is likely to be due to the combined NPY-induced hyperinsulinemia/hypercorticosteronemia (1).

It should be noted that the NPY-elicited effects are very marked when exogenous NPY is chronically infused i.c.v., resulting in high central concentrations of the neuropeptide. Physiologically, however, it is thought that these changes are modest, occurring via the spontaneous fluctuations of hypothalamic NPY levels, which transiently change nutrient partitioning toward fat accretion and decreased oxidation processes. This situation persists until leptin is secreted into the blood as a result of

hormonal changes such as transient hyperinsulinemia in response to meal taking. Secreted leptin reaches the brain and decreases hypothalamic NPY levels by exerting its negative feedback inhibition on the expression and amount of this neuropeptide (20–22). Experiments have shown, however, that in addition to NPY, other brain neuropeptidic systems play a role in the regulation of food intake. Thus, in transgenic mice made deficient in NPY, the expected decrease in both food intake and body weight fails to occur (23,24). Transgenic mice lacking the NPY-Y1 or Y5 receptor actually gain more weight, not less, than the controls. (25,26). This indicates that the regulation of food intake and body weight is redundant, i.e. that several pathways are implicated and that when one of them is knocked out, others take over to maintain a normal body weight homeostasis.

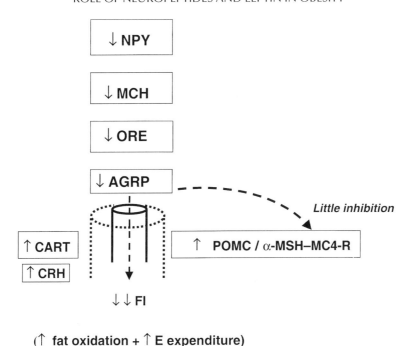

(↑ fat oxidation + ↑ E expenditure)

Figure 7.2   Diagram of the central effects of leptin on food intake. Leptin is depicted as decreasing the diameter of a tube relative to a normal one (dotted lines), due to its dual effect of reducing (↓) the expression or amount of neuropeptides that stimulate food intake (neuropeptide Y, NPY; melanin concentrating hormone, MCH; orexin, ORE; agouti-related protein, AGRP) and of increasing (↑) the expression or amount of neuropeptides that inhibit food intake (cocaine- and amphetamine-regulated transcript, CART; corticotropin-releasing hormone, CRH; the melanocortin system with proopiomelanocortin, POMC, α-MSH and the melanocortin-4 receptor, MC4-R). The effect of leptin on food intake (FI) is accompanied by increased fat oxidation and energy (E) expendidure, the three parameters together producing leanness

NPY and Obesity

When considering the hormono-metabolic changes produced by central NPY, one realizes that experimentally produced increases in central levels of this neuropeptide reproduce most of the abnormalities observed in experimental or genetic obesity syndromes (15,16), as well as in human obesity. The pathological relevance of increased hypothalamic NPY levels in mimicking obesity syndromes is supported by the observation that NPY expression and levels are indeed increased in the *ob/ob*, *db/db* obese mice and in the *fa/fa* obese rat (1,20–22). Increased NPY levels in *ob/ob* mice are due to the lack of synthesis and secretion of leptin in adipose tissue, the *ob* (leptin) gene being mutated. As a result of this mutation, plasma leptin levels are nil, leptin fails to exert its negative feedback on hypothalamic NPY levels which remain continually elevated maintaining, probably with other neuropeptides that are influenced by leptin, the obesity syndrome (1,27). In the *db/db* and the *fa/fa* obese rodents, the *ob* gene of

adipose tissue is normal, but the long form leptin receptor is mutated in its intracellular (*db/db*) (5) or extracellular (*fa/fa*) (28) domain. Even though leptin is overproduced by adipose tissue, bringing about a state of hyperleptinemia, it cannot act centrally and hypothalamic NPY levels remain high. The latter, probably in concert with other neuropeptides, maintain the obesity syndrome (29).

Effects of Melanin Concentrating Hormone (MCH)

MCH is a cyclic neuropeptide comprising 19 amino acids which is present in many areas of the brain, notably in the lateral hypothalamus (30). Its name derives from its ability to cause melanosome aggregation in fish skin, an action which is antagonized by α-MSH, the melanosome-dispersing factor. Recently, a role for MCH in the central regulation of food intake has been discovered, i.c.v. MCH administration increasing food intake in normal rats (31,32). As for the melanosome aggregation/dispersion system, the action of α-MSH is the opposite of that of MCH, resulting in decreased food intake (33). The antagonistic action of MCH and α-MSH extends to the regulation of the hypothalamo-pituitary-adrenal (HPA) axis, MCH decreasing plasma corticosterone and ACTH levels relative to controls, while α-MSH does the contrary, increasing plasma corticosterone and ACTH levels. (33).

I.c.v. administration of a single dose of MCH results in stimulation of food intake that is dose-dependent, lasts for about 6 hours (32,33), but is moderate in amplitude when compared to the effect of NPY (34). The feeding effect of central MCH administration is counteracted not only by α-MSH as just mentioned, but also by glucagon-like peptide (GLP-1) and neurotensin (34).

As is the case for NPY, central leptin administration decreases hypothalamic MCH expression and prevents MCH-induced increase in food intake (35,36). However, contrary to what is observed with NPY, long-term central MCH administration fails to produce sustained increases in food intake or in body weight gain, thus obesity (32). This is in contrast with the observation that, in the obese *ob/ob* mouse, hypothalamic MCH expression is increased and may participate in the final development of the obese phenotype (31).

To strengthen the physiological role of MCH in food intake regulation, mice carrying a targeted deletion of the MCH gene have been produced. When compared to controls, these mice are hypophagic, leaner, have decreased carcass lipids, and increased metabolic rate (37). Thus, MCH does represent an important hypothalamic pathway in the regulation of body weight homeostasis, a pathway further completed recently by the discovery of a 353 amino acid G-protein-coupled receptor, to which MCH specifically binds (38,39). Such a receptor is present in the hypothalamus and many other brain regions, in keeping with the several functions, beyond the feeding behavior, that are under the influence of MCH (38,39).

Effects of Orexins

Orexin A and B (from the Greek word for appetite) have been discovered recently and are also referred to as 'hypocretins' (due to their hypothalamic location and sequence analogy to secretin) (40,41). Orexin A (33 amino acids) and orexin B (28 amino acids) neurons are restricted to the lateral and posterior hypothalamus, whereas both orexin A and orexin B fibers project widely into different areas of the brain (42–45). The corresponding cloned receptors, OX1 and OX2, are found in the hypothalamus (ventromedial hypothalamic nucleus, paraventricular nucleus) a distribution that is receptor-specific (41,46).

The stimulatory effect of central administration of orexin on food intake is much weaker than that of NPY, and is smaller than that elicited by MCH. Orexin A is more potent than orexin B in eliciting feeding, and its effect is consistent, whereas that of orexin B is not (47, 48). When given peripherally, orexin A rapidly enters the brain by simple diffusion as it is highly lipophilic, while orexin B with its low lipophilicity is degraded, thus failing to reach the brain adequately (49). The fact that orexin B is easily inactivated by endopeptidases could be one of the reasons for its relative inefficiency in regulating food intake. In a way similar to what has been observed with NPY, some of the centrally elicited effects of orexin A, e.g. the stimulation of gastric acid secretion, are mediated by an activation of the parasympathetic nervous system, favoring anabolic processes (50).

Leptin administration produces a diminution of orexin A levels in the lateral hypothalamus (51), a finding that is in keeping with the observation of the presence of numerous leptin receptors on orexin-immunoreactive neurons in the lateral hypothalamus (52). Additional data must be gathered for the physiological role of the orexin system in food intake regulation to be better understood.

Effects of Opioids

The endogenous opioid system has long been known to play a role in the regulation of ingestive behavior. The opioid peptides exert their action via a complex receptor subtype system implicating kappa, mu and delta receptors for, respectively, dynorphin, β-endorphin and the enkephalins (53). The specific modulation of taste and food intake can be partly understood by the use of selective receptor subtype agonists and antagonists (54,55). Typically, the central administration of opioid agonists stimulates food intake, decreases the latency to feed, increases the number of interactions with the food, favors fat as well as sucrose ingestion, and increases body weight gain (54,56–60). In contrast, the central administration of opioid antagonists does the reverse, decreasing food intake and body weight (55,60–62).

The three major types of opioid receptors, mu, kappa, delta, have been cloned and belong to the G-protein-coupled family. Recently, another receptor highly homologous to the opioid receptors, but one that does not bind any opioid peptide with high affinity, has been cloned (63). This opioid receptor-like (ORL-1) is widely distributed within the central nervous system (CNS), the hypothalamus, hippocampus, and the amygdala, in particular (64). The endogenous ligand for this opioid-like orphan receptor has now been isolated (63). It is called nociceptin (as it increases pain responsiveness), or orphanin FQ. It is an 18 amino acid peptide which resembles dynorphin A and has a marked affinity for ORL-1 (63–65). Nociceptin and ORL-1 thus constitute a new peptidergic system within the CNS, a system of potential interest as it is present not only in rodents, but also in humans (64,65). When given centrally, nociceptin stimulates food intake in satiated rats, an effect that is blocked by an opioid antagonist, naloxone. As naloxone does not act at the level of ORL-1, this indicates that stimulation of food intake by nociceptin involves, at some ill-defined steps, the function of the 'classical' opioid system (65). Microinjection of nociceptin into two brain areas implicated in food intake (the ventromedial hypothalamic nucleus and the nucleus accumbens) also results in increased in food intake (64). The physiopathological implications of these findings will soon be unraveled.

Opioids and Obesity

The susceptibility to diet-induced obesity in the rat is strain dependent. For example, some strains of rats (e.g. Osborne-Mendel) overeat and become obese when fed a diet rich in fat. Other strains (e.g. S5B/P1) are resistant to high fat diet-induced obesity (66). In this context, it is interesting that central administration of a kappa opioid receptor antagonist decreases the intake of a high fat diet in the obesity-prone rats, while it does not do so in the obesity-resistant ones. In contrast, the central administration of a kappa opioid receptor agonist increases the intake of a high fat diet in obesity-prone rats, while it increases the intake of any type of diet in obesity-resistant animals (66). It is thus conceivable that the sensitivity to opioids differs from strain to strain, possibly from species to species. It is also possible that, within the brain areas constituting the opioid system, the distribution of the opioids, that of their receptors, may vary from strain to strain. This may lead to a strain-specific opioid dependency of the food intake process and evolution to obesity (66).

The likely importance of the opioid system in obesity is illustrated by the observation that the peripheral administration of compounds with potent opioid antagonistic activity to obese rats results in rapid, marked and sustained decreases in food intake and body weight gain (67,68).

ANOREXIGENIC PEPTIDES

Effects of Cocaine- and Amphetamine-Regulated Transcript (CART)

Cocaine- and amphetamine-regulated transcript (CART) is a recently discovered hypothalamic peptide which is regulated by leptin and is endowed with appetite-suppressing activity (69,70). In the rat, the CART gene encodes a peptide of either 129 or 116 amino acid residues (70). In contrast, only the short form of CART exists in humans (70). The mature peptide contains several potential cleavage sites and CART may be post-transcriptionally processed into several biologically active fragments. Thus, in most tissues studied, CART peptides are short, CART (42–89) being found in the rat hypothalamus (71). This tissue processing of CART resulting in neuropeptides of different lengths may indicate that different CART peptides have different biological functions (71).

Acute i.c.v. CART administration to normal rats produces a dose-dependent decrease in food intake (69,72). CART also transiently decreases the NPY-elicited feeding response in normal rats (69). Finally, CART appears to have a tonic inhibitory influence on food intake, as treatment of rats with anti-CART antiserum results in increased food intake (69).

CART is regulated, in part, by leptin as chronic

peripheral leptin administration to the leptin-deficient *ob/ob* mice results in a definite augmentation of the low expression of CART measured in the hypothalamic arcuate nucleus of these animals, an increase that is paralleled by the observed decrease in body weight. CART expression is also markedly reduced in the genetically obese leptin-resistant *fa/fa* rat, thus possibly playing a role in the hyperphagia of this animal (69). The physiological and pathological importance of CART has yet to be substantiated, although preliminary results with chronic infusion of the neuropeptide appear to indicate that it markedly reduces food intake and body weight of both normal and obese rats.

Effects of Corticotropin-releasing Hormone (CRH)

Apart from its role as controller of the hypothalamo-pituitary-adrenal (HPA) axis, CRH, a 41 amino acid neuropeptide, also functions as a central effector molecule that brings about a state of negative energy balance and weight loss. This is due to the ability of central CRH to decrease food intake (73), to increase the activity of the sympathetic nervous system and to stimulate thermogenesis (73–75). CRH also influences gastrointestinal functions, inhibiting gastric acid secretion and gastric emptying, processes that are controlled by the parasympathetic nervous system (76–79). Chronic i.c.v. CRH administration in normal (73), genetically obese *fa/fa* rats (80), as well as in monkeys (81), decreases food intake and body weight, partly by acting on energy dissipating mechanisms. Central microinjections of CRH were shown to inhibit NPY-induced feeding (82), in keeping with the notion that the locally released CRH could restrain the effect of NPY and/or of other orexigenic signals. Leptin administration results in transient increases in hypothalamic CRH levels, thus potentially favoring the CRH effects just mentioned (22). The leptin effect on CRH could occur via its increasing CRH type 2 receptor (CRHR-2) expression in the ventromedial hypothalamus, as these receptors are potentially responsible for the CRH-mediated decrease in food intake and sympathetic nervous system activation (83,84).

The Melanocortin System and Effects of α-Melanocyte-stimulating hormone (α-MSH)

Pro-opiomelanocortin (POMC) is the precursor of many different molecules, the melanocortins, among which are ACTH, β-endorphin, the melanocyte-stimulating hormones (α-,β-,γ-MSH). The α-melanocyte-stimulating hormone α-MSH is a 13 amino acid peptide which binds with different affinities to five different subtypes of G-protein-coupled receptors. An involvement of α-MSH in body weight homeostasis via an interaction with the melanocortin-4 (MC4), possibly the MC3 receptors, has been recently described. MC3 receptors are present mainly in the hypothalamus, MC4 receptors throughout the brain and in the sympathetic nervous system (85,86). When administered i.c.v. to normal rats, α-MSH decreases food intake (34), as does the central administration of a stable linear analog of α-MSH, NDP-MSH (87). The relationships existing between the melanocortins, their receptor subtypes and feeding have been illustrated by studying synthetic melanocortin receptor agonists and antagonists, amongst which are the compounds called MTII and SHU9119 (85,88). The i.c.v. administration of the agonist MTII markedly and dose-dependently inhibits food intake, while that of the antagonist SHU9119 markedly and dose-dependently stimulates food intake process (85,89). The co-injection of equal concentrations of the agonist and of the antagonist results in a food intake that is identical to that of control rats (85). In addition, MTII inhibits or suppresses, depending on the dose, the feeding response elicited by neuropeptide Y (85), in keeping with the observation that both MC3 and MC4 receptors are found in CNS sites in which NPY neurons are also present (90).

The effect of α-MSH in decreasing food intake is under the 'tonic' inhibitory influence from a melanocortin-receptor antagonist called 'agouti-related protein' (AGRP). When an active fragment of AGRP is administered i.c.v. to rats, an increased food intake is observed. Moreover, when α-MSH is similarly administered, the observed decrease in food intake is blocked by the further addition of AGRP (91).

The fundamental importance of the MC4 receptors has been highlighted by obtaining transgenic mice lacking the MC4 receptors (MC4-R-deficient mice). These mice (female and male) exhibit increased food intake and become obese. Both sexes have marked hyperinsulinemia, hyperleptinemia, with either normoglycemia (females) or hyperglycemia (males), plasma corticosterone levels being normal. These data support the view that MC4 receptors are essential in the cascade of events normally leading to decreased food intake and leanness (92). The decreased food intake produced by α-MSH and the subsequent cascade of events summarized above is accompanied by a change in the activity of the sympathetic nervous system. Thus, activation of the MC3/MC4-receptor system by the agonist MTII administered centrally results in a marked, specific, dose-dependent activation of the sympathetic nerves innervating the brown adipose tissue, as well as the renal and lumbar beds, while no change in blood pressure or heart rate is observed (93). The combination of decreased food intake and increased sympathetic activation with likely increase in energy dissipation suggests that the melanocortin system is well adapted to play a role in decreases in body weight.

Since the main central effects of leptin are to decrease food intake and body weight, and to increase energy dissipation, it has been postulated that this hormone could bring about these changes by influencing the melanocortin system. It is thus of interest to observe that the effect of leptin in decreasing food intake is blocked by a MC4 receptor antagonist (SHU9119), and that pretreatment with the antagonist is able to prevent the effects of leptin in decreasing both food intake and body weight. This effect is specific as the antagonist did not affect the decreased food intake produced by another peptide (GLP-1) (94). Thus, the MC4-receptor signaling is important in mediating the effects of leptin. In keeping with this finding is the observation that the MC4 receptor agonist, MTII, which decreases food intake in normal animals, also suppresses the hyperphagia of the leptin-deficient ob/ob mice. This suggests that leptin acts via MC4 receptors and that in the absence of leptin, i.e. in ob/ob mice, the lack of signaling through MC4 receptors would be responsible for the increased food intake (95), a viewpoint that remains to be fully validated (96).

When considering POMC (the precursor of melanocortins, of α-MSH) and AGRP (the antagonist of the MC4 receptor), it is of interest to observe that the lack of leptin in the ob/ob mouse (or

lack of leptin signaling in the db/db one) is accompanied by a decrease in POMC expression and an increase in that of AGRP (97–99). Moreover, leptin administration leads to an increase in POMC expression and a decrease in that of AGRP (100–103). It may thus be concluded that leptin decreases food intake and body weight, in part by favoring the action of melanocortin neuropeptide(s) at the MC4 receptor, while concomitantly preventing the inhibitory influence of AGRP on this same receptor, a concept excellently reviewed elsewhere (102). This specific effect of leptin is probably additive to its inhibitory one on hypothalamic NPY levels, NPY being one of the most potent food stimulators as described above, and being co-expressed with AGRP within the arcuate nucleus of the hypothalamus (104).

The Melanocortin System and Obesity

Obesity, as mentioned above, may result from altered functions of the MC4 receptors. This is illustrated in a global fashion by the observation that when the melanocortin receptor agonist (MTII) is administered i.c.v. to fasted–refed hyperphagic mice, to obese ob/ob mice, to yellow (Ay) obese mice, to NPY hyperphagic mice, their respective hyperphagia is largely canceled (95). In addition, it has been recently demonstrated that mice lacking POMC (hence lacking subsequent α-MSH synthesis and its inhibitory effect on feeding via its binding to MC4 receptors) overeat and become obese, a situation partly reversed by an α-MSH treatment (105).

The yellow obese mouse is an interesting animal model that underlines the potential importance of the melanocortin system. As reviewed recently, the pigment produced by melanocytes in the skin is under the regulation of α-MSH and a paracrine melanocyte signaling molecule called 'agouti' (from American Spanish 'aguti', meaning alternation of light and dark bands of colors in the fur of various animals). Agouti binds to MC1 receptors and decreases their signaling, resulting in decreased cAMP levels, thereby inducing melanocytes to synthesize a yellow pigment (pheomelanin). α-MSH binds to MC1 receptors and increases their signaling, resulting in increased cAMP, thereby stimulating the synthesis of a black pigment (eumelanin). The classical agouti hair color of many species appears brown, although the 'brown' hairs are in fact black-yellow-black banded hairs, due to the joint effects of agouti and α-MSH. The yellow mouse (A^y) is heterozygous for a mutation in the agouti gene. This mutation results in an ectopic expression of the agouti protein throughout the body, while the non-mutated gene induces the expression of the agouti protein only in hair follicles. The ectopic expression of agouti is at the origin of many different effects, i.e. yellow hairs, increased linear growth, decreased fertility, obesity. Within the brain, ectopic agouti functions as an antagonist of the MC4 receptor (with little effect on MC3-R), preventing the action of endogenous MC4 receptor agonists, with resulting obesity (102).

From a physiopathological viewpoint, the agouti protein turns out not to be as esoteric as it may sound. Indeed, a pathway very similar to that of the agouti in the skin has been described in the hypothalamus. Moreover, a novel gene called AGRP (agouti-related protein) or ART (agouti-related transcript) has been discovered in the hypothalamus of rodents as well as humans (97,98). It encodes a melanocortin (MC3, MC4) receptor antagonist comprising 132 amino acid residues which, as mentioned above, is the likely natural antagonist of the brain melanocortin system (97,98). The importance of the AGRP pathway is supported by the observation that over-expression of human AGRP in transgenic mice induces obesity without producing a yellow color of the fur, ARGP having no effect on MC1 receptors and therefore on the coat color (97,106).

CONCLUSION

From the description of the effects of the above-mentioned orexigenic and anorexigenic neuropeptides and their relationships with leptin, it is obvious that the regulation of food intake is complex, as is the evolution toward overeating and obesity. This complexity is even greater than described here, as additional factors have not been mentioned. For example, the role of glucocorticoids has not been discussed, although these hormones favor the occurrence of obesity through many different mechanisms, one of them being to inhibit the thinning action of leptin (107–109). Insulin, once within the brain after its passage though the blood–brain barrier, appears to participate in the regulation of energy homeostasis by decreasing food intake and

body weight gain in several animal species including monkeys (2). The hypothalamic neuropeptide galanin is associated with preference for dietary fats (110). Other factors described as being able to modulate food intake may, at the moment, be considered of lesser importance, although they may reemerge as being essential. Several additional neuropeptides will soon be discovered. Possibly the strongest candidates among current perceptions of the regulation of body weight homeostasis may be perceived differently in the months or years to come, and be superseded by others. Leptin appears to regulate many of the orexigenic and anorexigenic neuropeptides, and time will tell whether it can regulate all of them. Its pivotal importance in the modulation of food intake, body weight and energy expenditure is illustrated by the observation that it decreases the expression or content of many neuropeptides that favor food intake, while at the same time favoring that of other neuropeptides that inhibit these processes. Leptin thus appears to be strategically placed to modulate the dynamic equilibrium between neuropeptides with opposing final effects.

It should be noted that many of the genes and neuropeptides involved in the regulation of body weight homeostasis in animals mentioned above are also encountered in humans. Thus, families have been reported to have mutations in either the leptin gene or the leptin receptor gene (111,112). Other human mutations have an effect on orexigenic or anorexigenic neuropeptides and lead to obesity. These include mutation of the POMC gene (113–115), as well as the MC4 receptor gene (116). These rare cases provide support for the view that many of the pathways described here are likely to be present in humans. This is the basis of the view that, by the development of various antagonists or agonists, the correction of at least some aspects of human obesity is within reach.

ACKNOWLEDGEMENTS

The present work was carried out with grant No 31-53719.98 of the Swiss National Science Foundation (Berne), and by grants in aid of Eli Lilly and Company (Indianapolis, Indiana, USA) and of Novartis (Basle, Switzerland).

REFERENCES

1. Rohner-Jeanrenaud F, Cusin I, Sainsbury A, Zakrzewska KE, Jeanrenaud B. The loop system between neuropeptide Y and leptin in normal and obese rodents. *Horm Metab Res* 1996; **28**: 642–648.

2. Schwartz MW, Figlewicz DP, Baskin DG, Woods SC, Porte D Jr. Insulin in the brain: a hormonal regulator of energy balance. *Endocr Rev* 1992; **13**: 387–414.

3. Campfield LA, Smith FJ, Guisez Y, Devos R, Burn P. Recombinant mouse OB protein: evidence for a peripheral signal linking adiposity and central neural networks. *Science* 1995; **269**: 546–549.

4. Zhang Y, Proenca R, Maffei M, Barone M, Leopold L, Friedman JM. Positional cloning of the mouse obese gene and its human homologue. *Nature* 1994; **372**: 425–432.

5. Chen H, Charlat O, Tartaglia LA, Woolf EA, Weng X, Ellis SJ, Lakey ND, Culpepper J, Moore KJ, Breitbart RE, Duyk GM, Tepper RI, Morgenstern JP. Evidence that the diabetes gene encodes the leptin receptor: identification of a mutation in the leptin receptor gene in db/db mice. *Cell* 1996; **84**: 491–495.

6. Lee GH, Proenca R, Montez JM, Carroll KM, Darvishzadeh JG, Lee JI, Friedman JM. Abnormal splicing of the leptin receptor in diabetic mice. *Nature* 1996; **379**: 632–635.

7. Vaisse C, Halaas JL, Horvath CM, Darnell JE Jr, Stoffel M, Friedman JM. Leptin activation of Stat3 in the hypothalamus of wild-type and ob/ob mice but not db/db mice. *Nat Genet* 1996; **14**: 95–97.

8. Baumann H, Morella KK, White DW, Dembski M, Bailon PS, Kim H, Lai CF, Tartaglia LA. The full-length leptin receptor has signaling capabilities of interleukin 6-type cytokine receptors. *Proc Natl Acad Sci USA* 1996; **93**: 8374–8378.

9. Hakansson ML, Meister B. Transcription factor STAT3 in leptin target neurons of the rat hypothalamus. *Neuroendocrinology* 1998; **68**: 420–427.

10. Cusin I, Zakrzewska KE, Boss O, Muzzin P, Giacobino JP, Ricquier D, Jeanrenaud B, Rohner-Jeanrenaud F. Chronic central leptin infusion enhances insulin-stimulated glucose metabolism and favors the expression of uncoupling proteins. *Diabetes* 1998; **47**: 1014–1019.

11. Rohner-Jeanrenaud F. Neuroendocrine regulation of nutrient partitioning. *Annals of the New York Academy of Sciences* 1999; **892**: 261–271.

12. Weinberg DH, Sirinathsinghji DJ, Tan CP, Shiao LL, Morin N, Rigby MR, Heavens RH, Rapoport DR, Bayne ML, Cascieri MA, Strader CD, Linemeyer DL, MacNeil DJ. Cloning and expression of a novel neuropeptide Y receptor. *J Biol Chem* 1996; **271**: 16435–16438.

13. Gerald C, Walker MW, Criscione L, Gustafson EL, Batzl-Hartmann C, Smith KE, Vaysse P, Durkin MM, Laz TM, Linemeyer DL, Schaffhauser AO, Whitebread S, Hofbauer KG, Taber RI, Branchek TA, Weinshank RL. A receptor subtype involved in neuropeptide-Y-induced food intake. *Nature* 1996; **382**: 168–171.

14. Hu Y, Bloomquist BT, Cornfield LJ, DeCarr LB, Flores-Riveros JR, Friedman L, Jiang P, Lewis-Higgins L, Sadlowski Y, Schaefer J, Velazquez N, McCaleb ML. Identification of a novel hypothalamic neuropeptide Y receptor associated with feeding behavior. *J Biol Chem* 1996; **271**: 26315–26319.

15. Zarjevski N, Cusin I, Vettor R, Rohner-Jeanrenaud F, Jeanrenaud B. Chronic intracerebroventricular neuropeptide-Y administration to normal rats mimics hormonal and metabolic changes of obesity. *Endocrinology* 1993; **133**: 1753–1758.

16. Vettor R, Zarjevski N, Cusin I, Rohner-Jeanrenaud F, Jeanrenaud B. Induction and reversibility of an obesity syndrome by intracerebroventricular neuropeptide Y administration to normal rats. *Diabetologia* 1994; **37**: 1202–1208.

17. Sainsbury A, Rohner-Jeanrenaud F, Cusin I, Zakrzewska KE, Halban PA, Gaillard RC, Jeanrenaud B. Chronic central neuropeptide Y infusion in normal rats: status of the hypothalamo-pituitary-adrenal axis, and vagal mediation of hyperinsulinaemia. *Diabetologia* 1997; **40**: 1269–1277.

18. Billington CJ, Briggs JE, Grace M, Levine AS. Effects of intracerebroventricular injection of neuropeptide Y on energy metabolism. *Am J Physiol* 1991; **260**: R321–327.

19. Bray GA. Peptides affect the intake of specific nutrients and the sympathetic nervous system. *Am J Clin Nutr* 1992; **55**(1 Suppl): 265S–271S.

20. Stephens TW, Basinski M, Bristow PK, Bue-Valleskey JM, Burgett SG, Craft L, Hale J, Hoffmann J, Hsiung HM, Kriauciunas A *et al.* The role of neuropeptide Y in the antiobesity action of the obese gene product. *Nature* 1995; **377**: 530–532.

21. Cusin I, Rohner-Jeanrenaud F, Stricker-Krongrad A, Jeanrenaud B. The weight-reducing effect of an intracerebroventricular bolus injection of leptin in genetically obese fa/fa rats. Reduced sensitivity compared with lean animals. *Diabetes* 1996; **45**: 1446–1450.

22. Schwartz MW, Seeley RJ, Campfield LA, Burn P, Baskin DG. Identification of targets of leptin action in rat hypothalamus. *J Clin Invest* 1996; **98**: 1101–1106.

23. Erickson JC, Clegg KE, Palmiter RD. Sensitivity to leptin and susceptibility to seizures of mice lacking neuropeptide Y. *Nature* 1996; **381**: 415–421.

24. Erickson JC, Hollopeter G, Palmiter RD. Attenuation of the obesity syndrome of ob/ob mice by the loss of neuropeptide Y. *Science* 1996; **274**: 1704–1707.

25. Marsh DJ, Hollopeter G, Kafer KE, Palmiter RD. Role of the Y5 neuropeptide Y receptor in feeding and obesity. *Nat Med* 1998; **4**: 718–721.

26. Pedrazzini T, Seydoux J, Kunstner P, Aubert JF, Grouzmann E, Beermann F, Brunner HR. Cardiovascular response, feeding behavior and locomotor activity in mice lacking the NPY Y1 receptor. *Nat Med* 1998; **4**: 722–726.

27. Maffei M, Halaas J, Ravussin E, Pratley RE, Lee GH, Zhang Y, Fei H, Kim S, Lallone R, Ranganathan S, Kern PA, Friedman JM. Leptin levels in human and rodent: measurement of plasma leptin and ob RNA in obese and weight-reduced subjects. *Nat Med* 1995; **1**: 1155–1161.

28. Chua SC Jr, White DW, Wu-Peng XS, Liu SM, Okada N, Kershaw EE, Chung WK, Power-Kehoe L, Chua M, Tartaglia LA, Leibel RL. Phenotype of fatty due to Gln269Pro mutation in the leptin receptor (Lepr). *Diabetes* 1996; **45**: 1141–1143.

29. Cusin I, Rohner-Jeanrenaud F. Boucle régulatrice entre le neuropeptide Y et la leptine et son altération chez le ron-

geur obèse. *Med/Sci* 1998; **14**: 907–913.

30. Skofitsch G, Jacobowitz DM, Zamir N. Immunohistochemical localization of a melanin concentrating hormone-like peptide in the rat brain. *Brain Res Bull* 1985; **15**: 635–649.

31. Qu D, Ludwig DS, Gammeltoft S, Piper M, Pelleymounter MA, Cullen MJ, Mathes WF, Przypek R, Kanarek R, Maratos-Flier E. A role for melanin-concentrating hormone in the central regulation of feeding behaviour. *Nature* 1996; **380**: 243–247.

32. Rossi M, Choi SJ, O'Shea D, Miyoshi T, Ghatei MA, Bloom SR Melanin-concentrating hormone acutely stimulates feeding, but chronic administration has no effect on body weight. *Endocrinology* 1997; **138**: 351–355.

33. Ludwig DS, Mountjoy KG, Tatro JB, Gillette JA, Frederich RC, Flier JS, Maratos-Flier E. Melanin-concentrating hormone: a functional melanocortin antagonist in the hypothalamus. *Am J Physiol* 1998; **274**: E627–633.

34. Tritos NA, Vicent D, Gillette J, Ludwig DS, Flier ES, Maratos-Flier E. Functional interactions between melanin-concentrating hormone, neuropeptide Y, and anorectic neuropeptides in the rat hypothalamus. *Diabetes* 1998; **47**: 1687–1692.

35. Sahu A. Leptin decreases food intake induced by melanin-concentrating hormone (MCH), galanin (GAL) and neuropeptide Y (NPY) in the rat. *Endocrinology* 1998; **139**: 4739–4742.

36. Sahu A, Kalra SP. Absence of increased neuropeptide Y neuronal activity before and during the luteinizing hormone (LH) surge may underlie the attenuated preovulatory LH surge in middle-aged rats. *Endocrinology* 1998; **139**: 696–702.

37. Shimada M, Tritos NA, Lowell BB, Flier JS, Maratos-Flier E. Mice lacking melanin-concentrating hormone are hypophagic and lean. *Nature* 1998; **396**: 670–674.

38. Saito Y, Nothacker HP, Wang Z, Lin SH, Leslie F, Civelli O. Molecular characterization of the melanin-concentrating-hormone receptor. *Nature* 1999; **400**: 265–269.

39. Chambers J, Ames RS, Bergsma D, Muir A, Fitzgerald LR, Hervieu G, Dytko GM, Foley JJ, Martin J, Liu WS, Park J, Ellis C, Ganguly S, Konchar S, Cluderay J, Leslie R, Wilson S, Sarau HM. Melanin-concentrating hormone is the cognate ligand for the orphan G-protein-coupled receptor SLC-1. *Nature* 1999; **400**: 261–265.

40. de Lecea L, Kilduff TS, Peyron C, Gao X, Foye PE, Danielson PE, Fukuhara C, Battenberg EL, Gautvik VT, Bartlett FS 2nd, Frankel WN, van den Pol AN, Bloom FE, Gautvik KM, Sutcliffe JG. The hypocretins: hypothalamus-specific peptides with neuroexcitatory activity. *Proc Natl Acad Sci USA* 1998; **95**: 322–327.

41. Sakurai T, Amemiya A, Ishii M, Matsuzaki I, Chemelli RM, Tanaka H, Williams SC, Richarson JA, Kozlowski GP, Wilson S, Arch JR, Buckingham RE, Haynes AC, Carr SA, Annan RS, McNulty DE, Liu WS, Terrett JA, Elshourbagy NA, Bergsma DJ, Yanagisawa M. Orexins and orexin receptors: a family of hypothalamic neuropeptides and G protein-coupled receptors that regulate feeding behavior. *Cell* 1998; **92**: 573–585.

42. Date Y, Ueta Y, Yamashita H, Yamaguchi H, Matsukura S, Kangawa K, Sakurai T, Yanagisawa M, Nakazato M. Orexins, orexigenic hypothalamic peptides, interact with

autonomic, neuroendocrine and neuroregulatory systems. *Proc Natl Acad Sci USA* 1999; **96**: 748–753.

43. Broberger C, De Lecea L, Sutcliffe JG, Hokfelt T. Hypocretin/orexin- and melanin-concentrating hormone-expressing cells form distinct populations in the rodent lateral hypothalamus: relationship to the neuropeptide Y and agouti gene-related protein systems. *J Comp Neurol* 1998; **402**: 460–474.

44. Peyron C, Tighe DK, van den Pol AN, de Lecea L, Heller HC, Sutcliffe JG, Kilduff TS. Neurons containing hypocretin (orexin) project to multiple neuronal systems. *J Neurosci* 1998; **18**: 9996–10015.

45. Mondal MS, Nakazato M, Date Y, Murakami N, Yanagisawa M, Matsukura S. Widespread distribution of orexin in rat brain and its regulation upon fasting. *Biochem Biophys Res Commun* 1999; **256**: 495–499.

46. Trivedi P, Yu H, MacNeil DJ, Van der Ploeg LH, Guan XM. Distribution of orexin receptor mRNA in the rat brain. *FEBS Lett* 1998; **438**: 71–75.

47. Edwards CMB, Abusnana S, Sunter D, Murphy KG, Gathei MA, Bloom SR. The effect of the orexins on food intake: comparison with neuropeptide Y, melanin-concentrating hormone and galanin. *J Endocrinol* 1998; **160**: R7–R12.

48. Sweet DC, Levine AS, Billington CJ, Kotz CM. Feeding response to central orexins. *Brain Res* 1999; **821**: 535–538.

49. Kastin AJ, Akerstrom V. Orexin A but not orexin B rapidly enters brain from blood by simple diffusion. *J Pharmacol Exp Ther* 1999; **289**: 219–223.

50. Takahashi N, Okumura T, Yamada H, Kohgo Y. Stimulation of gastric acid secretion by centrally administered orexin-A in conscious rats. *Biochem Biophys Res Commun* 1999; **254**: 623–627.

51. Beck B, Richy S. Hypothalamic hypocretin/orexin and neuropeptide Y: divergent interaction with energy depletion and leptin. *Biochem Biophys Res Commun* 1999; **258**: 119–122.

52. Hakansson M, De Lecea L, Sutcliffe JG, Yanagisawa M, Meister B. Leptin receptor- and STAT3-immunoreactivities in Hypocretin/Orexin neurones of the lateral hypothalamus. *J Neuroendocrinol* 1999; **11**: 653–663.

53. Bodnar RJ. Opioid receptor subtype antagonists and ingestion. In: Cooper SJ, Clifton PG (eds) *Drug Receptor Subtypes and Ingestive Behaviour*. London: Academic Press, 1996: 127–146.

54. Leibowitz SF, Hoebel BG. Behavioral neuroscience of obesity.In: Bray GA, Bouchard C, James WPT (eds) *Handbook of Obesity* M. Dekker, Inc., New York: Basel, Hong Kong, 1997: 313–358.

55. Gosnell BA, Levine AS. Stimulation of ingestive behaviour by preferential and selective opioid agonists. In: Cooper SJ, Clifton PG (eds). *Drug Receptor Subtypes and Ingestive Behavior* London: Academic Press, 1996: 147–166.

56. Badiani A, Leone P, Noel MB, Stewart J. Ventral tegmental area opioid mechanisms and modulation of ingestive behavior. *Brain Res* 1995; **670**: 264–276.

57. Ruegg H, Yu WZ, Bodnar RJ. Opioid-receptor subtype agonist-induced enhancements of sucrose intake are dependent upon sucrose concentration. *Physiol Behav* 1997; **62**: 121–128.

58. Noel MB, Wise RA. Ventral tegmental injections of a selec-

tive mu or delta opioid enhance feeding in food-deprived rats. *Brain Res* 1995; **673**: 304–312.

59. Giraudo SQ, Kotz CM, Billington CJ, Levine AS. Association between the amygdala and nucleus of the solitary tract in mu-opioid induced feeding in the rat. *Brain Res* 1998; **802**: 184–188.

60. Giraudo SQ, Billington CJ, Levine AS. Effects of the opioid antagonist naltrexone on feeding induced by DAMGO in the central nucleus of the amygdala and in the paraventricular nucleus in the rat. *Brain Res* 1998; **782**: 18–23.

61. Cole JL, Leventhal L, Pasternak GW, Bowen WD, Bodnar RJ. Reductions in body weight following chronic central opioid receptor subtype antagonists during development of dietary obesity in rats. *Brain Res* 1995; **678**: 168–176.

62. Cole JL, Berman N, Bodnar RJ. Evaluation of chronic opioid receptor antagonist effects upon weight and intake measures in lean and obese Zucker rats. *Peptides* 1997; **18**: 1201–1207.

63. Meng F, Taylor LP, Hoversten MT, Ueda Y, Ardati A, Reinscheid RK, Monsma FJ, Watson SJ, Civelli O, Akil H. Moving from the orphanin FQ receptor to an opioid receptor using four point mutations. *J Biol Chem* 1996; **271**: 32016–32020.

64. Stratford TR, Holahan MR, Kelley AE. Injections of nociceptin into nucleus accumbens shell or ventromedial hypothalamic nucleus increase food intake. *Neuroreport* 1997; **8**: 423–426.

65. Pomonis JD, Billington CJ, Levine AS. Orphanin FQ, agonist of orphan opioid receptor ORL1, stimulates feeding in rats. *Neuroreport* 1996; **8**: 369–371.

66. Ookuma K, Barton C, York DA, Bray GA. Differential response to kappa-opioidergic agents in dietary fat selection between Osborne-Mendel and S5B/P1 rats. *Peptides* 1998; **19**: 141–147.

67. Mitch CH, Leander JD, Mendelsohn LG, Shaw WN, Wong DT, Cantrell BE, Johnson BG, Reel JK, Snoddy JD, Takemori AE *et al.* 4-Dimethyl-4-(3-hydroxyphenyl)piperidines: opioid antagonists with potent anorectant activity. *J Med Chem* 1993; **36**: 2842–2850.

68. Shaw WN. Long-term treatment of obese Zucker rats with LY255582 and other appetite suppressants. *Pharmacol Biochem Behav* 1993; **46**: 653–659.

69. Kristensen P, Judge ME, Thim L, Ribel U, Christjansen KN, Wulff BS, Clausen JT, Jensen PB, Madsen OD, Vrang N, Larsen PJ, Hastrup S. Hypothalamic CART is a new anorectic peptide regulated by leptin. *Nature* 1998; **393**: 72–76.

70. Thim L, Kristensen P, Larsen PJ, Wulff BS. CART, a new anorectic peptide. *Int J Biochem Cell Biol* 1998; **30**: 1281–1284.

71. Thim L, Kristensen P, Nielsen PF, Wulff BS, Clausen JT. Tissue-specific processing of cocaine- and amphetamine-regulated transcript peptides in the rat. *Proc Natl Acad Sci USA* 1999; **96**: 2722–2727.

72. Vrang N, Tang-Christensen M, Larsen PJ, Kristensen P. Recombinant CART peptide induces c-Fos expression in central areas involved in control of feeding behaviour. *Brain Res* 1999; **818**: 499–509.

73. Arase K, York DA, Shimizu H, Shargill N, Bray GA. Effects of corticotropin-releasing factor on food intake and brown adipose tissue thermogenesis in rats. *Am J Physiol* 1988;

255: E255–259.

74. Rothwell NJ. Central effects of CRF on metabolism and energy balance. *Neurosci Biobehav Rev* 1990; **14**: 263–271.

75. Egawa M, Yoshimatsu H, Bray GA. Effect of corticotropin releasing hormone and neuropeptide Y on electro-physiological activity of sympathetic nerves to interscapular brown adipose tissue. *Neuroscience* 1990; **34**: 771–775.

76. Tache Y, Gunion M. Corticotropin-releasing factor: central action to influence gastric secretion. *Fed Proc* 1985; **44**: 255–258.

77. Tache Y, Maeda-Hagiwara M, Turkelson CM. Central nervous system action of corticotropin-releasing factor to inhibit gastric emptying in rats. *Am J Physiol* 1987; **253**: G241–245.

78. Konturek SJ, Bilski J, Pawlik W, Thor P, Czarnobilski K, Szoke B, Schally AV. Gastrointestinal secretory, motor and circulatory effects of corticotropin releasing factor (CRF). *Life Sci* 1985; **37**: 1231–1240.

79. Broccardo M, Improta G. Pituitary-adrenal and vagus modulation of sauvagine- and CRF-induced inhibition of gastric emptying in rats. *Eur J Pharmacol* 1990; **182**: 357–362.

80. Rohner-Jeanrenaud F, Walker CD, Greco-Perotto R, Jeanrenaud B. Central corticotropin-releasing factor administration prevents the excessive body weight gain of genetically obese (fa/fa) rats. *Endocrinology* 1989; **124**: 733–739.

81. Glowa JR, Gold PW. Corticotropin releasing hormone produces profound anorexigenic effects in the rhesus monkey. *Neuropeptides* 1991; **18**: 55–61.

82. Heinrichs SC, Menzaghi F, Pich EM, Hauger RL, Koob GF. Corticotropin-releasing factor in the paraventricular nucleus modulates feeding induced by neuropeptide Y. *Brain Res* 1993; **611**: 18–24.

83. Richard D, Rivest R, Naimi N, Timofeeva E, Rivest S. Expression of corticotropin-releasing factor and its receptors in the brain of lean and obese Zucker rats. *Endocrinology* 1996; **137**: 4786–4795.

84. Nishiyama M, Makino S, Asaba K, Hashimoto K. Leptin effects on the expression of type-2 CRH receptor mRNA in the ventromedial hypothalamus in the rat. *Neuroendocrinology* 1999; **11**: 307–314.

85. Murphy B, Nunes CN, Ronan JJ, Harper CM, Beall MJ, Hanaway M, Fairhurst AM, Van der Ploeg LH, MacIntyre DE, Mellin TN. Melanocortin mediated inhibition of feeding behavior in rats. *Neuropeptides* 1998; **32**: 491–497.

86. Mountjoy KG, Wong J. Obesity, diabetes and functions for proopiomelanocortin-derived peptides. *Mol Cell Endocrinol* 1997; **128**: 171–177.

87. Brown KS, Gentry RM, Rowland NE. Central injection in rats of alpha-melanocyte-stimulating hormone analog: effects on food intake and brain Fos. *Regul Pept* 1998; **78**: 89–94.

88. Cone RD, Lu D, Koppula S, Vage DI, Klungland H, Boston B, Chen W, Orth DN, Pouton C, Kesterson RA. The melanocortin receptors: agonists, antagonists, and the hormonal control of pigmentation. *Recent Prog Horm Res* 1996; **51**: 287–317.

89. Giraudo SQ, Billington CJ, Levine AS. Feeding effects of hypothalamic injection of melanocortin 4 receptor ligands. *Brain Res* 1998; **809**: 302–306.

90. Mountjoy KG, Mortrud MT, Low MJ, Simerly RB, Cone

RD. Localization of the melanocortin-4 receptor (MC4-R) in neuroendocrine and autonomic control circuits in the brain. *Mol Endocrinol* 1994; **8**: 1298–1308.

91. Rossi M, Kim MS, Morgan DG, Small CJ, Edwards CM, Sunter D, Abusnana S, Goldstone AP, Russell SH,Stanley SA, Smith DM, Yagaloff K, Ghatei MA, Bloom SR. A C-terminal fragment of Agouti-related protein increases feeding and antagonizes the effect of alpha-melanocyte stimulating hormone in vivo. *Endocrinology* 1998; **139**: 4428–4431.

92. Huszar D, Lynch CA, Fairchild-Huntress V, Dunmore JH, Fang Q, Berkemeier LR, Gu W, Kesterson RA, Boston BA, Cone RD, Smith FJ, Campfield LA, Burn P, Lee F. Targeted disruption of the melanocortin-4 receptor results in obesity in mice. *Cell* 1997; **88**: 131–141.

93. Haynes WG, Morgan DA, Djalali A, Sivitz WI, Mark AL. Interactions between the melanocortin system and leptin in control of sympathetic nerve traffic. *Hypertension* 1999; **33**: 542–547.

94. Seeley RJ, Yagaloff KA, Fisher SL, Burn P, Thiele TE, van Dijk G, Baskin DG, Schwartz MW. Melanocortin receptors in leptin effects. *Nature* 1997; **390**: 349.

95. Fan W, Boston BA, Kesterson RA, Hruby VJ, Cone RD. Role of melanocortinergic neurons in feeding and the agouti obesity syndrome. *Nature* 1997; **385**: 165–168.

96. Boston BA, Blaydon KM, Varnerin J, Cone RD. Independent and additive effects of central POMC and leptin pathways on murine obesity. *Science* 1997; **278**: 1641–1644.

97. Ollmann MM, Wilson BD, Yang YK, Kerns JA, Chen Y, Gantz I, Barsh GS. Antagonism of central melanocortin receptors in vitro and in vivo by agouti-related protein. *Science* 1997; **278**: 135–138.

98. Shutter JR, Graham M, Kinsey AC, Scully S, Luthy R, Stark KL. Hypothalamic expression of ART, a novel gene related to agouti, is up-regulated in obese and diabetic mutant mice. *Genes Dev* 1997; **11**: 593–602.

99. Mizuno TM, Kleopoulos SP, Bergen HT, Roberts JL, Priest CA, Mobbs CV. Hypothalamic proopio-melanocortin mRNA is reduced by fasting and in ob/ob and db/db mice, but is stimulated by leptin. *Diabetes* 1998; **47**: 294–297.

100. Wilson BD, Bagnol D, Kaelin CB, Ollmann MM, Gantz I, Watson SJ, Barsh GS. Physiological and anatomical circuitry between Agouti-related protein and leptin signaling. *Endocrinology* 1999; **140**: 2387–2397.

101. Schwartz MW, Seeley RJ, Woods SC, Weigle DS, Campfield LA, Burn P, Baskin DG Leptin increases hypothalamic pro-opiomelanocortin mRNA expression in the rostral arcuate nucleus. *Diabetes* 1997; **46**: 2119–2123.

102. Wilson BD, Ollmann MM, Barsh GS. The role of agouti-related protein in regulating body weight. *Mol Med Today* 1999; **5**: 250–256.

103. Thornton JE, Cheung CC, Clifton DK, Steiner RA. Regulation of hypothalamic proopiomelanocortin mRNA by leptin in ob/ob mice. *Endocrinology* 1997; **138**: 5063–5066.

104. Hahn TM, Breininger JF, Baskin DG, Schwartz MW. Co-expression of Agrp and NPY in fasting-activated hypothalamic neurons. *Nat Neurosci* 1998; **1**: 271–272.

105. Yaswen L, Diehl N, Brennan MB, Hochgeschwender U. Obesity in the mouse model of pro-opiomelanocortin deficiency responds to peripheral melanocortin. *Nat Med* 1999; **5**: 1066–1070.

106. Graham M, Shutter JR, Sarmiento U, Sarosi I, Stark KL. Overexpression of Agrt leads to obesity in transgenic mice. *Nat Genet* 1997; **17**: 273–274.

107. Zakrzewska KE, Cusin I, Sainsbury A, Rohner-Jeanrenaud F, Jeanrenaud B. Glucocorticoids as counterregulatory hormones of leptin: toward an understanding of leptin resistance. *Diabetes* 1997; **46**: 717–719.

108. Zakrzewska KE, Sainsbury A, Cusin I, Rouru J, Jeanrenaud B, Rohner-Jeanrenaud F. Selective dependence of intracerebroventricular neuropeptide Y-elicited effects on central glucocorticoids. *Endocrinology* 1999; **40**: 3183–3187.

109. Zakrzewska KE, Cusin I, Stricker-Krongrad A, Boss O, Ricquier D, Jeanrenaud B, Rohner-Jeanrenaud F. Induction of obesity and hyperleptinemia by central glucocorticoid infusion in the rat. *Diabetes* 1999; **48**: 365–370.

110. Akabayashi A, Koenig JI, Watanabe Y, Alexander JT, Leibowitz SF. Galanin-containing neurons in the paraventricular nucleus: a neurochemical marker for fat ingestion and body weight gain. *Proc Natl Acad Sci USA* 1994; **91**: 10375–10379.

111. Montague CT, Farooqi IS, Whitehead JP, Soos MA, Rau H, Wareham NJ, Sewter CP, Digby JE, Mohammed SN, Hurst JA, Cheetham CH, Earley AR, Barnett AH, Prins JB, O'Rahilly S. Congenital leptin deficiency is associated with severe early-onset obesity in humans. *Nature* 1997; **387**: 903–908.

112. Clement K, Vaisse C, Lahlou N, Cabrol S, Pelloux V, Cassuto D, Gourmelen M, Dina C, Chambaz J, Lacorte JM, Basdevant A, Bougneres P, Lebouc Y, Froguel P, Guy-Grand B. A mutation in the human leptin receptor gene causes obesity and pituitary dysfunction. *Nature* 1998; **392**: 398–401.

113. O'Rahilly S, Gray H, Humphreys PJ, Krook A, Polonsky KS, White A, Gibson S, Taylor K, Carr C. Brief report: impaired processing of prohormones associated with abnormalities of glucose homeostasis and adrenal function. *N Engl J Med* 1995; **333**: 1386–1390.

114. Jackson RS, Creemers JW, Ohagi S, Raffin-Sanson ML, Sanders L, Montague CT, Hutton JC, O'Rahilly S. Obesity and impaired prohormone processing associated with mutations in the human prohormone convertase 1 gene. *Nat Genet* 1997; **16**: 303–306.

115. Krude H, Biebermann H, Luck W, Horn R, Brabant G, Gruters A. Severe early-onset obesity, adrenal insufficiency and red hair pigmentation caused by POMC mutations in humans. *Nat Genet* 1998; **19**: 155–157.

116. Vaisse C, Clement K, Guy-Grand B, Froguel P. A frameshift mutation in human MC4R is associated with a dominant form of obesity. *Nat Genet* 1998; **20**: 113–114.

8

Regulation of Appetite and the Management of Obesity

John E. Blundell

University of Leeds, Leeds, UK

Appetite control implies a control over energy intake. Some researchers argue that it only requires a habitual addition of 20–30 kilocalories per day to lead over a number of years to significant body weight increases which, in turn, leads to an epidemic of obesity. If human beings are the most intelligent life force on this planet, why is it that they cannot adjust their (eating) behaviour by the very small amounts which would be required for weight stability rather than weight escalation? Some explanation for this may be found through an examination of the processes involved in the regulation of appetite.

WHAT IS THE RELATIONSHIP BETWEEN APPETITE AND OBESITY?

There are clear logical reasons for believing that the expression of appetite—reflected in the pattern of eating and overall energy intake—makes a large contribution to the maintenance of a healthy weight. The impact of appetite on obesity is a time-dependent process and will occur at least over many months and usually years. The relationship between appetite and weight gain is therefore part of a developmental, or ageing, process and this perspective is important (1).

Appetite fits into an energy balance model of weight regulation but it is not necessary to believe that appetite control is an outcome of the regulation of energy balance. Appetite is separately controlled and is relevant to energy balance since it modulates the energy intake side of the equation. This happens because appetite includes various aspects of eating patterns such as the frequency and size of eating episodes (gorging versus nibbling), choices of high fat or low fat foods, energy density of foods consumed, variety of foods accepted, palatability of the diet and variability in day-to-day intake. All of these features can play a role in encouraging energy intake to exceed energy expenditure thereby creating a positive energy balance. If this persists then it will lead to weight gain. However, there appears to be no unique pattern of eating or forms of energy intake that will exclusively or invariably lead to an excess of energy intake over expenditure. Nevertheless, some characteristics of the expression of appetite do render individuals vulnerable to over-consumption of food—these characteristics can be regarded as risk factors. These *risk factors* and other modulating features of the expression of appetite will be disclosed by an analysis of how appetite is regulated.

CAN APPETITE BE CONTROLLED FOR THE MANAGEMENT OF OBESITY?

It is widely accepted that body weight control and, by implication, a lack of control arises from an

International Textbook of Obesity. Edited by Per Björntorp.

interaction between biology and the environment—particularly the food supply reflected in the nutritional environment. The link between the two domains is eating behaviour and the associated subjective sensations which make up the expression of appetite. It is this eating behaviour which transmits the impact of biological events into the environment, and which also mediates the effects of the nutrient environment on biology. Appetite is not nutrition, rather it is the expression of appetite which allows nutrition to exert an effect on biology, and vice versa. Consequently, adjustments in the processes regulating the expression of appetite should have a significant impact on body weight regulation.

Of course obesity can be managed by direct changes in the environment itself—to enforce an increase in physical activity or to coercively prevent food consumption. Equally, pharmacological or surgical interventions can be made directly in biology to prevent the assimilation of food or to alter the energy balance. In addition, adjustments in the environment and biology have the potential to influence body weight *indirectly* by altering food intake—often by acting on the signals involved in processes regulating appetite. The details of these actions will be apparent as the regulation of appetite is examined.

Consequently, in principle, appetite can be controlled for the management of obesity. We can envisage interventions either in specific foods which influence biology which in turn adjusts eating behaviour or through a direct and deliberate cognitive control of behaviour. There are many reasons to believe that an adjustment to the expression of appetite is the best chance we have to prevent the persistent surfeit of energy consumed over energy expended which is currently characterizing much of the world's population. At the end of this chapter we should be better informed about the possible strategies for regulating appetite to prevent further escalation of the obesity epidemic.

BASIC CONCEPTS IN APPETITE CONTROL

As a first step to recognizing how appetite can contribute to the prevention of obesity, it is useful to outline some basic principles which explain how the

expression of appetite can be understood. This conceptual approach will indicate how the detailed mechanisms and processes contribute to the global picture.

THE PSYCHOBIOLOGICAL SYSTEM OF APPETITE CONTROL

It is now accepted that the control of appetite is based on a network of interactions forming part of a psychobiological system. The system can be conceptualized on three levels (Figure 8.1). These are the levels of psychological events (hunger perception, cravings, hedonic sensations) and behavioural operations (meals, snacks, energy and macronutrient intakes); the level of peripheral physiology and metabolic events; and the level of neurotransmitter and metabolic interactions in the brain (2). Appetite reflects the synchronous operation of events and processes in the three levels. When appetite is disrupted as in certain eating disorders, these three levels become desynchronised. Neural events trigger and guide behaviour, but each act of behaviour involves a response in the peripheral physiological system; in turn, these physiological events are translated into brain neurochemical activity. This brain activity represents the strength of motivation to eat and the willingness to refrain from feeding.

The lower part of the psychobiological system (Figure 8.1) illustrates the appetite cascade which prompts us to consider the events which stimulate eating and which motivate organisms to seek food. It also includes those behavioural actions which actually form the structure of eating, and those processes which follow the termination of eating and which are referred to as post-ingestive or post-prandial events.

Even before food touches the mouth, physiological signals are generated by the sight and smell of food. These events constitute the cephalic phase of appetite. Cephalic-phase responses are generated in many parts of the gastrointestinal tract; their function is to anticipate the ingestion of food. During and immediately after eating, afferent information provides the major control over appetite. It has been noted that 'afferent information from ingested food acting in the mouth provides primarily positive feedback for eating; that from the stomach and small intestine is primarily negative feedback' (3).

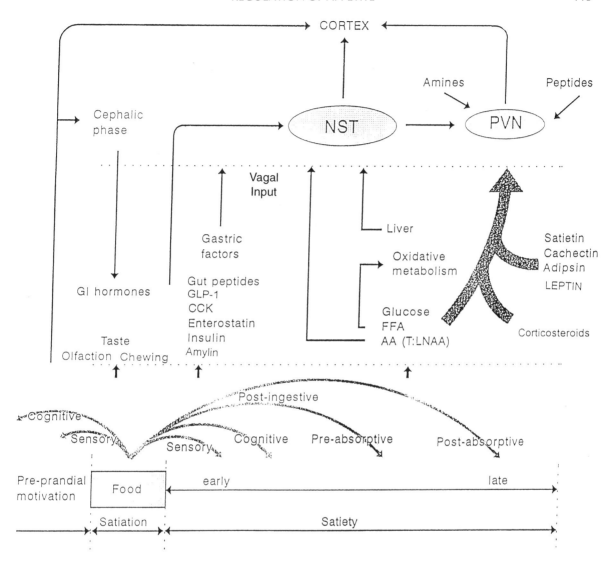

Figure 8.1 Diagram showing the expression of appetite as the relationship between three levels of operations: the behavioural pattern, peripheral physiology and metabolism, and brain activity. PVN, paraventricular nucleus; NST, nucleus of the tractus solitarius; CCK, cholecystokinin; FFA, free fatty acids; T:LNAA, tryptophan: large neutral amino acids; GLP-1, glucagon-like peptide 1. (See Blundell (2) for detailed diagram)

SATIETY SIGNALS AND THE SATIETY CASCADE

Scientifically important components of the appetite system are those physiological events which are triggered as responses to the ingestion of food and which form the inhibitory processes that first of all stop eating and then prevent the re-occurrence of eating until another meal is triggered. These physiological responses are termed satiety signals, and can be represented by the satiety cascade (Figure 8.2).

Satiation can be regarded as the complex of processes which brings eating to a halt (cause meal termination) whilst *satiety* can be regarded as those events which arise from food consumption and which serve to suppress hunger (the urge to eat) and maintain an inhibition over eating for a particular

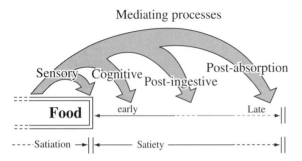

Figure 8.2   The satiety cascade illustrating the classes of events which constitute satiety signals arising from food consumption

period of time. This characteristic form of an eating pattern (size of meals, snacks etc.) is therefore dependent upon the coordinated effects of satiation and satiety which control the size and frequency of eating episodes.

Initially the brain is informed about the amount of food ingested and its nutrient content via sensory input. The gastrointestinal tract is equipped with specialized chemo- and mechano-receptors that monitor physiological activity and pass information to the brain mainly via the vagus nerve (4). This afferent information constitutes one class of 'satiety signals' and forms part of the pre-absorptive control of appetite. It is usual to identify a post-absorptive phase that arises when nutrients have undergone digestion and have crossed the intestinal wall to enter the circulation. These products, which accurately reflect the food consumed, may be metabolized in the peripheral tissues or organs or may enter the brain directly via the circulation. In either case, these products constitute a further class of metabolic satiety signals. Additionally, products of digestion and agents responsible for their metabolism may reach the brain and bind to specific chemoreceptors, influence neurotransmitter synthesis or alter some aspect of neuronal metabolism. In each case the brain is informed about some aspects of the metabolic state resulting from food consumption.

It seems likely that chemicals released by gastric stimuli or by food processing in the gastrointestinal tract are involved in the control of appetite (5). Many of these chemicals are peptide neurotransmitters, and many peripherally administered peptides cause changes in food consumption (6). There is evidence for an endogenous role for cholecystokinin (CCK), pancreatic glucagon, bombesin and somatostatin. Much recent research has confirmed

the status of CCK as a hormone mediating meal termination (satiation) and possibly early phase satiety. This can be demonstrated by administering CCK intravenously (the mouth cannot be used since CCK would be inactivated as soon as it reached the stomach) and measuring changes in food intake and hunger. CCK will reduce meal size and also suppress hunger before the meal; these effects do not depend on the nausea that sometimes accompanies an intravenous infusion (7). Food consumption (mainly protein and fat) stimulates the release of CCK (from duodenal mucosal cells) which in turn activates CCK-A type receptors in the pyloric region of the stomach. This signal is transmitted via afferent fibres of the vagus nerve to the nucleus tractus solitarius (NTS) in the brainstem. From here the signal is relayed to the hypothalamic region where integration with other signals occurs. The components of this system are set out in Figure 8.3.

Other potential peripheral satiety signals include peptides such as enterostatin (8), neurotensin and glucagon-like peptide 1 (GLP-1) (9).

APPETITE AND THE DRIVE TO EAT

For years the focus of investigations of appetite control has centred upon the termination of eating. This is because the termination of an eating episode—being the endpoint of a behavioural act—was perceived to be an unambiguous event around which empirical studies could be organized. Consequently satiety came to be the concept which formed the basis for accounts of appetite.

However, some 50 years ago there was an equal emphasis on the excitatory or drive features of appetite. This was embodied in Morgan's 'central motive state' and in Stellar's location of this within the hypothalamus (10). One major issue was to explain what gave animals (and humans) the energy and direction which motivated the seeking of food. These questions are just as relevant today but the lack of research has prevented much innovative thinking. In the light of knowledge about the physiology of energy homeostasis, and the utilization of different fuel sources in the body, it is possible to make some proposals. One source of the drive for food arises from the energy used to maintain physiological integrity and behavioural adaptation.

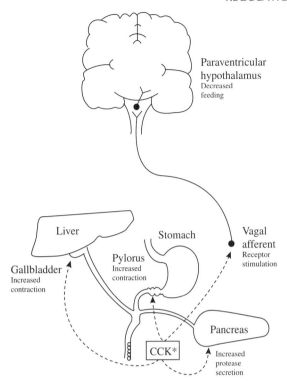

Figure 8.3 Peripheral–brain circuit indicating the postulated mode of action of CCK (cholecystokinin) as a satiety signal mediating the inhibition of eating

Consequently, there is a drive for food generated by energy expenditure. Approximately 60% of total energy expenditure is contributed by the resting metabolic rate (RMR). Consequently RMR provides a basis for drive and this resonates with the older concept of 'needs translated into drives'. In addition, through adaptation, it can be envisaged that other components of energy expenditure would contribute to the drive for food. The actual signals that help to transmit this energy need into behaviour could be reflected in oxidated pathways of fuel utilization (11), abrupt changes in the availability of glucose in the blood (12) and eventually brain neurotransmitters such as neuropeptide Y (NPY) which appears to be linked to metabolic processes. Leptin is also likely to play a role via this system.

In turn this drive to seek food—arising from a need generated by metabolic processing—is given direction through specific sensory systems associated with smell, but more particularly with taste. It is logical to propose that eating behaviour will be directed to foods having obvious energy value. Of particular relevance to the current situation are the characteristics of sweetness and fattiness of foods. In general most humans possess a strong liking for the sweet taste of foods and for the fatty texture. Both of these commodities indicate foods which have beneficial (energy yielding) properties.

Accordingly, appetite can be considered as a balance between excitatory and inhibitory processes. The excitatory processes arise from bodily energy needs and constitute a drive for food (which in humans is reflected in the subjective experience of hunger). The most obvious inhibitory processes arise from post-ingestive physiological processing of the consumed food—and these are reflected in the subjective sensation of fullness and a suppression of the feeling of hunger. However, the sensitivity of both the excitatory and inhibitory processes can be modulated by signals arising from the body's energy stores.

It should be noted that the drive system probably functions in order to ensure that energy intake at least matches energy expenditure. This has implications for the maintenance of obesity since total energy expenditure is proportional to body mass. This means that the drive for food may be strong in obese individuals in order to ensure that a greater volume of energy is ingested to match the raised level of expenditure. At the same time whilst there is a process to prevent energy intake falling below expenditure, there does not seem to be a strong process to prevent intake rising above expenditure. Consequently, any intrinsic physiological disturbance which leads to a rise in excitatory (drive) processes or a slight weakening of inhibitory (satiety) signals would allow consumption to drift upwards without generating a compensatory response. For some reason a positive energy balance does not generate an error signal that demands correction. Consequently the balance between the excitatory and inhibitory processes has implications for body weight regulation and for the induction of obesity.

SIGNALS FROM ADIPOSE TISSUE: LEPTIN AND APPETITE CONTROL

One of the classical theories of appetite control has involved the notion of a so-called long-term regulation involving a signal which informs the brain about the state of adipose tissue stores. This idea

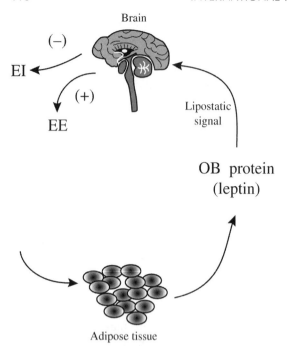

Figure 8.4 Diagram indicating the proposed role of the OB protein (leptin) in a signal pathway linking adipose tissue to central neural networks. It has been postulated that leptin interacts with neuropeptide Y in the brain (see text) to exert effects on food intake (and indirectly on adipose tissue) and on the pancreas (release of insulin). The leptin link between adipose tissue and the brain is only a part of a much more extensive peripheral–central circuit. EE, energy expenditure; EI, energy intake

the peripheral circulation. The identification and synthesis of the protein made it possible to evaluate the effects of experimental administration of the protein either peripherally or centrally (14). Because the OB protein caused a reduction in food intake (as well as an increase in metabolic energy expenditure) it has been termed 'leptin'. There is some evidence that leptin interacts with NPY, one of the brain's most potent neurochemicals involved in appetite, and with melanocortin-4 (MC4). Together these and other neuromodulators may be involved in a peripheral–central circuit which links an adipose tissue signal with central appetite mechanisms and metabolic activity (Figure 8.4).

In this way the protein called leptin probably acts in a similar manner to insulin which has both central and peripheral actions; for some years it has been proposed that brain insulin represents a body weight signal with the capacity to control appetite.

At the present time the precise relationship between the OB protein and weight regulation has not been determined. However, it is known that in animals and humans which are obese the measured amount of OB protein in the plasma is greater than in lean counterparts. Indeed there is always a very good correlation between the plasma levels of leptin and the degree of bodily fatness (15). Therefore although the OB protein is perfectly positioned to serve as a signal from adipose tissue to the brain, high levels of the protein obviously do not prevent obesity or weight gain. However, the OB protein certainly reflects the amount of adipose tissue in the body. Since the specific receptors for the protein (namely OB receptor) have been identified in the brain (together with the gene responsible for its expression) a defect in body weight regulation could reside at the level of the receptor itself rather than with the OB protein. It is now known that a number of other molecules are linked in a chain to transmit the action of leptin in the brain. These molecules are also involved in the control of food intake, and in some cases a mutation in the gene controlling these molecules is known and is associated with the loss of appetite control and obesity. For example, the MC4-R mutation (melanocortin-4 receptor) leads to an excessive appetite and massive obesity in children, just like the leptin deficiency (16).

These findings lead to a model of appetite control based on the classic two-process idea involving the stimulation (drive) to eat, and a quick-acting short-term inhibition of food consumption which decays

has given rise to the notion of a lipostatic or ponderstatic mechanism (13). Indeed this is a specific example of a more general class of peripheral appetite (satiety) signals believed to circulate in the blood reflecting the state of depletion or repletion of energy reserves which directly modulate brain mechanisms. Such substances may include satietin, adipsin, tumour necrosis factor (TNF or cachectin—so named because it is believed to be responsible for cancer induced anorexia) together with other substances belonging to the family of neural active agents called cytokines.

In 1994 a landmark scientific event occurred with the discovery and identification of a mouse gene responsible for obesity. A mutation of this gene in the *ob/ob* mouse produces a phenotype characterized by the behavioural trait of hyperphagia and the morphological trait of obesity. The gene controls the expression of a protein (the OB protein) by adipose tissue and this protein can be measured in rapidly. The drive for food would be reflected in high levels of hunger which are normally subjected to episodic inhibitory (satiety) signals. There are strong logical reasons why the drive (need) for food should be related to energy expenditure of metabolism and physical activity. Evidence suggests a role for NPY (which produces excessive food intake in animal studies) and leptin (whose absence releases the hunger drive in humans). This interpretation of leptin action is consistent with the suggestion of a dual role of leptin (24). Within the interaction between excitatory (drive) and inhibitory (satiety) processes there is ample room for the operation of a large number of mediating 'orexic' or 'anorexic' neuro-modulators (2).

LEPTIN DEFICIENCY AND APPETITE CONTROL

It seems clear that for the majority of obese people, the OB protein (leptin) system is not a major cause of rapid or massive weight gain.

However, for certain individuals very low levels of leptin (or the absence of leptin) may constitute a major risk factor. Recently a number of individuals have come to light. For example, two young cousins have been studied who displayed marked hyperphagia from a very early age. This hyperphagia took the form of a constant hunger accompanied by food cravings and a continuous demand for food (17). The eldest of the two cousins had reached a body weight of more than 90 kg by the age of 9. Her serum leptin level (like that of the cousin) was very low, and subsequently a mutation in the gene for leptin was revealed. This finding seems to implicate leptin (OB protein) in the control of the drive for food; that is, in the expression of hunger and active food seeking rather than with satiety or the short-term inhibition over eating. Leptin therefore appears to modulate the tonic signal associated with the translation of need into drive; when leptin levels are low or absent then the drive is *unleashed* and results in voracious food seeking. The MC4 receptor is also part of the same system and the absence of this receptor also abolishes restraint over appetite leading to massive hyperphagia. This phenomenon is quite different from the removal of a single satiety signal which would lead only to an increase in meal size or a modest increase in meal frequency.

FAT PREFERENCE AS AN APPETITE RISK FACTOR

It is clear that the expression of appetite—the willingness of people to eat or to refrain from eating—reflects an interaction between biology and the environment (particularly the presence of salient food-related stimuli). The tendency of this eating to lead to a positive or negative energy balance will be strongly influenced by the energy density of the foods selected. Considering over-consumption, the high energy density of fatty foods means that dietary fat intake is likely to lead to a positive energy (and fat) balance, and in turn to weight gain (18,19).

Evidence for the effect of dietary fat on appetite and weight gain arises from many different forms of investigation including epidemiological surveys, nutrient balance studies in calorimeters, short-term interventions on food intake and experiments on fat substitutes (20). One important issue in assessing the effects of fat ingestion is the difference between satiation and satiety (see Figure 8.1). Satiation is the process in operation while foods are being eaten; satiety is the state engendered as a consequence of consumption. In considering dietary fat as a risk factor in over-consumption, the effect on satiation is likely to be much more important than that on post-ingestive satiety.

The experimental evidence has led to the disclosure of two phenomena—termed 'passive over-consumption' and the 'fat paradox'. Use of an experimental procedure called concurrent evaluation has indicated that, when people eat to a state of comfortable fullness from a range of either high fat or high carbohydrate foods, they consume much greater quantities of energy from the fatty diet. This has been termed high fat hyperphagia or passive over-consumption. The effect is almost certainly due, in large part, to the high energy density of the high fat foods; hence it can be regarded as passive rather than active eating. However, the term passive means only that there is no deliberate intention on the part of the eater to over-consume, and does not mean that the phenomenon occurs without the mediation of mechanisms. Evidence indicates that people can consume very large amounts of fat in single meals and over a whole day (20). This is due to a weak effect of fat on satiation and a disproportionately weak effect of fat on satiety (21). Some studies have shown that human subjects obliged to

Table 8.1 Postulated interactions between behavioural risk factors and the obesigenic environment which generate a tendency for over-consumption

Biological vulnerability (behavioural risk factor)	Environmental influence	Potential for over-consumption
Preference for fatty foods	Abundance of high fat (high energy-dense)	↑ fat intake
Weak satiation (end of meal signals)	Large portion size	↑ meal size
Oro-sensory responsiveness	Availability of highly palatable foods with specific sensory-nutrient combinations	↑ amount eaten ↑ frequency
Weak post-ingestive satiety	Easy accessibility to foods and presence of potent priming stimuli	↑ frequency of eating ↑ tendency to re-initiate eating

eat a high fat diet for 3 weeks actually *increased* their hunger and decreased feelings of fullness before a test meal (22). This finding resonates with animal studies showing that when mice are fed a high fat diet there is a consequent decrease in leptin signalling in the hypothalamus. Therefore a high fat diet may weaken any inhibition over the tonic signal which translates needs into hunger drive.

The capacity of some people to consume very large quantities of fat creates a paradox. On one hand fat in the intestine generates potent satiety signals (5). On the other hand, exposure to a high fat diet leads to over-consumption (of energy) suggesting that fat has a weak effect on satiety (21). The resolution of this paradox is revealed by the evidence that although individuals—in the experimental situation—eat greater energy from the high fat foods, they may consume a smaller volume or weight of food. Since the function of a satiety signal is to limit the amount of food people put into the mouth, the signal has done its job but is overwhelmed by the speed with which the large amount of energy (from the high fat foods) can be delivered to the stomach. This dietary override of physiological satiety signals has a number of implications.

However, although there is a compelling correlation between dietary fat and obesity, the relationship does not constitute a *biological inevitability*. Some people eat a habitual high fat diet and remain lean.

RISK FACTORS FOR APPETITE CONTROL

Most researchers do not have any trouble accepting the idea that the state of a person's metabolism constitutes a major risk for developing weight gain and becoming obese. However, as obesity develops, metabolic characteristics change so that the state of obesity itself is associated with a different metabolic profile to that accompanying the process of weight gain. This makes it important to do longitudinal studies (whilst weight is increasing) as well as cross-sectional studies (comparing lean and obese subjects). Recently, Ravussin and Gautier (23) have drawn attention to this issue and have outlined those metabolic and physiological factors associated with weight gain and with the achievement of obesity.

The tendency to gain weight is associated with a low basal metabolic rate, low energy cost of physical activity, a low capacity for fat oxidation (relatively high respiratory quotient—RQ), high insulin sensitivity, low sympathetic nervous system activity and a low plasma leptin concentration. In the state of obesity itself many of these risk factors (or predictors of weight again) are reversed.

Just as certain metabolic variables (risk factors) can lead to a positive energy balance, so we can envisage certain behaviourally mediated processes which themselves constitute the *risk factors* leading to hyperphagia or 'over-consumption' (high energy intake leading to a positive energy balance). These processes may be patterns of eating behaviour, the sensory or hedonic events which guide behaviour, or sensations which accompany or follow eating. For convenience this cluster of events can be referred to as behavioural risk factors. These events may include a preference for fatty foods, weakened satiation (end of meal signals), relatively weak satiety (post-ingestive inhibition over further eating), strong oro-sensory preferences (e.g. for sweetness combined with fattiness in foods), a binge potential, and a high food-induced pleasure response. In turn, these events may be subdivided to describe more specific components leading to a risk of over-consumption.

These behavioural risk factors can be regarded as biological dispositions which create a vulnerability for weight gain and which manifest themselves through behavioural acts themselves, or through physiological processes which promote or permit changes in behaviour.

However, such risk factors alone would be unlikely to lead to a positive energy balance in a benign environment, i.e. one in which the food supply and the cultural habits worked against excessive consumption. In most of today's societies, however, the food environment exploits biologically based dispositions and this promotes the achievement of a high energy intake. This conceptualization is set out in Table 8.1.

INDIVIDUAL VARIABILITY IN APPETITE CONTROL: THE HIGH FAT PHENOTYPE

The concept of fat as an environmental risk factor is reflected in a general agreement that the increased energy intake which occurs on high fat diets is reflected in body weight gain and increasing obesity. When individuals in a large national survey were classified according to dietary fat intake, obesity (BMI > 30) among high fat consumers was 19 times that found in the low fat consumers (25). Consequently, this supports the view that, in general, a high intake of dietary fat tends to increase the likelihood of weight gain. However it is also clear that obesity resulting from a high fat diet is not a biological inevitability. In all databases we have examined, some high fat eaters remain normal weight or lean. This observation has led to a characterization of people based on the nature of their habitual dietary intake.

Comparisons between groups characterized by the amount of fat consumed in the diet has revealed quite diverse responses to nutrient challenges and to energy loading. The degree of hunger experienced and the behavioural responses were different (26). These features are present in individuals (in this case young male adults) indistinguishable in terms of their BMIs, percentage body fat, age and general lifestyle. In an extension of these investigations certain physiological features have been examined. The outcome indicates that the high fat (high energy) consumers with similar body weights to low fat consumers have lower respiratory quotients (RQs—the respiratory quotient reflects the oxidation of fat or carbohydrate), as expected, but also have higher resting metabolic rates (Table 8.2).

Taken together these two features would constitute physiological processes offering protection against the weight-inducing potential of a high fat diet. This cluster of behavioural and physiological features suggests the existence of a distinct phenotype. That is, a particular type of individual with the physiological capacity to retain a stable lean body. A further interesting feature of the high fat phenotype is the presence of a high level of plasma leptin. However, it is possible that the high circulating leptin may not be translated into an effective hypothalamic signal.

In addition, the investigation of the consequences of the habitual consumption of a particular diet has drawn attention to the interplay between biology and the environment. The relationship is not 100% predictable. In general it is clear that a high fat diet will favour the generation of a positive energy balance and weight gain, but some individuals who are physiologically protected (through genetic disposition or adaptation) will respond differently. The fact that the relationship between dietary fat and body weight is not a biological inevitability means that correlations from epidemiological studies (between dietary fat and obesity) can be expected to be weak. The interpretation of these weak correlations is made even more confusing because of the huge

Table 8.2 Characteristics of male high and low fat phenotypes

	High fat phenotype (HF)	Low fat phenotype (LF)
Age (years)	20.5	20.6
Body Mass Index	22.6	22.1
% body fat	9.9	9.8
Dietary fat (g/day)	158.8	80.8*
(% energy)	44.3	32.0*
Basal metabolic rate (kcal/day)	1624	1455*
Resting respiratory quotient	0.84	0.89*
Plasma leptin (ng/ml)	2.92	1.79*

* Significant difference between HF and LF, $P < 0.05$ (2-tail).

problem of mis-reporting food intake in large-scale surveys (27).

FAT INTAKE AND ADIPOSITY IN CHILDREN

Exposure to a diet containing high fat foods constitutes a risk factor for body weight gain but this relationship does not constitute a 'biological inevitability'. How does this relationship manifest itself in children?

First, evidence suggests the existence of a relationship between parental obesity and obesity in the offspring (28). In a retrospective cohort study of 854 subjects born between 1965 and 1971, obesity (defined as a BMI of 27.8 for men and 27.3 for women) in later adulthood was compared with the medical records of the parents. Among those who were obese during childhood, the chance of obesity in adulthood ranged from 8% (for 1- to 2-year-olds without obese parents) to 79% (for 10- to 14-year-olds with at least one obese parent). Therefore obese children under 3 years of age without obese parents are at low risk for obesity in adulthood, but among older children, obesity is an increasingly important predictor of adult obesity. In this study, parental obesity more than doubled the risk of adult obesity among children under 10 years of age.

One mediating factor (and possibly a mechanism) in the development of adult obesity from childhood involves the so-called 'adiposity rebound' (AR). This is the name given to the second augmentation of BMI after birth, and there is an inverse relationship between adult BMI and the age of AR. In a longitudinal study of Czech children, followed from 1 month of age to adulthood, the heaviest adults had an AR around 5 years and the leanest at 7.6 (29).

A number of studies have also examined the dietary fat intake of children and both the diet composition and adiposity of the parents. In one study, a high-risk group of children (one or two overweight parents) was compared with a low-risk group (no parent overweight) at 4.5 years of age. The high-risk group was consuming a higher percentage of fat in their diet and a smaller percentage of carbohydrate (30). In an unselected sample of 4- to 7-year-old children (35 girls, 36 boys) there was an influence of maternal adiposity on dietary fat intake in the children, and, for the boys a correlation between their own fat mass and fat intake (31). These data suggest that mothers may contribute more strongly than fathers to the development of obesity in children by influencing their dietary fat intake. Moreover, it is known that young children's preferences for particular foods are powerful predictors of consumption when self-selection is permitted (32). Interestingly, it has been demonstrated that the fat preferences (and fat consumption) of 3- to 5-year-old children are related to parental adiposity (33). The fat intake from 18 children was obtained from 30 h weighed food intake records and compared with the body composition measures of children and parents. Children's fat intakes were correlated with preferences for high fat foods and to their triceps skinfold measurements. In addition, there were strong correlations between the children's fat preferences and fat intakes and the BMIs of the parents. Children of heavier parents had stronger preferences for (and higher consumption of) fatty foods. In a further study of 9- to 10-year-old children, the fattest children consumed significantly more energy from fat than the lean children (34).

These findings strongly support an environmental impact of the habitual diet upon the development of weight gain and obesity. However, the data could also suggest a biological influence over the preferences for those high fat foods which form part of the habitual diet. This scenario, which focuses attention on the energy intake side of the energy balance equation, should not obscure the role of physical activity and energy expenditure. One major factor in the ever-increasing frequency of sedentary behaviours is television viewing. In a representative cohort of 746 youths aged 10–15 years there was a strong dose–response relationship between the prevalence of overweight and the hours of television viewed (35). The incidence of obesity was 8.3 times greater in those youths watching more than 5 hours of television per day compared with those watching 0 to 2 hours. As is the case with adults (36), overweight in children appears to be strongly influenced by the environmental factors of low physical activity (high frequency of sedentary activities) and exposure to a high energy-dense (high fat) diet. However, we should be wary of assuming that the effect of TV watching is necessarily due to sedentarism since viewing also provides an opportunity for further eating. Consequently, in children appetite control can play a significant role in weight gain and obesity. It is very obvious in cases of major gene mutations (leptin and MC4 receptor) that these forms of childhood obesity are driven exclusively by loss of restraint over appetite.

THE OBESITY EPIDEMIC: WHAT CAN WE LEARN FROM APPETITE CONTROL?

In simple terms it can be said that the increased prevalence of worldwide obesity arises largely from the excess of energy intake over energy expenditure. This can be driven to happen, or allowed to happen, through the defects in single major genes or by multiple genes with lower effects acting together. It can also arise because of the 'obesigenic' nature of the environment (37); and it can also occur through the mediation of some intrinsic modulation of the excitatory or inhibitory processes involved in appetite control (described earlier). There exists a simple formula indicating that the amount of excess energy intake (above expenditure), required for weight gain over years, is very small—perhaps between 20 and 40 kilocalories. However, the simplicity of this equation, and the apparent ease with which it seems possible for an individual to make the necessary correction to achieve weight stability, is illusory. This is because the expression of appetite displays a high degree of individual variability, and because the processes are complex. Therefore the volitional control over appetite required to make minimal savings in energy on a daily basis is, in practice, extremely difficult. A small deliberate adjustment can be swamped by uncontrollably large swings in day-to-day or intra-day consumption (particularly of dietary fat). In part, this explains why appetite control is difficult to maintain in the long term.

However, the control of appetite is clearly central to the containment of obesity and certain factors arise from an analysis of the field. These factors can be considered as principles to guide our understanding of appetite in relation to obesity.

- Emerging relationships between the nutritional environment and biological vulnerability (metabolic and behavioural risk factors) form the basis for a modern psychobiological approach to appetite control.
- Understanding the processes which permit overconsumption leading to a positive energy balance can inform a public health approach to prevent the further escalation of the obesity epidemic.
- The actions of specific nutrients on processes of preference and satiety can form the basis of a science of functional foods for appetite control.
- A pharmacological approach to obesity treatment can be formulated on drugs directed to specific molecules which influence drive and food seeking, food preferences and rewards, satiety signals and lipostatic hunger mechanisms.

In these ways, an understanding of appetite control can help to combat the epidemic of obesity.

REFERENCES

1. Blundell JE, King NA. Overconsumption as a cause of weight gain: behavioural–physiological interactions in the control of food intake (appetite). In: Chadwick DJ, Cardew G (eds) *The Origins and Consequences of Obesity*. Chichester: John Wiley, 1996: 138–158.
2. Blundell JE. Pharmacological approaches to appetite suppression. *Trends Pharmacol Sci* 1991; **12**: 147–157.
3. Smith GP, Greenberg D, Corp E, Gibbs J. Afferent information in the control of eating. In: Bray GA, Liss AR (eds) *Obesity: Towards a Molecular Approach*. New York: Alan R. Liss, 1990: 63–79.
4. Mei N. Intestinal chemosensitivity. *Physiol Rev* 1985; **65**: 211–237.
5. Read NW. Role of gastrointestinal factors in hunger and satiety in man. *Proc Nutr Soc* 1990; **51**: 7–11.
6. Smith GP, Gibbs J. Peripheral physiological determinants of eating and body weight. In: Brownell KD, Fairburn CG (eds) *Eating Disorders and Obesity: A Comprehensive Handbook*. New York: Guildford Publications, 1995: 8–12.
7. Greenough A, Cole G, Lewis J, Lockton A, Blundell J. Untangling the effects of hunger, anxiety, and nausea on energy intake during intravenous cholecystokinin octapeptide (CCK-8) infusion. *Physiol Behav* 1998; **65**(2): 303–310.
8. Erlanson-Albertsson C, Larson A. The activation peptide of pancreatic procolipase decreases food intake in rats. *Regul Pep* 1988; **22**: 325–331.
9. Blundell JE, Naslund E. Invited Commentary: Glucagon-like peptide-1, satiety and appetite control. *Br J Nutr* 1999: **81**: 259–260.
10. Stellar E. The physiology of motivation. *Psychol Rev* 1954: **61**: 5–22.
11. Friedman MI, Rawson NE. Fuel metabolism and appetite control. In: Fernstrom JD, Miller GD (eds) *Appetite and Body Weight Regulation*. Boca Raton, FL: CRC Press, 1994: 63–76.
12. Campfield LA, Brandon P, Smith FJ. On-line continuous measurement of blood glucose and meal pattern in free feeding rats: the role of glucose in meal initiation. *Brain Res Bull* 1985; **14**: 605–616.
13. Weigle, D. Appetite and the regulation of body composition.

J Fed Am Soc Exp Biol 1994; **8**: 302–310.

14. Campfield LA, Smith FJ, Guisez Y, Devos R, Burn P. Recombinant mouse OB Protein: evidence for a peripheral signal linking adiposity and central neural networks. *Science* 1995; **269**: 546–549.

15. Maffei M, Halaas J, Ravussin E *et al*. Leptin levels in human and rodent: measurement of plasma leptin and ob RNA in obese and weight reduced subjects. *Nat Med* 1995; **1**: 1155–1161.

16. Hinney A, Schmidt A, Nottebom K, Heibült O, Becker I, Ziegler A, Gerber G, Sina M, Görg T, Mayer H, Siegfried W, Fichter M, Remschmidt H, Hebebrand J. Several mutations in the melanocortin-4 receptor gene including a nonsense and a frameshift mutation associated with dominantly inherited obesity in humans. *J Clin Endocrinol Metab* 1999; **84**: 1483–1486.

17. Montague CT, Farcoqi IS, Whitehead JP *et al*. Congenital leptin deficiency is associated with severe early onset obesity in humans. *Nature* 1997; **387**: 903–908.

18. Golay A, Bobbioni E. The role of dietary fat in obesity. *Int J Obes* 1997; **21**(Suppl 3): S2–S11.

19. Ravussin E, Swinburn BA. Pathophysiology of obesity. *Lancet* 1992; **340**: 404–408.

20. Blundell JE, Macdiarmid JI. Passive overconsumption: fat intake and short-term energy balance. *Ann N Y Acad Sci* 1997; **827**: 392–407.

21. Lawton CL, Burley VJ, Wales JK, Blundell JE. Dietary fat and appetite control in obese subjects: weak effects on satiation and satiety. *Int J Obes* 1993; **17**: 409–416.

22. French SJ, Murray B, Rumsay RDE, Fadzlin R, Read NW. Adaptation to high fat diets: effects on eating behaviour and plasma cholecystokinin. *Br J Nutr* 1995; **73**: 179–189.

23. Ravussin E, Gautier JF. Metabolic Predictors of weight gain. *Int J Obes* 1999; **23**: 37–41.

24. Caro JF, Kolaczinski JW, Zhang PL *et al*. Leptin: the tale of an obesity gene. *Diabetes* 1996; **45**: 1455–1462.

25. Macdiarmid JI, Cade JE, Blundell JE. High and low fat consumers, their macronutrient intake, and body mass index: further analysis of the National Diet and Nutrition Survey of British Adults. *Eur J Clin Nutr* 1996; **50**: 505–512.

26. Cooling J, Blundell JE. Are high-fat and low-fat consumers distinct phenotypes? Differences in the subjective and behavioural response to energy and nutrient challenges. *Eur J Clin Nutr* 1998; **52**: 193–201.

27. Blundell JE. What foods do people habitually eat? A dilemma for nutrition, an enigma for psychology. *Am J Clin Nutr* 2000; **71**: 3–5.

28. Whitaker RC, Wright JAS, Pepe MS, Seidel KD, Dietz WH. Predicting obesity in young adulthood from childhood and parental obesity. *N Engl J Med* 1997; **337**: 869–873.

29. Prokopec M, Bellisle F. Adiposity in Czech children followed from 1 month of age to adulthood: analysis of individual BMI patterns. *Ann Hum Biol* 1993; **206**: 517–525.

30. Eck LH, Klesges RC, Hanson CL, Slawson D. Children at familial risk for obesity: an examination of dietary intake, physical activity and weight status. *Int J Obes* 1991; **16**: 71–78.

31. Nguyen VT, Larson DE, Johnson RK, Goran MI. Fat intake and adiposity in children of lean and obese parents. *Am J Clin Nutr* 1996; **63**: 507–513.

32. Birch LL. Preschool children's food preferences and consumption patterns. *J Nutr Educ* 1979; **11**: 189–192.

33. Fisher JO, Birch LL. Fat preferences and fat consumption of 3- to 5-year-old children are related to parental adiposity. *J Am Diet Assoc* 1995; **95**: 759–764.

34. Tucker LA, Seljaas MS, Hager RL. Body fat percentage of children varies according to their diet composition. *J Am Diet Assoc* 1997; **97**: 981–986.

35. Gortmaker SL, Must A, Sobol AM, Peterson K, Colditz GA, Dietz WH. Television viewing as a cause of increasing obesity among children in the United States, 1986–1990. *Arch Paediatr Adolesc Med* 1996; **150**: 356–362.

36. Prentice AM, Jebb SA. Obesity in Britain: gluttony or sloth? *BMJ* 1995; **311**: 437–439.

37. Egger G, Swinburn B. An 'ecological' approach to the obesity pandemic. *BMJ* 1997; **315**: 477–480.

Physiological Regulation of Macronutrient Balance

Susan A. Jebb[1] and Andrew M. Prentice[2]

[1]*MRC Human Nutrition Research, Cambridge and* [2]*MRC International Nutrition Group, London*

BACKGROUND

For centuries the concept of energy balance has provided the bedrock for research into the mechanisms controlling body weight. However, in recent years there has been growing interest in the regulation of the individual macronutrients that combine to determine the energy status of an individual. Thus the classical energy balance equation can be more accurately represented as the integrated sum of each individual macronutrient (Figure 9.1). This chapter will discuss the evidence for the physiological regulation of macronutrient balance and the implications for the prevention and treatment of obesity.

MACRONUTRIENT METABOLISM

Digestion of food is macronutrient-specific from the moment of its ingestion. This raises the possibility that differences in the absorption, processing or storage of nutrients may provide a potential mechanism to explain a macronutrient-specific effect on body weight.

Digestion

In the first instance the efficiency of absorption of energy from individual macronutrients is variable.

Approximately 96% of the energy from fat is absorbed, 91% from protein and a variable proportion from carbohydrate, depending on the relative content of 'available' carbohydrate and resistant starch. However, knowing the composition of the diet, the availability of energy is largely predictable (1). Moreover, except in pathological malabsorption syndromes, it is extremely consistent between individuals, which makes this an unlikely cause of individual susceptibility to weight gain.

The effect of macronutrients on diet-induced thermogenesis DIT) is also variable. When consumed individually as the only source of nourishment, short-term experiments indicate that less energy is dissipated in the processing of fat (6%) compared to carbohydrate (12.5%) or protein (21%) (2). However, measurements made over the whole day in a whole-body calorimeter indicate very little difference in overall energy expenditure on diets with radically different ratios of fat to carbohydrate. For example, in a study in which individuals were fed isoenergetic diets with constant protein content and either 9 or 79% energy as carbohydrate, with reciprocal changes in fat intake, daily energy expenditure measured on two separate occasions in a whole-body calorimeter was not significantly different (3). Similar results have been obtained in groups of lean and obese men and women (4).

Major changes in the proportion of protein in the

International Textbook of Obesity. Edited by Per Björntorp.

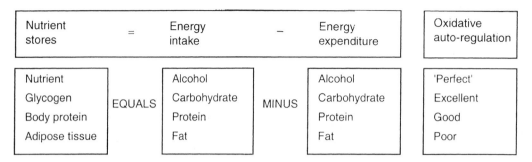

Figure 9.1   The oxidative hierarchy of macronutrients

diet do seem to lead to noticeable differences in diet-induced thermogenesis, but again the effect on 24-hour energy expenditure is negligible. For example, Westerterp *et al.* (5) showed that on a high protein/high carbohydrate/low fat diet (30: 60: 10% by energy) diet-induced thermogenesis represented 14.6% of the total intake and 24-hour energy expenditure was 9.2 MJ. Whilst on the low protein/ low carbohydrate/high fat diet (10: 60: 30% by energy), diet-induced thermogenesis represented only 10.5% of total energy intake ($P = 0.01$) and while there was a trend towards a lower energy expenditure over 24 hours (8.9 MJ), the difference was not statistically significant ($P = 0.08$) (5).

Macronutrient Oxidation

Once assimilated into the body a nutrient may be oxidized or stored. This process of nutrient partitioning is a key regulatory point in macronutrient metabolism and recent studies have shown a precise hierarchy in which macronutrients are recruited for oxidation. Since total energy expenditure is essentially constant, except for limited (and predictable) thermogenesis, the oxidation of any one nutrient will tend to suppress the oxidation of others. Alcohol dominates oxidative pathways, since it is a toxin and must be eliminated from the body as quickly as possible (6). Carbohydrate and protein also show a linkage between intake and oxidation. Numerous short-term studies have shown that the addition of carbohydrate to a meal will induce an increase in carbohydrate oxidation and likewise for protein (7,8). However, no such auto-regulatory process exists for fat oxidation. The addition of fat to a meal

does not stimulate fat oxidation. Indeed the oxidation of fat is ultimately dependent on the intake of the other macronutrients, since fat oxidation accounts for the difference between the energy requirements of the individual and the combined energy content of the ingested alcohol, carbohydrate and protein (9). The addition or subtraction of carbohydrate from the diet causes a parallel increase or decrease in carbohydrate oxidation, with reciprocal changes in fat oxidation. However, when fat is added or subtracted from the diet the effect on substrate oxidation is negligible (10).

The impressive flexibility in carbohydrate oxidation rates in response to changes in intake is shown in Figure 9.2. Here, during profound overfeeding, subjects were receiving 150% of their baseline energy requirements including 539 g/day carbohydrate. Carbohydrate oxidation increased immediately and after 4–5 days carbohydrate oxidation closely matched intake so that carbohydrate balance was re-established, although at a higher level of glycogen stores. Conversely during underfeeding, when subjects received only 3.5 MJ/day, with 83 g/ day carbohydrate, the oxidation of carbohydrate was suppressed and balance was again virtually re-established. The small persistent negative carbohydrate balance probably reflects a gradual depletion of muscle glycogen stores in response to this period of profound under-nutrition. Thus there is sufficient flexibility in carbohydrate oxidation to match intake over the range of about 80–540 g/day in adult men. Throughout this period the change in fat oxidation were counter-regulatory (Figure 9.3). During overfeeding the excess energy was stored primarily as fat, with a marked positive fat balance, and during underfeeding the energy deficit was met by the oxidation of endogenous fat, leading to nega-

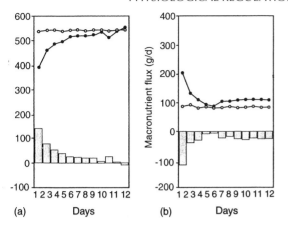

Figure 9.2 Carbohydrate flux during overfeeding (a) and underfeeding (b). Open circles, carbohydrate intake; closed circles, carbohydrate oxidation; hatched bars, net carbohydrate balance. Data from Jebb *et al.* (9)

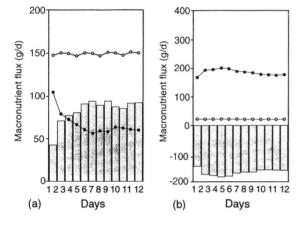

Figure 9.3 Fat flux during overfeeding (a) and underfeeding (b). Open circles, fat intake; closed circles, fat oxidation; hatched bars, net fat balance. Data from Jebb *et al.* (9)

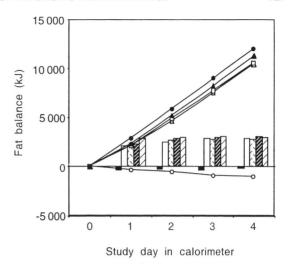

Study day in calorimeter

Figure 9.4 Daily and cumulative changes in fat balance during intentional overfeeding by fat or different carbohydrates. Solid bars and circles, control diet; open bars and open triangles, 50% overfeeding by fructose; stippled bars and open squares, 50% overfeeding by sucrose; heavy hatched bars and solid triangles, 50% overfeeding by glucose; light hatched bars and solid circles, 50% overfeeding by fat. Data from McDevitt *et al.* (11)

The cumulative increase in fat balance did not differ significantly between treatments involving overfeeding by fat, sucrose, glucose or fructose.

If individuals eat to energy balance, the pattern of macronutrient oxidation will closely match the dietary composition (i.e. respiratory quotient = food quotient). However, in conditions of energy imbalance the oxidative hierarchy predicts that fat will be the macronutrient most likely to be mobilized or stored to balance the body's energy budget in the medium to long term.

Macronutrient Storage

The biochemical potential for the inter-conversion of macronutrients has aroused considerable interest, particularly in relation to *de novo* synthesis of fat from dietary carbohydrate. In energetic terms this is a very inefficient process, in which approximately 20–30% of the energy is dissipated as heat, whilst dietary fat can be stored with the loss of only 4% of its energy (12). A propensity towards *de novo* lipogenesis is a plausible 'energy wasting' strategy which may help some individuals to remain slim in the face of excess food. However, detailed studies

tive fat balance. Changes in protein oxidation during both over- and underfeeding were modest, but with a trend towards auto-regulation (9).

Experiments investigating whether different primary sources of carbohydrate have variable effects on this carbohydrate-driven system of fuel selection have revealed no detectable differences between glucose, fructose and sucrose (11). When various energy sources are fed under controlled conditions (i.e. which exclude effects of appetite) fats and carbohydrates have a very similar effect on fat balance. This can be seen in Figure 9.4, which illustrates changes in fat balance when subjects are intentionally overfed in a whole-body calorimeter for 4 days.

using stable isotopes suggest that this process is quantitatively unimportant in humans (13), except under conditions of profound overfeeding (14). This does not preclude an effect of other macronutrients on fat storage, an effect which is achieved by their suppression of the utilization of dietary fat.

MACRONUTRIENT EFFECTS ON INTAKE

Short-term studies of the effects of macronutrients on energy intake have often used a preload/test-meal paradigm. Subjects are given a 'preload' of known or unknown composition and after a fixed interval are offered one or more 'test-meals', at which they can eat *ad libitum*, but consumption is monitored. During the intervening periods they may also be asked to complete visual analogue scales indicating hunger or satiety. Similar studies have also been conducted to assess food intake over 1–3 days after a specific macronutrient manipulated meal or meals.

There are relatively few studies to address the specific effect of protein on subsequent intake. However, most data would suggest that in isoenergetic quantities, protein is probably the most satiating macronutrient (15–17). Whether this leads to differences in prospective consumption is more debatable. For example in a study of breakfasts high in protein, fat or carbohydrate followed by *ad libitum* consumption at lunch 5 hours later and thereafter, Stubbs *et al.* found that the high protein breakfast suppressed self-reported hunger to a greater extent over the entire 24-hour period (18). However, it was not translated into any difference in 24-hour energy intake or balance. Similarly in an extended 3-day study there was no difference in intake on days 2 and 3 following a high protein diet on day 1, relative to isoenergetic diets high in fat or carbohydrate (19). However, in most diets, protein is a much smaller constituent than fat or carbohydrate, which probably limits its overall contribution to the regulation of energy intake.

Instead most of the preload studies have focused on the relative roles of fat and carbohydrate by providing a constant proportion of protein and thus allowing reciprocal changes in fat and carbohydrate. For example, in a study where subjects were given a standard breakfast as a preload, or the same meal supplemented with 1520 kJ of fat or carbohydrate, *ad libitum* intake was measured at a subsequent test meal or snack (20). Visual analogue scores showed that the carbohydrate supplement suppressed hunger and the desire to eat, whereas the fat supplement had no effect relative to the control. By 4 hours later this difference had disappeared and there was no difference in energy intake at the test lunch consumed 4.5 hours after breakfast. In a subsequent study in which preloads were followed by an *ad libitum* snack 90 minutes later, when the difference in the hunger scores between preloads was still evident, there was a significant suppression of the snack intake after the carbohydrate-supplemented preload, whilst intake followed the fat-supplemented preload did not differ from the control.

The different results obtained by altering the interval between preload and test meal (20,21) or by varying the size or composition of foods (22) preclude total consensus in the interpretation of these studies. A further confounding factor in the analysis of these studies is the effect of the subjects' state of knowledge. Overt manipulations of the fat to carbohydrate content of foods may produce contradictory results to covert studies. For example, Shide and Rolls showed that following a covert low fat preload, subjects consumed less at an *ad libitum* lunch than following a high fat preload. However, when information about the fat content of the preload was provided, the intake at lunch was greater following the low fat preload (23). In some cases the individual characteristics of the subjects may further distort the interpretation. Some studies have suggested that the degree of dietary restraint will influence intake at a test meal (24), although others have failed to find a difference between restrained and unrestrained eaters (23). However, it is generally agreed that dietary carbohydrate initiates a much stronger satiety signal than dietary fat and in so doing may limit prospective food consumption.

The concept that dietary carbohydrate may be more satiating than fat is consistent with the hypothesis of Flatt (7). Flatt argues that the quantity of carbohydrate oxidized each day is similar to the body's storage capacity for carbohydrate, whereas the storage capacity for fat is considerably greater than day-to-day consumption or oxidation of this macronutrient. Thus day-to-day fluctuations in carbohydrate stores are proportionally very much larger than for fat. This confers a much greater sensitivity to changes in the pool size for carbohydrate, than for fat, and Flatt argues that this modulates later consumption in order to restore the equilibrium. Based on this hypothesis the status of the body's carbohydrate store is critical in determining intake and implies that individuals eat sufficient food to defend their carbohydrate stores. Thus on a diet with a low carbohydrate:fat ratio the total amount of energy consumed in order to provide sufficient carbohydrate will be greater than when consuming a diet with a high carbohydrate:fat ratio. This scenario must inevitably lead to fat deposition which will persist until such time as the substrate mixture being oxidized matches that of the habitual diet (i.e. RQ = FQ). Fat accumulation is thus interpreted as a response to a high fat diet (25).

Evidence for this theory comes from prolonged feeding trials in mice (7). Specifically there was a negative correlation between changes in carbohydrate stores and the subsequent day's *ad libitum* intake, yet no association between net energy balance on one day and intake the next. However, extensive testing of this model in human studies has largely failed to support this early conjecture. This is clearly demonstrated in a study where glycogen stores were perturbed by feeding isoenergetic extremes of fat to carbohydrate intake (9 vs. 79% carbohydrate) on a 'manipulation' day and observing *ad libitum* intake on the following 'outcome' day (3). These studies were conducted within a whole-body calorimeter such that macronutrient balance could be ascertained relative to a nominal zero at the start of each phase of the study. Despite a difference in carbohydrate balance of 327 g between the high and low carbohydrate manipulations there was no significant difference in intake the following day. Subsequent studies have examined the impact of macronutrient manipulations which also include changes in energy balance on subsequent energy intake (26). Here an energy deficit of approximately 15% was created by the removal of either dietary fat or carbohydrate. The macronutrient manipulations produced significant differences in substrate oxidation, which were predictable from the oxidative hierarchy, but there was no evidence of any macronutrient-specific effects on subsequent intake. In each case, energy balance was restored after 1 day of *ad libitum* eating. These studies suggest that the net flux of all macronutrients may be better able to explain the pattern of subsequent energy intake

than nutrient-specific models. In the light of this, Friedman has proposed a theoretical framework in which the stimulus to food intake is derived at the level of oxidative phosphorylation and adenosine triphosphate (ATP) production (27). However, to date there is relatively little direct experimental evidence in support of this model.

IMPLICATIONS FOR OBESITY

Macronutrients and Weight Gain

The integrated impact of the differential regulation of macronutrient intake, digestion, absorption, storage and oxidation generally supports the hypothesis that dietary fat may be particularly associated with weight gain. This has been examined in a number of studies conducted over several days or weeks. Here the period of study must be related to the precision of the measurements of changes in macronutrient balance. Tightly controlled experimental studies performed in calorimeters, where changes in fat stores can be measured to ± 9 g fat/day, can be conducted over just a few days, whereas measurements made in free-living conditions, using *in vivo* body composition measurements require a period of several weeks or even months, since the precision is of the order of ± 1 kg fat (28). Community studies, which rely solely on changes in body weight as an index of changes in fat stores, must be conducted over several months in order to provide a reliable indicator of long-term changes in fat stores, rather than acute fluctuations caused by shifts in water or carbohydrate balance.

Other studies have investigated the regulation of macronutrient balance using hour-by-hour measurements of the subjects' self-selected intake and subsequent substrate oxidation whilst continuously confined to a whole body calorimeter. In one experiment six lean young healthy men were studied on three occasions in which each individual meal and snack was covertly manipulated to provide approximately 13% dietary energy as protein, 20, 40 or 60% energy as fat and the remainder as carbohydrate (29). Hence diets which were relatively high in fat were low in carbohydrate, with a high energy density and vice versa. On the 60% fat diet subjects were in marked positive energy and fat balance, but there was no significant change in carbohydrate balance. Body weight increased by 0.9 kg over 7 days. On the 20% fat diet energy and fat balance was negative, although there was a modest positive carbohydrate balance. Despite the negative energy balance subjects gained 0.2 kg over 7 days, due to the increase in glycogen stores.

In a subsequent study conducted under free-living conditions absolute energy balance was lower on each dietary treatment, probably reflecting the greater energy needs of subjects outside the confines of the calorimeter. However, the inter-treatment effect was remarkably similar (30). Here the 20% fat diet elicited spontaneous weight loss of 0.74 kg in 14 days, relative to a gain of 0.09 kg on the 60% fat diet, despite eating *ad libitum*. This is consistent with a study in women, who lost 0.4 kg in 2 weeks on a 15–20% fat diet, but gained 0.32 kg over a similar period on a diet providing 45–50% fat (31).

This phenomenon of 'high fat hyperphagia' is a plausible explanation for the association of high fat diets with obesity (see Chapter 10). It is a robust and readily reproducible effect that is observed across different groups of subjects and in different laboratories. Given the increasing prevalence of obesity, a number of strategies have been considered to counterbalance the effect of high-fat diets. In a public health context physical activity offers an attractive option which will also provide independent health benefits. In experimental studies subjects who are confined to a calorimeter with a sedentary protocol, readily over-eat on high fat diets relative to high carbohydrate diets. However, a recent study has shown that the imposition of 3×40 minute periods of cycling, designed to raise the physical activity level (TEE/BMR) from 1.25 to 1.61, resulted in a significant reduction in energy balance, relative to the high fat–sedentary protocol. This was attributable to both an increase in energy needs and a reduction in intake (32) (Figure 9.5). This interaction between macronutrient and physical activity was also observed in the epidemiological analysis of the Gothenburg (Göteborg) Women's Study where the risk of weight gain was significantly increased only in those women consuming a high fat diet who were also classified as sedentary (33).

In a clinical setting pharmacotherapy has been proposed to curb hyperphagia. In a study of six obese women offered either a 25 or 50% fat diet, along with either a centrally acting appetite suppressant (dexfenfluramine) or placebo, the drug reduced energy intake on the high fat diet relative to

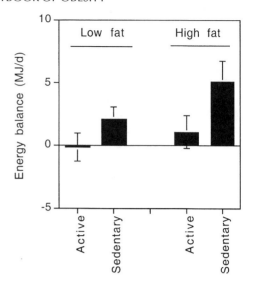

Figure 9.5 Interactions between the fat content of the diet and physical activity in the regulation of fat balance. Data from Murgatroyd *et al.* (32)

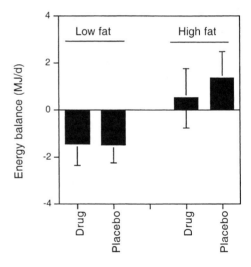

Figure 9.6 Interactions between the fat content of the diet and an appetite suppressant (dexfenfluramine) in the regulation of fat balance. Data from Poppitt *et al.* (34)

the placebo by 10%, but it did not significantly decrease intake on the low fat diet. It is noteworthy, however, that the effect of decreasing the fat content of the diet was more than three times greater than the impact of the drug (34) (Figure 9.6).

One of the most convincing mechanisms to explain the phenomenon of high fat hyperphagia relates to the energy density of fat (39 kJ/g), which is disproportionately high relative to carbohydrate (16 kJ/g) or protein (23 kJ/g). In studies where the energy density of the diets was held constant in the face of macronutrient manipulations the high fat hyperphagia is frequently abolished. For example, in a crossover study using predominantly liquid diets of similar energy density but containing either 24 or 47% fat, there was no difference in energy intake over a 2-week period (35). In the studies of Stubbs and colleagues described above, it was apparent that subjects had consumed a similar bulk of food on each occasion, despite the macronutrient manipulation (29,30). Thus the hyperphagia observed on high fat diets may be viewed as 'passive over-consumption', i.e. increases in energy intake in the absence of increases in the volume of food consumed. This was investigated further in a study where the energy density of the diets was fixed, whilst still providing 20, 40 or 60% energy as fat (36). Here high fat hyperphagia was not observed, although it is notable that there was a persistent decrease in energy intake on the high carbohydrate/ low fat diet, suggesting that the suppressive effect of carbohydrate on food intake is over and above its effects on the energy density of the food.

The importance of the energy density of food as a determinant of energy intake has previously been reviewed in detail (37). Traditional high fat foodstuffs frequently have a higher energy density than low fat/high carbohydrate foods. However, the advent of new food processing methods means that an increasing number of items may be low in fat but retain an energy density comparable to the high fat variety. Their effects on body weight regulation are unclear. Likewise the role of non-caloric sweeteners (38) and fat substitutes in the relation of macronutrient balance in children (39) and adults remains controversial with conflicting results obtained using different experimental paradigms (40–42).

The primary conclusion of the experimental studies described above is that diets containing a high proportion of fat disrupt the physiological processes that regulate macronutrient balance and frequently result in positive fat balance and weight gain. In contrast, in less controlled studies, especially in the community, it is the balance between physiological processes and external and/or cognitive influences which determines the overall effect. Here the effects of macronutrients on energy intake cannot be easily segregated from other factors controlling appetite (see Chapter 8). Accordingly it does not inevitably follow that low fat diets lead to weight loss.

Macronutrients and Weight Loss

There is currently a clear divide in scientific opinion regarding the merits of low fat/high carbohydrate diets in the context of weight loss (43,44). We conclude that although there is evidence of spontaneous weight loss associated with low fat diets relative to high fat control diets, most intervention studies have shown only a small reduction in body weight (up to 0.6 kg/month). Moreover this loss occurs mostly in the first 3–6 months, after which weight may be gradually regained. This precludes the use of low fat diets as the sole strategy for weight reduction.

Nonetheless it is pertinent to note that most *ad libitum*, low fat intervention studies currently in the literature were not primarily designed to examine the impact of macronutrient manipulations on body weight. Indeed most subjects were not overweight and may therefore be more likely to protect their body weight, through either physiological or cognitive processes. Some studies gave specific advice to subjects to increase carbohydrate intake to maintain body weight (45) or advised on other nonspecific strategies to equalize energy intake to control values (46,47). Some studies used a low fat diet as part of a broader management plan (48,49) including advice to stop smoking, which would tend to lead to weight gain. The notable exception is the study of Ornish, in which there is a decrease of 11.5 kg in weight (relative to controls) over 1 year (48). These patients were mostly overweight and angiographic evidence of coronary artery disease, which may have provided a very significant motivational factor to enhance compliance to the comprehensive management programme.

In studies of the treatment of obese patients there is little evidence of any macronutrient-specific effects on weight loss (50–53). Here the rate of weight loss is closely related to the energy deficit that is achieved, suggesting that the macronutrient effects are more subtle than gross differences in energy intake. However, low fat diets are an effective method to decrease total energy intake and two studies have shown that subjects in the low fat group perceived the diet to be more palatable and showed significant improvements in quality of life scores which may increase the likelihood of greater compliance in the longer term (50,51). Two studies have assessed the value of *ad libitum* low fat diets, relative to energy-restricted diets for weight maintenance over 1 year following acute weight loss. Schlundt found no significant difference between groups in terms of weight regain, while Toubro and Astrup demonstrated significantly enhanced weight maintenance in the low fat group (54,55).

These studies raise a number of general issues regarding the efficacy of low fat diets in community studies. Firstly, compliance to the low fat regime is obviously a prerequisite for effective weight loss. An individual's perception of their personal fat intake relative to the population average does not correlate well with actual fat intake (56). Indeed in one survey and when questioned, most people tend to believe that they eat less fat than the average person! Thus subjects who routinely incorporate some low fat products in their diet (e.g. low fat milks or spreads) may believe that they have reduced their fat intake, yet consciously or subconsciously compensate, by consuming additional fat in other items. In studies in the UK the majority of consumers report that in recent years they have reduced their personal fat intake (57), yet estimates of fat consumption from the National Food Survey have remained rather constant (58). In a study which incorporated independent estimates of compliance, using ^{13}C-labelled glucose and subsequent measurement of ^{13}C in expired air, there was a positive relationship between individual adherence to the low fat diet and the extent of weight loss (59). This confirms that different level of compliance is a major determinant of the success of low fat interventions.

Secondly, the actual change in dietary fat intake may be less than reported by dietary surveys. This is difficult to assess since self-reporting of food intake is notoriosly unreliable and dietary education may increase any bias in the reported macronutrient intake. Attempts to educate subjects how to *consume* less fat may also serve to educate subjects how to *report* less fat. Alternatively subjects may accurately report their intake on specific measurement days, when they may closely adhere to the dietary prescription, but this may be a poor reflection of their typical eating habits (60).

Finally, there is growing concern that subjects may reduce their fat intake but not necessarily reduce their total energy intake. Even in one of the most effective of the intervention studies where there was a striking reduction in dietary fat from 31.5 to 6.8%, this was accompanied by only a 0.6 MJ/day decrease in energy intake over one year (48). Apparently three-quarters of the decrease in fat was counterbalanced by increases in energy from other dietary constituents. This compensation may represent a physiological system which recognizes the fall in energy intake and endeavours to restore the *status quo* by stimulating consumption (26). Even if subjects adhere to the low fat prescription, weight loss may be attenuated by increases in other macronutrients. The overt nature of a study where subjects must self-select their own food (unlike the mostly covert laboratory manipulations) may trigger unpredictable cognitive responses, as observed in the preload/test meal paradigms (23). Covert manipulations may therefore be more effective in producing spontaneous weight loss because there is no obstructive cognitive response. However, the effect of reductions in dietary energy density on innate appetite control systems are insufficient to overcome total dietary disinhibition. The emphasis on low fat foods may contribute to a perception that such foods will not cause weight gain regardless of the amount consumed, thus liberating subjects from exerting any dietary restraint (61). Low fat foods which *substitute* for the high fat equivalent will tend to lead to a cut in energy intake, but the *addition* of low fat foods to the diet will simply increase energy intake.

The rather limited impact of reductions in the proportion of fat in the diet on body weight is in contrast with the effect of increases in protein, where the community data is generally stronger than derived from the laboratory studies described previously. In observational studies of food intake over a 9-day period, dietary protein was the most efficient macronutrient at suppressing subsequent intake, independent of its contribution to net energy intake (62). In a larger study of 160 women with 16 days of weighed food records over a 1-year period the energy consumed as protein was inversely related to total energy intake (63). Most convincingly, in a dietary intervention study for the treatment of obesity two groups were randomized to a 30% fat diet. A high protein group consumed 25% energy as protein and 45% energy as carbohydrate, whilst a high carbohydrate group consumed 12% as protein and 58% as carbohydrate. Over a 6-month period the mean weight loss in the high protein group was

8.9 kg compared to only 5.1 kg in the high carbohydrate group ($P < 0.0001$) (64). The principal mechanism of this effect appeared to be a greater reduction in overall energy intake in the high protein group, which would be consistent with increased satiety reported previously following high protein preloads. However, further research is required to assess the long-term impact of high protein diets on morbidity and mortality before high protein diets can be considered as a viable public health intervention for the control of macronutrient balance and body weight.

CONCLUSIONS

There is clear evidence of physiological processes that regulate macronutrient balance in humans. However, the continuing rise in obesity suggests that these processes are also readily over-ridden. Specifically dietary fat is associated with passive over-consumption as a consequence of its relatively high energy density and weak effects on both satiation and satiety. Moreover dietary fat does not stimulate its own oxidation and its submissive position in the oxidative hierarchy ensures its preferential storage over and above carbohydrate, thus minimizing the potential for oxidative feedback signals.

The seemingly logical extension of this physiological regulation of macronutrient balance would imply that strategies to decrease dietary fat would be associated with successful weight control and possibly weight loss. However, the key question is whether the macronutrient-specific effects on appetite are sufficient to promote a decrease in energy intake in the face of other physiological mechanisms designed to maintain body weight and energy balance. The lesser effects of macronutrient manipulations seen in overt interventions, versus covert studies, suggest that potent cognitive factors are at work which are able to overcome the physiological differences between macronutrients in the control of body weight. Reductions in dietary fat may reduce the risk of passive over-consumption, but will do nothing to limit active over-consumption.

In spite of significant differences between macronutrients in digestion, oxidation, storage and appetite control the physiological regulation of macronutrient balance is at best only one aspect of the aetiology of obesity and its effective management.

REFERENCES

1. Southgate DAT, Durning JVGA. Calorie conversion factors: an experimental reassessment of the factors used in the calculation of the energy value of human diets. Br J Nutr 1970; 24: 517–535.
2. Swaminathan R, King RFGJ, Holmfiled J et al. Thermic effect of feeding carbohydrate, fat, protein and mixed meal in lean and obese subjects. Am J Clin Nutr 1985; 42: 177–181.
3. Shetty PS, Prentice AM, Goldberg GR et al. Alterations in fuel selection and voluntary food intake in response to isoenergetic manipulation of glycogen stores in humans. Am J Clin Nutr 1994; 60: 534–543.
4. Thomas CD, Peters JC, Reed GW et al. Nutrient balance and energy expenditure during ad libitum feeding of high fat and high-carbohydrate diets in humans. Am J Clin Nutr 1992; 55: 934–942.
5. Westerterp KR, Wilson SAJ, Rolland V. Diet induced thermogenesis measured over 24h in a respiration chamber: effect of diet composition. Int J Obes 1999; 23: 287–292.
6. Sonko BJ, Prentice AM, Murgatroyd PR, Goldberg GR, van de Ven MLHM, Coward WA. Effect of alcohol on post-meal fat storage. Am J Clin Nutr 1994; 59: 619–625.
7. Flatt J-P. The difference in storage capacities for carbohydrate and for fat and its implications for the regulation of body weight. Ann N Y Acad Sci 1987; 499: 104–123.
8. Bingham S, Cummings J. Urine nitrogen as an independent validatory measure of dietary intake: a study of nitrogen balance in individuals consuming their normal diet. Am J Clin Nutr 1985; 42: 1276–1289.
9. Jebb SA, Prentice AM, Goldberg GR, Murgatroyd PR, Black AE, Coward WA. Changes in macronutrient balance during over- and under-nutrition assessed by 12-d continuous whole-body calorimetry. Am J Clin Nutr 1996; 64: 259–266.
10. McNeill G, Morrison DC, Davidson L, Smith JS. The effect of changes in dietary carbohydrate v. fat intake on 24-h energy expenditure and nutrient oxidation in post-menopausal women. Proc Nutr Soc 1992; 51: 91A.
11. McDevitt RM, Poppitt SD, Murgatroyd PR, Prentice AM. Macronutrient disposal during controlled overfeeding by glucose, fructose, sucrose or fat in lean and obese women. Am J Clin Nutr 2000; 72: 369–377.
12. Blaxter K. Energy Metabolism in Animals and Man. Cambridge: Cambridge University Press, 1989.
13. Hellerstein MK, Christiansen M, Kaempler S et al. Measurement of de novo hepatic lipogensis in humans stable isotopes. J Clin Investi 1991; 87: 1841–1852.
14. Acheson KJ, Schutz Y, Bessard T, Anantharaman K, Flatt J-P, Jequier E. Glycogen storage capacity and de novo lipogenesis during massive carbohydrate overfeeding in man. Am J Clin Nutr 1988; 48: 240–247.
15. Rolls BJ, Hetherington M, Burley VJ. The specificity of satiety: the influence of different macronutrient contents on the development of satiety. Physiol Behav 1988; 43: 145–153.
16. Hill AJ, Blundell JE. Comparison of the action of macronutrients on the expression of appetite in lean and obese humans. Ann N Y Acad Sci 1990; 597: 529–531.
17. Barkeling B, Rossner S, Bjorvell H. Effects of a high protein meal (meat) and a high-carbohydrate meal (vegetarian) on

satiety measured by automated computerised monitoring of subsequent food intake, motivation to eat and food preferences. *Int J Obes* 1990; **14**: 743–751.

18. Stubbs RJ, Wyk MCWV, Johnstone AM, Harbron CG. Breakfasts high in protein, fat or carbohydrate: effect on within-day appetite and energy balance. *Eur J Clin Nutr* 1996; **50**: 409–417.

19. Johnstone A, Stubbs R, Harbron C. Effect of overfeeding macronutrients on day-to-day food intake in man. *Eur J Clin Nutr* 1996; **50**: 418–430.

20. Blundell J, Burley V, Cotton J, Lawton C. Dietary fat and the control of energy intake: evaluating the effects of fat on meal size and postmeal satiety. *Am J Clin Nutr* 1993; **57**: 772S–778S.

21. Rolls B, Kim S, McNelis A, Fischma M, Foltin R, Moran T. Time course of effects of preloads high in fat or carbohydrate on food intake and hunger ratings in humans. *Am J Physiol* 1991; **260**: R756–R763.

22. de Graaf C, Hulshof T, Westrate J, Jas P. Short-term effects of different amounts of protein, fats and carbohydrates on satiety. *Am J Clin Nutr* 1992; **55**: 33–38.

23. Shide D, Rolls B. Information about the fat content of preloads influences energy intake in healthy women. *J Am Dietet Assoc* 1995; **95**: 993–998.

24. Lowe M, Whitlow J, Bellwoar V. Eating regulation: the role of restraint, dieting and weight. *Int J Eating Disord* 1991; **10**: 461–471.

25. Astrup A, Western P, Toubro S, Raben A, Buemann B, Christensen NJ. Obesity as an adaptation to a high fat diet: evidence from a cross-sectional study. *Am J Clin Nutr* 1994; **59**: 350–355.

26. Goldberg GR, Murgatroyd PR, Mckenna APM, Heavey PM, Prentice AM. Dietary compensation in response to covert imposition of negative energy balance by removal of fat or carbohydrate. *Br J Nutr* 1998; **80**: 141–147.

27. Friedman MI. Fuel partitioning and food intake. *Am J Clin Nutr* 1998; **67**(Suppl): 513S–538S.

28. Jebb SA, Elia M. Techniques for the measurement of body composition: a practical guide. *Int J Obes* 1993; **17**: 611–621.

29. Stubbs RJ, Harbron CG, Murgatroyd PR, Prentice AM. Covert manipulation of dietary fat and energy density: effect on substrate flux and food intake in men eating ad libitum. *Am J Clin Nutr* 1995; **62**: 316–329.

30. Stubbs RJ, Ritz P, Coward WA, Prentice AM. Covert manipulation of the ratio of dietary fat to carbohydrate and energy density: effect on food intake and energy balance in free-living men eating ad libitum. *Am J Clin Nutr* 1995; **62**: 330–337.

31. Lissner L, Levitsky DA, Strupp BJ, Kalkwarf JJ, Roe DA. Dietary fat and the regulation of energy intake in human subjects. *Am J Clin Nutr* 1987; **46**: 886–892.

32. Murgatroyd PR, Goldberg, GR, Leahy FE, Gilsenan MB, Prentice AM. Effects of inactivity and diet composition on human energy balance. *Int J Obes* 1999; **23**: 1269–1275.

33. Lissner L, Heitmann BL, Bengtsson C. Low-fat diets may prevent weight gain in sedentary women: Prospective observations from the Population Study of Women in Gothenburg, Sweden. *Obes Res* 1997; **5**: 43–48.

34. Poppitt SD, Murgatroyd PR, Tanish KR, Prentice AM. Effect of dexfenfluramine on energy and macronutrient balance on high-fat and low-fat diets. *Int J Obes* 1997; **21**: 197.

35. Stratum PV, Lussenburg R, van Wezel L, Vergroesen A, Cremer H. The effect of dietary carbohydrate:fat ratio on energy intake by adult women. *Am J Clin Nutr* 1978; **31**: 206–212.

36. Stubbs RJ, Harbron CG, Prentice AM. Covert manipulation of the dietary fat to carbohydrate ratio of isoenergetically dense diets: effect on food intake in feeding men ad libitum. *Int J Obes* 1996; **20**: 651–660.

37. Poppitt SD, Prentice AM. Energy density and its role in the control of food intake: Evidence from metabolic and community studies. *Appetite* 1996; **26**: 153–174.

38. Anderson GH. Sugars, sweetness and food intake. *Am J Clin Nutr* 1995; **62**(Suppl): 195S–202S.

39. Birch LL, Johnson SL, Jones MB, Peters JC. Effects of a non-energy fat substitute on children's energy and macronutrient intake. *Am J Clin Nutr* 1993; **58**: 326–333.

40. Rolls B, Piraglia P, Jones M, Peters J. Effects of olestra, a noncaloric fat substitute, on daily energy and fat intakes in lean men. *Am J Clin Nutr* 1992; **56**: 84–92.

41. Cotton JR, Weststrate JA, Blundell JE. Replacement of dietary fat with sucrose polyester: effects on energy intake and appetite control in non-obese males. *Am J Clin Nutr* 1996; **63**: 891–896.

42. Hill JO, Seagle HM, Johnson SL et al. Effects of 14 d of covert substitution of olestra for conventional fat on spontaneous food intake. *Am J Clin Nutr* 1998; **67**: 1178–1185.

43. Katan M, Grundy S, Willett W. Beyond low-fat diets. *N Engl J Med* 1997; **337**: 563–566w.

44. Conner W, Conner S. The case for a low-fat, high carbohydrate diet. *N Engl J Med* 1997; **337**: 562–563.

45. Black H, Herd J, Goldberg L et al. Effect of a low-fat diet on the incidence of actinic keratosis. *N Engl J Med* 1994; **330**: 1272–1275.

46. Sheppard L, Kristal A, Kushi L. Weight loss in women participating in a randomised trial of low-fat diets. *Am J Clin Nutr* 1991; **54**: 821–828.

47. Hunninghake D, Stein E, Dujovne C et al. The efficacy of intensive dietary therapy alone or combined with lova-statin in outpatients with hypercholesterolemia. *N Engl J Med* 1993; **328**: 1213–1291.

48. Ornish D, Brow S, Scherwitz L et al. Can lifestyle changes reverse coronary heart disease? The Lifestyle Heart Trial. *Lancet* 1990; **336**: 129–133.

49. Singh R, Rostogi S, Verma R et al. Randomised controlled trial of cardioprotective diet in patients with recent acute myocardial infarction: results of one year follow-up. *Br Med J* 1992; **304**: 1015–1019.

50. Shah M, McGovern P, French S, Baxter J. Comparison of a low-fat, ad libitum complex-carbohydrate diet with a low-energy diet in moderately obese women. *Am J Clin Nutr* 1994; **59**: 980–984.

51. Jeffrey R, Hellerstedt W, French S, Baxter J. A randomised trial of counselling for fat restriction versus calorie restriction in the treatment of obesity. *Int J Obes* 1995; **19**: 132–137.

52. Golay A, Allaz A, Morel Y, Tonnac Nd, Tankova S, Reaven G. Similar weight loss with low or high carbohydrate diets. *Am J Clin Nutr* 1996; **63**: 174–178.

53. Lean M, Han T, Prvan T, Richmond P, Avenell S. Weight loss with high and low carbohydrate 1200 kcal diets in free living women. *Eur J Clin Nutr* 1997; **51**: 243–248.

54. Schundt D, Hill J, Pope-Cordle J, Arnold D, Virts K, Katan

M. Randomised evaluation of a low fat ad libitum carbohydrate diet for weight reduction. *Int J Obes* 1993; **17**: 623–629.

55. Toubro S, Astrup A. Randomised comparison of diets for maintaining obese subjects' weight after major weight loss: ad lib, low fat high carbohydrate diet v fixed energy intake. *BMJ* 1997; **314**: 29–34.

56. Mela D. Understanding fat preference and consumption: applications of behavioural sciences to a nutritional problem. *Proc Nutr Soc* 1995; **54**: 453–464.

57. Lloyd H, Paisley C, Mela D. Changing to a low fat diet: Attitudes and beliefs of UK consumers. *Eur J Clin Nutr* 1993; **47**: 361–373.

58. MAFF. *Household Food Consumption and Expenditure.* London: HMSO, 1940–1995.

59. Lyon X-H, Vetta VD, Milton H, Jequier E, Schutz Y. Compliance to dietary advice directed towards increasing the carbohydrate to fat ratio of the everyday diet. *Int J Obes* 1995; **19**: 260–269.

60. Black AE, Goldberg GR, Jebb SA, Livingstone MBE, Prentice AM. Critical evaluation of energy intake data using fundamental principles of energy physiology 2. Evaluating the results of dietary surveys. *Eur J Clin Nutr* 1991; **45**: 583–599.

61. Allred JB. Too much of a good thing? *J Am Diet Assoc* 1995; **95**: 417–418.

62. DeCastro J. Macronutrient relationships with meal patterns and mood in the spontaneous feeding behaviour of humans. *Physiol Behav* 1987; **39**: 561–569.

63. Bingham SA, Gill C, Welch A *et al.* Comparison of dietary assessment methods in nutritional epidemiology: weighed records vs 24-h recalls, food frequency questionnaires and estimated diet records. *Br J Nutr* 1994; **72**: 619–643.

64. Skov AR, Toubro S, Ronn B, Holm L, Astrup A. Randomised trial on protein vs carbohydrate in ad libitum fat reduced diet for the treatment of obesity. *Int J Obes* 1999; **23**: 528–536.

10

Fat in the Diet and Obesity

Berit Lilienthal Heitmann[1] and Lauren Lissner[2]

[1]Glostrup and Copenhagen University Hospital, Copenhagen, Denmark and [2]Department of Community Medicine, Göteborg Univesity Hospital, Göteborg, Sweden

TRENDS IN FAT INTAKE

During recent decades, trends of declining fat intake have been reported for most countries. However, both diet surveys and food disappearance data suggest that for most countries, fat intake is still above the recommended 30% of total energy. Countries like the USA and Norway have reported particular success in reduction of dietary fat intake (1,2). In the USA, for instance, a reduction in energy from fat from about 40% to 33% was achieved between 1960 and 1995 (1). In Norway, fat intake was reduced from 40% to 34% in only 15 years (2), making Norwegians a role model for the other Nordic countries, where a high fat consumption is the tradition. Finland (3) has followed this trend, and now reports patterns of decreasing fat intake similar to those in the USA and Norway. However, some countries, like Denmark and Sweden, still displayed intake figures for fat consumption as high as 39–43% until the late 1980s, and only recently have decreases been reported (4–6).

INCONSISTENT TRENDS IN OBESITY AND FAT INTAKE

Although trends in fat intake have been found to correlate closely with trends in cardiovascular disease, several studies have demonstrated that obesity is increasing at the same time that fat intake is decreasing (7). In fact, some of the countries that have experienced a substantial decrease in fat intake have noted the most dramatic increases in obesity prevalences. In Finland, for instance, prevalence of obesity rose from 10% to 14% in men and from 10% to 11% in women between the late 1970s and early 1990s (8) while at the same time fat intake decreased from approximately 38% to 34% (3). In the USA, data from the National Health and Nutrition Examination Survey (NHANES) show that while fat intake was decreasing, prevalences of severe obesity increased from 10% to 20% in men and from 15% to 25% in women (9). Although the possibility of ecological fallacy must be considered when interpreting such results, it cannot be excluded that the secular trends in obesity may have been even more dramatic if not for the decrease in fat intake.

Figure 10.1 shows trends in fat intake and obesity among adult Americans (9,10).

There are at least three interpretations for this paradox of opposite trends for fat intake and obesity. One is that people are decreasing their energy intake but also becoming less active. Another is that people are maintaining their energy intake despite the reduction in fat intake. A third explanation, is that fat intakes are not as low as reported. With regard to the first alternative, data from England have implicated sedentary activity as the most plausible explanation. For instance, trends in number of cars, or number of televisions per household, were more closely associated with the dramatic increase in severe obesity seen in England

International Textbook of Obesity. Edited by Per Björntorp.
© 2001 John Wiley & Sons, Ltd.

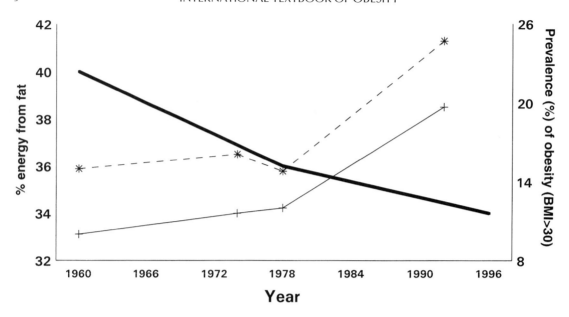

Figure 10.1 Trends in fat intake and obesity among adult Americans. Bold line, fat intake; +, obese men; *, obese women

over the past two decades, than were trends in fat or energy intake (11). With regard to the second alternative, it has been suggested that total energy may well remain high, despite the proliferation of low fat products on the market. This may be due to the misperception that low fat products can be consumed without restraint (12). Finally, with regard to the third alternative, social desirability bias may cause people increasingly to report false low fat intakes, as official recommendations and public health campaigns to reduce fat intake are intensified and disseminated.

BIAS IN DIET SURVEYS

In dietary surveys, there is a great potential for bias deriving from a tendency for obese subjects to underreport their food intake to a greater extent than normal weight individuals (13,14). In addition, it was recently demonstrated that the obese underreport total energy more than energy from protein, suggesting that the other energy-yielding nutrients must have been underreported disproportionately (15) (Figure 10.2). This is in general agreement with the assumption that obese individuals underreport socially undesirable foods such as those rich in fat and/or simple carbohydrate. The consequence of both specific and non-specific underreporting by

the obese is that the diet–obesity and diet–health associations may be distorted (16). In addition, diet–obesity associations found in dietary surveys may not reflect those found in the general population, since non-responders generally are more likely to be obese, more likely to be smokers, more likely to have a low educational level (17), and may have a different dietary consumption pattern than responders. Finally, older food databases may not sufficiently capture nutrient composition of these new low fat products, and hence, add to the creation of biased diet–obesity relationships.

EVIDENCE LINKING FAT TO OBESITY

Cross-sectional evidence from studies linking intake data to degree of obesity clearly suggests that dietary fat is associated with overweight. In a recent review, Lissner and Heitmann (18) found that in more than 80% of the cross-sectional studies reviewed, dietary fat intake was associated with obesity. The diet of obese subjects has been found to contain 5–8% more fat than the diet of the normal weight control groups (19), and this is likely to be a conservative estimate if obesity-related underreporting of fat occurs. Furthermore, most experimental studies provide evidence that, compared to a covert low fat diet, spontaneous energy intake is

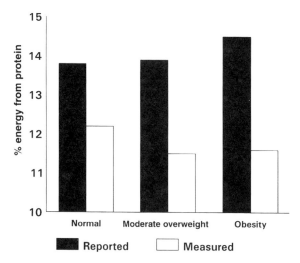

Figure 10.2 Reported and measured energy from protein among normal weight (BMI <25), moderately overweight (BMI 25–30) and obese (BMI >30) Danish men and women

Table 10.1 Evidence linking fat intake to obesity

The evidence for:

- The majority of cross-sectional surveys display a positive association between fat intake and obesity.
- These associations are likely to be underestimated due to social desirability biases
- Experimental studies suggest that spontaneous energy intake is increased following ingestion of a high fat meal compared to a low fat meal.
- Randomized short-term dietary intervention trials show weight loss, although modest, on calorically unrestricted low fat diets.
- Animal experiments show obesity development in rats fed equi-caloric high fat diets, compared to low fat diets

The evidence against:

- Secular trends for fat intake and obesity are in opposite directions in most countries.
- Inconsistent results from prospective observational studies linking fat intake to subsequent weight gain.
- No long-term clinical trials have supported promotion of weight gain from high fat hyperphagia.
- Experimental studies with equalization of energy density suggest the fat content per se is unrelated to subsequent energy intake.

increased following ingestion of a high fat diet (20–22). In addition, a number of studies have suggested that appetite control is dissociated from fat since energy intake of a subsequent meal was not suppressed by adding up to 60 g fat (2.3 MJ) to the previous meal (for review see Astrup and Raben (19)). Likewise, one study demonstrated that 2-year maintenance of weight loss was more successful on an *ad libitum* low fat diet than on calorie counting (23). Finally, randomized dietary fat intervention studies consistently show that weight is lost on a calorically unrestricted low fat diet, although rates of weight loss per day are modest (ranges between 17 g and 37 g per day) (18).

The specific mechanism for dietary fat in obesity development is generally believed to depend on passive over-consumption on the high fat diet, due mainly to its high energy density and also palatability related factors. However, the effect is likely to vary under different circumstances. For instance, fat intake has been reported to predict weight gain in sedentary, but not inactive women, suggesting that certain subgroups of the population may be particularly sensitive to over-consumption of a high fat diet (24). The hypothesis that genetic factors determine the identity of fat-sensitive individuals will be discussed in more detail later.

A possible energy independent effect of the fat related to a lower satiating power has also been suggested (25,26). Oscai *et al.* (27) demonstrated

that rats developed obesity when fed fat-rich, but not low fat equi-caloric diets. Other mechanisms include a particular storage preference (28) and/or a lower thermic effect of fat compared to carbohydrate (29) or protein. Proposed mechanisms linking fat to obesity development are given in Table 10.1 (29).

EVIDENCE UN-LINKING FAT FROM OBESITY

A number of observational studies have suggested that the role of fat in obesity development may be exaggerated, and suggest that the population differences in weight do not appear to be due primarily to the fat intake (30). For instance, in a recent literature review, it was found that short-term hypophagia on low fat diets is compensated in the longer term (18). A report from the National Centre for Health Statistics has shown that Americans today eat less fat but more calories than earlier, a finding that may explain the rise in obesity, but acquits the role of fat (31). In addition, results from prospective observational studies give inconsistent results, and do not support the relation between a high fat intake and subsequent weight gain. Klesges *et al.* (32), for instance, found a clear positive association between dietary fat and subsequent weight changes, while Colditz *et al.* (33), using the same dietary instrument, and Kant *et al.* (34), using a different instrument, could not find such an association. Other studies have also shown inconsistent results (35–37). Indeed, Katan (38) recently reviewed the literature on long-term fat trials, and found that low fat diets in these trials had resulted in decreases in body weight of only 0.4–2.6 kg relative to control diets. Based on this, he concluded that the evidence from the long-term trials could not support the idea that a high proportion of fat in the diet could be responsible for the 10–15 kg weight gain that people in affluent societies experienced between adolescence and middle age.

Results from feeding studies in humans, with covert manipulation of energy density in the diet, suggest that increase in the fat content does not result in an increase in energy intake, when density is constant (39). Also Stubbs *et al.* (40,41) manipulated macronutrient intake in iso-caloric diets and found that the energy density of the diet was dissociated from the fat content, since spontaneous energy intake remained unchanged as the fat increased from 20% to 60%.

In experimental animals, Ramirez and Friedman (42) demonstrated that increasing the energy density of the chow food led to an increase in energy intake, but did not affect the weight of the food eaten. Results like these suggest that fat is only less satiating than carbohydrate if the energy density is tied to the fat content, and hence, challenge the specific role that has been attributed to fat in obesity development. Rather, results like these imply that it is the bulk, or the weight, of food that controls satiety. Indeed, Westerterp *et al.* (43) recently demonstrated that change in the fat content of the diet resulted in change in body composition only when energy intake was simultaneously changed, and several studies have found the weight of food eaten to be more constant than daily energy intake (20,22,44). Hence, an increasing energy density may result in passive over-consumption only because individuals habitually eat a constant weight of food per day (40,41).

Finally, it has been suggested that the benefits of decreasing the density of one meal, by removing selected high fat items from the diet, may be compensated by the inclusion of high fat items in a later meal (45). On the other hand, this leaves a greater potential for diluting diets, for instance with fibre. In fact, it may be argued that the benefits of a low fat diet with regard to obesity may depend not on the low fat per se, but on the accopanying high fibre content (Table 10.1).

A SPECIFIC ROLE FOR GENES?

Genetic susceptibility for weight gain may be influenced by dietary factors, such as fat intake (46). Indeed, a few studies have indicated that development of obesity is, in part, due to differential effects of fat in the diet for those who are genetically predisposed, compared to those who are not (47–49). In this context, studies in both animals and humans have demonstrated that food intake seems to play a specific role for obesity development in association with a predisposition to obesity (37,50,51). For instance, Sclefani and Assimon (52) found that obesity prone mice ate more high fat, but less sugar-rich foods than leanness prone mice. In addition, obesity prone mice have been found to gain weight at a much faster rate than wild-type mice fed the same high fat diets (50), suggesting a gene–environment interaction between the high fat diet and the subsequent weight gain. Furthermore, compared to non-obese controls, impaired ability to increase the fat/carbohydrate oxidation ratio in response to a high fat diet has been suggested in post-obese women (51), implying that this obesity prone group is particularly susceptible to weight gain on such a diet. Although not all studies have been able to document gene–environment interactions relating a high fat intake to weight gain (53,54), a study using identical twins found that weight gain in response to controlled overfeeding was more similar within identical twin pairs than between pairs of twins, suggesting a specific genetic influence (47). Finally, the specific role of fat in obesity development may be restricted to those who are predisposed, only. This was the case in one study where women with a familial history of obesity had a stronger risk of major weight gain compared to women without such a predisposition, when consuming a high fat diet (37).

Several genes have been proposed, for instance

Table 10.2 Evidence for and against a genetic component

- Obesity prone mice have been found to prefer high fat diets.
- Weight gain in obesity prone mice is higher than in wild type mice fed the same high fat diets
- Subjects with a familial predisposition to obesity seem to have an impaired ability to increase the fat/carbohydrate oxidation ratio in response to a high fat diet.
- One study found that women with a familial history of obesity had a stronger risk of dietary fat-related weight gain compared to women without such a predisposition.
- Two studies found no evidence of a genetic predisposition for dietary fat-related weight gain.

the family of uncoupling proteins, apparently used by cells to convert excess calories to heat. These may provide insight into identifying subjects predisposed for obesity, since this gene is thought to be involved in overall metabolic rate. It may be that rodents with this gene have the ability to burn off excess calories, while animals without the gene store the extra calories. Furthermore, the gene seems to be activated by dietary fat, and the fat intake seems to play a differential role for activation of the gene in different strains of mice (55).

Lean and obese/obesity prone individuals seem to vary in their response to fat manipulation, since obese individuals have been found to compensate less well than lean unrestrained individuals for energy intake in response to preloads of varying energy densities (56). Furthermore, not only do obese subjects generally report liking high fat foods more so than lean subjects (57,58) they also may not be as sensitive to the satiety value of fat as lean subjects (20,59). Indeed, the literature suggests that the selection of macronutrients is, in part, heritable (60). For instance, obese rodents have been found to avoid sweets compared to their lean littermates, and genus that mediate the consumption of sugar have been mapped, and are being isolated and characterized. For sweet taste preference, major gene effects have been described, mapping studies of genetic loci have been published, and single-gene mutants have been discovered. However, only a few studies have assessed the role of genetic variability in dietary fat preference, but so far no genes have been characterized (60,61). In addition, it has been proposed that the development of obesity may be viewed as a regulatory mechanism by which the impaired lipid oxidation rate in the body is raised to match the dietary fat intake (27). This capacity to increase lipid oxidation after consumption of a high fat diet may vary greatly among individuals, and may depend on both physiological and genetic factors.

Finally, the genetically determined ability to taste bitter substances relates to obesity and may also be associated to fat preferences. Obese subjects are less sensitive to the bitterness of phenylthiocarbamide, and hence, the gene that determines this bitter taste polymorphism may either have effects on both dietary fat perception and body weight, or be linked to genes contributing to these phenotypes (60) (Table 10.2).

CONCLUSION

In summary, the epidemiological evidence linking fat intake to obesity must be considered together with evidence that obese individuals underreport food intake in general, and may underreport fat intake in particular. Such reporting biases would imply that studies finding that obese individuals consume more dietary fat than non-obese are likely to have underestimated the difference in intake. Furthermore, these reporting biases may distort the fat–obesity associations in unpredicable ways, creating both spurious and conservative associations (16,62). However, obesity related social desirability bias may not explain the opposing secular trends between fat intake and obesity prevalence at the population level, since these recent dietary trends are often based on aggregate-level food disappearance data, rather than reported diets.

Although the available epidemiologal studies indicate that dietary fat does not play the leading aetiological role in the epidemic of obesity, the likelihood that the data are systematically biased makes it impossible to speculate on the true magnitude of any such effect. Thus, methodological constraints necessitate cautious interpretations of epidemiological data. However, the evidence from experimental research, linking fat intake to obesity, seems to suggest that energy density, and not fat intake, is the most likely mechanism here. However, the distinction between fat and energy density is somewhat artificial, since these dietary properties tend to be parallel.

Although the role of restricting dietary fat has been advocated in both prevention and treatment for obesity for a number of years, the data available today suggest that dietary fat is probably one small part of a multifactorial aetiology. In this regard, there is some evidence that a low fat diet may be protective to specific subgroups of the population, and hence, be more relevant to obesity in a preventive than a treatment perspective. One such group may be subjects with a propensity to weight gain, who may be identified by their familial clustering of obesity. Another group may include the physically inactive, who could benefit from an extra margin of safety provided by a low fat diet in protection against positive energy balance. Other subgroups who might benefit are ex-smokers, during the initial quitting period, and consumers who are able to use fat-reduced products in a rational way. However, it must be kept in mind that low fat diets offer no panacea, since individuals with a predisposdition for overeating appear to learn how to do so, even on fat-reduced diets.

In conclusion, focusing on total fat intake may be beneficial to some individuals, but should not remove the focus from total energy balance. The vast amount of studies on dietary fat intake and obesity may have created a misperception that as long as a food is low in fat, there is no limit to the amount that can be consumed without gaining weight.

REFERENCES

1. Department of Agriculture, Agricultural Research Service. Data tables: results from USDA's 1995 continuing survey: CSFI/DHKS 1995. Riverdale, Md.: Food Surveys Research Group, 1995 (CD-ROM).
2. Johansson L, Drevon CA, Bjørneboe GEA. The Norwegian diet during the last hundred years in relation to coronary heart disease. *Eur J Clin Nutr* 1996; **50**: 277–283.
3. Fogelholm M, Männistö S, Vartiainen E, Pietinen P. Determinants of energy balance and overweight in Finland 1982 and 1992. *Int J Obes* 1996; **20**: 1097–1104.
4. Osler M, Heitmann BL. Food patterns associated with intakes of fat, carbohydrate and dietary fibre in a cohort of Danish adults followed for six years. *Eur J Clin Nutr* 1997; **51**: 354–361.
5. *Journal of Agricultural Economics* (ed. Löfdahl E) 1996; **58**: 303–305.
6. Levnedsmiddelstyrelsen. *Danskernes kostvaner 1995 – Hovedresultater*. Dept of Health, 1996: 235.
7. Katan MB, Grundy SM, Willett WC. Beyond low fat diets. *N Engl J Med* 1997; **337**: 563–566.
8. Seidell JS, Rissanen AM. Time trends in the worldwide prevalence of obesity. In: Bray GA, Bouchard C, James WPT (eds) *Handbook of Obesity*. New York: Marcel Dekker, 1998: 79–91.
9. WHO. Obesity-preventing and managing the global epidemic. Report of a WHO Consultation on Obesity, Geneva, 3–5 June 1997. WHO publications: Geneva, 1997.
10. Americans eat less fat, more calories. *Morbidity and Mortality Weekly Report*. CDC, 1994.
11. Prentice AM, Jebb SA. Obesity in Britain: gluttony or sloth? *BMJ* 1995; **311**: 437–439.
12. Rolls BJ, Miller DL. Is the low-fat message giving people a license to eat more? *J Am Coll Nutr* 1997; **16**: 535–543.
13. Black AE, Goldberg GR, Jebb SA *et al*. Critical evaluation of energy intake data using fundamental principles of energy physiology. 2. Evaluating the results of published surveys. *Eur J Clin Nutr* 1991; **45**: 583–599.
14. Heitmann BL. The influence of fatness, weight change, slimming history and other lifestyle variables on diet reporting in Danish men and women aged 35–65 years. *Int J Obes* 1993; **17**: 329–336.
15. Heitmann BL, Lissner L. Dietary underreporting by obese individuals—is it specific or non-specific? *BMJ* 1995; **311**: 986–989.
16. Lissner L, Heitmann BL, Lindroos AK. Measuring intake in free-living human subjects: a question of bias. *Proc Nutr Soc* 1998; **57**: 1–8.
17. Price GM, Paul AA, Cole TJ. Nonresponders in a prospective national survey in the United Kingdom. *Am J Clin Nutr* 1997; **65**(suppl): 1341S–1342S.
18. Lissner L, Heitmann BL. Dietary fat and obesity: evidence from epidemiology. *Eur J Clin Nutr* 1995; **49**: 79–90.
19. Astrup A, Raben A. Obesity: an inherited metabolic deficiency in the control of macronutrient balance? *Eur J Clin Nutr* 1992; **46**: 611–620.
20. Lissner L, Levitsky DA, Strupp BJ, Kalfwarf HJ, Roe DA. Dietary fat and the regulation of energy intake in human subjects. *Am J Clin Nutr* 1987; **46**: 886–892.
21. Kendall A, Levitsky DA, Strupp BJ, Lissner L. Weight loss on a low-fat diet: consequence of the imprecision of the control of food intake in humans. *Am J Clin Nutr* 1991; **53**: 1124–1129.
22. Tremblay A, Lavallee N, Aæmeras N, Allard L, Despres J, Bouchard C. Nutritional determinants of the increase in energy intake associated with a high-fat diet. *Am J Clin Nutr* 1991; **53**: 1134–1137.
23. Toubro S, Astrup A. Randomised comparison of diets for maintaining obese subject's weight after major weight loss: ad lib, low fat, high carbohydrate diet *v* fixed energy intake. *BMJ* 1997; **314**: 29–34.
24. Lissner L, Heitmann BL, Bengtsson C. Low-fat diets may prevent weight gain in sedentary women: prospective observations from the population study of women in Gothenburg, Sweden. *Obes Res* 1997; **5**: 43–48.
25. Blundell JE, Burley VJ, Cotton JR, Lawton CL. Dietary fat and the control of energy intake: evaluating the effects of fat on meal size and postmeal satiety. *Am J Clin Nutr* 1993; **57**: 7772–7778.
26. van Amelsvoort JMM, van Stratum P, Kraal JH, Lussenburg RN, Houtsmuller UMT. Effects of varying the carbohydrate:fat ratio in a hot lunch on postprandial variables in male volunteers. *Br J Nutr* 1989; **61**: 267–283.
27. Oscai LB, Brown MM, Miller WC. Effect on dietary fat on food intake, growth and body composition in rats. *Growth* 1984; **48**: 415–424.
28. Flatt JP. The difference in the storage capacities for carbohy-

drate and for fat, and its implications in the regulation of body weight. *Ann N Y Acad Sci* 1987; **499**: 104–123.

29. Lean MEJ, James PT. Metabolic effects of isoenergetic nutrient exchange over 24 years in relation to obesity in women. *Int J Obes* 1988; **12**: 15–27.

30. Lissner L, Heitmann BL. The dietary fat:carbohydrate ratio in relation to body weight. *Current Opinion in Lipidology* 1995; **6**: 8–13.

31. Allred JB. Too much of a good thing? *J Am Diet Assoc* 1995; **95**: 417–418.

32. Klesges RC, Klesges LM, Haddock CK, Eck LH. A longitudinal analysis of the impact of dietary intake and physical activity on weight change in adults. *Am J Clin Nutr* 1992; **55**: 818–822.

33. Colditz GA, Willett WC, Stampfer MJ, London SJ, Segal MR, Speizer FE. Patterns of weight change and their relation to diet in a cohort of healthy women. *Am J Clin Nutr* 1990; **51**: 1100–1105.

34. Kant AK, Graubard BI, Schatzkin A, Ballard-barbash R. Proportion of energy intake from fat and subsequent weight change in the NHANES I Epidemiologic Follow-up Study. *Am J Clin Nutr 1995;* **61**: 11–17.

35. Rissanen AM, Heliövaara M, Knekt P, Reunanen A, Aromaa A. Determinants of weight gain and overweight in adult Finns. *Eur J Clin Nutr* 1991; **45**: 419–430.

36. Pudel V, Westenhoefer J. Dietary and behavioural principles in the treatment of obesity. International Monitor on Eating Patterns and Weight Control (Medicom/Servieer) 1992; **1**: 2–7.

37. Heitmann BL, Lissner L. Sørensen TIA, Bengtsson C. Dietary fat intake and weight gain in women genetically predisposed for obesity. *Am J Clin Nutr* 1995; **61**: 1213–1217.

38. Katan MB. High-oil compared with low-fat, high-carbohydrate diets in the prevention of ischemic heart disease. *Am J Clin Nutr* 1997; **66**(Suppl): 974S–979S.

39. van Stratum P, Lussenburg RN, van Wezel LA, Vergroesen AJ, Cremer HD. The effect of dietary carbohydrate:fat ratio on energy intake by adult women. *Am J Clin Nutr* 1978; **31**: 206–212.

40. Stubbs RJ, Harbron CG, Murgatroyd PR, Prentice AM. Covert manipulation of dietary fat and energy density: effect on substrate flux and food intake in men eating ad libitum. *Am J Clin Nutr* 1995; **62**: 316–329.

41. Stubbs RJ, Ritz P, Coward WA, Prentice AM. Covert manipulation of the ratio of dietary fat to carbohydrate and energy density: effect on food intake and energy balance in free living men, eating ad libitum. *Am J Clin Nutr* 1995: **62**: 330–337.

42. Ramirez I, Friedman MI. Dietary hyperphagia in rats: role of fat, carbohydrate and energy content. *Physiol Behav* 1990; **47**: 1157–1163.

43. Westerterp KR, Verboeket-van de Venne, WPHG, Westerterp-Plantenga MS, Velthuis-te Wierik EJM, de Graaf C, Weststrate JA. Dietary fat and body fat: an intervention study. *Int J Obes* 1996; **20**: 1022–1026.

44. Duncan KH, Bacon JA, Weinsier RL. The effects of high and low energy density diets on satiety, energy intake, and eating time of obese and nonobese subjects. *Am J Clin Nutr* 1983; **37**: 763–767.

45. Poppit SD, Prentice AM. Energy density and its role in the control of food intake: evidence from metabolic and community studies. *Appetite* 1996; **26**: 153–174.

46. Bouchard C (ed) *The Genetics of Obesity.* Boca Raton, FL: CRC Press, 1994.

47. Bouchard C, Tremblay A, Després JP, Nadeau A, Lupien PJ, Thériault G, Dussault J, Moorjani S, Pinault S, Fournier G. The response to long-term overfeeding in identical twins. *N Engl J Med* 1990; **322**: 1477–1482.

48. Price RA, Ness R, Sørensen TIA. Change in commingled body mass index distributions associated with secular trends in overweight among Danish young men. *Am J Epidemiol* 1991; **133**: 501–510.

49. Price RA, Stunkard AJ. Commingling analysis of obesity in twins. *Hum Hered* 1989; **39**: 121–135.

50. West D, Boozer CN, Moody DL, Atkinson R. Dietary obesity in nine inbred mouse strains. *Am J Physiol* 1992; **262**: R1025–1032.

51. Astrup A. Dietary composition, substrate balances and body fat in subjects with a predisposition to obesity. *Int J Obes* 1993; **17**(Suppl): S-32–36.

52. Sclefani A, Assimon SA. Influence of diet type and maternal background on dietary-obesity in the rat: A preliminary study. *Nutr Behav* 1985; **2**: 139–147.

53. Jørgensen LM, Sørensen TIA, Schroll M, Larsen S. Influence of dietary factors on weight change assessed by multivariate graphical models. *Int J Obes* 1995; **19**: 909–915.

54. Lindroos AK, Lissner L, Carlsson B, Carlsson L, Torgersson J, Karlsson C, Stenlöf K, Sjöström, L. Familial predisposition for obesity may modify the predictive value of serum leptin concentrations for long-term weight change in obese women. *Am J Clin Nutr* 1998; **67**: 1119–1123.

55. Fleury C, Neverova M, Collins S, Raimbault S, Champigny O, LeviMeyreuis C, Bouillaud F, Seldin MF, Surwitt RS, Ricquier D, Warden CH. Uncoupling protein-2: a novel gene linked to obesity and hyperinsulinemia. *Nat Gen* 1997; **15**: 269–272.

56. Rolls BJ, Pirraglia PA, Jones MB, Peters JC. Effects of olestra, a noncaloric fat substitute, on daily energy and fat intakes in lean men. *Am J Clin Nutr* 1992; **56**: 84–92.

57. Drewnowski A, Kurth C, Holden-Wiltse J, Saari J. Food preferences in human obesity: carbohydrates versus fats. *Appetite* 1992; **18**: 207–221.

58. Mela DJ, Sacchetti DA. Sensory preferences for fats: relationships with diet and body composition. *Am J Clin Nutr* 1991; **53**: 908–915.

59. Rolls BJ, Kim-Harris S, Fischman MW, Foltin RW, Moran TH, Stoner SA. Satiety after preloads with different amounts of fat and carbohydrate: implications for obesity. *Am J Clin Nutr* 1994; **60**: 476–487.

60. Reed DR, Bachmanov AA, Beauchamp GK, Tordoff MG, Price RA. Heritable variation in food preferences and their contribution to obesity. *Behav Genet* 1997; **27**: 373–884.

61. Smith BK, West DB, York DA. Carbohydrate vs fat preference: evidence of differing patterns of macronutrient selection in two inbred mouse strains. *Obes Res* 1995; **3**(Suppl 3): 411s–411s.

62. Heitmann BL. Social desirability bias in dietary self-report may compromise the validity of dietary intake measures. Implications for diet disease relationships. *Int J Epidemiol* 1996; **25**: 222–223.

11

Energy Expenditure at Rest and During Exercise

Björn Ekblom

Karolinska Institute, Stockholm, Sweden

ENERGY METABOLISM

Alactacid Energy Metabolism—Adenosine Triphosphate

The immediate source for muscle contraction is delivered from splitting of adenosine triphosphate (ATP) to adenosine diphosphate (ADP) and a 'free' phosphate ion (P). This reaction is very fast and does not normally limit energy turnover and muscle performance. However, the ATP stores in the muscles are very limited. The whole ATP pool would be emptied in only a few seconds of muscle contraction. Therefore ATP has to be continuously regenerated through other energy systems.

These supporting energy systems are very effective and can keep the ATP concentration unchanged or only marginally lowered, even during heavy exercise. In essence, there are four such systems, with different speeds of reaction and capacities, which release energy for active phosphorylation of ADP to restore the ATP pool. They are (1) creative phosphate, (2) lactacid anaerobic metabolism, (3) aerobic metabolism and (4) adenylate kinase reactions.

Creatine Phosphate

The most immediate energy system to restore ATP from rephosphorylation of ADP is creatine phosphate (CrP). CrP is stored in the muscle for immediate use, but it can also be regarded as an energy transport system between the mitochondria and the myofibrillar system as well as an 'energy buffer' for phosphorylation of ATP, when the capacity and speed of the other energy regeneration systems cannot keep up with an acceptable ATP concentration in the myofibrillar system. Phosphorylation of ADP from CrP (CrP + ADP to Cr + ATP) is fast. The total CrP pool can be used up by several seconds of heavy exercise.

At rest and during light submaximal exercise the CrP concentration is not different from resting concentration due to continuous rephosphorylation of Cr in the mitochondria. During normal dynamic heavy exercise the CrP pool may be lowered to 50% or less of resting and completely emptied during extreme exercise conditions.

The amount of CrP in the muscle as well as ATP and ADP concentrations can only be measured by sophisticated laboratory methods.

Lactacid Anaerobic Metabolism

In this energy pathway the chemically bound energy in carbohydrates, mainly muscle glycogen, can be utilized for ATP regeneration during stepwise degradation of glycogen or glucose to lactate (Hla) and hydrogen ions. No oxygen is used. This reaction is fairly fast but normally limited by the

International Textbook of Obesity. Edited by Per Björntorp.
© 2001 John Wiley & Sons, Ltd.

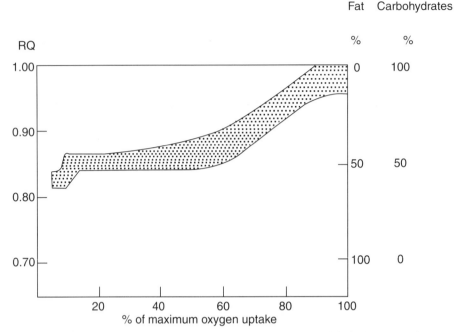

Figure 11.1   Metabolism of fat and carbohydrate at rest and during submaximal exercise, and during heavy exercise

formation of hydrogen ions which decrease the muscle pH and impair muscle performance in several ways.

If muscle glycogen stores are more or less empty this anaerobic energy system is impaired due to the reduced substrate availability. For each molecule of glucose or glycogen two and three ATP, respectively, are formed. This energy system is activated only during heavy exercise. Measurements of lactate concentration in blood are only able to indicate a qualitative involvement of this anaerobic energy system during physical stress. It is not possible to make quantitative calculations of the lactacid anaerobic energy yield during exercise from measurements of lactate concentrations in the blood due to dilution and transport of lactate in different water compartments in the body, elimination of lactate in the metabolism and other factors.

Aerobic Metabolism

Quantitatively the most important energy system during exercise is the breakdown and splitting of the energy-rich fat and carbohydrate molecules. Fat is stored in large amounts in fat cells all over the body but also in the muscle, which is very important. Glucose is stored as glycogen in the liver and muscles. Small but important amounts of glucose are also found in the plasma.

During aerobic conditions—when oxygen is available at the site of the mitochondria—fatty acids and glucose in combination are metabolized to carbon dioxide and water. For each molecule of glucose 38 or 39 ATP can be formed depending on whether glucose or glycogen is the substrate. For each fatty acid about 130 ATP can be formed. The latter figure varies depending on the type of fatty acid that is metabolized.

Since oxygen is a prerequisite for this reaction it is possible to calculate how much energy has been converted at rest and during exercise by measuring oxygen consumption. This is done at the level of pulmonary ventilation—see below. When fatty acids are used as substrate 19.3 kJ (4.7 kcal) is transformed for each litre of oxygen used. Corresponding value for glucose is 21.0 kJ (5.0 kcal) and for protein 18.8 kJ (4.5 kcal). However, for most calculations of energy expenditure at rest and during exercise a figure of 21 kJ (5 kcal) for each litre of oxygen can be used.

Respiratory quotient (RQ) is the volume of carbon dioxide formed divided by the volume of oxygen used—for measurements see below. Since fat oxidation has a RQ of 0.7 and glucose 1.0 it is possible using RQ determinations to evaluate the relative contribution of fat and carbohydrate, respectively, in energy metabolism. At rest and during submaximal exercise RQ is normally about 0.80 to 0.85 and reaches 1.0 during heavy exercise. Thus, at rest and during submaximal exercise, fat and carbohydrate are combusted to about an equal extent while during heavy exercise, when RQ is about 1.0, only carbohydrates are metabolized (Figure 11.1). It should be emphasized that carbohydrate- or fat-rich diets alter the RQ at rest and during submaximal exercise.

The aerobic reaction of fat and carbohydrate metabolism is slower than other energy systems. On the other hand, the stores are very large for fat and intermediate for glycogen. The stores of glycogen both in the liver and in the muscles can be increased by carbohydrate-rich diets. Supplementation with solutions containing carbohydrates but not fatty acids increases physical and mental endurance during prolonged exercise.

The limitation of the aerobic energy system is the maximal availability of oxygen at the site of the mitochondria, delivered through the oxygen transport system—see below. Endurance, defined as the capacity to carry out prolonged submaximal exercise, is to a large extent limited by the glycogen stores in the muscles and liver.

Adenylate Kinase Reaction

This special energy pathway is not very well investigated but is believed to be used only during extreme physical stress conditions. In this reaction two ADP react to form one mole of ATP and one mole of AMP (aminomonophosphate) in an attempt to produce ATP very quickly and to reduce the amount of ADP in the muscle. To keep this reaction going forward AMP has to be degraded by deamination. In several subsequent degrading reaction steps uric acid will be formed and can be used as a marker for the net loss of ATP. But more importantly, during this last reaction step oxygen free radicals can be formed, which may negatively influence cell membranes, several biochemical and other functions and structures in the muscle. Under normal conditions this reaction is of little value in the total energy output.

Summary

The energy metabolism for generating ATP to the muscle contraction is complex and not fully understood. It includes reactions which can deliver energy very fast—such as the adenylate kinase reaction, creatine phosphate and glucose/glycogen spliting. The negative aspects of these reactions are the limited stores and negative effects of the reactions. Aerobic breakdown of fat and carbohydrates provides a more patient and durable energy metabolism. The aerobic energy systems are fairly slow but stores are large. The metabolites of these reactions have hardly any negative effects. In the discussion of energy balance and weight maintenance it is only the aerobic metabolism that is of interest.

MEASUREMENTS OF ENERGY METABOLISM

Oxygen Consumption

Oxygen in the ambient air is transported by the pulmonary ventilation and in the main circulation to the muscle capillaries, from which through diffusion it reaches the muscle mitochondria. To quantify the amount of oxygen involved in metabolism in the mitochondria, the oxygen uptake is measured at the site of the pulmonary ventilation using the Douglas bag method or automatic analysis systems. The volume of expired air and the oxygen and carbon dioxide concentration in the expired air are measured. Since the oxygen and carbon dioxide in the inspired air normally is 20.94 and 0.03%, respectively, it is easy to calculate the amount of oxygen that has been taken up and carbon dioxide that has been produced in litres per minute, both at rest and during exercise (1). The error in measuring oxygen uptake during submaximal and maximal exercise with these methods is now less than 2%.

At rest oxygen uptake in a normal trained or untrained young man with body mass 70 to 75 kg is about 0.25 litres per minute. Corresponding value for a young woman of the same age is somewhat less due to smaller body mass. With increasing age resting oxygen uptake decreases mainly due to decreasing muscle mass. During exercise oxygen uptake normally increases linearly with increasing rate of work up to maximal exercise.

Table 11.1 Maximal aerobic power and energy expenditure during 1 hour of exercise

	$\dot{V}O_{2max}$ (litres per minute)	kJ per hour
Untrained women		
25 years	2.3	1400
50 years	1.9	1200
75 years	1.4	900
Untrained men		
25 years	3.3	2100
50 years	2.7	1700
75 years	2.0	1300
Endurance athletes		
women	4.0–4.5	4200–4800
men	5.0–7.4	5400–7800

The maximal aerobic power is defined as the peak oxygen uptake during dynamic exercise with large muscle groups under normal atmospheric conditions. In order to ensure that the maximal oxygen uptake has been reached the linear relation between oxygen uptake and submaximal work load should 'level off' at maximal oxygen uptake. High values for blood lactate concentration and heart rate can only be used as indications that maximal oxygen uptake have been reached. Maximal aerobic power in most healthy mean and women is limited by the capacity of the heart to pump blood during maximal exercise (maximal cardiac output). However, maximal oxygen uptake can be modified by many factors such as lowered oxygen carrying capacity in the blood (anaemia), medication and other factors. Values of maximal oxygen uptake in trained and untrained men and women are given in Table 11.1.

Direct measurements of oxygen uptake can only be done with specialized laboratory or field test equipment. Furthermore, in some activities such as prolonged work or in many work situations direct measurements of oxygen uptake are more or less impossible. Therefore, energy expenditure must usually be evaluated by other methods.

Heart Rate

Measurement of heart rate during physical activity is one possible way to estimate oxygen consumption and energy expenditure. The background for

this is that there is roughly a linear relationship between oxygen uptake and heart rate for most types of physical work under normal conditions (1).

However, it must be emphsized that the heart rate for a given absolute and even relative (per cent of maximum) oxygen uptake can vary extensively, for example with age, different peak heart rates, training status, diseases, psychological status and stress, medication (beta-blockers) and many other factors. Therefore, each estimation of energy expenditure from heart rate recordings should be done individually, taking all these variations into consideration.

The estimation of energy expenditure from heart rate recordings is done first by establishing the relationship between heart rate and oxygen uptake during increasing rates of work on a cycle ergometer, treadmill or the type of exercise that the subject is performing. The energy expenditure can thereafter be estimated by interpolation from heart rate recordings during the actual activity.

If all these measurement are done properly, the error of the method for estimation of energy expenditure from heart rate recordings during the actual work is in the range of $\pm 15\%$. However, this method is less accurate than the direct measurement of oxygen uptake due to the temporary variation in heart rate caused by static work, psychological stress etc. Therefore, estimations of energy expenditure from heart rate recordings must be done with great caution.

Core Temperature

Determination of core temperature during or immediately after exercise can also be used for estimation of energy expenditure during dynamic exercise. The background is that there is a close relationship between core temperature and the relative oxygen uptake (1). Thus, if the exercise has persisted for longer than 15 to 20 minutes and has been performed under normal conditions (e.g. within the air temperature range of approximately from 5 to 35°C), a core temperature of 38.0°C indicates a relative energy expenditure of about 50% of maximal aerobic power. At an average energy expenditure of 75% of maximal aerobic power the core temperature is approximately 38.8°C. These figures are consistent for men and women, irrespective of whether the individual is untrained or well trained or has a maximal aerobic power of 3 or 6 litres per minute.

This method has its limitations, such as the inertia of the core temperature with time and changes in energy expenditure. Furthermore, core temperature rises for a given energy expenditure during hypohydrated conditions, with extreme adiposity and some other conditions. Nevertheless, this method may be very useful in some situations, such as during intermittent exercise, in which the rate of work changes rapidly and also during physical exercise with high levels of psychological stress. In this latter situation the heart rate is increased due to the effect of catecholamines and, thus, the normal relation between heart rate and oxygen uptake is changed and not valid. In this and some other situations measurements of core temperature may be the best method to estimate the relative energy expenditure during exercise. In addition, maximal aerobic power must be measured or estimated.

Double Labelled Water

The doubly labelled water method is one of the best and in many situations the only possible method for estimation of energy expenditure over long periods (2). The method makes it possible to measure the total energy expenditure during periods up to 2 weeks under free-living conditions with a minimum of inconvenience for the individual. At the start the individual drinks water containing two isotopes ($^2H_2$ and ^{18}O). The two isotopes will then be diluted in the total body water pool. Both leave the body as water but in addition the oxygen also disappears as carbon dioxide as a result of the energy metabolism. By measuring the concentration of $^2H_2$ and ^{18}O in urine at the start and after some time the total energy expenditure during the period can be estimated. The only drawback of this method is the high cost of the isotopes and analysis, so that it is only feasible for studies with a small number of subjects.

Dietary Intake

If total body mass and its composition is unchanged over time, then energy expenditure must equal energy intake. Thus, measuring dietary intake may be one possibility to estimate total energy turnover over a prolonged period (weeks). However, under- and overreporting is very common, especially in obese subjects (3). Furthermore, there are normal variations in body weight of ± 1–$2\,kg$ even over fairly short periods of time. One kilo body mass change due to for instance body water shifts can indicate a fat mass change of about $27\,MJ$ ($6500\,kcal$), which equals more than 2 days' normal free-living energy expenditure in most individuals. Therefore, one must be cautious about making assumptions based on estimations of energy expenditure from individually reported dietary intakes.

Summary

Energy expenditure is best estimated by measuring oxygen consumption, since direct calorimetry is not a practical method. For calculation of energy expenditure for a fairly short period of time aerobic power times duration can simply be used. However, this procedure is not useful and possible in many practical situations outside laboratory settings. Therefore, calculations of energy expenditure from indirect estimations of oxygen consumption by heart rate recordings and core temperature measurements during and after physical activity, respectively, are well-accepted methods. For calculations of energy expenditure for longer periods of time (days and weeks) only the diary intake and doubly labelled water methods are valid and possible. In all these methods there are many different possibilities for erroneous recordings and calculations. Therefore these methods must be used with caution.

ENERGY EXPENDITURE AT REST

In general medicine and medical practice the interest in energy metabolism is often focused on basal metabolism. This is easy to understand because variations in basal metabolic rate (BMR) can be in the range of 30–40%. This variation can account for large increases and decreases in body weight, especially if they persist for a long period of time. The reason for the inter- but also intra-individual variations in BMR can only partly be explained by variations in active body mass—mainly muscle mass. Therefore, a mitochondria protein—the uncoupling protein (UCP), found in the mitochondria in the brown adipose tissue—is of great interest in this respect.

Brown adipose tissues have many mitochondria. The energy released in the brown fat cells is to a lesser degree than in other cells used for active phosphorylation of ADP to ATP and more for thermogenesis. Recently, proteins which have structures very like the UCP ones in brown adipose tissue have also been found in muscle tissue. Although there are many questions to be answered regarding the presence of the UCP-like protein in the muscle (exact function, regulation etc.), it can be speculated that this protein might explain why only about half of the oxygen used in metabolism in the muscles is used for active phosphorylation of ADP at rest (4). The consequence could be that some part of the energy taken in is not stored in the body, if the energy released in the metabolism is not used for mechanical events in the muscle but only increases the thermogenesis. Of interest in this discussion is that it has been shown that there are differences between overweight and normal-weight individuals in how this UCP-like protein is expressed in mRNA (5).

Studies in rats have shown that regular endurance training decreases the mRNA linked to the UCP in muscles (6). On the other hand, after an endurance exercise session the activity of UCP is increased (7), which might explain part of the increased post-exercise oxygen consumption. Regular physical training increases muscle and mitochondrial mass and as a consequence presumably also the amount of UCP. Thus, both acute and chronic exercise is of importance for the BMR and consequently the energy balance in both normal-weight and overweight individuals.

If UCP is downregulated by physical activity then its activity should increase with physical inactivity, leading to an increased BMR per kilo lean body mass. On the other hand, muscle mass is reduced as a result of physical inactivity. In any case, when studying changes in body weight, diet and eating habits and level of physical exercise in individuals, in groups and also in population investigations, it is obvious that the energy turnover both during and after exercise as well as the influence of exercise on BMR must be considered. Thus, level of physical exercise is therefore of vital importance in the discussion of energy balance in humans.

Summary

About two-thirds of the energy expenditure over 24 hours amounts to the resting energy metabolism. New findings regarding the uncoupling protein can shed new light on BMR and might to some extent explain the variations in BMR between individuals and perhaps also changes in BMR with time and ageing.

ENERGY EXPENDITURE DURING EXERCISE

Intensity and Duration

One cannot apply strict mathematical principles to biological systems, but when analysing energy balance for longer periods of time, energy metabolism during and after exercise must be taken into account. It is obvious that both the intensity and the duration are the main determinants of energy expenditure during exercise. However, many factors may modify the energy expenditure for a given rate of work and the total cost for certain activities. For this reason it is difficult to give exact figures for the energy cost of exercise. Therefore the discussion of energy expenditure should be based on individual conditions and values given for certain activities or for groups of subjects are subject to large uncertainties.

During short-term (a few minutes) hard dynamic muscular exercise carried out with large muscle groups, the energy metabolism may increase to 10–15 times the BMR in untrained subjects and 25–30 times the BMR in well-trained athletes from endurance events. However, due to muscle fatigue during heavy exercise the duration of exercise is often fairly short. In such cases the total energy expenditure is relatively low. On the other hand, low-intensity exercise, which may require half or two-thirds of the individual's maximal aerobic power, can be performed for a very long time even by an untrained individual. In this case total energy turnover can be fairly high.

Variations in Energy Expenditure During Submaximal Exercise

Variations in energy expenditure for a given sub-

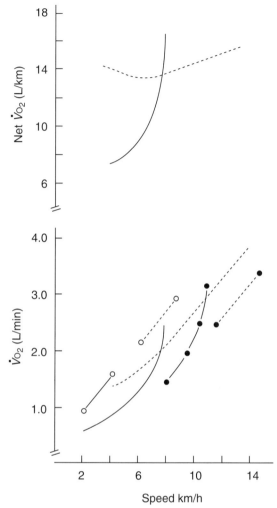

Figure 11.2 Energy expenditure (as measured by oxygen uptake) during walking and running

than walking in both these aspects. The upper panel of the figure also shows that the net energy cost for running per kilometre is more or less independent of speed. For a normal man with a body mass of 70 to 75 kg the energy expenditure during running is about 280 to 300 kJ per kilometre independent of speed, while walking for the same man may cost between 150 and 350 kJ per kilometre depending on speed. It must be emphasized that well-trained male and female racewalkers and long-distance runners have much lower values for energy expenditure both per minute and net per kilometre than normal, untrained individuals.

Women and children have lower energy cost for a given speed in walking and running due to their lower body mass. However, energy expenditure calculated per kilo body mass is the same for men and women whereas children have higher values. The energy expenditure also increases with body weight. Overweight individuals can have 50% and higher energy expenditure for a given walking speed. For example, during uphill treadmill walking (4–5 km per hour, 4° elevation) the oxygen uptake in an untrained overweight woman with a BMI of 35–40 may be maximal. Thus, for a given low walking speed the variation in energy expenditure can be up to 100% in a normal population.

The energy expenditure at a given speed varies also with different conditions such as surface, uphill and downhill walking and running, wind resistance etc. People with joint disease, an amputation or other physical handicaps have decreased locomotion economy, that is the oxygen uptake for a given submaximal rate of work is increased.

In some types of exercise in which technique is very important, such as swimming, the energy expenditure at a given speed may vary by more than 100% for poor and good swimmers for the same swimming stroke but also for different swimming strokes in the same individual. On the other hand, the energy expenditure for submaximal cycling is about the same for well-trained cyclists and as it is for runners for instance.

In high speed activities in which wind resistance increases, the energy expenditure increases curvilinearly. In addition, the style, position and/or equipment can influence the energy expenditure for a given speed. This is particularly true in cycling but also for running. For example, running behind another runner may save up to 6% in energy cost because of the wind protection.

maximal rate of work are due both to individual variations in economy of locomotion, such as different technique and body mass, and to temporary interindividual factors, such as changes in core temperature and choice of substrate.

Energy expenditure (as evaluated from oxygen consumption) during walking and running is illustrated in Figure 11.2. At low speeds—2–5 km per hour—walking costs less than running; that is oxygen uptake during walking is less than in running at the same speed. This is true for both energy expenditure per minute of exercise and net cost of energy per kilometre covered. However, at speeds greater than 6 to 8 km per hour running is more effective

There are situations in which the energy expenditure for a given submaximal rate of work is increased such as in hypothermia due to shivering, in very cold climates due to resistance of cold, stiff clothes and when for instance running technique is impaired for various reasons. However, in most such situations the magnitude of the increased energy expenditure for a given rate of work is of little quantitative importance. On the other hand, in many situations the energy expenditure for a given rate of work does not change. There are no major changes in energy expenditure for a given rate of work with variations in hot or moderately cold climate (except for shivering), in moderate altitude compared to sea-level, in anaemia and most diseases including most types of medication, although in these conditions the physical performance can be severely impaired. It should also be emphasized that although the energy expenditure at submaximal work is not changed, the total energy expenditure may be reduced due to the individual becoming fatigued earlier.

The average energy expenditures for different activities performed for more than 10–15 minutes by a man aged 20–30 years are given in Table 11.2. It must be emphasized that these values are subject to large interindividual variations, as discussed above.

Substrate Use During Exercise and Physical Training

As stated above, fatty acids and carbohydrates in combination are used during submaximal exercise. A common question in this discussion of substrate utilization is: Which is the best way to burn fat during exercise?

From Figure 11.1 it can be seen that the RQ for an untrained person (upper part of the shadowed area) is about 0.85 to 0.88 at exercise intensities from about 25 to 60% of maximal aerobic power. This means that the fat and carbohydrate contribution to the energy expenditure is 45 and 55%, respectively. From these data the substrate use during exercise can be calculated.

The total fatty acid contribution to the exercise expenditure is highest at around 60% of maximal aerobic power, which is a pace that even an untrained person can exercise at for some time. This means that for an untrained individual with a maxi-

Table 11.2 Average energy cost for different activities for a 20- to 30-year-old man

	kJ per minute
Complete rest	4–7
Sitting	6–8
Standing	7–9
Standing, light activity	9–13
Light housework	13–30
Gardening activities	15–45
Walking	
3 km per hour	15–30
5 km per hour	20–40
7 km per hour	30–60
Running	
7 km per hour	30–50
9 km per hour	40–70
11 km per hour	50–90

mal aerobic power of about 3.3 litres per minute, 0.50 g of fat is used per minute at this intensity. Suppose that this individual through physical training increases his/her maximal aerobic power by 0.5 litres per minute, which is possible in 4 to 5 months of endurance training. Compared to the situation before the training period, two observations can be mentioned regarding the fat and carbohydrate contribution to the energy expenditure. Firstly, for a given submaximal relative but also absolute rate of work the RQ is lowered (lower part of the shadowed area in Figure 11.1). Thus, more fatty acids are used and the stores of carbohydrate are utilized less. Secondly, the intensity for peak fatty acid contribution to the energy expenditure has increased from 60% to about 70% of maximal aerobic power. This means that the peak contribution of fatty acids in this individual has increased due to the training effects from 0.50 to 0.75 g per minute. In addition, the individual can probably be active for longer periods of time after the training period and, thus, increase the fatty acid turnover still more. For instance, if she/he increases the exercise time from 30 minutes before to 45 minutes after the training period at the exercise intensity at which she/he can exercise fairly easily, then the fatty acid breakdown increases from 15 g to 30 g for the exercise period. The increased use of fatty acids at a given rate of work and the higher speed of exercise may be of interest not only in conditioning exercise such as jogging and cycling but also in the everyday 'behaviour' type of exercise (climbing stairs, walking short distances etc.) as part of the energy expenditure in the discussion of energy balance.

Maximal Exercise

Variations in maximal power are due to age, genetic endowment, body size, physical activity and some other factors and can partly explain differences in total energy expenditure for different reasons. Individuals with high maximal aerobic power will more likely walk distances or climb stairs than use cars and elevators. They can more easily carry loads and they may in general be more physically active in normal life. In addition, due to increased energy intake when physically active they also have increased intake of essential nutrients. But the total daily need and turnover for essential nutrients increases less than the increased total daily energy need and turnover when a person becomes more physically active. Therefore the difference between intake and turnover of essential nutrients widens with increasing levels of physical activity under the assumption that the individual is in energy balance while trained and untrained.

Total Energy Expenditure

As stated above, duration of exercise may be more important than intensity for total energy expenditure. In Table 11.1 the total energy expenditure is given for one hour of exercise such as walking in uneven terrain, cycling or playing a game of tennis, volleyball or table tennis in a moderate fashion. The intensity of these types of physical activities is on average about 50 to 60% of maximal aerobic power when carried out as free-chosen physical activity. The rate of work of 50 to 60% is easily performed even by an untrained person for one hour. The individual maximal oxygen uptake values for untrained men and women at different ages and endurance athletes are also given in Table 11.1.

The table shows that one hour of leisure time exercise yields an energy expenditure in an untrained person which corresponds to about one-quarter of 24 hour BMR, which is 7 MJ for men and 5–6 MJ for women. The importance of these types of regular physical exercise is illustrated when discussing body mass changes over time. It is not uncommon that body fat mass in many individuals increases 2 kg in one year. This corresponds to a daily energy imbalance of about 150 kJ. Unless net energy intake is increased this corresponds to an extra 10 minutes of walking per day. Furthermore, in order to maximize the beneficial effects of physical activity on health, and in prevention of diseases that are related to physical inactivity, the Surgeon General in the USA has recommended accumulated low-intensity physical activity of at least 30 minutes per day (8). Thus, regular low-intensity physical activity such as walking and cycling to work two times 15–20 minutes a day may be a good base for energy balance, body weight maintenance and good health.

Sporting activities can generate quite a large total energy expenditure. In male elite soccer matchplay the heart rate is on average some 25 to 30 beats per minute lower than peak heart rate obtained during maximal exercise. Core temperature after the game is above 39 °C as an average for the players in the team. Blood lactate concentration measured several times during the match varies between 4 and 10 mM. Thus, from these figures it can be calculated that the average energy expenditure during the game amounts to 75 to 80% of maximal aerobic power. For an average male elite player with a maximal oxygen uptake of 4.5 litres per minute the total energy expenditure for a whole game including some warm-up can be calculated to be about 7.5 MJ (1800 kcal) which is about the same as the BMR for 24 hours. Corresponding values for total energy expenditure for a female elite player are some 20% less (9).

The energy cost of a marathon race (42 km) for a 30- to 40-year-old man who performs the race in 4 hours is about 12–15 MJ (3000–3500 kcal). However, in order to be able to carry out the race in 4 hours the training during the preceding 6 months can be calculated to be about 400 MJ. It is obvious that regular physical training for sport is of importance for energy balance and body weight control.

Summary

Energy for physical activity is generated though several complicated systems of which the aerobic splitting of fat and glucose is the most important one. For most people physical activity amounts to about 30–40% of the total energy expenditure during 24 hours. The amount of exercise energy expenditure during 24 hours is dependent on intensity and duration but many other factors can influence energy expenditure.

In the population physical activity can be divided into four main parts. The difference between them is often not very clear. The lowest one is spontaneous activity, which is trivial activities such as moving arms and legs, take small steps etc. The energy needed for this type of activity is fairly small but for people who seldom sit still or move regularly the whole day the total amount can reach some volume.

The physical stress in most jobs is nowadays much lower than 20–30 years ago. Office work has very low energy demands. In industrial work monotonous and low energy expenditure physical exercise gives rise to overuse problems. On the other hand, other jobs such as construction work can reach a daily total average energy expenditure of 12 000–13 000 kJ or more. In general, physical activity in most work places does not add enough physical activity to the daily physical activity.

The next part is the 'behaviour' physical exercise, i.e. climbing stairs, walking a few blocks instead of taking a bus or car, often doing physically active things inside or outside the home. This type of activity is very important for energy balance. Over the day such activity can easily use 1000 kJ in extra energy expenditure. Of particular importance is the way that the person travels to work. In many countries it is common to ride a bicycle or walk 15–20 minutes to reach the workplace. This type of physical activity is of utmost importance for good health and body mass maintenance as well as for weight reduction in overweight individuals.

Physical conditioning can, if carried out on regular basis, create a daily energy expenditure well above 3000 kJ and, thus, well above the level for good health and body mass maintenance. Elite athletes often have a daily energy expenditure of 14 000–16 000 kJ (3500–4000 kcal); in some sports it may be even higher. In addition to energy expenditure during exercise, the effect of regular physical activity on resting metabolic rate is of interest.

Thus physical activity is very important for body mass maintenance. All its different parts must be considered when discussing energy balance.

REFERENCES

1. Åstrand PO, Rodahl K. *Textbook of Work Physiology.* New York: McGraw-Hill, 1986.
2. Speakman JR. *Doubly-labelled Water: Theory and Practice.* London: Chapman and Hall, 1997.
3. Bandini LG, Schoeller DA, Cyr HN, Dietz WH. Validity of reported energy intake in obese and nonobese adolescents. *Am J Clin Nutr* 1990; **52**: 421–425.
4. Brand MD, Chien LF, Ainshow EK, Rolfe DF, Porter RK. The causes and functions of mitochondrial proton leak. *Biochim Biophys Acta* 1994; **1187**: 132–139.
5. Nordfors L, Hoffstedt J, Nyberg B, Thörne A, Arner P, Schalling M, Lönnqvist F. *Diabetologia* 1998; **41**: 935–939.
6. Boss O, Samec S, Despplanches D, Mayet MH *et al.* Effect of endurance training on mRNA expression of uncoupling proteins 1, 2 and 3 in the rat. *FASEBJ* 1998; **12**: 335–339.
7. Tonkonogi M, Harris B, Sahlin K. Mitochondrial oxidative function in human saponin.skinned muscle fibres: effect of prolonged exercise. *J Physiol* 1998; **510**: 279–286.
8. US Department of Health and Human Services (1996) *Physical Activity and Health. A Report of the Surgeon General.* GA. Superintendent of Documents. PO Box 371954. PA 15250-7954, S/N 017-023-00196-5, USA.
9. Ekblom B (ed.) *Handbook of Sports Medicine and Science—Football (Soccer).* Oxford: Blackwell Scientific Publications, 1994..

12

Exercise and Macronutrient Balance

Angelo Tremblay and Jean-Pierre Després

Laval University, Ste-Foy, Quebec, Canada

INTRODUCTION

Reduced physical activity represents one of the most significant changes in lifestyle that has been observed during the twentieth century. Our sedentary lifestyle and the reduced energy requirements of the majority of our jobs has been a source of comfort in a business world where efficiency and productivity are sought. The impact of the transition from a traditional to a modern lifestyle on daily energy needs can be estimated by various means. By using the doubly labelled water technique and indirect calorimetry, Singh *et al.* (1) showed that the energy cost of living at the peak labor season was as high as 2.35 × resting metabolic rate (RMR) in Gambian women. When this value is compared to results usually obtained in women living in industrialized countries, 1.4 to 1.8 × RMR (2,3), it can be estimated that for a given body weight, a modern lifestyle may have reduced the energy cost of living by as much as 1 to 4 MJ/day. Accordingly, a recent analysis by Prentice and Jebb (4) has emphasised the contribution of sedentariness to the increased prevalence of overweight in the United Kingdom.

Despite these observations, the contribution of exercise to the prevention and treatment of obesity is still perceived as trivial by many health professionals. The perception of many of them was recently well summarized by Garrow (5) who stated that exercise is a remarkably ineffective means of

achieving weight loss in obese people, mainly because their exercise tolerance is so low that the level of physical activity that they can sustain makes a negligible contribution to total energy expenditure. When one looks at the currently available literature, it is difficult to disagree with this statement. Indeed, numerous studies have demonstrated that when exercise is used alone to treat obesity, body weight loss is generally small (6). In addition, the further weight loss generated by adding an exercise program to a reduced-calorie diet is also often small if not insignificant (7).

Traditionally, the study of the impact of exercise on body weight control has focused on its energy cost and on the hope that the body energy loss will be equivalent to the cumulative energy cost of exercise sessions. In practical terms, this means for instance that if a physical activity program induces an excess of energy expenditure of 2000 kcal/week, a similar energy deficit should be expected in the active obese individual. Recent experimental data show that such a view is not realistic since it does not take into account the compensations in other components of energy balance which may either attenuate or amplify the impact of exercise on body energy stores. It thus appears preferable to consider exercise as a stimulus affecting regulatory processes which can ultimately affect all the components of energy balance instead of only focusing on its energy cost. The objective of this chapter is to

International Textbook of Obesity. Edited by Per Björntorp.

summarize recent developments in knowledge pertaining to the effects of exercise on energy balance. Clinical implications of these notions are also addressed.

EXERCISE AND MACRONUTRIENT BALANCE

The maintenance of body weight stability depends on one's ability to match energy intake to expenditure. This principle is one of the most accepted axioms of science and represents the main guideline for health professionals treating obesity. However, even if energy balance is a central issue in body weight control, it does not necessarily imply that matching energy intake to expenditure is the primary target of mechanisms involved in the regulation of body energy stores.

Flatt (8) reported convincing evidence showing that energy balance is linked to macronutrient balance. His research and that of other scientists have also clearly established that the regulation of the balance of each macronutrient is not performed with the same precision. Of particular interest for obesity research is the fact that fat balance is the component of the macronutrient balance that is the most prone to large variations. This is probably explained by some of the following factors:

- The weak potential of dietary fat to promote a short-term increase in its oxidation (9–11).
- The weak potential of high fat foods to favor satiety without overfeeding (12–15).
- The inhibiting effect of the intake of other energy substrates on fat oxidation (16,17).
- The absence of a metabolic pathway other than lipogenesis to buffer a significant fraction of an excess fat input (excess dietary fat intake and/or fat synthesized from other substrates).
- The greater dependence of fat oxidation on sympathoadrenal stimulation (18).

The fact that fat balance appears as the 'Achilles tendon' of the macronutrient balance system is probably compatible with the importance of maintaining body homeostasis. Indeed, it is probably less toxic and damaging for the body to store a large amount of triglycerides as opposed to an equicaloric storage of alcohol and glycogen. However, in the long run, a large body accumulation of fat

Table 12.1 Effects of leptin and insulin (euglycemia) on energy balance

Variables	Leptin	Insulin
Energy intake	↓	↓
Energy expenditure	↑	↑
Activity level	↑	?
Neuropeptide Y	↓	↓
Sympathetic nervous system activity	↑	↑

causes metabolic complications which worsen health status. For the exercise physiologist, the question raised by this argument is whether the exercise stimulus can facilitate the regulation of fat balance, i.e. can favor fat balance without relying on body fat gain to promote macronutrient balance.

REGULATION OF FAT BALANCE: FAT GAIN OR EXERCISE?

Many years ago, Kennedy (19) proposed a lipostatic theory stipulating that variables related to adipose tissue contribute to the long-term control of food intake. Accordingly, studies performed under different experimental conditions provided evidence suggesting that fat cell size (20), plasma glycerol (21), fat cell lipolysis (22), and fat oxidation (23) may be related to fat and energy balance and to the long-term stability of body weight. More recently, the discovery of leptin (24) represented an important step in the investigation of the role of adipose tissue on the regulation of fat and energy balance. As shown in Table 12.1, leptin exerts many functions and its most documented role has been to favor a negative energy balance or at least to promote the stabilization of body weight in a context of overfeeding by reducing food intake (25). This table also indicates that variations in plasma insulin without changes in glycemia produce effects which are similar to those of leptin. Since the clearance of insulin is modulated by the hepatic exposure to free fatty acid (FFA) flux (26), which itself partly depends on fat cell size, it is reasonable to associate changes in adiposity with the effects of changes in insulinemia on fat and energy balance.

To summarize, these observations demonstrate that adipose tissue is not passive when one experiences long-term underfeeding or overfeeding. It rather behaves like an organ actively involved in the

Table 12.2 Opposite (A) and concordant (B) effects of physical activity and metabolic cardiovascular syndrome related to fat gain

	Physical activity effect	Variables	Metabolic cardiovascular syndrome
A	↓	Blood pressure	↑
	↓	Plasma glucose	↑
	↓	Plasma insulin	↑
	↓	Plasma triacylglycerols	↑
	↓	Plasma total cholesterol	↑
	↑	Plasma HDL cholesterol	↓
	↓	Plasma apoB[a]	↑
	↓	Plasma cholesterol: HDL cholesterol	↑
	↑	LDL particle size[a]	↓
B	↑	SNS activity	↑
	↑	Energy expenditure	↑
	↑	Fat oxidation	↑

[a]Additional atherogenic features of the metabolic cardiovascular syndrome (31).
HDL, high density lipoprotein; LDL, low density lipoprotein; SNS, sympathetic nervous system; apoB, apolipoprotein B.

recovery of fat and energy balance and of body weight stability.

Research conducted over the last decades has shown that exercise can also affect many of the above referenced variables. It has been demonstrated that exercise stimulates adipose tissue lipolysis and that trained individuals are more sensitive to the lipolytic effects of catecholamines (27,28). Furthermore, Turcotte et al. (29) reported that for any given plasma FFA concentration, trained individuals would utilize more fat during exercise than their untrained controls. With respect to leptinemia, recent data tend to show that for a given level of body fat, trained individuals display reduced plasma leptin levels compared to sedentary controls (30).

We can therefore suggest from the above observations that both fat gain and exercise represent strategies which may contribute to the regulation of fat and energy balance. However, these results also indicate that physically active individuals have a major advantage over sedentary individuals as they may regulate their fat balance more efficiently, i.e. with less substrate gradient and reduced hormone concentrations. In other words, trained persons are expected to rely to a lesser extent on variations in adiposity to maintain fat balance under free-living conditions. The main corollary of this phenomenon is depicted in Table 12.2, which reminds us there is also, unfortunately, a price to be paid in taking advantage of the regulatory impact of fat gain on fat and energy metabolism. Indeed, body fat gain, particularly in the visceral fat compartment, is associated with an increase in blood pressure and

plasma glucose and insulin as well as with an atherogenic dyslipidemic plasma profile (32,33). This cluster of atherogenic and diabetogenic metabolic abnormalities is seldom formed among non-obese physically active individuals.

EXERCISE, FAT BALANCE AND BODY WEIGHT CONTROL

The evidence summarized above suggests that the exercise-trained individual can maintain a reduced level of adiposity because of an increased sensitivity and overall better performance of mechanisms involved in the regulation of fat balance. If this beneficial adaptation can be reproduced in the obese individual undertaking a physical activity program, this response would favor a metabolic context facilitating body weight loss. Accordingly, recent data demonstrate that the effects of exercise favorably influence components of fat and energy balance.

Exercise and Fat Oxidation

Exercise-trained individuals are characterized by an increased level of fat oxidation despite the fact that their adiposity is generally lower than that of untrained subjects (34–37). In the post-exercise state, the increase in fat oxidation is explained by an increase in resting metabolic rate and/or by an increased relative fat content of the substrate mix oxidized. Moreover, evidence suggests that the enhanced fat oxidation characterizing trained individuals is at least partly explained by acute effects of exercise (38–40).

The mechanisms underlying the exercise-induced increase in fat oxidation are not clearly established but experimental data suggest that it is related to an increase in sympathetic nervous system activity (35) that seems to be mediated by beta adrenoreceptors (36). Other recent data emphasize the possibility that the impact of exercise on fat utilization is mainly determined by a change in glycogen stores and/or glucose availability (41,42). This observation is concordant with our recent finding that when exercise is immediately followed by a liquid supplementation compensating for carbohydrate and lipid oxidized during exercise, essentially no change in post-exercise fat oxidation is found (43).

For the obese individual who displays limitations in the ability to perform prolonged vigorous exercise, the above findings open new therapeutic perspectives. For instance, they raise the possibility that combining exercise and food-related sympathomimetic agents could produce a substantial increase in fat oxidation. One of these agents is capsaicin, which was recently found to significantly increase fat oxidation in the postprandial state (44). In addition, the possibility that the stimulating effect of exercise on fat oxidation depends on glucose availability raises the hypothesis that performing exercise in the postabsorptive state exerts a greater enhancing effect on total fat oxidation than an exercise bout performed in the fed state. From a clinical standpoint, these hypotheses are important since the ability to burn fat with exercise is a significant correlate of post-exercise energy and fat balance (45).

Exercise and Fat Intake

Excess dietary fat is known to affect spontaneous energy intake considerably. In humans tested under conditions mimicking free-living conditions, the intake of high fat foods is associated with a large increase in daily energy intake (12–15). This is concordant with studies demonstrating a significant positive relationship between habitual dietary fat intake and adiposity (15,46–48). When the enhancing effect of a high fat diet on energy intake is considered in the context of exercise practice, high

Table 12.3 Energy intake, expenditure and balance over 2 days under high or low fat conditions following a moderate intensity exercise session

	Post-exercise period	
Variables	Low fat diet	High fat diet
Energy intake (MJ)	25.7 ± 3.3	32.2 ± 5.1
Energy expenditure (MJ)	29.9 ± 7.3	29.1 ± 6.2
Energy balance (MJ)	-4.2	3.1

Adapted from Tremblay *et al.* (49).

fat feeding is expected to inhibit the impact of exercise on energy balance. As shown in Table 12.3, we found that when subjects have free access to high fat foods after having performed a 60-minute vigorous exercise, they overfeed to a level that does not permit exercise to induce a negative energy balance (49). In contrast, a substantial energy deficit is achieved when exercise is followed by free access to low fat foods. This is in agreement with other recently reported data showing that high fat feeding favors an increase in the post-exercise compensation in energy intake (50).

In another recent study, we examined the impact of combining exercise and *ad libitum* intake of low fat foods on daily energy balance in heavy men (51). These subjects were tested twice in a respiratory chamber under either a sedentary condition with *ad libitum* intake of a mixed diet or an exercise condition with a low fat diet. As expected, daily energy balance was considerably reduced (1.6 MJ) under the latter condition. This finding and the evidence summarized above suggest that it is of primary importance to take into account diet composition to optimize the daily energy deficit which can be achieved with exercise.

Recent studies have been designed to test the hypothesis that exercise per se can modify macronutrient preferences. This has been examined by Verger *et al.* (52) who reported an increased preference for carbohydrate after prolonged exercise. In a subsequent study, these authors did not reproduce this finding but rather noted an increased preference for proteins after prolonged exercise (53). Another recent study performed in our laboratory revealed that vigorous exercise in untrained subjects did not selectively modify the preference for any macronutrient (54). On the other hand, Westerterp-Plantenga *et al.* (55) obtained results demonstrating that exercise may increase the preference for carbohydrates.

In summary, diet composition seems to be an important determinant of the potential of exercise to induce an overall negative energy balance. However, it remains uncertain whether a change in macronutrient preferences can be spontaneously driven by exercise or should be the result of a voluntary change in food selection.

CLINICAL IMPLICATIONS

The literature summarized above suggests that combining exercise and a reduced dietary fat intake should favor spontaneous body weight loss in obese individuals. In obese women, this combination was found to induce a mean decrease in body weight of 16% that was associated with a normalization of the metabolic risk profile (7). In a more recent study, we used the exercise–low fat diet combination as a follow-up of a treatment of obesity consisting of drug therapy and low calorie diet (56). In this context, exercise and low fat diet accentuated the fat loss induced by the first phase of treatment up to a mean cumulative weight loss of 14% and 10% of initial values in men and women, respectively. In addition, the exercise–low fat diet follow-up was again associated with a normalization of the metabolic risk profile. As shown in Table 12.4, these observations are consistent with a recent study demonstrating that the regular physical activity and adherence to a low fat dietary regimen are the main features of the lifestyle of ex-obese individuals maintaining a large weight loss on a long-term basis (57).

Even if the combination of exercise and low fat diet can induce a considerable body energy deficit under free-living conditions, it is likely that adipose tissue-related regulatory factors of energy and fat balance will over time favor the restabilization of body weight. These factors, which are associated with resistance to further loss of weight in the reduced-obese individual, are probably the same ones that promote the achievement of a new body weight plateau in the context of overfeeding. Thus, as discussed above, the decrease in sympathetic nervous system activity and in plasma FFA, leptin, and insulin probably contributes to resistance to losing more fat after having experienced success with exercise and a low fat diet. In this context of increased

Table 12.4 Characteristics of individuals maintaining a weight loss of at least 30 pounds (13.6 kg) for at least one year

Body weight loss	30.1 kg
Duration of maintenance	5.7 years
Relative fat intake	25% of total energy intake
Physical activity participation[a]	11 847 kJ/week

[a]Including strenuous physical activities.
Adapted from McGuire et al. (57).

vulnerability towards a fattening lifestyle, the ex-obese person obviously must maintain his/her new exercise–low fat diet lifestyle to prevent further weight regain.

CONCLUSIONS

The combination of exercise and a low fat diet is an effective way to induce a spontaneous negative energy and fat balance. In the context of a weight-reducing program, this represents a strategy that focuses on lifestyle changes instead of directly targeting caloric restriction. The amount of body fat loss expected under these conditions probably corresponds to what the body does not need anymore to regulate macronutrient balance. This model considers adipose tissue as an active organ whose impact on energy balance can be at least partly replaced by a healthy lifestyle characterized by healthy food habits and regular exercise.

REFERENCES

1. Singh J, Prentice AM, Diaz E, Coward WA, Ashford J, Sawyer M, Whitehead RG. Energy expenditure of Gambian women during peak agricultural activity measured by doubly-labeled water method. *Br J Nutr* 1989; **62**: 315–329.
2. Prentice AM, Black AE, Coward WA, Cole TJ. Energy expenditure in overweight and obese adults in affluent societies: an analysis of 319 doubly-labelled water measurements. *Eur J Clin Nutr* 1996; **50**: 93–97.
3. Prentice AM, Davies HL, Black AE, Ashford J, Coward WA, Murgatroyd PR, Goldberg GR, Sawyer M, Whitehead RG. Unexpectedly low levels of energy expenditure in healthy women. *Lancet* 1985; June: 1419–1422.
4. Prentice AM, Jebb SA. Obesity in Britain: gluttony or sloth? *Br Med J* 1995; **311**: 437–439.
5. Garrow JS. Treatment of obesity. *Lancet* 1992; **340**: 409–413.
6. Ballor DL, Keesey RE. A meta-analysis of the factors affecting exercise-induced changes in body mass, fat mass and fat-free mass in males and females. *Int J Obes* 1991; **15**:

717–726.

7. Tremblay A, Després J-P, Maheux J, Pouliot MC, Nadeau A, Moorjani PJ, Lupien PJ, Bouchard C. Normalization of the metabolic profile in obese women by exercise and a low fat diet. *Med Sci Sports Exerc* 1991; **23**: 1326–1331.

8. Flatt JP. Dietary fat, carbohydrate balance, and weight maintenance: effects of exercise. *Am J Clin Nutr* **45**: 296–306.

9. Flatt JP, Ravussin E, Acheson KJ, Jéquier E. Effects of dietary fat on post-prandial substrate oxidation and on carbohydrate and fat balances. *J Clin Invest* 1985; **76**: 1119–1124.

10. Schutz Y, Bessard T, Jéquier E. Diet-induced thermogenesis measured over a whole day in obese and non-obese women. *Am J Clin Nutr* 1984; **40**: 542.

11. Schutz Y, Flatt JP, Jéquier E. Failure of dietary fat intake to promote fat oxidation: a factor favoring the development of obesity. *Am J Clin Nutr* 1989; **50**: 307–314.

12. Lissner L, Levitsky DA, Strupp BJ, Kalkwarf HJ, Roe, DA. Dietary fat and regulation of energy intake in human subjects. *Am J Clin Nutr* 1987; **46**: 886–892.

13. Stubbs JR, Harbon GH, Murgatroyd PR, Prentice AM. Covert manipulation of dietary fat and energy density: effect on substrate flux and food intake in men eating ad libitum. *Am J Clin Nutr* 1995; **62**: 316–329.

14. Tremblay A, Lavallée N, Alméras N, Allard L, Després JP, Bouchard C. Nutritional determinants of the increase in energy intake associated with a high fat diet. *Am J Clin Nutr* 1991; **53**: 1134–1137.

15. Tremblay A, Plourde G, Després JP, Bouchard C. Impact of dietary fat content and fat oxidation on energy intake in humans. *Am J Clin Nutr* 1989; **49**: 799–805.

16. Jéquier E. Carbohydrates as a source of energy. *Am J Clin Nutr* 1994; **59**(Suppl): 682S–685S.

17. Suter PM, Schutz Y, Jéquier E. The effect of ethanol on fat storage in healthy subjects. *N Engl J Med* 1992; **326**: 983–987.

18. Acheson K, Jéquier E, Wahren J. Influence of beta-adrenergic blockade on glucose-induced thermogenesis in man. *J Clin Invest* 1983; **72**: 981–986.

19. Kennedy GC. The role of depot fat in the hypothalamic control of food intake in the rat. *Proc R Soc* (London) 1952; **140B**: 578–592.

20. Björntorp P, Carlgren G, Isaksson B, Krotkiewski M, Larsson B, Sjostrom L. Effect of an energy-reduced dietary regimen in relation to adipose tissue cellularity in obese women. *Am J Clin Nutr* 1975; **28**: 445–452.

21. Wirtshafter D, Davis JD. Body weight: reduction by long-term glycerol treatment. *Science* 1977; **198**: 1271–1274.

22. Tremblay A, Després JP, Bouchard C. Adipose tissue characteristics of ex-obese long-distance runners. *Int J Obes* 1984; **8**: 641–648.

23. Schutz Y, Tremblay A, Weinsier RL, Nelson KM. Role of fat oxidation in the long-term stabilization of body weight in obese women. *Am J Clin Nutr* 1992; **55**: 670–674.

24. Zhang Y, Proenca R, Maffei M, Barone M, Leopold L, Friedman JM. Positional cloning of the mouse obese gene and its human homologue. *Nature* 1994; **372**: 425–432.

25. Halaas JL, Gajiwala KS, Maffei M, Cohen SL, Chait BT, Rabinowitz D, Lallone RL, Burley SK, Friedman JM. Weight-reducing effects of the plasma protein encoded by the obese gene. *Science* 1995; **269**: 543–546.

26. Svedberg J, Stromblad G, Wirth A, Smith U, Bjortorp P. Fatty acids in portal vein of the rat regulate hepatic insulin clearance. *J Clin Invest* 1991; **88**: 2054–2058.

27. Crampes F, Beauville M, Riviere D, Garrigues M. Effect of physical training in humans on the response of isolated fat cells to epinephrine. *J Appl Physiol* 1986; **61**: 25–29.

28. Després JP, Bouchard C, Savard R, Tremblay A, Marcotte M, Thériault G. The effect of a 20-week endurance training program on adipose tissue morphology and lipolysis in men and women. *Metabolism* 1984; **33**: 235–239.

29. Turcotte L, Richter EA, Kiens B. Increased plasma FFA uptake and oxidation during prolonged exercise in trained vs. untrained humans. *Am J Physiol* 1992; **262**: E791–E799.

30. Pasman WJ, Westerterp-Plantenga MS, Saris WHM. The effect of exercise training on leptin levels in obese males. *Am J Phys* 1998; **274**: E280–E286.

31. Lamarche B, Tchernof A, Mauriège P, Cantin B, Dagenais GR, Lupien PJ, Després J-P. Fasting insulin and apolipoprotein B levels and low-density lipoprotein particle size as risk factors for ischemic heart disease. *JAMA* 1998; **279**: 1955–1961.

32. Després JP, Moorjani S, Lupien PJ, Tremblay A, Nadeau A, Bouchard C. Regional distribution of body fat, plasma lipoproteins and cardiovascular disease. *Arteriosclerosis* 1990; **10**: 497–511.

32. Verger P, Lanteaume MT, Louis-Sylvestre J. Human intake and choice of foods at intervals after exercise. *Appetite* 1992; **18**: 93–99.

33. Després J-P, Lamarche B. Low-intensity endurance training, plasma lipoproteins, and the risk of coronary heart disease. *J Intern Med* 1994; **236**: 7–22.

34. Poehlman ET, Danforth E. Endurance training increases metabolic rate and norepinephrine appearance rate in older individuals. *Am J Physiol* 1991; **261**: E233–E239.

35. Poehlman ET, Gardner AW, Arciero PJ, Goran MI, Calles-Escandon J. Effects of endurance training on total fat oxidation in elderly persons. *J Appl Physiol* 1994; **76**: 2281–2287.

36. Tremblay A, Coveney JP, Després JP, Nadeau A, Prud'homme D. Increased resting metabolic rate and lipid oxidation in exercise-trained individuals: evidence for a role of beta adrenergic stimulation. *Can J Physiol Pharmacol* 1992; **70**: 1342–1347.

37. Tremblay A, Després JP, Bouchard C. The effects of exercise-training on energy balance and adipose tissue morphology and metabolism. *Sports Med* 1985; **2**: 223–233.

38. Bahr R, Ingnes I, Vaage O, Sejersted OM, Newsholme EA. Effect of duration of exercise on excess postexercise O_2 consumption. *J Appl Physiol* 1987; **62**: 485–490.

39. Bielinski R, Schutz Y, Jequier E. Energy metabolism during the postexercise recovery in man. *Am J Clin Nutr* 1985; **42**: 69–82.

40. Tremblay A, Nadeau A, Fournier G, Bouchard C. Effect of a three-day interruption of exercise training on resting metabolic rate and glucose-induced thermogenesis in trained individuals. *Int J Obes* 1988; **12**: 163–168.

41. Coyle EF, Jeukendrup AE, Wagenmakers AJM, Saris WHM. Fatty acid oxidation is directly regulated by carbohydrate metabolism during exercise. *Am J Physiol* 1997; **273**: E268–E275.

42. Schrauwen P, Lichtenbelt WD, Saris WH, Westerterp KR. Fat balance in obese subjects: role of glycogen stores. *Am J*

Physiol 1998; **274**: E1027–1033.

43. Dionne I, VanVugt S, Tremblay A. Postexercise macronutrient oxidation: a factor dependent on postexercise macronutrient intake. *Am J Clini Nutr* 1999; **69**: 927–930.

44. Yoshioka M, St-Pierre S, Suzuki M, Tremblay A. Effects of red pepper added to high-fat and high-carbohydrate meals on energy metabolism and substrate utilization in Japanese women. *Br J Nutr* 1998; **80**: 503–510.

45. Alméras N, Lavallée N, Després JP, Bouchard, C, Tremblay A. Exercise and energy intake: effect of substrate oxidation. *Physiol Behav* 1995; **57**: 995–1000.

46. Dreon DM, Frey-Hewitt B, Ellsworth N, Williams PT, Terry RB, Wood PD. Dietary fat: carbohydrate ratio and obesity in middle-aged men. *Am J Clin Nutr* 1988; **47**: 995–1000.

47. Romieu I, Willett WC, Stampfer MJ, Colditz GA, Sampson L, Rosner B, Hennekens CH, Speizer FE. Energy intake and other determinants of relative weight. *Am J Clin Nutr* 1988; **47**: 406–412.

48. Tucker LA, Kano M. Dietary fat and body fat: a multivariate study of 205 adult females. *Am J Clin Nutr* 1992; **56**: 616–622.

49. Tremblay A, Alméras N, Boer J, Kranenbarg EK, Després JP. Diet composition and postexercise energy balance. *Am J Clin Nutr* 1994; **59**: 975–979.

50. King NA, Blundell JE. High-fat foods overcome the energy expenditure due to exercise after cycling and running. *Eur J Clin Nutr* 1995; **49**: 114–123.

51. Dionne I, White M, Tremblay A. Acute effects of exercise and low-fat diet on energy balance in heavy men. *Int J Obes* 1997; **21**: 413–416.

53. Verger P, Lanteaume MT, Louis-Sylvestre J. Free food choice after acute exercise in men. *Appetite* 1994; **22**: 159–164.

54. Imbeault P, Saint-Pierre S, Almeras N, Tremblay A. Acute effects of exercise on energy intake and feeding behaviour. *Br J Nutr* 1997; **77**: 511–521.

55. Westerterp-Plantenga MS, Ijedema MJ, Wijckmans NE, Saris WH. Acute effects of exercise or sauna on appetite in obese and nonobese men. *Physiol Behav* 1997; **62**: 1345–1354.

56. Doucet E, Imbeault P, Alméras N, Tremblay A. Physical activity and low-fat diet: Is it enough to maintain weight stability in the reduced-obese individual following weight loss by drug therapy and energy restriction? *Obes Res* 1999; **7**: 323–333.

57. McGuire MT, Wing RR, Klem ML, Seagle HM, Hill JO. Long-term maintenance of weight loss: do people who lose weight through various weight loss methods use different behaviors to maintain their weight? *Int J Obes* 1998; **22**: 572–577.

Part IV

Pathogenesis and Types of Obesity

13

The Specificity of Adipose Depots

Caroline M. Pond

The Open University, Milton Keynes, UK

INTRODUCTION

For human and veterinary medicine, the main issue in adipose tissue biology is obesity and its associated metabolic complications. So much attention is devoted to finding ways of reducing the mass of adipose tissue and correcting complications such as hyperglycaemia and hyperlipidaemia, that its positive contributions to other metabolic functions are often overlooked. This chapter is mainly concerned with the involvement of adipose tissue in roles other than as a whole-body energy storage. Students of obesity should be aware of these specialized functions, as they could be jeopardized by indiscriminate suppression of the growth or metabolism of adipose tissue, or by its surgical removal. It is also possible that their failure or modification contributes to obesity by emancipating other adipocytes from their normal controls.

The persistent lack of interest in alternative metabolic roles for adipose tissue can be attributed to firmly established traditions in techniques and materials used to study it, as well as to the way in which theories about its functioning have developed. Early studies of human starvation, mammalian hibernation and bird migration all showed that adipose tissue's main role is provisioning muscles and other bulk users of lipid for oxidation as fuel. 'Energy balance' became the byword for all research into adipose tissue metabolism, and is undoubtedly still an important concept for many kinds of investigation. The discovery of leptin as the mediator of satiety signals between adipocytes and the brain has reinforced the notion that adipose tissue is a single, uniform organ that, for its own perverse and perhaps irrelevant reasons, just happens to be dispersed into many depots widely scattered throughout the body.

Adipose tissue's role in storing and releasing lipids for oxidation by muscles and other active tissues became so firmly established that little thought was given to the possibility that it could also supply specific fatty acids for structural or informational roles, or precursors of protein synthesis. So, although rat adipose tissue was found to contain unexpectedly high levels of glutamine more than 35 years ago (1), its involvement in amino acid metabolism has only recently been studied in humans (2,3). If adipocytes' only function is to supply fuels to the bloodstream, then site-specific differences in the triacylglycerol fatty acid composition of human superficial adipose tissue can only be interpreted as metabolically trivial and unworthy of further study (4). The findings that adipocytes associated with lymph nodes in guinea-pigs contain consistently more polyunsaturated fatty acids than those remote from nodes, and that within-depot differences persist after major change in composition of dietary lipids, suggest local provisioning of immune cells that has nothing to do with serving as a whole-body energy store (5).

Another problem for the evolution of concepts about adipose tissue function is the long-standing 'habit' of using murid rodents as animal models of obesity. Young rats are quite lean unless subjected to surgical, genetic or dietary manipulation, and

International Textbook of Obesity. Edited by Per Björntorp.
© 2001 John Wiley & Sons, Ltd.

only the perirenal, inguinal and gonadal depots (especially the epididymal in males) provide enough tissue for most biochemical procedures. As explained below, these depots turn out to be only minimally involved in non-storage roles. The spectacular achievements in the selective 'knocking out' of particular genes in mice have reinforced this habit: this species is so small that only these large depots contain enough adipose tissue to work with. In all practical biology, what one finds depends upon where one looks, as well as upon what is sought, and concentrating research on the major depots precludes the chance revelation of features that might suggest additional or alternative roles.

Site-specific properties of vertebrate tissues have been most thoroughly studied in the nervous system and the musculature. While the arrangements and physiological capacities of muscle fibres are easily explained as adaptations to their roles in the particular species under investigation, the functional interpretation of the anatomical location of specialized regions of the brain and spinal cord leaves much to be desired, necessitating chiasmata and very long spinal and cranial nerves. Very thorough comparative studies starting in the mid-nineteenth century and encompassing everything from agnathan fish to modern humans, have explained, and therefore 'forgiven', many of these anomalies as the products of gradualistic evolutionary change (6). Common explanations account satisfactorily for both the tissue's site-specific properties and its anatomical location.

Unfortunately, all adipocytes look similar under the microscope with conventional fixation and staining techniques, and their abundance varies erratically between individuals. The lack of easily recognized internal structure or a fixed relationship to external 'landmarks' undermines confidence in the reliability of identifying homologous samples even in clearly delimited adipose depots such as the mesentery or popliteal. The task was seen as hopeless in overlapping and irregularly shaped depots such as inguinal, or superficial abdominal. Consequently, for many years, adipose tissue was believed to 'have no anatomy': its arrangement was regarded as not amenable to the functional or phylogenetic interpretations that had proved so successful for characterizing the details of the anatomy of nearly all other tissues. Although site-specific properties are now widely recognized in humans as well as in laboratory animals (7,8), we still do not have the

information with which to determine whether adipose tissue with certain properties is found in a particular location because it interacts with adjacent tissues, because of its blood supply, or simply because the site is convenient for storage (9).

Lack of interest in the functional anatomy of adipose tissue also tended to suppress discussion about the validity of extrapolating concepts based on the study of the epididymal depot of rats and mice to the much more widely distributed adipose mass of humans. For obvious reasons, the sites for taking biopsies of human adipose tissue are chosen for their surgical accessibility, and do not include depots homologous to those most widely studied in rats. As well as these practical considerations, the relative abundance of the major adipose depots in primates is different from that of rodents: in humans, lemurs and monkeys, the epididymal depots are minimal but these species have substantial quantities of adipose tissue on the inner and outer sides of the abdominal wall, with the latter often expanding to form the massive 'paunch' depot, but there is almost none in the homologous sites in rodents (10,11).

Consequently, while many 'differences' between sample sites have been reported, they are not sufficiently comprehensive, and the homologies between depots are not accurate enough for the data to be integrated into generalizations from which the biological principles behind the organization can be established. We should be aiming to develop a synthetic theory that accounts for the distribution and anatomical relations of adipose tissue in all mammals (12). Such a concept would be a basis for identifying and interpreting sex and species differences in the normal arrangement and provide a standard against which deviations could be assessed.

Although enormous amounts of information about 'fat patterning' in humans have been amassed, there is very little corresponding data for wild animals. The primary aim of the human studies was to establish correlations between anatomical features and metabolic variables as a means of predicting pathological states, rather than to explain the anatomy in terms of the normal physiology. By concentrating on humans, scientists made their task even more difficult than it really is: modern people are not only much fatter than most other mammals, but the distribution of their adipose tissue is complicated by sexual and age difference. The tissue's more clear-cut and consistent anatomy in wild animals more readily suggests hypotheses about the primary determinants of its distribution. But testing these ideas experimentally requires a large laboratory animal that has sufficient tissue for experimental study in at least some of the minor depots.

The purpose of this chapter is to show that there is no reason beyond traditional scepticism why the organization of adipose tissue cannot be as explainable in terms of adaptation to function or phylogeny as that of other vertebrate tissues.

THE ADIPOSE TISSUE AROUND LYMPH NODES

Reptiles and amphibians have just a few adipose depots, mostly in the abdomen or around the tail. This arrangement is clearly practical for tissue whose sole function is storage because the adipose tissue can undergo large changes in mass without affecting the adjacent organs. In contrast, mammalian adipose tissue is always split into a few large and numerous small depots scattered over much of the body. In many of the minor depots, including 'yellow' bone marrow, the omentum and many intermuscular and perivascular sites, adipocytes are intimately associated with lymphoid tissue (13). Thorough studies of wild animals (9,12,14) show that the major depots, such as the perirenal and the posterior superficial depots, undergo large changes in mass, like adipose depots in lower vertebrates, while many of those associated with lymphoid tissue, such as the politeal, do not alter much even in massive obesity or emaciation. The popliteal has also been extensively studied in humans, because part of it is clearly visible over the gastrocnemius muscle of the lower leg. Its mass changes only slightly, in spite of large changes in body composition, so people with bulging thighs may have slim calves (15). This peculiar and almost universal feature of mammals remains to be explained convincingly.

Most mammalian adipose depots contain one or more lymph nodes, though the exact number varies between conspecific individuals, posing further obstacles to quantitative study. Some adipose depots, such as the mesentery and omentum, have dozens of lymph nodes embedded in them, but others, including the popliteal depot, contain only one or a few, and they may be concentrated into one corner. The microscopic structure of the adipose tissue surrounding lymph nodes has not been investigated in detail since the work of Suzuki (16): standard histological techniques revealed no site-specific differences other than adipocyte size, and by the time immunocytochemical methods became available, interest in the microscopic anatomy of adipose tissue had waned. Many such depots are small, itself a disincentive to study, both because those of laboratory rodents offer very little tissue for experimental study, and because their reduction in humans would have little impact on obesity.

Lymph nodes as major sites of proliferation and dissemination of lymphocytes are a special feature of mammals: a few similar structures are found in certain birds but they are absent from lower vertebrates. They almost always occur embedded in adipose tissue, although most anatomical illustrations and models tend to conceal rather than emphasize the fact. Immunologists habitually begin all histological and physiological studies by 'cleaning' the adipose tissue off the node (17,18). The fact that lymph nodes and ducts are embedded in adipose tissue is disregarded in biochemical studies of lymph flow (19). The lymph ducts run through the adipose tissue and divide into numerous fine branches as they approach the node, thereby generating points of entry over much of its surface, and coming into contact with a large proportion of the adipocytes that immediately surround it. The adipose tissue associated with some nodes represents such a tiny fraction of the total that it is difficult to suppose that it could make a significant contribution to whole-body lipid supply. So why is it present at all?

The need to swell when fighting infection was, until recently presented as the main, if not the sole, reason for the anatomical association between adipose tissue and lymph nodes (17). However, adipocytes embedded in their network of collagen are not very compressible. It is difficult to see why adipose tissue should be preferred as a container for expandable nodes over a mainly extracellular, genuinely extensible material such as connective tissue (12). The lymphoid tissue of birds and lower vertebrates also expands when activated, but it is not closely associated with adipose tissue. In many species it could not be, because adipose tissue is confined to a few centrally located fat bodies, instead of, as in mammals, being partitioned into numerous small depots, where it can be associated with lymph nodes.

Since 1994, we have been exploring an alternative hypothesis: major lymph nodes occur in association with adipose tissue because the latter is specialized to serve as a regulatory and 'nurse' tissue. A simple experiment enables the lymphoid cells themselves to point out which kinds of adipose tissue they interact with most strongly (20). A standard mixture of lymphoid cells from the large cervical lymph nodes was incubated with or without a mitogen for several days with explants of adipose tissue taken from near to and away from nodes of various depots of the same animal. The number of new lymphocytes formed was estimated from incorporation of labelled thymidine, and lipolysis by the glycerol concentration in the incubation medium. Mature guinea-pigs of a large strain were used for this investigation: there is simply not enough adipose tissue in the node-containing depots of rats or mice to supply well-controlled experiments.

The presence of adipose tissue always curtails both spontaneous and mitogen-stimulated proliferation of lymphocytes, but the extent of inhibition depends greatly upon the source of the sample. In all the eight depots studied that contain one or more lymph nodes, but especially the mesentery, omentum, forearm, popliteal and cervical depots, the samples taken from near to a lymph node suppressed the formation of new lymphocytes more strongly than those taken from elsewhere in the same depot. The least effective samples were those from the perirenal, which in guinea-pigs (and most other mammals) do not contain any lymph nodes.

The same experiments revealed that lymphoid cells consistently induce more lipolysis in adipose tissue from near to nodes than in samples from elsewhere in the same depot, especially in the small intermuscular popliteal and cervical depots, and the omentum and mesentery (Figure 13.1). Co-incubation with lymphoid cells causes lipolysis to rise by more than threefold in perinodal samples, a greater increase than is observed when isolated adipocytes are stimulated with large doses of noradrenaline. Such effects are highly localized: adipose tissue from 1–2 mm around major lymph nodes may respond twice as much as neighbouring samples from just a centimetre away. Lipolysis from the perirenal is higher than all the other samples when they are incubated alone, but the presence of lymphoid cells stimulates a rise of less than 5%, a negligible increase compared to that observed in explants from the node-containing depots.

The gross anatomy of these nodes and their surrounding adipose tissue suggests an explanation for the strong local interactions. The mesenteric nodes, being the first to come into contact with material absorbed through the gut, are in the front line of defence against pathogens invading through the intestine. The omentum also contains a great deal of lymphoid tissue and is believed to remove debris from the abdominal cavity. The popliteal lymph node is the most distal of the lower limb nodes, and lymphoid cells arising from it protect the whole of the hindlimb below the knee. The cubital lymph node (in the 'forearm' adipose depot) is also located as 'the end of the line', and performs similar functions for the distal part of the forelimb.

Hands and feet (and paws and hooves) are continually exposed to abrasion and assaults from parasites and pathogens, so the nodes that serve them are nearer 'the front line' in dealing with local, minor injuries, infections and inflammations than the more centrally located inguinal and axillary ('behind arm') nodes. The popliteal depots are small, representing less than 5% of the total adipose mass in guinea-pigs and most other mammals (12), but they contain relatively large nodes. The popliteal 'space' contains a little adipose tissue around the node in all eutherian mammals, even in very lean wild animals in which nodeless depots are depleted completely, and in seals in which most of the adipose tissue is specialized as superficial blubber. Enclosing these important lymph nodes may be their main role: they do not enlarge with fattening as much as the large superficial and intra-abdominal depots, and seem to be conserved in starvation (9,10,14,15).

Perirenal adipocytes respond satisfactorily to all other known local and blood-borne stimulants of lipolysis, and indeed this depot is often taken as a representative of the adipose mass as a whole, but as Figure 13.1 shows, it is atypical as far as interactions with the lymphocytes and macrophages are concerned. In guinea-pigs and many other mammals, the perirenal is among the largest of all depots and undergoes extensive changes in size as total fatness changes. Its lack of interaction with lymphoid cells may arise from the fact that it normally contains no lymph nodes, so would be unable to participate in local interactions with lymphoid cells, or may simply be a necessary corollary of its role as an energy store for the body as a whole.

The other, smaller depots expand and shrink less

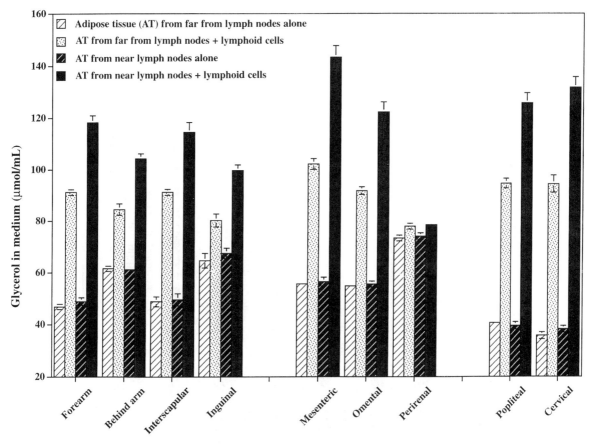

Figure 13.1 Site-specific differences in spontaneous and lymphoid cell-stimulated glycerol release (20). Means ± SE of glycerol in the medium after incubation with the mitogen, lipopolysaccharide for 48 h and an explant of adipose tissue. Explants were taken from far from (light bars) or near to (dark bars) lymph node(s) (or, in the case of perirenal, a knot of blood vessels) of four superficial (left group of bars), three intra-abdominal (centre) and two intermuscular (right) adipose depots with (shaded bars) or without (striped bars) lymphoid cells. All values are means of data from 10 mature adult guinea-pigs

readily because part of their adipose tissue is conserved for special, local functions. Adipocytes prepared from the small quantity of adipose tissue surrounding lymph nodes are insensitive to fasting: as Figure 13.2 shows, spontaneous lipolysis in such adipocytes excised from guinea-pigs after 16–17 hours of food deprivation is much lower than in those from the perirenal or epididymal depots of the same animals (21). Somehow, these adipocytes have not responded to the endocrine conditions of fasting, although as these data show, they are perfectly capable of large increases in lipolysis. The perinodal adipocytes are more sensitive to noradrenaline applied alone and in combination with tumour necrosis factor-α (TNFα) or interleukin-6 (IL-6), and their maximum rate of lipolysis is much higher than that

of the nodeless depots, and significantly higher than that of adipocytes from elsewhere in node-containing depots.

Incubation with mixtures of cytokines and noradrenaline reveals even larger within-depot differences in the control of lipolysis. Adipocytes taken from sites within the same depot as little as 5 mm apart release glycerol at widely different rates under the same conditions (20). Figure 13.3 shows such data from the poplineal samples. Corresponding samples from the mesentery and omentum produce a similar picture. High doses of noradrenaline combined with 24 h of incubation with TNFα or IL-6 stimulated lipolysis, while other combinations of cytokines suppress the process to below the control values. These properties indicate that in the *in vivo*

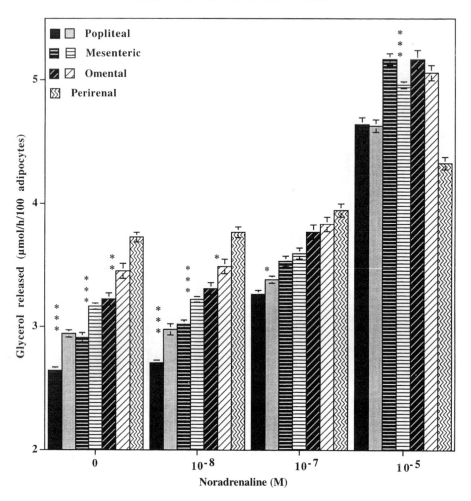

Figure 13.2   Means ± SE of spontaneous and noradrenaline-stimulated release of glycerol from adipocytes from near to lymph node(s) (dark bars) and far from lymph node(s) (light bars) on the first day of the experiment, without any prior treatment (21). Shaded bars: popliteal; horizontally striped bars: mesenteric; diagonally striped bars: omental; wavy bars: perirenal; $n = 12$ guinea-pigs, body mass 1096 ± 35 g, age 16.0 ± 0.2 months, fasted for 16–17 hours. Asterisks denote significant differences (Student's t-test) between pairs of samples from the same depot under the same conditions: *** significantly different at $P < 0.001$; ** significantly different at $P < 0.01$; * significantly different at $P < 0.05$

situation, lymphoid cells could regulate lipolysis in adipocytes located in the vicinity of their node over a wide range of values and very precisely.

Human subcutaneous adipose tissue (presumably not associated with lymph nodes) releases small quantities of IL-6 (22), and cytokines from such sources may somehow be involved in the slow development of chronic disease (23). But in the short term, cytokines secreted in and around lymph nodes that 'leaked' into the bloodstream would have little effect on the large, nodeless depots that contain the great majority of the body's lipid stores: lipolysis in adipocytes from the perirenal and

gonadal depots was unaltered by these mixtures of cytokines (21).

Noradrenaline also stimulates the smooth muscle of lymph vessels (24,25). The application of regular electrical pulses to the lumbar sympathetic ganglion produced a threefold increase in the flow of lymphocytes out of the popliteal ganglion of a sheep (26). This (and many other) lymph nodes are supplied by numerous very fine afferent lymph vessels that branch from the main afferent vessel and enter the node over almost its entire surface (27,28). Such tiny vessels are permeable to large molecules and even some kinds of small cells (29). Although the

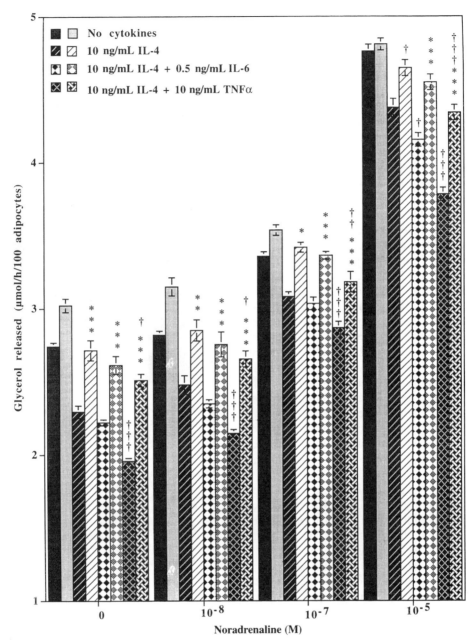

Figure 13.3 The effect of pre-incubation with 10 ng/mL IL-4 alone and with 0.5 ng/mL interleukin-6, or 10 ng/mL TNFα on spontaneous and noradrenaline-stimulated release of glycerol from adipocytes from near (darker bars) and far from (light bars) lymph nodes in the popliteal depot of the same guinea-pigs as for Figure 13.2 (21). All measurements were made on the second day post mortem. Asterisks denote significant differences from the corresponding sample incubated without cytokines: *** significantly different at $P<0.001$; ** significantly different at $P<0.01$; * significantly different at $P<0.05$. For clarity, symbols indicating within-depot differences, and those indicating that all the values from 'near node' adipocytes are significantly different at $P<0.001$ from those from the corresponding control samples incubated without cytokines, are *not* shown. Daggers denote significant differences between incubation with two cytokines and the corresponding sample incubated with IL-4 alone: ††† significantly different at $P<0.001$; †† significantly different at $P<0.01$; † significantly different at $P<0.05$

authors of these studies do not mention the adipose tissue, the consequences of these anatomical arrangements and physiological properties *in vivo* would be to bring lymphoid cells and the adipocytes immediately surrounding the node into close proximity, enabling them to exchange metabolites.

The observations on multiple samples taken from large adult guinea-pigs summarized in Figures 13.1–13.3 highlight the limitations of conclusions based only on the perirenal or epididymal depots or on 3T3 adipocyte cell lines, from which no site-specific information can be obtained. In particular, they challenge the long-held assumption that all adipocytes in an anatomically defined depot respond equally to blood-borne and neural stimuli, and each adipocyte makes a small but equal contribution to the concentration of metabolites in the blood. The data in Figures 13.1 and 13.3 suggest that a small fraction of the total adipose mass responds strongly to cytokines, and the rest very little or not at all. In brief, most of the 'hard work' of responding rapidly to the fluctuating state of lymphoid cells in a lymph node is performed by a few adipocytes, while the others, which unfortunately are the ones most widely studied, respond more slowly to stronger and more persistent stimuli. This concept should be considered when comparing levels of blood metabolites with the properties of samples of adipocytes *in vitro*. Inappropriately chosen samples can sometimes produce misleading data (30).

In the popliteal depot of the rat, receptors for TNFα are much more abundant on the adipocytes that enclose the lymph node in a shell approximately 1 mm (= 10–15 adipocytes) thick (31). Type II (p75) receptors are continuously present on perinodal adipocytes, as well as on many of the lymphoid cells within it and endothelial cells. Type I (p60) appear on adipocytes surrounding the popliteal lymph node within 30 minutes of a stimulated immune challenge to the region of the lower leg drained by this node (Figure 13.4), and on the homologous adipocytes of the unchallenged leg within 24 h. These receptors cannot be seen on adipocytes elsewhere in the popliteal lymph node, although if the signal gets as far as the other leg, it presumably also reaches the rest of the adipose depot. On a longer time scale, this simulated immune stimulus also increases vascularization of the activated adipose tissue (32). These observations indicate that adipocytes around lymph nodes are

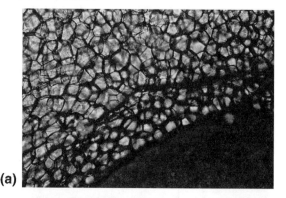

(a)

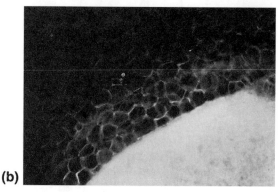

(b)

Figure 13.4 Immunofluorescent visualization of receptors for tumour necrosis factor-α on adipocytes around the popliteal depot of a rat. The field of a view is a little over 1 mm wide. (a) Bright-field view of a thick section (120 μm) through the popliteal adipose depot and the lymph node enclosed therein (bottom right) that has been stained with FITC-labelled antibody to type II receptors for tumour necrosis factor-α. All the adipocytes appear similar. (b) The same section illuminated with ultraviolet light. The antibody binds to cells in the lymph node itself and to adipocytes surrounding it, but those more than 0.5 mm remote from the node remain unstained. The blood vessel visible as a nearly horizontal black line in (a) also picks up stain. (Courtesy of H. MacQueen (31))

equipped to amplify their capacity to respond to lymphoid cells within a few hours of their activation.

This concept is confirmed by *in vivo* studies. When a single popliteal lymph node is activated by the long-established procedure of injecting a small quantity of lipopolysaccharide into the tissues that it drains, lipolysis in the adipocytes immediately surrounding it increases within an hour, and remains elevated for at least 9 hours before declining almost to baseline (33). Adipocytes thus activated also become more sensitive to noradrenaline, a synergism that suggests that the adipose tissue around the lymph nodes may be a forum for interactions between sympathetic stimulants such as stress and exercise, and immune function. These effects can be amplified simply by incubating excised adipose tissue explants in tissue culture medium for 24 h, strongly implicating paracrine and/or auto-crine interactions in perpetuating the response to the immune stimulus after it has been removed from contact with the activated lymph node.

Cytokines generally seem to act locally in a paracrine or autocrine manner, with only small quantities reaching all organs via the general circulation (34). Paracrine interactions between adipocytes are becoming more widely recognized (35). There would be good reason for keeping cytokine-mediated interactions between adipose tissue and lymphoid cells local and transient. High levels in the blood cause severe malfunction of the lungs, kidneys and other vital organs, leading to septic shock syndrome. Moderate blood levels of this cytokine for long periods are associated with abrupt, sustained depletion of adipose tissue lipids and muscle wasting, leading to cachexia, a common complication of cancer and chronic bacterial disease, and possibly at lower concentration to insulin resistance (30).

To find out more about what lymph node lymphoid cells might be getting by stimulating lipolysis in the adipose tissue around them, we compared the fatty acid composition of triacylglycerols in adipose tissue from different parts of depots that contain lymph nodes (Figure 13.5) (5). In all those examined, but especially in the intermuscular, omental and mesenteric depots, there were fewer saturated fatty acids, and more polyunsaturates in the triacylglycerols found in the adipose tissue 1–2 mm around the nodes than elsewhere in the depot.

The adipose tissue from around lymph nodes that *in vitro* interacts most strongly with lymphoid cells, and has the largest responses to TNFα and the interleukins, also contains a greater proportion of the very fatty acids that these cells need for their proliferation and integrated function, and cannot make for themselves. Selective release and retention of certain fatty acids has been demonstrated in adipocytes *in vitro* (36,37), suggesting how such site-specific differences could arise. The processes measured in Figures 13.2–13.4 suggest some reasons why they exist: selective, local stimulation of lipolysis

from the adipocytes near the nodes would maximize supplies of polyunsaturated fatty acids to the activated lymphoid cells. Lipolysis from these adipocytes is not strongly stimulated by fasting (Figure 13.2), so these local controls determine fatty acid release regardless of fever, anorexia or other whole body state that the larger 'general storage' depots (e.g. perirenal, inguinal) readily respond to. These observations are also consistent with the reports that lymphocyte function is more strongly modulated by polyunsaturated fatty acids than by monounsaturates or saturates both *in vitro* (38) and *in vivo* (39).

While many of the fatty acids so released were probably oxidized, some would have been incorporated into membrane phospholipid and/or serve as precursors for lipid-based messenger molecules for the proliferating lymphocytes. The increase in proportion of polyunsaturated fatty acids in rat liver lipids following 10 days of chronic infusion of TNFα has been attributed to changes in liver metabolism (40). But such 'new' fatty acids could equally come from triacylglycerols in the adipose tissue around lymph nodes, in which lipolysis is especially sensitive to this cytokine (21), and polyunsaturated fatty acids are more abundant (Figure 13.5). This concept of local provision of fatty acids should be considered for investigations into effects of diet on lipids in lymphoid tissue (41), and the relationship between dietary lipids, adipocyte composition and breast cancer (42).

Certain adipose depots also have significant capacity for the synthesis and release of glutamine (3), that activated lymphoid cells use in large quantities (43). Provision of glutamine to support protein synthesis in lymphoid cells may be another way in which adipose tissue supplies the immune system during periods of anorexia and cachexia, when external sources are greatly reduced, and competition with other tissues such as muscle may be strong.

Such site-specific differences in the composition of the storage lipids came as a surprise—previous investigators had assumed that continuous lipolysis and re-esterification of triacylglycerols would eventually homogenize the entire store. The only other example of site-specific differences in fatty acid composition of triacylglycerols hitherto described were the extremities and superficial adipose tissue of some cold-adapted mammals (12,44) which, although similar in principle, differ in some important details. The adaptations of adipose tissue triacyl-

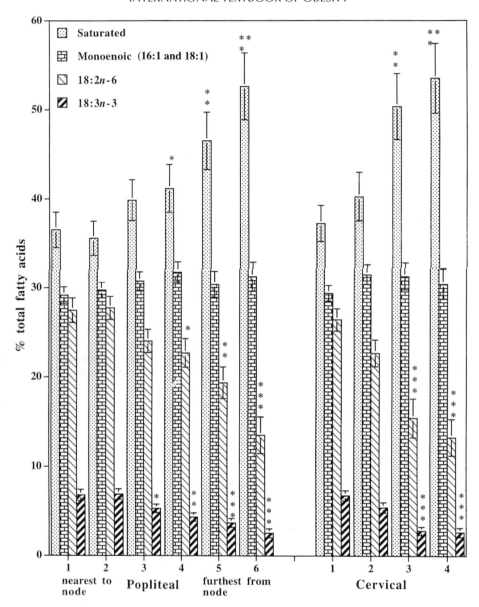

Figure 13.5 Means ± SE of the proportions of saturated FAs, monounsaturated FAs, linoleic acid (18:2n-6) and α-linolenic acid (18:3n-3) extracted from the triacylglycerols in samples of adipose tisue from six sites in the popliteal depot and four sites in the intermuscular cervical depot between the neck muscles (5). Popliteal samples 1 and 2 were from as near as possible to the node on the distal and proximal sides; 3 and 4 from the middle of the depot near where the sciatic nerve runs through it towards the gastrocnemius muscle, respectively about 4 mm and 6 mm anterior to the node; sample 5 was from as far as possible from the node going towards the anterior, behind the knee joint; sample 6 was from as far as possible from the node going dorsally. Cervical sample 1 was from near the large central node; 2 near the group of smaller nodes near the dorsal edge of the adipose depot; 3 and 4 from opposite sides of the depot, as far away as possible from lymph nodes. $n = 17$ adult guinea-pigs fed on plain chow. Asterisks refer to differences between the composition of sample 1 and others from the same depot, assessed using Student's t-test: *** Significantly different at $P < 0.001$; ** significantly different at $P < 0.01$; * significantly different at $P < 0.05$

glycerols to cooler conditions mainly involve substituting saturated fatty acids with monounsaturates. In this case (Figure 13.5), the saturates decrease as the relative abundance of the polyunsaturates increase, with the proportions of monounsaturates remaining constant.

WITHIN-DEPOT SITE-SPECIFIC PROPERTIES AND OBESITY

These data together clearly show that certain adipocytes have properties that are minimal or absent in samples from the standard perirenal or epididymal depots. Although indistinguishable in histological appearance from typical adipocytes, those around major lymph nodes are equipped to participate in local interactions with lymphoid cells, and seem to be at least partially exempt from contributing to whole-body supply during fasting. Bone marrow is another site where adipocytes are contiguous with lymphoid cells, and the combination is known to be capable of functioning like lymph nodes (45). At least in non-ruminants, these marrow adipocytes retain their storage lipid, and even the capacity to accumulate more, during prolonged starvation when those in the 'typical' depots are almost totally depleted (46). The mammalian immune system seems to have organized its own local supplies of the polyunsaturated fatty acids (and perhaps of other metabolites), thereby avoiding the need for their transportation through the general circulation, and competition with other tissues. Paracrine interactions between perinodal adipocytes and lymphoid cells would also allow ready access to large quantities of fatty acids, without the need for their accumulation inside rapidly dividing, metabolically active lymphocytes; this concept recalls that of Unger et al. (47) who suggested that adipocytes protect pancreatic islets (and by implication other types of cell) from toxic accumulation of triacylglycerols in obesity.

Converting adipocytes from fatty acid retention and controlled secretion to lipid oxidation is being considered as a therapy for obesity (48). If the interaction between lymph nodes and surrounding adipose tissue proves to be an integral part of the normal immune response, and I firmly believe that it is, drastic alteration of the metabolism of these adipocytes may not be physiologically desirable. By making immune responses slower or less efficient,

such manipulation could make the animal or person more susceptible to infection and perhaps cancer.

Nothing is known of how permanent this specialized population of cells is, or how it is affected by expansion of the rest of the adipose tissue. There are indications that the lipid composition of the diet affects the interaction between lymphoid cells and adipocytes. In guinea-pigs (5), the capacity of lymphoid cells to stimulate lipolysis in adipose tissue from around lymph nodes is significantly reduced after small quantities of suet (rich in saturated and monoenoic fatty acids) were added to the normal chow for several weeks, while spontaneous lipolysis from similar explants incubated alone is unaltered (Figure 13.6). The ability of adipose tissue explants to curtail mitogen-stimulated proliferation of lymphocytes is even more severely impaired (Figure 13.7), although the basic pattern of site-specific differences in triacylglycerol fatty acid composition remains unchanged. In assessing the roles of dietary lipids in immune function (49), the possibility that adipose tissue is intervening to sequester or release certain fatty acids selective cannot be disregarded.

Guinea-pigs are grazers, whose natural diet is very low in fat, and contains mostly unsaturated fatty acids, so this minor modification of the diet probably induced a major departure from the normal situation. These data suggest that circulating lipids affect local interactions between adipose tissue and lymphoid cells, though the mechanism remains unknown. A high fat diet or hyperlipidaemia may impair local immune responses, and reduce the sensitivity of adipocytes to cytokines. Such properties could be relevant to known associations between high fat diet, obesity and certain forms of cancer (42,50,51).

What lessons do these concepts have for the study of human obesity? In naturally lean wild animals, depots associated with lymph nodes are not readily depleted and are relatively massive and conspicuous. The omentum, mesentery and popliteal remain surprisingly small, even in very obese specimens, possibly because their specialized functions would be impaired by too little, or too much, 'whole-body storage'. In contrast to humans, the additional adipose tissue in naturally obese species such as polar bears, and subspecies of reindeer and arctic foxes accumulates in the perirenal and in superficial depots not associated with lymph nodes (9,12,44).

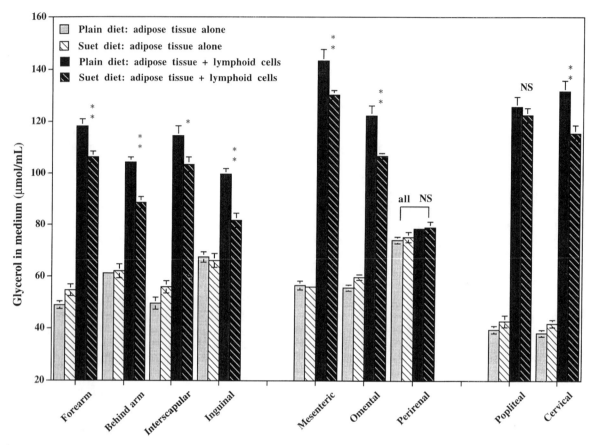

Figure 13.6 Means ± SE of glycerol in the medium after incubation for 48 h of explants of adipose tissue taken from near a lymph node (or, in the case of perirenal, a knot of blood bessels) of four superficial (left group of bars), three intra-abdominal (centre) and two intermuscular (right) adipose depots of guinea-pigs fed on normal chow (plain bars; $n = 10$ guinea-pigs) or suet-enriched chow (striped bars; $n = 7$ guinea-pigs), either alone (pale bars) or with lipopolysaccharide-stimulated lymphoid cells (darker bars) (5). Asterisks refer to differences between measurements from incubations under similar conditions of homologous explants from guinea-pigs on the two different diets. *** Significantly different at $P < 0.001$; ** significantly different at $P < 0.01$; * significantly different at $P < 0.05$. Horizontal bracket refers to differences between homologous explants incubated with or without lymphoid cells. NS, not significant

The synergism between certain cytokines and the sympathetic nervous system agonist noradrenaline (Figure 13.3), and the fact that stimulation of the perinodal adipose tissue in one popliteal depot induces detectable changes in the mesenteric and omental adipose tissue (33), suggest that a pathway by which frequent activation of the immune system could promote lipolysis in the intra-abdominal depots. Repeated activation over many years could contribute to the development of intra-abdominal obesity, as does chronic overstimulation of the hypothalamo-pituitary-adrenal endocrine axis (52).

The omentum contains a large amount of lymphoid tissue intimately interspersed with adipose tissue and has a high capacity for glutamine metab-

olism (3). Lipolysis in omental adipocytes is strongly influenced by lymphoid cells (Figures 13.1, 13.2 and 13.6), and amino acid metabolism may be as well. Its physiological functions are not firmly established, but in middle-aged people, especially men, living in Europe and the USA the omentum is often hypertrophied. Explanation for this effect, which can lead to metabolic disorders as well as being cosmetically unsatisfactory, relate mainly to lipid metabolism and endocrinological abnormalities (51). Digby (3) suggested that abnormalities of amino acid metabolism, perhaps triggered by the high protein content of the Western diet and/or excessive activation of omental lymphoid tissues, may also make an important contribution. This

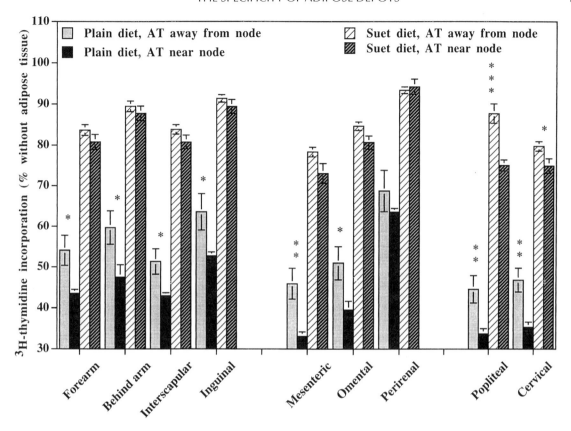

Figure 13.7 Site-specific differences in the effects of adipose tissue (AT) explants from guinea-pigs fed on unmodified chow (plain bars: $n = 10$, $100\% = 17\,541 \pm 470$ d.p.m.) or suet-enriched chow (striped bars: $n = 7$, $100\% = 18\,754 \pm 219$ d.p.m.) on lipopolysaccharide-stimulated proliferation of their lymphoid cells in culture (5). Means $\pm$ SE of cell proliferation, measured as incorporation of ^{3}H-thymidine (% counts in aliquots cells from the same source incubated under identical conditions without any adipose tissue) into lymphocytes incubated with one explant of adipose tissue taken from away from lymph node(s) or, in the case of the perirenal depot, away from knots of blood vessels (light bars) and from near to lymph node(s) or near to knots of blood vessels (dark bars). Sets of samples were taken from four superficial (left group of bars), three intra-abdominal (centre) and two intermuscular (right) adipose depots. Asterisks refer to differences between data from incubations with adipose explants from 'near to' or 'away from' lymph nodes of the same depot of the same specimens. *** Significantly different at $P < 0.001$; ** significantly different at $P < 0.01$; * significantly different at $P < 0.05$

suggestion again shifts the emphasis from energy storage and blood metabolites to specialized properties of certain regions of the adipose mass.

CONCLUSIONS

The investigations discussed here show that small groups of adipocytes of unexceptional microscopical appearance prove to have unusual biochemical properties that are minimal or absent in the larger, more widely studied depots. In some cases, the site-specific physiological and biochemical properties can be related to the adipocytes' anatomical relations with other tissues, suggesting a functional explanation for a combination of characters that is not concerned only, or even mainly, with energy storage. Such specialized properties not only help to explain why the adipose mass is dispersed in mammals, it also suggests novel mechanisms for disturbance of lipid metabolism and obesity, and signals a warning that drastic manipulation of adipose tissue may produce unforeseen consequences for other physiological systems.

ACKNOWLEDGEMENTS

I thank Dr Hilary MacQueen for providing Figure 13.4. Several aspects of the research discussed in this chapter were carried out in collaboration with C.A. Mattacks and supported by a consumables grant from The Leverhulme Trust.

REFERENCES

1. Christophe J, Wodon C. Composition en acides aminés du tissue adipeux épididymaire du rat nomal. *Arch Int Biochem Physiol* 1963; **71**: 720–740.
2. Frayn KN, Khan K, Coppack SW, Elia M. Amino acid metabolism in human subcutaneous adipose tissue in vivo. *Clin Sci* 1991; **80**: 471–474.
3. Digby JE. The roles of different adipose depots in glutamine metabolism following feeding, fasting and exercise in the guinea-pig. PhD thesis, The Open University, 1998.
4. Phinney SD, Stern JS, Burke KE, Tang AB, Miller G, Holman RT. Human subcutaneous adipose tissue shows site-specific differences in fatty acid composition. *Am J Clin Nutr* 1994; **60**: 725–729.
5. Mattacks CA, Pond CM. The effects of feeding suet-enriched chow on site-specific differences in the composition of triacylglycerol fatty acids in adipose tissue and its interactions *in vitro* with lymphoid cells. *Br J Nutr* 1997; **77**: 621–643.
6. Goodrich ES. *Studies on the Structure and Development of Vertebrates*. New York: Dover Publications, 1958.
7. Cousin B, Casteilla L, Dani C, Muzzin P, Revelli JP. Adipose tissues from various anatomical sites are characterized by different patterns of gene expression and regulation. *Biochem J* 1993; **292**: 873–876.
8. Björntorp P. The regulation of adipose tissue distribution in humans. *Int J Obes* 1996; **20**: 291–302.
9. Pond CM. An evolutionary and functional view of mammalian adipose tissue. *Proc Nutr Soc* 1992; **51**: 367–377.
10. Pond CM, Mattacks CA. The anatomy of adipose tissue in captive *Macaca* monkeys and its implications for human biology. *Folia Primatol* 1987; **48**: 164–185.
11. Pereira ME, Pond CM. Organization of white adipose tissue in lemuridae. *Am J Primatol* 1995; **35**: 1–13.
12. Pond CM. *The Fats of Life*. Cambridge: Cambridge University Press, 1998.
13. Pond CM. Physiological specialisation of adipose tissue. *Progr Lipid Res* 1999; **38**: 225–248.
14. Pond CM. The structure and organization of adipose tissuee in naturally obese non-hibernating mammals. In: Ditschuneit H, Gries FA, Hauner H, Schusdziarra V, Wechs-ler JG (eds) *Obesity in Europe '93, Proceedings of the 5th European Congress of Obesity*. London: J. Libbey, 1994: 419–426.
15. Abe T, Sakurai T, Kurata J, Kawakami Y, Fukunaa T. Subcutaneous and visceral fat distribution and daily physical activity: Comparison between young and middle aged women. *Br J Sport Med* 1996; **30**: 297–300.
16. Suzuki T. Histological studies on lymphatic apparatus in human adipose tissue. *Acta School Med Univ Kyoto* 1952; **30**: 174–182.
17. Henry K, Farrer-Brown G. *A Colour Atlas of the Thymus and Lymph Nodes*. London: Wolfe Medical Publications, 1981.
18. Kowala MC, Schoefl GI. The popliteal lymph node of the mouse: internal architecture, vascular distribution and lymphatic supply. *J Anat* 1986; **148**: 25–46.
19. Ikomi F, Zweifach BW, Schmid-Schonbein GW. Fluid pressures in the rabbit popliteal afferent lymphatics during passive tissue motion. *Lymphology* 1997; **30**: 113–123.
20. Pond CM, Mattacks CA. Interactions between adipose tissue around lymph nodes and lymphoid cells in vitro. *J Lipid Res* 1995; **36**: 2219–2231.
21. Mattacks CA, Pond CM. Interactions of noradrenalin and tumour necrosis factor-α, interleukin-4 and interleukin-6 in the control of lipolysis from adipocytes around lymph nodes. *Cytokine* 1999; **11**: 334–346.
22. Mohamed-Ali V, Goodrick S, Rawesh A, Katz DR, Miles JM, Yudkin JS, Klein S, Coppack SW. Subcutaneous adipose tissue releases interleukin-6, but not tumor necrosis factor-alpha, in vivo. *J Clin Endocrinol Metab* 1997; **82**: 4196–4200.
23. Yudkin JS, Stehouwer CDA, Emeis JJ, Coppack SW. C-reactive protein in healthy subjects: associations with obesity, insulin resistance, and endothelial dysfunction—A potential role for cytokines originating from adipose tissue? *Arterioscler Thromb Vasc Biol* 1999; **19**: 972–978.
24. van Helden DF. Pacemaker potentials in lymphatic smooth muscle of the guinea-pig mesentery. *J Physiol* 1993; **471**: 465–479.
25. McHale NG. Role of the lymph pump and its controls. *News Physiol Sci* 1995; **10**: 112–117.
26. McHale NG, Thornbury KO. Sympathetic stimulation causes increased output of lymphocytes from the popliteal node in anaesthetised sheep. *Exp Physiol* 1990; **75**: 847–850.
27. Heath T, Brandon R. Lymphatic and blood vessels of the popliteal node in sheep. *Anat Rec* 1983; **207**: 461–472.
28. Lowden S, Heath T. Lymphatic drainage from the distal small intestine in sheep. *J Anat* 1993; **183**: 13–20.
29. Shields JW. Lymph, lymph glands and homeostasis. *Lymphology* 1992; **25**: 147–153.
30. Grünfeld C, Gulli R, Moser AH, Gavin LA, Feingold KR. Effect of tumour necrosis factor administration in vivo on lipoprotein lipase activity in various tissues of the rat. *J Lipid Res* 1989; **30**: 579–585.
31. MacQueen HA, Pond CM. Immunofluorescent localization of tumour necrosis factor-α receptors on the popliteal lymph node and the surrounding adipose tissue following simulated immune challenge. *J Anat* 1998; **192**: 223–231.
32. MacQueen HA, Waights V, Pond CM. Vascularisation in adipose depots surrounding immune-stimulated lymph nodes. *J Anat* 1999; **194**: 33–38.
33. Pond CM, Mattacks CA. *In vivo* evidence for the involvement of the adipose tissue surrounding lymph nodes in immune responses. *Immunol Lett* 1998; **63**: 158–167.
34. Memon RA, Feingold KR, Grünfeld C. The effects of cytokines on intermediary metabolism. *Endocrinologist* 1994; **4**: 56–63.
35. Mohamed-Ali V, Pinkney JH, Coppack SW. Adipose tissue as an endocrine and paracrine organ. *Int J Obes* 1998; **22**:

1145–1158.

36. Gavino VC, Gavino GR. Adipose hormone-sensitive lipase preferentially releases polyunsaturated fatty acids from triglycerides. *Lipids* 1992; **27**: 950–954.

37. Raclot T, Langin D, Lafontan M, Groscolas R. Selective release of human adipocyte fatty acids according to molecular structure. *Biochem J* 1997; **324**: 911–915.

38. Calder PC, Bond JA, Bevan SJ, Hunt SV, Newsholme EA. Effect of fatty acids on the proliferation of concanavalin A-stimulated rat lymph node lymphocytes. *Int J Biochem* 1991; **23**: 579–588.

39. Calder PC, Newsholme EA. Polyunsaturated fatty acids suppress human peripheral blood lymphocyte proliferation and interleukin-2 production. *Clin Sci* 1992; **82**: 695–700.

40. Rainia N, Matsui J, Cunnane SC, Jeejeebhoy KN. Effect of tumour necrosis factor-α on triglyceride and phospholipid content and fatty-acid composition of liver and carcass in rats. *Lipids* 1995; **30**: 713–718.

41. Guimaraes ARP, Kuga E, Torres RP, Colquhoun A, Curi R, Mancini J. Composition of fatty acids in the liver and lymphoid organs of rats fed fatty acid-rich diets. *Biochem Mol Biol Int* 1995; **36**: 451–461.

42. Petrek JA, Hudgins LC, Ho MN, Bajorunas DR, Hirsch J. Fatty acid composition of adipose tissue, an indication of dietary fatty acids, and breast cancer prognosis. *J Clin Oncol* 1997; **15**: 1377–1384.

43. Ardawi MS, Newsholme EA. Glutamine metabolism in lymphocytes of the rat. *Biochem J* 1983; **212**: 835–842.

44. Pond CM, Mattacks CA, Colby RH, Tyler NJC. The anatomy, chemical composition and maximum glycolytic capacity of adipose tissue in wild Svalbard reindeer (*Rangifer tarandus platyrhynchus*), in winter. *J Zool, Lond* 1993; **229**: 17–40.

45. Tripp RA, Topham DJ, Watson SR, Doherty PC. Bone marrow can function as a lymphoid organ during primary immune response under conditions of disrupted lymphocyte trafficking. *J Immunol* 1997; **158**: 3716–3720.

46. Bathija A, Davis S, Trubowitz S. Bone marrow adipose tissue: response to acute starvation. *Am J Haematol* 1979; **6**: 191–198.

47. Unger RH, Zhou YT, Orci L. Regulation of fatty acid homeostasis in cells: Novel role of leptin. *Proc Natl Acad Sci* 1999; **96**: 2327–2332.

48. Zhou YT, Wang ZW, Higa M, Newgard CB, Unger RH. Reversing adipocyte differentiation: Implications for treatment of obesity. *Proc Natl Acad Sci* 1999; **96**: 2391–2395.

49. Calder PC. *n*-3 Polyunsaturated fatty acids and cytokine production in health and disease. *Ann Nutr Metab* 1997; **41**: 203–234.

50. London SJ, Sacks FM, Stampfer MJ, Henderson IC, Maclure M, Tomita A, Wood WC, Remine S, Robert NJ, Dmochowski JR, Willett WC. Fatty acid composition of the subcutaneous adipose tissue and risk of proliferative benign breast disease and breast cancer. *J Natl Cancer Inst* 1993; **85**: 785–793.

51. Stoll BA. Obesity and breast cancer. *Int J Obes* 1996; **20**: 389–392.

52. Björntorp P. Body fat distribution, insulin resistance, and metabolic diseases. *Nutrition* 1997; **9**: 795–803.

14

Causes of Obesity and Consequences of Obesity Prevention in Non-human Primates and Other Animal Models

Barbara C. Hansen

*University of Maryland,
Baltimore, Maryland, USA*

INTRODUCTION

Obesity develops slowly and spontaneously in some rodent strains and in non-human primates, with peak body weight reached in 'middle-age' or in older age. The animal models of obesity may be classified as: (a) spontaneous naturally occurring (of unknown genetic and physiologic cause(s)); (b) specific genetic models of known or unknown single gene mutations occurring spontaneously (and selected for by breeding), or produced by transgenic approaches; (c) dietary or nutritionally induced obesity usually by high fat and/or highly palatable diets in rodents (a form of obesity which is likely to be polygenic), or by high fat diets or forced overfeeding in non-human primates; and (d) neuroendocrine disorders causing obesity, such as via hypothalamic lesions or chemical infusions (e.g. the injection of gold thioglucose into mice), as detailed in Table 14.1. The present review will focus principally upon the spontaneously occurring form of obesity in non-human primates and in rodents, the form(s) of obesity that are highly likely to be directly relevant to most human obesity.

OBESITY AS A DISEASE OF AGING IN PRIMATES: THE NATURAL HISTORY OF CHANGES IN BODY ADIPOSITY

Obesity has been identified in many primate species, including orangutans, gorillas (1), chimpanzees (2), baboons (*Papio ursinus*) (3), vervet monkeys (*Cercopithecus aethiops*) (4), cynomolgus monkeys (*Macaca fascicularis*) (5), bonnet macaques (*Macaca radiata*) (6), pigtail macaques (*Macaca nemistrina*) (7), squirrel monkeys (8), and the Celebes ape (*Macaca nigra*) (9), although the species most studied is the rhesus monkey (*Macaca mulatta*) (10–12). Several rodent species develop a similar adult-onset obesity, including the Sprague-Dawley rat (13), the gerbil (*Psammomys obesus*, Israeli desert sand rat) (14), the New Zealand Obese mouse, the

Table 14.1 Animal models of obesity and diabetes

Classification of animal models of obesity and diabetes	Examples of models/methods
Spontaneous, naturally occurring-of unknown genetic/physiologic causes	Probable genetic Gene–gene interactions Gene–environment interactions Aging-associated e.g. non-human primates, aging Sprague-Dawley rats
Specific genetic models of single gene mutations of known or unknown function (spontaneous, bred, or transgenic)	*Ob/ob* mouse *Db/db* mouse *Fa/fa* rat *Tub* mouse *Ay mouse* Others
Dietary induced obesity	High fat diet fed rodents 'Cafeteria' (highly palatable) diet fed rodents
Neuroendocrine disorders	Hypothalamic or related brain area lesions or stimulation (including electrolytic, knife cut, chemical, viral)

BSB mouse (*Mus spretus* and other strains), and the spiny mouse (*Acomys caharinus*). Spontaneous obesity also develops in some cats (15) and dogs, as well as in many other species, when the individuals are maintained in an unfettered environment.

Spontaneous adult-onset obesity develops in primates and rodents in an environment that is either permissive of, or facilitative to, weight gain. The usual laboratory setting of *ad libitum* food availability and of protection from predators and disease is sufficient to produce adult-onset obesity in many, but not all, non-human primates (16,17). (Some 20–30% remain lean all of their lives despite a facilitative environment, and further, among the obese, the amount of excess weight and fat varies widely.) The peak body weight in these laboratory housed monkeys is usually not reached until about 15 years of age ('middle-age'), with the weight gained after age 7 being composed primarily of adipose tissue. Thus, obesity in non-human primates must be considered to be a disease of aging. Although primates are able to reproduce by about the age of 4 years, no spontaneously obese younger monkeys (under the age of 6 years) have ever been described, and thus, primates do not provide a model for childhood-onset obesity in humans.

Does obesity occur in primates living in their natural environment? The best evidence comes from the identification of obese monkeys in the protected environment offered by the island of Cayo Santiago off the coast of Puerto Rico (18). On that island, large colonies of monkeys are provi-

sioned with primate chow to provide *ad libitum* intake in a free-ranging, but predator-free, environment. In a reported survey of these monkeys, the obese monkeys ranged from 9 to 16 years of age (19). In some matrilines, the prevalence of obesity ranged as high as 20% in these free-living monkeys (20). Obesity has also been observed in other freely feeding and protective environments, including in some zoological collections. The relationship between obesity, diabetes and aging in monkeys has been reviewed recently (21).

Fat Mass and Distribution: Abdominal or Central Obesity

Obesity in humans and monkeys develops very gradually and progressively in 'middle-age'. Specifically, percent body fat begins to increase in monkeys after about the age of 7 years, and continues, in some monkeys, to increase into late maturity. This increase in fat mass can be detected widely in subcutaneous tissue and also in intra-abdominal adipose mass. Its distribution is heavily abdominal in both males and females (22,23). The abdominal circumference shows a consistent increase with increasing body weight in middle age (age 7 to 20 in monkeys), as shown in Figure 14.1 for one monkey (D-7), and as previously described for a large group of monkeys (24).

In many monkeys, this change in body fat com-

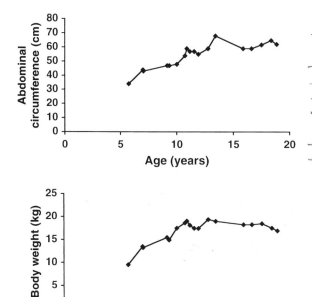

Figure 14.1 Longitudinal changes in abdominal circumference and in body weight of a monkey (D-7) followed from age ∼5 to age ∼20 years

position is accompanied by a progressive series of changes in fasting plasma glucose and insulin, as shown for monkey A-7 in Figure 14.2. Also shown is the later decline in insulin sensitivity (M rate, or glucose uptake rate as measured by a euglycemic hyperinsulinemic clamp), and the slight later decline in glucose tolerance as measured by an intravenous glucose tolerance test.

Figure 14.3 summarizes the overall pattern or sequence of events seen in a large group of monkeys, arrayed by phase, or stage in the progression from young lean adult (phase 1) to overt severe diabetes (phase 9).

OBESITY AS A GENETIC DISORDER

Genetic and metabolic factors in the development of obesity have received increasing attention since the identification of the protein product of the *ob* gene—leptin, and its receptor. Clearly there are cases among humans, as well as in strains of rodents, in which a single gene mutation has been identified as the direct and specific cause of obesity. That obesity is a genetic disorder is rarely disputed today. What remains under discussion is the relative magnitude of the contribution of genes to body weight compared to the contributions of excessive ingestion of calories due to environmental considerations. Excessive ingestion of food and reduced energy expenditure, both of which may be exacerbated by an enriched environment, are sometimes considered to be the primary culprits.

Concerning obesity in humans, just as it may be difficult to get a genie back in a bottle, so it may be difficult to 'demodernize' the environment of humans, or to otherwise alter it so as to mitigate the 'New World syndrome' (25). This is confirmed by the modest success of most weight control programs, and suggests that the forces aligned against weight loss and weight loss maintenance are indeed powerful and poorly susceptible to the combination of environmental manipulations and volitional changes among humans with excess weight.

We have found the same to be true in non-human primates. For example, forced weight reduction by limitation of available calories provided to obese monkeys produces weight loss. However, the recidivism when the monkeys are returned to a nonrestrained calorie regimen is 100%. This occurs despite the use of a high fiber, low fat chow diet which is not highly palatable. What might be the nature of these 'forces' that mitigate against significant weight loss for most middle-aged persons, and that promote weight regain or recidivism in most of those who have successfully lost weight? Are these 'forces' present in animals as well?

The strong familial aggregation of risk for obesity in humans provides evidence for a powerful familial component to the development of obesity. Some suggest that this is a combination of shared environment and shared genetic propensities. Both quantitative trait loci in rodent models and family linkage studies in humans have identified a number of chromosome areas which may carry obesity promoting genes. However, at this time these remain only promising regions, some of which may contain candidate genes for further study.

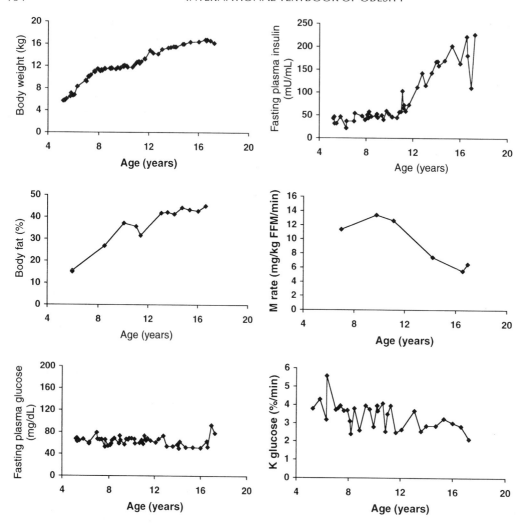

Figure 14.2 Longitudinal data from a single monkey (A-7), beginning at sexual maturity (young lean adult age 5) through the progressive development of obesity followed through age 17. Panels show sequential changes in body weight, % body fat determined by tritiated water dilution, fasting plasma glucose, fasting plasma insulin (and progressive hyperinsulinemia), M or glucose uptake rate during a euglycemic hyperinsulinemic clamp (a measure of whole body insulin sensitivity which declined over time) and K glucose or glucose disappearance rate during an intravenous glucose tolerance test (which showed a slow declining function)

Single Gene Mutations in Animal Models

Candidate Genes for Human Obesity

Lessons for human obesity can be learned from animal models of genetic obesity. First, single gene mutations can and do cause obesity in both rodent models and in humans—this is indisputable. In rodents such mutations have been identified in at least five genes, including the *ob* gene for the circulating adipose tissue-secreted factor leptin, the *db* gene for the receptor of leptin (and in rats, the *fa* gene), the *agouti yellow* (*Ay/a*) mutation which controls the production of melanin pigments controlling skin color in mice (with its human equivalent agouti signaling protein gene), the *fat* mutation in the carboxipeptidase E gene which is a prohormone processing enzyme, and the *tub* mutation which is still under study to determine its function, but which may be a protein involved in insulin signaling (26). Other genes which have been implicated in body

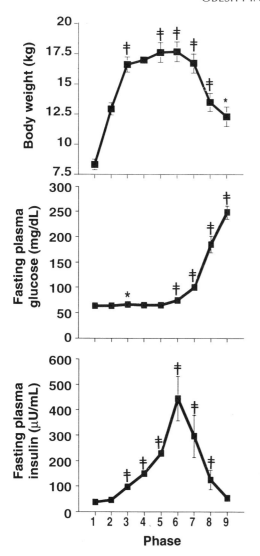

Figure 14.3 Progressive changes in body weight, fasting plasma glucose, and fasting plasma insulin as monkeys progress from lean normal (phase 1) to heavier and older (phase 2), following which some monkeys continue through a series of phases reaching overt diabetes (phase 8) and severe diabetes (phase 9)(Redrawn from Hansen (101)). Others remain in phase 2 all of their lives. * $P \leq 0.05$;† ≤ 0.01; = $P \leq 0.001$ (in comparison to phases 1 and 2)

suppressor of obesity, the mahogany protein, which may be a signaling protein or receptor similar to the proteoglycan receptors. Although extensive efforts have been made to identify mutations in these and in other candidate genes for obesity in humans, to date, only a handful of individuals have been identified with mutations in any of the genes which have produced obesity in rodents.

Mutations of the ob *Gene in Rodents and Humans*

Based on the observations of food intake and body weight in parabiotic obese and lean rodents, a circulating product of the adipose tissue had long been suspected of being involved in body weight regulation (28,29). Cross circulation studies in non-human primates, by contrast, did not support the idea that a circulating factor might be involved in feeding regulation in any dominant or major way (30). Interestingly, both studies now appear to be confirmed.

The specific genes and their mutations implicated in the early rat parabiosis studies were identified only a few years ago (31,32). The cloning of these genes, the identification of their mutations in obese rodents, and the identification of the circulating gene product (leptin) and its receptor (32) led to the hope that the genetic basis for human obesity might soon become clear. The *ob* genes in humans (33) and in monkeys (34) were cloned and sequenced. The deduced amino acid sequence of the human OB protein coding region was found to be 84% identical to that of mice, 83% identical to rats, and 91% identical to that of the rhesus monkey. The genes of many obese persons and monkeys have been searched for defects in the *ob* or leptin gene and its receptor. As noted, only a handful of patients and no monkeys have been identified with mutations in either of these genes (35–37).

Variations in the Circulating Product of the ob *Gene, leptin*

With the identification of the peptide released from adipose tissue, animal models as well as humans were examined for characteristics associated with variations in plasma leptin levels. Both monkeys and humans have been reported to show strong correlations between body weight and plasma leptin levels, and between body fat and leptin levels, as

weight regulation include the melanocortin-4 receptor (MC4-R) (27), and its other isoforms, melanin-concentrating hormone, receptors mediating leukocyte adhesion (deficiency in intercellular adhesion molecule-1 or in its receptor, leukocyte integrin alpha M beta2 (Mac-1)), and the possible

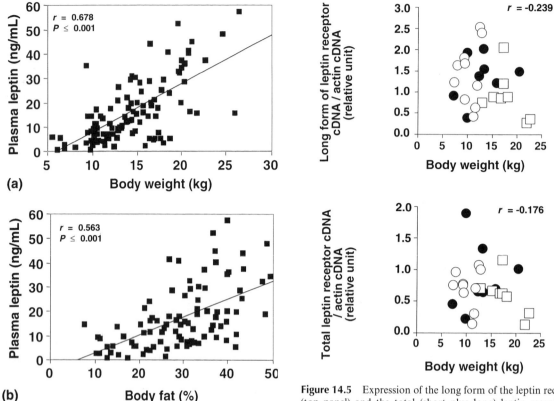

Figure 14.4 Both body weight (a) and body fat (b) were highly correlated to plasma leptin levels (*P* as shown) in a large group of rhesus monkeys (expanded from Hotta *et al.* (34))

Figure 14.5 Expression of the long form of the leptin receptor (top panel) and the total (short plus long) leptin receptor in adipose tissue of monkeys ranging widely in body weight. Open circles are normal monkeys, open squares are obese hyperinsulinemic, and solid circles are overtly diabetic monkeys. (Reproduced with permission from Hotta *et al.* (37))

shown in Figure 14.4 for rhesus monkeys (38). It was immediately noticed that while lean subjects generally have low leptin levels, not only was there an increase in leptin levels with increasing adiposity, but the variability increased greatly, such that obese subjects could be identified with normal to extremely elevated levels, e.g. 5- to 10-fold higher than normal. No explanation for these large variations has been established, since all plasma samples were obtained consistently under overnight fasted conditions. What is clear is that leptin is not released and does not circulate in a simple ratio to fat mass. This is in contrast to the observation that, in rats, the leptin–body fat ratio is a constant for a particular strain (39). Circulating levels are altered significantly by fasting and refeeding, and by many other factors.

The possibility that these large variations in circulating leptin levels might indicate important differences in the receptors for leptin has also been closely examined in rhesus monkeys. No leptin re-

ceptor mutations were identified, and expression levels as determined by polymerase chain reaction (PCR) of the two principal isoforms of the receptor, the long form and the short form, were not associated with body weight as shown in Figure 14.5. There was also no association between expression of the forms of the leptin receptor and fasting plasma insulin, plasma glucose, or circulating plasma leptin levels.

Insulin and the Insulin Receptor Genes

Rare genetic defects in either the insulin molecule or the insulin receptor have been identified in humans and associated with insulin resistance and obesity (40). In non-human primates, which have circulating plasma insulin levels five-fold or more higher than in humans, no defects in either have been found to account for the apparent insulin resistance.

The insulin molecule in monkeys is identical to that of humans (41), and sequencing of the insulin receptor has shown it to be remarkably similar to that of humans (42). Molecular examination of the few amino acid substitutions in the monkey insulin receptor compared to that of humans failed to show why monkeys have such elevated insulin levels relative to humans (43).

The insulin receptor is expressed in two isoforms in humans and in monkeys. One form is expressed in higher proportions in obese, hyperinsulinemic prediabetic monkeys (and similarly in humans), and this proportion reverts to normal in diabetes (44,45). Whether the relative proportion of these isoforms plays a role in the progression of obesity to diabetes is unknown. The hyperinsulinemia of obese monkeys is not associated with any difference in food intake relative to similarly obese normoinsulinemic monkeys (46).

Many transgenic animal models of obesity are under study at this time. However, they will not be discussed in this review, which focuses upon spontaneous models of the human condition.

Mendelian Syndromes of Obesity not Identified in Animal Models

There is a large group of Mendelian syndromes in which obesity is a component, including Prader–Willi, Bardet–Biedl, Alstrom, Carpenter, Cohen, Wilson–Turner and others. However, these lack specific animal models. These genetic disorders are rare in humans, and family studies do not suggest that the genes responsible for these syndromes are involved in the common form(s) of human obesity. For more than 99% of all obese humans, and 100% of all obese non-human primates, the genetic basis of the obesity is unknown.

Adipose Gene Expression

In animal models, adipose tissue has been the focus of numerous studies aimed at understanding its physiological and genetic regulation and the differential expression of various genes that might regulate adipose tissue mass. In non-human primates the possibility that the obese may differ in the expression of the genes that regulate adipocyte differentiation has been explored. The peroxisome prolif-

erator-activated receptor γ (PPARγ) has been the specific focus of much study since its identification as the receptor for the insulin sensitizer class of pharmaceutical agents, the thiazolidinediones (see below), and its very early expression during adipose cell differentiation. There are two isoforms of PPARγ, (γ1 and γ2), and both have been cloned and sequenced in the rhesus monkey (47). The latter is highly expressed in adipocytes, while PPARγ1 is expressed widely in many tissues. The ratio of the PPARγ2 mRNA to total PPARγ mRNA was significantly related to body weight and to fasting plasma insulin, while neither total PPAR γ nor its two isoforms individually were related to obesity or to insulin levels (47). This is in contrast to the finding in rats of increased PPARγ mRNA levels in the white adipose tissue of obese rats (48).

Other genes expressed during adipocyte differentiation include: CCAAT/enhancer binding protein α (C/EBP α), lipoprotein lipase (LPL), phosphoenolpyruvate carboxykinase (PEPCK), and the glucose transporter gene (GLUT 4). As shown in Figure 14.6, in a study of normal weight, obese, and diabetic monkeys, none of the best known regulators of adipose differentiation were associated with body weight in any of the three groups, nor in the total group (47). They were, however, found to be associated with aging (49).

A newly identified adipocytokine, adiponectin (an adipose-specific protein abundantly expressed and released into the circulation), is paradoxically decreased in human and in monkey obesity. Its circulating levels are inversely correlated with plasma leptin levels. Adiponectin has been sequenced in both humans and monkeys and found to have 98% identity (50). There was no relationship between body weight or obesity and adiponectin mRNA, suggesting posttranscriptional regulation by adiposity, a regulation which was disturbed when diabetes developed.

Genetic Susceptibility and Gene–Environment Interactions

Linkage studies and extensive candidate gene studies give presumptive evidence that multiple genes may be involved in the susceptibility to obesity in both humans and in animals, with each gene contributing in small measure to the propensity or sus-

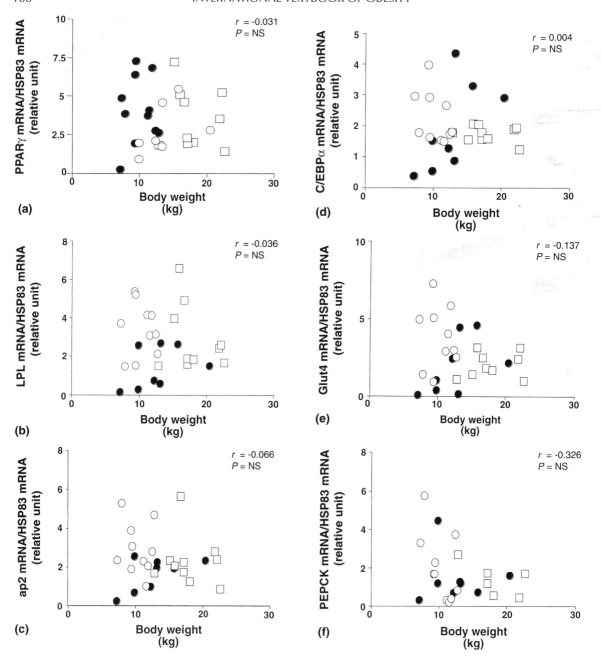

Figure 14.6   Genes implicated in adipose cell differentiation were examined in normal (open circles), obese (open squares) and diabetic (solid circles) monkeys. The expression levels of PPARγ (a), LPL (b), aP2 (c), CEBPα (d), Glut 4 (e), and PEPCK (f) mRNA measured by slot blot hybridization were not associated with body weight or total body fat, but, with the exception of aP2 and PEPCK, they were highly coordinately regulated with each other. (Redrawn from Hotta *et al.* (47))

ceptibility to develop obesity. This likelihood may contribute heavily to the difficulty in isolating the specific genetic contributions within a family or group where a single gene mutation is not known to be present.

Studies both in animals and in humans support the contention that individuals differ in their susceptibility to weight gain and to overt obesity under conditions in which the environment is facilitative or non-constraining. For example, a high fat diet fed to some strains of mice results in significantly more excess body fat than when fed to other strains; indeed there are strains that are resistant to the obesifying effects of a high fat diet (51). A high fat diet also induces obesity in adult rabbits (52). Similarly, in humans differences in susceptibility to weight gain have been identified (53,54).

Efforts are continuing to identify the genetic and molecular basis of obesity or of the 'obesities'. The likely outcome in the future is the identification of many genes, and, within those gene coding regions or in nearby regions that affect gene expression, many different mutations or variants which are responsible for the heavy genetic burden of obesity in humans and in non-human primates. Combinations of these genes are likely to increase susceptibility to weight gain and obesity when the environment is permissive or culpatory. The direct effects of these interacting genes may be to alter metabolic rate or nutrient partitioning, to alter lipid metabolism or adipose tissue function, to alter lean mass, to alter the hormonal milieu, and/or to regulate feeding behavior and appetite. Polygenic as well as major gene effects may be acting to produce the complex phenotype of obesity and its associated disorders in primates. The current state of this understanding for human obesity has been reviewed extensively (55). In addition, many of these genes are likely to interact with each other and with the environment for both humans and animals, thus further increasing the challenge for the future understanding of the mechanisms underlying the physiological basis of obesity.

Obesity as a Nutritionally Induced Disorder

It is clear that obesity results from an imbalance of energy input and energy output, and that in some animal models it can be induced by dietary methods. For example, the *Psammomys obesus* or Israeli desert gerbil or sand rat exhibits obesity only under nutritional conditions that this species does not see in the wild (14). Susceptibility of various animal models to nutritionally induced obesity appears to differ across strains and even within a single strain of rodents, and is a characteristic which some investigators have used in selective breeding (51). The mechanism which underlies this susceptibility to dietary obesity is unclear, but in the sand rat is suspected to relate to impaired activation of the insulin receptor and compromised tyrosine kinase activation, which interestingly, is reversible with calorie restriction (see below for further discussion of calorie restriction in obesity). High fat feeding produces many changes in metabolism, as illustrated by the recent finding of increased uncoupling protein 3 (UCP3) levels in brown adipose tissue and reduced skeletal muscle UCP3 in dietary obese rats (56). High fat diets in monkeys have produced significant weight gain, increased body fat, and increases in triglycerides and low density lipoprotein (LDL) and high density lipoprotein (HDL) cholesterol (57).

Viral Models

Viruses have been suspected of being involved in obesity in humans (58), and have been shown to be capable of producing obesity in rodents (59). Whether this is an important mechanism for the induction of obesity is, as yet, unclear.

Adipose Tissue Metabolism During the Development of Obesity

Although insulin sensitivity at the whole body level generally declines as obesity develops, as shown above for monkey A-7, it is seldom appreciated that this longitudinal change at the whole body level is not associated with a similar decline in the sensitivity of isolated adipocytes to insulin actions. Generally, it is believed that whole body insulin action, as measured by a euglycemic hyperinsulinemic clamp, is principally determined by glucose uptake into muscle, with a small contribution of adipose tissue and other organs. At the level of the

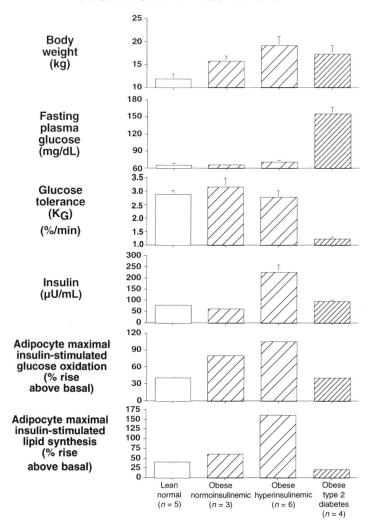

Figure 14.7   Insulin action on adipocytes obtained from the abdominal subcutaneous tissue of four groups of monkeys whose characteristics are differentiated in the top four panels: lean normal monkeys, obese normoinsulinemic monkeys, obese hyperinsulinemic monkeys, and obese with overt type 2 diabetes. Differences in body weights, fasting plasma glucose, intravenous glucose tolerance, and fasting plasma insulin are shown in the top four panels. Panel 5 is the effect of insulin to increase glucose oxidation in isolated adipocytes and panel 6 is the effect of insulin to increase lipid synthesis, both in isolated subcutaneous abdominal adipocytes. (Redrawn with permission from Hansen *et al.* (60))

adipocyte, the action of insulin, as measured in biopsies obtained both cross-sectionally and longitudinally from rhesus monkeys during the development of obesity and progression to diabetes, shows *increased* ability of insulin to stimulate glucose oxidation and to stimulate lipid synthesis in obese animals compared to normals (60). The deterioration in insulin action at the adipocyte is a late event accompanying the development of diabetes, as shown in Figure 14.7.

RELATIONSHIP BETWEEN OBESITY AND TYPE 2 DIABETES MELLITUS

Glucose Tolerance in Obesity

Animal models of obesity are highly associated with observations of reduced glucose tolerance (61), and in the non-human primate this glucose intolerance precedes overt type 2 diabetes, as recently reviewed (62). Glucose tolerance to an intravenous glucose infusion ranged in monkeys from a glucose disappearance rate of 5 %/min to 2%/min without any change in fasting plasma glucose. When tolerance dropped below 2%, fasting plasma glucose began to be elevated (61). Thus, there is a powerful compensatory response which, despite declining glucose uptake rates, maintains plasma glucose at normal levels in the obese non-human primate.

Hepatic Glucose Production

Longitudinal *in vivo* studies in rhesus monkeys have shown that as obese monkeys begin to make the final transition from impaired insulin sensitivity and impaired glucose tolerance at the whole body to overt type 2 diabetes, increasing fasting plasma glucose very closely parallels increasing basal hepatic glucose production (63). In a related event, as hyperinsulinemia progresses to high levels, hepatic extraction of insulin (the proportion of the insulin presented to the liver which is removed by the liver) declines (64).

Insulin Secretion and Insulin Sensitivity

Beta cell insulin secretion is minimally affected during the early stages of obesity, as shown by the comparison of changes in body fat and in fasting plasma insulin for monkey A-7 illustrated in Figure 14.2. Insulin sensitivity, measured at the whole body by the euglycemic hyperinsulinemic clamp, remained normal during that period as well, while fat mass more than doubled. The increase in insulin secretion and the decline in insulin sensitivity that took place in this monkey after age 12 were closely related, and have been observed in a larger group of monkeys (65). Thus, changes in adiposity per se were not directly associated with changes in insulin secretion or insulin sensitivity. In most monkeys and in most humans, increased adiposity appears play a role as an apparent facilitator or permissive factor for the declines in whole body insulin action and the increase in insulin output. Both basal fasting levels of insulin and β cell responsiveness to a glucose stimulus increase in the early stages of the transition from 'simple' obesity to insulin-resistant prediabetic obesity (66). Insulin secretion subse-

quently generally declines as fasting plasma glucose begins to rise in the early stages of overt diabetes (notably shown in Figure 14.4) (67). Nevertheless, at the time of diagnosis of diabetes, insulin levels are usually still elevated above normal, and β cell responsiveness to glucose is completely absent, as recently reviewed (62).

Under basal fasting conditions in both monkeys and humans, insulin is secreted with a 10 to 14 minute oscillating periodicity (68, 69), and the amplitude of this periodic secretory output increases with obesity and hyperinsulinemia. This amplification of the secretory output in obesity may play a protective role, or alternatively, may signal disturbed β cell functioning and regulation in the prodrome to diabetes. Further, this periodic secretory pattern is completely disrupted by 48 hours of fasting or by the development of diabetes, even when basal insulin levels are above or within the normal range (70). Oscillations are also lost by an exogenous infusion of glucose raising glucose levels to about 6 mmol (71). The presence of oscillations in plasma levels of insulin may thus be viewed as a reflection of a 'contented' beta cell (71).

Insulin Resistance

Tissue Specificity in the Sequence of Appearance of Defective Insulin Action

There is a wide range of insulin sensitivity in monkeys with normal glucose tolerance (24,72), including obese monkeys with or without insulin resistance.

We tend to think of insulin sensitivity, or its converse, insulin resistance, as a single entity, regardless of how or where it is measured. This is unfortunate and has resulted from the paucity of studies in which whole body insulin-resistance and resistance at each of the major insulin sensitive tissues have been measured simultaneously. Most commonly, so-called 'normals' (usually age and/or weight matched) are compared to so-called diabetics (individuals with significant hyperglycemia). Under these groupings, normals are normal in both whole body and tissue determinations and diabetics are 'resistant' at both the whole body and at various tissues. More detailed analysis has shown in rhesus monkeys that whole body insulin resistance, probably principally reflective of skeletal muscle insulin resistance, develops in obesity in parallel with hyperinsulinemia (72), and well before the appearance of insulin resistance at adipose tissue and at liver (63). Resistance in the latter two tissues seems to be directly associated with the progression of individuals from obese with hyperinsulinemia to overtly diabetic.

Insulin Action on Glycogen Metabolism in Skeletal Muscle, Adipose Tissue, and Liver

Obese hyperinsulinemic monkeys had a significant decline in insulin-mediated change in glycogen synthase activity in skeletal muscle (73). This defect appeared early at about the same time as the increasing insulin secretion noted above, that is, at the same time as β cell hyper-responsiveness developed. Obese and insulin resistant monkeys also had significantly higher insulin stimulated glucose 6-phosphate concentrations compared to normal monkeys, suggesting that a step distal to glucose 6-phosphate is a major contributor to reduced insulin-mediated glucose disposal and reduced insulin action on glycogen synthase activity (74).

In adipose tissue, by contrast, both basal and insulin-stimulated total activities of both glycogen synthase and glycogen phosphorylase were increased above normal in obese hyperinsulinemic monkeys (75). Insulin action to increase glycogen synthase independent activity was reduced in obese hyperinsulinemic monkeys compared to the normal monkeys. Specifically, in normal monkeys insulin stimulation induced a 100% increase in glycogen synthase independent activity over basal levels compared to a 50% increase in obese hyperinsulinemic monkeys (and no increase in diabetic monkeys) (75).

At the liver of monkeys, a different picture of defects in insulin action with obesity has emerged. Glycogen synthase activation and glycogen phosphorylase inactivation by insulin (in a reciprocal fashion) were significant in the liver of both normal lean monkeys (76) and obese hyperinsulinemic monkeys under the condition of a euglycemic hyperinsulinemic clamp (76). In obese insulin-resistant monkeys, under the same conditions, glycogen synthase (GS) total activity was lower under basal conditions compared to the lean young animals. Nevertheless, total GS activity was significantly increased by insulin stimulation in the liver of insulin-resistant monkeys. Both the basal GS independent activity and the insulin-stimulated independent activity of the insulin-resistant monkeys were higher in the latter group compared to the lean animals (77). Thus, insulin action at the liver was found to be strong in monkeys that were otherwise determined to be insulin resistant at muscle and adipose tissue, as well as resistant at the whole body level. This would accord with the normal hepatic glucose production of insulin-resistant obese monkeys (increased only in diabetics where insulin's suppression of hepatic glucose production is significantly impaired (63)).

PREVENTION OF OBESITY: LESSONS FROM ANIMAL MODELS

The Need for Obesity Prevention

Although the causes of obesity in the vast majority of humans (99%) and in all obese non-human primates are unknown, studies in rodents and in non-human primates have unequivocally demonstrated that calorie restraint, sufficient to prevent significant increase in total body fat, prevents obesity (by definition), but more importantly, prevents most obesity-associated diseases. Excess body fat or altered energy balance clearly plays a facilitative role in many of the comorbidities of obesity. While we continue the search for the underlying causes of obesity, animal models show that even without knowing the causes, interventions to reduce the degree of obesity can have very strong positive consequences for many obesity-associated diseases, as well as for overall reduction in mortality and extension of life span.

Trowell and Burkitt's studies of epidemiological changes in modernizing societies showed that obesity is the first of the 'diseases of civilization' to emerge in the longitudinal picture (78). As such obesity is clearly the earliest target for intervention to halt a wide range of non-communicable diseases of modern and modernizing societies. Gracey has termed this defined cluster of diseases the New World syndrome (79), and has included within its sphere obesity, type 2 diabetes, hypertension, dyslipidemia, and cardiovascular disease (also termed the metabolic syndrome X (80)) (with the addition of cigarette smoking and alcohol abuse).

The World Health Organization has commented

extensively on the societal factors which have accompanied or induced the changes leading to the New World syndrome, and which have led to identification of obesity as a global epidemic (25). The WHO Report cited such components of modernization as the development of market economies, reliance on imported non-traditional foods, increasing urbanization, changing occupational structures, increasing socioeconomic status, increases in animal fat and animal protein intake, decreases in vegetable fat and vegetable protein intake, reduction in total and specifically complex carbohydrates, and increases in sugar intake. The net effect of these factors might be viewed as providing an unrestrained environment in which genetic potential becomes fully expressed. Alternatively, the environment may be interacting in such a way as to be detrimental to 'normal' gene expression.

As noted below, evidence from animal models strongly indicates that these diseases are not independent. As in diseases of human civilization, the sequence of the appearance in animals starts with obesity. The prevention of obesity can prevent or greatly reduce all of the others, and as a further consequence, greatly reduce morbidity and mortality. Because the benefits of obesity prevention have to date been difficult to attain in humans, examination of the data from animal models of obesity prevention can be informative for the human condition and the potential importance of obesity mitigation.

Primary prevention includes all measures aimed at reducing the incidence or preventing the occurrence of a disease and its complications or of reducing the risk of disease. Secondary prevention includes the measures introduced to mitigate the consequences of a disease, slow its progression, and reduce its associated morbidities following the early diagnosis of the disease. For example, primary prevention of obesity in animals is achieved when the development of increased body fat is completely prevented, usually by calorie restriction, while secondary prevention is introduced when weight reduction or body fat ablation of an already obese animal has been instituted.

Successful prevention interventions rely upon an understanding of the natural history of a disease, together with the identification of sufficiently powerful and successful methods for preventing the disease. In the case of obesity prevention in humans a significant number of risk factors for obesity have

been identified, and a modest amount is known about the natural history of obesity (as established in this volume). In humans, however, only a few methods of limited applicability (primarily surgical approaches) have been identified which truly modify the course of the disease, generally mitigating its consequences after obesity has reached severe stages (81). In rodents and in non-human primates, by contrast, deeper understanding of the aging-related changes in body composition and of the factors increasing risk for obesity have been developed. In addition, the usual laboratory environment, with its readily available constraints and manipulability, has enabled the introduction of powerful non-surgical approaches to obesity prevention, thus allowing assessment of its consequences and its likely implications for humans. Current efforts in humans are principally limited to identification of high-risk individuals for 'lifestyle' changes, and environmental manipulations. The power of these interventions is extremely limited at this time. Nevertheless, studies in non-human primates demonstrate that the successful prevention of obesity has far-reaching consequences and extraordinarily high potential for positive impact on human health.

Efficacy of Primary Prevention of Obesity in Rodents and Non-human Primates

Extension of Average Life Expectancy

The longest ongoing study of calorie restriction in non-human primates, initiated when the monkeys were fully adult at about age 10, continues at this time and has already shown the powerful effects of obesity prevention in preventing or greatly postponing morbidity and increasing average lifespan. Further, simply instituting primary prevention of obesity (by calorie titration on an individual animal basis) has provided the most powerful means known to prevent the development of overt diabetes (82). In the restricted animals, there is no diabetes, while in the *ad libitum* fed animals diabetes rate exceeds 30%, and the obesity rate exceeds 50% (82). Calorie restriction also results in the prevention or significant postponement of many features that normally contribute to cardiovascular risk, including many diabetes-associated metabolic dysfunctions, such as reduced dyslipidemia, and improved blood pressure profile (83). As a result of this disease prevention, there appears to be excellent potential to extend maximal lifespan as well. This, however, must await further extension of the study as the monkeys are now in their late 20s and the maximal reported lifespan in captivity for the rhesus monkey is 40 years (83).

Anti-aging Properties of Obesity Prevention

The extension of average life expectancy and the potential for extension of maximal lifespan raise the possibility that, as in rodents, calorie restriction in non-human primates exerts an anti-aging effect which is separate from and in parallel with the anti-disease effects so clearly already demonstrated (83). The mechanisms by which such anti-aging effects of obesity prevention are achieved are, as yet, unknown. However, several such potential mechanisms are under study in rodents as well as in non-human primates. In rodents, a reduction in mitochondrial oxidative damage during aging has been found with calorie restriction (84). Examination of differential gene expression in rodents with and without calorie restriction has indicated a marked reduction in the stress response and a lower expression of a number of metabolic genes in the calorie-restricted group (85).

Body Fatness Required to Reduce Disease

Improvement in glucose tolerance, dyslipidemia and blood pressure, and prevention of diabetes do not appear to require maximal leanness. In one reported study, body fatness in calorie-restricted monkeys has been maintained at levels ranging from 10 to 22%, a normal range for non obese adult monkeys (83). Whether levels below this (excessive leanness) will further improve health or will in fact be detrimental to health will await the reports of other studies of calorie restriction in non-human primates (86).

Fat distribution may also be playing a role, as calorie restriction in non-human primates results in improved body fat distribution (reduced fat in the abdominal region) which is directly associated with the reduced overall body fat content (87).

Prevention of Hyperleptinemia

The hyperleptinemia associated generally with obesity in humans and monkeys as noted above (38)

is prevented by calorie restriction with the prevention of obesity, and the normalization of leptin levels could potentially be advantageous, although this is speculative at this point.

Prevention of Obesity: Effects on Glucoregulation, Insulin Secretion, and Insulin Action

Regulation of Plasma Glucose and Glucose Tolerance

In rodents as well as in rhesus monkeys, calorie restriction results in maintenance of normal fasting plasma glucose levels, and normal glucose tolerance (82). Both fasting plasma glucose and fasting plasma insulin are lower relative to control *ad libitum* fed monkeys, but are not reduced relative to normal lean young adult monkeys (88,89).

Insulin Sensitivity

In monkeys, dietary restriction produces significantly higher *in vivo* insulin action compared to *ad libitum* fed monkeys of the same age (90). Aging and obesity-associated insulin resistance appear to be mitigated by long-term restraint on calories in monkeys, and the same is likely to be true in humans. The development of type 2 diabetes that is prevented by calorie restriction and obesity prevention may be accomplished by this sustaining of insulin action (82), presumably particularly in skeletal muscle.

Glycogen Synthesis and Glycogen Synthase Activity

In non-human primates, glycogen synthase activity in skeletal muscle is increased by calorie restriction (91). The mechanism by which this effect is achieved is unknown. In some of those monkeys, however, there was an unexpected decrease in glycogen synthase fractional activity with insulin stimulation, a greater increase in skeletal muscle glucose 6-phosphate, and the greatest increase in glycogen phosphorylase activity with insulin. These unusual responses were associated with a relatively lower whole body glucose uptake rate compared to the other calorie-restricted monkeys. There was an unexpected increase in the glucose 6-phosphate K_a of skeletal muscle glycogen synthase, indicating phosphorylation (rather than dephosphorylation) of glycogen synthase in response to insulin (91). These changes may be involved in the anti-diabetogenic properties of caloric restriction.

Obesity, Dyslipidemia, and its Prevention by Calorie Restriction

Dyslipidemia: Hypertriglyceridemia and Low HDL Cholesterol

Monkeys, like humans, frequently develop dyslipidemia in middle age, including hypertriglyceridemia and reduced HDL cholesterol levels (92), and this dyslipidemia is highly associated with the presence of obesity, with or without diabetes. Pharmaceutical agents which alter dyslipidemia in humans do so in monkeys as well (93,94).

Prevention of Dyslipidemia by Calorie Restriction to Prevent Obesity

Abnormalities in plasma lipid levels are virtually entirely prevented by calorie restriction in non-human primates (95,96). Both the reduction in plasma triglyceride levels relative to *ad libitum* fed controls, and the increase in the HDL2b subfraction, which is associated with reduction in atherosclerotic risk, were principally accounted for by the reduction in body mass and the associated improvement in glucoregulation noted above (96). Calorie restriction in rhesus monkeys, while producing no change in plasma LDL cholesterol concentrations, reduced the molecular weight of the LDL particles, and reduced their triglyceride and phospholipid content, together with reduced proteoglycan binding (97).

Restraining Calories to Prevent Obesity: Effects on Energy Expenditure

Energy Expenditure

When rhesus monkeys were studied after 10 years of adult onset calorie restriction with long-term stabilized body weight, total daily energy expenditure was reduced compared to *ad libitum* fed monkeys, as shown in Figure 14.8. Note that the regression

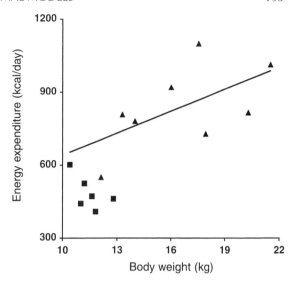

Figure 14.8 Energy expenditure determined by the doubly labeled water method in 6 calorie restricted monkeys (solid squares) and in 8 ad libitum fed 'control' monkeys (solid triangles) Straight line is regression line for controls only. (Reproduced with permission from Delaney *et al.* (98))

line shown is for the *ad libitum* monkeys only. This reduced energy expenditure was present even when the energy expenditure rate was adjusted for differences in body weight, body surface area, or lean body mass (98).

Thyroid Hormone

In the same study of long-term calorie restriction in adult rhesus monkeys, thyroxine (T4) was reduced and the free thyroxine index tended to be lower, without change in triiodothyronine (T3).

Body Temperature

Calorie restraint in adult monkeys has been reported to result in lower body temperature (99). However, this was not observed in a group of long-term older calorie-restricted monkeys (98).

Physical Activity

Physical activity of the calorie-restricted monkeys was greater than of the similar aged *ad libitum* monkeys (who were considerably fatter), but activity did not differ between calorie-restricted older monkeys and similar body weight younger adult animals (98).

The reduced energy expenditure during calorie restriction is therefore not due to a reduced activity level as might have been suspected.

Secondary Prevention or Weight Reduction in Obesity

Secondary prevention, or mitigation of already existing obesity for the purpose of reducing the negative health consequences of obesity, is also important. Behavioral and environmental manipulations are widely applied but only modestly successful. Surgical treatments are of limited application. Pharmacological approaches are expanding and currently animal models are contributing to the examination of new anti-obesity agents.

New Pharmacological Studies in Animal Models of Obesity

Beta 3 Adrenergic Receptor Agonists to Increase Energy Output from Adipose Tissue and Reduce Fat Mass

Although β adrenergic agonists have been under study in rodents for more than 20 years, only in the past several years has the uniqueness of the primate (human and non-human) $\beta3$ receptor been identified. Currently, $\beta3$ agents under study are specific for the human receptor and are being extensively tested in non-human primates whose $\beta3$ receptor is very similar the human sequence(100). The $\beta3$ receptor sequence in the rhesus monkey is shown in Figure 14.9. Studies of $\beta3$ agonists in monkeys have been reviewed recently (101). Such agonists have been shown to be active at the non-human primate receptor (102), acutely producing lipolysis and metabolic rate elevation and increased UCP1 expression in brown adipose tissue. To date, however, none has been reported to produce a reduction in body weight. This may be due to an insufficient number of $\beta3$ receptors on the adipose tissue of humans. Recent studies have shown an increase in the expression of the mitochondrial uncoupling proteins (UCP2 and 3), and possible increase in the number of brown adipocytes (103). These agonists also seem to have lipid-lowering and insulin-sensitizing effects. In young rats a $\beta3$ agent has led to reduced

body mass and adiposity which was blunted in older rats (104).

Glucose-lowering and Insulin-sensitizing Agents

GLP-1 and exendin-4. GLP-1 (glucagon-like polypeptide-1) has been studied in non-human primates (101), but its short half-life has precluded it from being considered for clinical use. Another amino acid peptide with 53% sequence similarity to GLP-1, exendin-4, has been shown to have prolonged glucose lowering action *in vivo* in obese non-human primates and in rodent models of obesity and diabetes (105).

Thiazolidinediones. Thiazolidinediones, a class of insulin sensitizers, have been examined in animal models of obesity and of diabetes, including application to non-human primates (101). In general they improve insulin sensitivity and lower plasma glucose levels in some, but not all prediabetic and diabetic subjects (106). They also reduce hypertriglyceridemia. Recently a new mechanism of action of this class has been reported, the enhancement of glycogen synthase activity in skeletal muscle, possibly accounting for some of the apparent insulin-sensitizing effects observed in the whole body (107). Figure 14.10 shows the results of a study in which the thiazolidinedione R-102380 was administered for 6 weeks with measurements made before and at the end of the dosing period. Glycogen synthase activity was measured in skeletal muscle biopsies obtained under basal and insulin-stimulated conditions (before and during a euglycemic clamp). All four monkeys studied showed an increase in insulin action to increase glycogen synthase independent activity as well as fractional activity (independent divided by total activity). Insulin-sensitizers are likely to continue to be a focus of expanded efforts to mitigate the health consequences of obesity and to slow or prevent the development of diabetes.

Products Secreted from Adipose Tissue

Leptin administration. The administration of leptin to either rodents or to humans with leptin deficiency has been shown to reverse this form of obesity (108). The leptin-deficient obese subjects lost significant adipose tissue mass, and reproductive function was restored (108). When administered

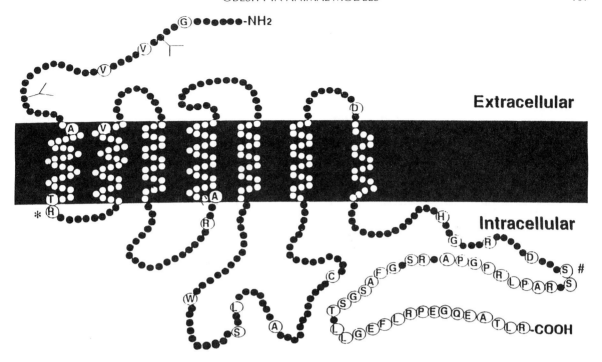

Figure 14.9 Sequence of the β3 adrenergic receptor in the monkey. Differences from the human sequence are shown in the white circles. The asterisk identifies the arginine substitution at codon 64 found in all monkeys examined (100)

to non-human primates without any abnormality in the leptin axis, peripheral leptin had no effect on food intake or body weight (109). However, when leptin was administered to the normal monkeys intracerebroventricularly there appeared to be a delayed reduction in food intake the next day. Leptin administered to the obese *Psammomys obesus* sand rat failed to affect body weight, body fat, or adipose gene expression (110), although there were some gene expression changes induced by leptin in lean control animals.

Further studies of possible central mechanisms of leptin action are needed, but the hope for a quick 'obesity fix' is unlikely to be realized by the administration of leptin to most obese persons.

CONCLUSIONS

Is It Time to Enhance Investigation of the Means to Prevent Obesity?

Sufficient data currently exist from studies of animal models to demonstrate unequivocally the extraordinary power of obesity prevention to per-

manently alter the trajectory of a wide range of diseases, including but not limited to heart disease, type 2 diabetes, hypertension, cancer, and other aging-associated chronic diseases.

Public health approaches have to date proven to be too weak in efficacy to provide for strong positive cost–benefit conclusions related to widespread obesity treatment. Behavioral modification has had a small measure of success in a very limited number of humans, and the likelihood of strengthening these behavioral or environmental manipulations to a level sufficient to impact overall incidence of obesity is low. Biomedical approaches may, in the future, offer the potential power to alter the obesity trajectory and to change the negative health consequences of this extraordinarily prevalent disease.

Non-human primates in the study of obesity have offered numerous pointers to the human condition, some of which have been reviewed here. Together these findings offer an optimistic view of the future benefits of obesity mitigating efforts.

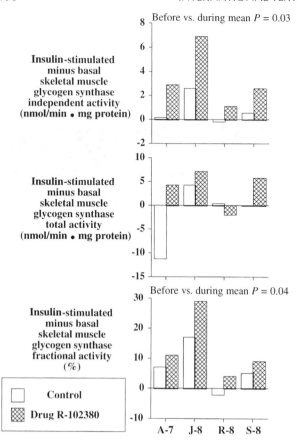

Figure 14.10 An insulin sensitizer of the thiazolidinedione class (R-102380) administered to four monkeys for more than 6 weeks induced a significant increase in the change in glycogen synthase activity induced by insulin (before and during a eu-glycemic hyperinsulinemic clamp). Both the glycogen synthase independent activity and the fractional activity of glycogen synthase were significantly increased (107)

REFERENCES

1. Hruban Z, Meehan T, Wolff P, Wollmann RL, Glagov S. Aortic dissection in a gorilla. *J Med Primatol* 1986; **15**: 287–293.
2. Steinetz BG, Randolph C, Cohn D, Mahoney CJ. Lipo-protein profiles and glucose tolerance in lean and obese chimpanzees. *J Med Primatol* 1996; **25**: 17–25.
3. Venter CS, Nel CJ, Vorster HH, *et al.* Soluble-fibre concentrate lowers plasminogen activator inhibitor-1 in baboons (*Papio ursinus*). *Br J Nutr* 1997; **78**: 625–637.
4. Fincham JE, Seier JV, Verster A, *et al.* Pleural Mesocesto-ides and cardiac shock in an obese vervet monkey (*Cercopithecus aethiops*). *Vet Pathol* 1995; **32**: 330–333.
5. Wagner JD, Carlson CS, O'Brien TD, Anthony MS, Bullock BC, Cefalu WT. Diabetes mellitus and islet

6. Rosenblum LA, Smiley J. Weight gain in bonnet and pigtail macaques. *J Med Primatol* 1980; **9**: 247–253.
7. Walike BC, Goodner CJ, Koerker DJ. Assessment of obesity in pigtailed monkeys (*Macaca nemestrina*). *J Med Primatol* 1977; **6**: 151–162.
8. Ausman LM, Rasmussen KM, Gallina DL. Spontaneous obesity in maturing squirrel monkeys fed semipurified diets. *Am J Physiol* 1981; **241** (Regulatory): R316–321.
9. Howard CF, Jr, Yasuda M, Wolff J. Hyperinsulinemia in *Macaca nigra*: precession to obesity and/or diabetes? *Diabetes Res* 1990; **13**: 163–168.
10. Hamilton CL, Ciaccia P. The course of development of glucose intolerance in the monkey (*Macaca mulatta*). *J Med Primatol* 1978; **7**: 165–173.
11. Hansen BC. Prospective study of the development of diabetes in spontaneously obese monkeys. In: Berry EM, Blondheim SH, Eliahou HE, Shrafrir E (eds) *Recent Advances in Obesity Research V.* London: John Libbey, 1987: 33–41.
12. Hansen BC. Obesity and diabetes in monkeys. In: Björntorp P, Brodoff BN (eds) *Obesity.* New York: JB Lippincott, 1992: 256–265.
13. Lauterio TJ, Davies MJ, DeAngelo M, Peyser M, Lee J. Neuropeptide Y expression and endogenous leptin concentrations in a dietary model of obesity. *Obes Res* 1999; **7**: 498–505.
14. Shafrir E, Ziv E. Cellular mechanism of nutritionally induced insulin resistance: the desert rodent *Psammomys obesus* and other animals in which insulin resistance leads to detrimental outcome. *J Basic Clin Physiol Pharmacol* 1998; **9**: 347–385.
15. Cohn LA, Dodam JR, McCaw DL, Tate DJ. Effects of chromium supplementation on glucose tolerance in obese and nonobese cats. *Am J Vet Res* 1999; **60**: 1360–1363.
16. Wolden-Hanson T, Davis GA, Baum ST, Kemnitz JW. Insulin levels, physical activity, and urinary catecholamine excretion of obese and non-obese rhesus monkeys. *Obes Res* 1993; **1**: 5–17.
17. Jen K-LC, Hansen BC, Metzger BL. Adiposity, anthropometric measures, and plasma insulin levels of rhesus monkeys. *Int J Obes* 1985; **9**: 213–224.
18. Howard CF, Kessler MJ, Schwartz S. Carbohydrate impairment and insulin secretory abnormalities among *Macaca mulatta* from Cayo Santiago. *J Med Primatol* 1986; **11**: 147–146.
19. Schwartz SM, Kemnitz JW. Age-and gender-related changes in body size, adiposity, and endocrine and metabolic parameters in free-ranging rhesus macaques. *Am J Physical Anthro* 1992; **89**: 109–121.
20. Schwartz SM, Kemnitz JW, Howard CF. Obesity in free-ranging rhesus macaques. *Int J Obes* 1993; **17**: 1–10.
21. Hansen BC, Ortmeyer HK. Obesity, diabetes and aging: Lessons from life-time studies in monkeys. In: Guy-Grand B, Ailhaud G (eds) *Progress in Obesity Research.* London: John Libbey, Inc, 1999, pp. 525–544.
22. Kemnitz J, Francken G. Characteristics of spontaneous obesity in male rhesus monkeys. *Physiol Behav* 1986; **38**: 477–483.
23. Kemnitz JW, Goy RW, Flitsch TJ, Lohmiller JJ, Robinson JA. Obesity in male and female rhesus monkeys: fat dis-

tribution, glucoregulation, and serum androgen levels. *J Clin Endocrinol Metab* 1989; **69**: 287–293.

24. Bodkin NL, Hannah JS, Ortmeyer HK, Hansen BC. Central obesity in rhesus monkeys: association with hyperinsulinemia, insulin resistance, and hypertriglyceridemia? *Int J Obes* 1993; **17**: 53–61.

25. WHO Consultation on Obesity. *Obesity: Preventing and Managing the Global Epidemic*. Geneva: World Health Organization, 1998.

26. Kapeller R, Moriarty A, Strauss A, *et al.* Tyrosine phosphorylation of tub and its association with Src homology 2 domain-containing proteins implicate tub in intracellular signaling by insulin. *J Biol Chem* 1999; **274**: 24980–24986.

27. Ohman M, Oksanen L, Kainulainen K, *et al.* Testing of human homologues of murine obesity genes as candidate regions in Finnish obese sib pairs. *Eur J Hum Genet* 1999; **7**: 117–124.

28. Coleman DL, Hummel KP. Effects of parabiosis of normal with genetically diabetic mice. *Am J Physiol* 1969; **217**: 1298–1304.

29. Coleman DL. Effects of parabiosis of obese with diabetes and normal mice. *Diabetologia* 1973; **9**: 294–298.

30. Walike BC, Smith OA. Regulation of food intake during intermittent and continuous cross circulation in monkeys (*Macaca mulatta*). *J Comp Physiol Psychol* 1972; **80**: 372–381.

31. Zhang Y, Proenca R, Maffei M, Barone M, Leopold L, Friedman JM. Positional cloning of the mouse *obese* gene and its human homologue. *Nature* 1994; **372**: 425–432.

32. Tartaglia LA, Dembski M, Weng X, *et al.* Identification and expression cloning of a leptin receptor, OB-R. *Cell* 1995; **83**: 1263–1271.

33. Green ED, Maffei M, Braden VV, *et al.* The human obese (OB) gene: RNA expression pattern and mapping on the physical, cytogenetic, and genetic maps of chromosome 7. *Genome Res* 1995; **5**: 5–12.

34. Hotta K, Gustafson TA, Ortmeyer HK, Bodkin NL, Nicolson MA, Hansen BC. Regulation of *obese (ob)* mRNA and plasma leptin levels in rhesus monkeys: Effects of insulin, body weight and diabetes. *J Biol Chem* 1996; **271**: 25327–25331.

35. Montague CT, Farooqi IS, Whitehead JP, *et al.* Congenital leptin deficiency is associated with severe early-onset obesity in humans. *Nature* 1997; **387**: 903–908.

36. Farooqi S, Rau H, Whitehead J, O'Rahilly S. Ob gene mutations and human obesity. *Proc Nutr Soc* 1998; **57**: 471–475.

37. Hotta K, Gustafson TA, Ortmeyer HK, Bodkin NL, Hansen BC. Monkey leptin receptor mRNA: Sequence, tissue distribution, and mRNA expression in the adipose tissue of normal, hyperinsulinemic and type 2 diabetic rhesus monkeys. *Obes Res* 1998; **6**: 353–360.

38. Bodkin NL, Nicolson M, Ortmeyer HK, Hansen BC. Hyperleptinemia: Relationship to adiposity and insulin resistance in the spontaneously obese rhesus monkey. *Horm Metab Res* 1996; **28**: 674–678.

39. Greenberg JA, Boozer CN. The leptin–fat ratio is constant, and leptin may be part of two feedback mechanisms for maintaining the body fat set point in non-obese male Fischer 344 rats. *Horm Metab Res* 1999; **31**: 525–532.

40. Taylor SI, Kadowaki T, Kadowaki H, Accili D, Cama A,

41. Naithani VK, Steffens GJ, Tager HS. Isolation and amino-acid sequence determination of monkey insulin and proinsulin. *Hoppe-Seyler's Z Physiol Chem* 1984; **365**: 571–575.

McKeon C. Mutations in insulin-receptor gene in insulin-resistant patients. *Diabetes Care* 1990; **13**: 257–279.

42. Huang Z, Hansen BC, Shuldiner AR. Characterization of the insulin receptor gene in the rhesus monkey, a diabetes-prone species. *Exp Clin Endocrinol* 1993; **101**: 358–360.

43. Fan Z, Kole H, Bernier M, *et al.* Molecular mechanism of insulin resistance in the spontaneously obese and diabetic rhesus monkey: site directed mutagenesis of the insulin receptor. *Endocrinology* 1995; **77**: 180.

44. Huang Z, Bodkin NL, Ortmeyer HK, Hansen BC, Shuldiner AR. Hyperinsulinemia is associated with altered insulin receptor mRNA splicing in muscle of the spontaneously obese diabetic rhesus monkey. *J Clin Invest* 1994; **94**: 1289–1296.

45. Huang Z, Bodkin NL, Ortmeyer HK, *et al.* Altered insulin receptor mRNA splicing in liver associated with deterioration of glucose tolerance in spontaneously obese and diabetic rhesus monkey: Analysis of controversy between monkey and human studies. *J Clin Endocrinol Metab* 1996; **81**: 1552–1556.

46. Hannah J, Hansen BC. Food intake and meal patterns in rhesus monkeys: Significance of chronic hyperinsulinemia. *Physiol Behav* 1990; **48**: 519–522.

47. Hotta K, Gustafson TA, Yoshioka S, Ortmeyer HK, Bodkin NL, Hansen BC. Relationships of PPARγ and PPARγ2 mRNA levels to obesity, diabetes and hyperinsulinemia in rhesus monkeys. *Int J Obes* 1998; **22**: 1000–1010.

48. Gorla-Bajszczak A, Siegrist-Kaiser C, Boss O, Burger AG, Meier CA. Expression of peroxisome proliferator-activated receptors in lean and obese Zucker rats. *Eur J Endocrinol* 2000; **142**: 71–78.

49. Hotta K, Gustafson TA, Yoshioka S, Ortmeyer HK, Bodkin NL, Hansen BC. Age-related adipose tissue mRNA expression ADD1, PPARγ, lipoprotein lipase and GLUT4 glucose transporter in rhesus monkeys. *J Gerontol: Biol Sc* 1999; **54A**: B1–B8.

50. Hotta K, Hansen BC, Bodkin NL, *et al.* Regulation of adiponectin expression in nondiabetic and type 2 diabetic rhesus monkeys. *Diabetologia* 2000; (in press).

51. West DB, Boozer CN, Moody DL, Atkinson RL. Dietary obesity in nine inbred mouse strains. *Am J Physiol* 1992; **262** (Regulatory Integrative Comp Physiol 31): R1025–1032.

52. Antic V, Tempini A, Montani JP. Serial changes in cardiovascular and renal function of rabbits ingesting a high-fat, high-calorie diet. *Am J Hypertens* 1999; **12**: 826–829.

53. Heitmann BL, Lissner L, Sorensen TIA, Bengtsson C. Dietary fat intake and weight gain in women genetically predisposed for obesity. *Am J Clin Nutr* 1995; **61**: 1213–1217.

54. Bouchard C. The response to long-term overfeeding in identical twins. *N Engl J Med* 1990; **322**: 1477–1482.

55. Perusse L, Chagnon YC, Weisnagel J, Bouchard C. The human obesity gene map: the 1998 update [In Process Citation]. *Obes Res* 1999; **7**: 111–129.

56. Corbalan MS, Margareto J, Martinez JA, Marti A. High-fat feeding reduced muscle uncoupling protein 3 expression in rats. *J Physiol Biochem* 1999; **55**: 67–72.

57. Gray DS, Sharma RC, Chin HP, Jiao Q, Kramsch DM.

Body fat and fat distribution by anthropometry and the response to high-fat cholesterol-containing diet in monkeys. *Exp Mol Pathol* 1993; **58**: 53–60.

58. Dhurandhar NV, Kulkarni PR, Ajinkya SM, Sherikar AA, Atkinson RL. Association of adenovirus infection with human obesity. *Obes Res* 1997; **5**: 464–469.

59. Bernard A, Cohen R, Khuth ST, *et al.* Alteration of the leptin network in late morbid obesity induced in mice by brain infection with canine distemper virus. *J Virol* 1999; **73**: 7317–7327.

60. Hansen BC, Jen K-L, Schwartz J. Changes in insulin responses and binding in adipocytes from monkeys with obesity progressing to diabetes. *Int J Obes* 1988; **12**: 391–401.

61. Metzger BL, Hansen BC, Speegle LM, Jen K-LC. Characterization of glucose intolerance in obese monkeys. *J Obes Wt Regul* 1985; **4**: 153–167.

62. Hansen BC. Primate animal models of type 2 diabetes. In: LeRoith D, Taylor SI, Olesfky JM (eds) *Diabetes Mellitus: A Fundamental and Clinical Text*. Philadelphia: Lippincott-Raven Publishers, 2000: 734–743.

63. Bodkin NL, Metzger BL, Hansen BC. Hepatic glucose production and insulin sensitivity preceding diabetes in monkeys. *Am J Physiol* 1989; **256** (Endocrinol Metab): E676–E681.

64. Hansen BC, Striffler JS, Bodkin NL. Decreased hepatic insulin extraction precedes overt noninsulin dependent (type 2) diabetes in obese monkeys. *Obes Res* 1993; **1**: 252–260.

65. Hansen BC, Bodkin NL. Heterogeneity of insulin responses: phases in the continuum leading to non-insulin-dependent diabetes mellitus. *Diabetologia* 1986; **29**: 713–719.

66. Hansen BC, Bodkin NL. β-cell hyperresponsiveness: earliest event in development of diabetes in monkeys. *Am J Physiol* 1990; **259** (Regulatory Integrative Comp Physiol 28): R612–R617.

67. Hansen BC, Bodkin NL, Schwartz J, Jen K-LC. Beta cell responses, insulin resistance and the natural history of non insulin dependent diabetes in obese rhesus monkeys. In: Shafrir E, Renold AE (eds) *Frontiers in Diabetes Research. Lessons from Animal Diabetes II*. London: John Libbey, 1988: 279–287.

68. Hansen BC, Jen K-LC, Pek S, Wolfe RA. Rapid oscillations of plasma insulin, glucagon, and glucose in obese and normal weight humans. *J Clin Endocrinol Metab* 1982; **54**: 785–792.

69. Hansen BC, Vinik AI, Jen K-LC. Fluctuations in basal levels and effects of altered nutrition on plasma somatostatin. *Am J Physiol* 1982; **242** (Endocrinol Metab 5): R289–R295.

70. Hansen BC, Jen K-LC, Koerker DJ, Goodner CJ, Wolfe RA. Influence of nutritional state on periodicity in plasma insulin levels in monkeys. *Am J Physiol* 1982; **242** (Regulatory Integrative Comp Physiol 15): R255–R260.

71. Matthews DR. Oscillatory insulin secretion: a variable phenotypic marker. *Diabet Med* 1996; **13**: S53–58.

72. Bodkin NL, Ortmeyer HK, Hansen BC. Diversity of insulin resistance in monkeys with normal glucose tolerance. *Obes Res* 1993; **1**: 364–370.

73. Ortmeyer HK, Bodkin NL, Hansen BC. Insulin-mediated glycogen synthase activity in muscle of spontaneously insulin-resistant and diabetic rhesus monkeys. *Am J Physiol* 1993; **265** (Regulatory Integrative Comp Physiol 34): R552–R558.

74. Ortmeyer HK, Bodkin NL, Hansen BC. Relationship of skeletal muscle glucose-6-phosphate to glucose disposal rate and glycogen synthase activity in insulin-resistant and non-insulin-dependent diabetic rhesus monkeys. *Diabetologia* 1994; **37**: 127–133.

75. Ortmeyer HK, Bodkin NL, Hansen BC. Adipose tissue glycogen synthase activation by in vivo insulin in spontaneously insulin-resistant and Type 2 (non-insulin-dependent) diabetic rhesus monkeys. *Diabetologia* 1993; **36**: 200–206.

76. Ortmeyer HK, Bodkin NL, Hansen BC. Insulin regulates liver glycogen synthase and glycogen phosphorylase activity reciprocally in rhesus monkeys. *Am J Physiol* (Endocrinol Metab) 1997; **272**: E133–E138.

77. Ortmeyer H, Bodkin N. Lack of defect in insulin action on hepatic glycogen synthase and phosphorylase in insulin-resistant monkeys. *Am J Physiol* (Gastrointest Liver) 1998; **274**: G1005–G1010.

78. Trowell HC, Burkitt DP. *Western Diseases: Their Emergence and Prevention*. Cambridge, MA: Harvard University Press, 1981.

79. Truett GE, Bahary N, Friedman JM, Leibel RL. Rat obesity gene *fatty (fa)* maps to chromosome 5: Evidence for homology with the mouse gene *diabetes (db)*. *Proc Natl Acad Sci USA* 1991; **88**: 7806–7809.

80. Hansen BC, Saye J, Wennogle LP (eds). *The Metabolic Syndrome X: Convergence of Insulin Resistance, Glucose Intolerance, Hypertension, Obesity, and Dyslipidemias-Searching for the Underlying Defects*. New York: New York Academy of Sciences, 1999.

81. Sjostrom CD, Lissner L, Sjostrom L. Long term effects of weight loss on hypertension and diabetes: the SOS intervention study. *Int J Obes* 1998; **22**: S78.

82. Hansen BC, Bodkin NL. Primary prevention of diabetes mellitus by prevention of obesity in monkeys. *Diabetes* 1993; **42**: 1809–1814.

83. Hansen BC, Bodkin NL, Ortmeyer HK. Calorie restriction in non human primates: mechanisms of reduced morbidity and mortality. *Toxicol Sci* 1999; **52**: 56–60.

84. Lass A, Sohal BH, Weindruch R, Forster MJ, Sohal RS. Caloric restriction prevents age-associated accrual of oxidative damage to mouse skeletal muscle mitochondria. *Free Radic Biol Med* 1998; **25**: 1089–1097.

85. Lee CK, Klopp RG, Weindruch R, Prolla TA. Gene expression profile of aging and its retardation by caloric restriction. *Science* 1999; **285**: 1390–1393.

86. Lane MA, Ingram DK, Roth GS. Calorie restriction in nonhuman primates: effects on diabetes and cardiovascular disease risk. *Toxicol Sci* 1999; **52**: 41–48.

87. Colman RJ, Ramsey JJ, Roecker EB, Havighurst T, Hudson JC, Kemnitz JW. Body fat distribution with long-term dietary restriction in adult male rhesus macaques. *J Gerontol A Biol Sci Med Sci* 1999; **54**: B283–290.

88. Kemnitz JW, Roecker EB, Weindruch R, Elson DF, Baum ST, Bergman RT. Dietary restriction increases insulin sensitivity and lowers blood glucose in rhesus monkeys. *Am J Physiol* 1994; **266** (Endocrinol Metab 29): E540–E547.

89. Lane M, Ball SS, Ingram DK, *et al.* Diet restriction in rhesus monkeys lowers fasting and glucose-stimulated glucoregulatory endpoints. *Am J Physiol* (Endocrinol. Metab. 31) 1995; **268**: E941–E948.

90. Bodkin NL, Ortmeyer HK, Hansen BC. Long-term dietary restriction in older-aged rhesus monkeys: effects on insulin resistance. *J Gerontol: Biol Sci* 1995; **50**: B142–B147.

91. Ortmeyer HK, Bodkin NL, Hansen BC. Chronic caloric restriction alters glycogen metabolism in rhesus monkeys. *Obes Res* 1994; **2**: 549–555.

92. Hannah JS, Verdery RB, Bodkin NL, Hansen BC, Anh-Le N, Howard BV. Changes in lipoprotein concentrations during the development of noninsulin dependent diabetes mellitus in obese rhesus monkeys (*Macaca mulatta*). *J Clin Endocrinol Metab* 1991; **72**: 1067–1072.

93. Winegar DA, Brown PJ, Wilkison WO, *et al.* Effects of fenofibrate on lipid parameters in obese rhesus monkeys. *Endocrinol* 1998; **216**: 466.

94. Hannah JS, Bodkin NL, Paidi MS, Anh-Le N, Howard BV, Hansen BC. Effects of acipimox on the metabolism of free fatty acids and VLDL triglyceride. *Acta Diabetol* 1995; **32**: 279–293.

95. Bodkin NL, Hansen BC. Prevention of Syndrome X by long-term dietary restriction (DR) in aged rhesus monkeys. *Gerontologist* 1995; **35**: 239.

96. Verdery RB, Ingram DK, Roth GS, Lane MA. Caloric restriction increases HDL_2 levels in rhesus monkeys (*Macaca mulatta*). *Am J Physiol* 1997; **273**: E714–719.

97. Edwards IJ, Rudel LL, Terry JG, Kemnitz JW, Weindruch R, Cefalu WT. Caloric restriction in rhesus monkeys reduces low density lipoprotein interaction with arterial proteoglycans. *J Gerontol A Biol Sci Med Sci* 1998; **53**: B443–448.

98. DeLany JP, Hansen BC, Bodkin NL, Hannah J, Bray GA. Long-term calorie restriction reduces energy expenditure in aging monkeys. *J Gerontol A Biol Sci Med Sci* 1999; **54**: B5–11.

99. Lane MA, Baer DJ, Rumpler WV, *et al.* Calorie restriction lowers body temperature in rhesus monkeys, consistent with a postulated anti-aging mechanism in rodents. *Proc Natl Acad Sci USA* 1996; **93**: 4159–4164.

100. Walston J, Lowe A, Silver K, *et al.* The β3-adrenergic receptor in the obesity and diabetes prone rhesus monkey is very similar to human and contains arginine at codon 64. *Gene* 1997; **188**: 207–213.

101. Hansen BC. Primates in the experimental pharmacology of obesity. In: Lockwood D, Heffner TG (eds) *Handbook of Experimental Pharmacology: Obesity—Pathology and Therapy.* Heidelberg: Springer-Verlag, 2000: 461–489.

102. Fisher MH, Amend AM, Bach TJ, *et al.* A selective human beta 3 adrenergic receptor agonist increases metabolic rate in rhesus monkeys. *J Clin Invest* 1998; **101**: 2387–2393.

103. Weyer C, Gautier JF, Danforth E, Jr. Development of beta 3-adrenoceptor agonists for the treatment of obesity and diabetes—an update. *Diabetes Metab* 1999; **25**: 11–21.

104. Kumar MV, Moore RL, Scarpace PJ. Beta3-adrenergic regulation of leptin, food intake, and adiposity is impaired with age. *Pflugers Arch* 1999; **438**: 681–688.

105. Young AA, Gedulin BR, Bhavsar S, *et al.* Glucose-lowering and insulin-sensitizing actions of exendin-4: studies in obese diabetic (*ob/ob, db/db*) mice, diabetic fatty Zucker rats and diabetic monkeys (*Macaca mulatta*). *Diabetes* 1999; **48**: 1026–1034.

106. Kemnitz JW, Elson DF, Roecker EB, Baum ST, Bergman RN, Meglasson MD. Pioglitazone increases insulin sensitivity, reduces blood glucose, insulin, and lipid levels, and lowers blood pressure, in obese, insulin-resistant rhesus monkeys. *Diabetes* 1994; **43**: 204–211.

107. Ortmeyer HK, Bodkin NL, Yoshioka S, Horikoshi H, Hansen BC. A thiazolidinedione improves in vivo insulin action on skeletal muscle glycogen synthase in insulin-resistant rhesus monkeys. *Int J Exp Diabetes Res* 2000; **1**: 195–202.

108. Farooqi IS, Jebb SA, Langmack G, *et al.* Effects of recombinant leptin therapy in a child with congenital leptin deficiency. *N Engl J Med* 1999; **341**: 879–884.

109. Tang-Christensen M, Havel PJ, Jacobs R, Larsen PJ, Cameron JL. Central administration of leptin inhibits food intake and activates the sympathetic nervous system in rhesus macaques. *J Clin Endocrinol Metab* 1999; **84**: 711–717.

110. Sanigorski A, Cameron-Smith D, Lewandowski P, *et al.* Impact of obesity and leptin treatment on adipocyte gene expression in *Psammomys obesus*. *J Endocrinol* 2000; **164**: 45–50.

15

Social Status, Social Stress and Fat Distribution in Primates

Carol A. Shively and Jeanne M. Wallace

Wake Forest University School of Medicine, Winston-Salem, North Carolina, USA

INTRODUCTION

The relationship between the stress associated with low social status and disease susceptibility is apparent in human and non-human primates. In human beings, low socioeconomic status is associated with increased mortality from all causes, increased coronary heart disease (CHD) morbidity and mortality, increased rates of depression, the prevalence of the metabolic syndrome, and central obesity (1). We have studied these relationships in female cynomolgus monkeys for many years. Like human beings, low social status (subordinate) female monkeys are more susceptible than their dominant counterparts to a number of pathological processes that result in disease, including depression and coronary artery atherosclerosis. This chapter will focus on the relationship between social status, fat distribution patterns, and two disease endpoints in adult female cynomolgus monkeys, coronary heart disease risk and depression.

A NONHUMAN PRIMATE MODEL OF CORONARY ARTERY ATHEROSCLEROSIS AND CHD RISK

Atherosclerosis (an accumulation of fatty, connective, and necrotic tissue) of the coronary arteries is the principal pathological process which causes CHD. Cynomolgus monkeys (*Macaca fascicularis*) are currently the only animal model of sex differences in susceptibility to diet-induced atherogenesis. Among Caucasians in Western society, men have about twice the incidence of CHD and twice as extensive coronary artery atherosclerosis as women (2–4). The male to female ratio of coronary artery atherosclerosis extent in cynomolgus monkeys is also about 2:1. Like women, female cynomolgus monkeys are protected against atherosclerosis relative to their male counterparts (5).

Female cynomolgus monkeys have menstrual cycles that are similar to those of women in terms of length and cyclic hormone fluctuations (6,7). Following bilateral ovariectomy, extensive coronary artery atherosclerosis develops in females in amounts that are indistinguishable from those of males (8). CHD risk is also increased in oophorectomized and postmenopausal women (9). Subcutaneous replacement of estradiol, or estradiol and progesterone in physiological doses protects against atherosclerosis in female monkeys (10), and hormone replacement therapy (HRT) is associated with decreased CHD risk in postmenopausal women (11). Thus, ovarian function, and in particular estradiol, is implicated in the phenomenon of female protection, both in women and in female cynomolgus macaques.

International Textbook of Obesity. Edited by Per Björntorp.

PSYCHOSOCIAL FACTORS THAT INFLUENCE CORONARY ARTERY ATHEROSCLEROSIS AND CHD RISK IN FEMALE MONKEYS

Social Status

Cynomolgus monkeys typically live in large social groups that are characterized by complex social relationships. Complex social living includes the possibility of social stress effects on health. A major social organizing mechanism of monkey society is the social status hierarchy (12). Female monkeys with low social status, or subordinates, are behaviorally and physiologically different from dominants.

The distinguishing behavioral characteristics of subordinates are depicted in Figure 15.1. Subordinate females are the recipients of about three times the hostility or aggression of their dominant counterparts. They are groomed less, i.e. they spend less time in positive affiliative behavior. They spend more time vigilantly scanning their social group than dominants. The purpose of the vigilant scanning appears to be to track and avoid dominants in order to avoid aggressive interactions. Subordinates also spend significantly more time alone than dominant females (13–15). Primates typically communicate non-verbally by touch, facial expressions and body language or postures. Although human primates also are able to communicate with language, they still rely heavily on non-verbal communication. When a female monkey spends time alone, it means that the monkey is not in physical contact or within touching distance of another monkey. Rather, the monkey is socially isolated. This is intriguing given the observations in human beings that suggest that social support is associated with reduced CHD risk, and observations in monkeys suggesting that social isolation increased coronary artery atherosclerosis and heart rate (16–18). Thus, it seems that subordinates are subject to hostility and have very little social support.

Physiological characteristics of subordinates that distinguish them from dominants include differences in measurements of adrenal function. Following dexamethasone suppression, the adrenal glands of subordinate females hypersecrete cortisol in response to an adrenocorticotropic hormone challenge, and are also relatively insensitive to cortisol

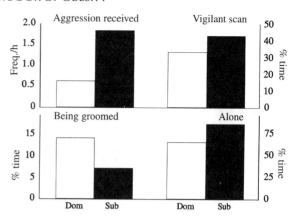

Figure 15.1 Behavioral characteristics of socially dominant (Dom; white bars) and subordinate (Sub; black bars) female monkeys. Subordinates receive more aggression, are groomed less—that is they spend less time in positive affiliative behavior, spend more time alone, and they spend more time vigilantly scanning their social group than dominants. Freq./h = frequency per hour; % time = percentage of time spent. (Based on data from Shively *et al.* (13,14))

negative feedback (15). Since the hypersecretion of cortisol is typically viewed as indicative of a stressed individual, these findings imply that, in general, subordinate females are stressed females.

Subordinate females also have a greater number of abnormal menstrual cycles than dominant females (8). Progesterone concentrations are lower during the luteal phase, and estradiol concentrations are lower in the follicular phase of the menstrual cycles of subordinate females. Moderately low luteal phase progesterone concentrations indicate that although ovulation may have occurred, the luteal phase was hormonally deficient. Very low luteal phase progesterone concentrations indicate an anovulatory cycle (19,20). Thus, stressed, subordinate females have poor ovarian function compared to dominants. Subordinate females with poor ovarian function have more coronary artery atherosclerosis than their dominant counterparts (Figure 15.2). Indeed, the coronary artery atherosclerosis extent in these subordinate, stressed females is comparable to that found in both ovariectomized females and males (5,8).

The effects of stress on ovarian function in women are difficult to evaluate because of the difficulties in characterizing menstrual cycle quality over long periods of time. However, the results of several studies are consistent with the hypothesis that stress can have a deleterious effect on ovarian function in women (21–23). Furthermore, mechan-

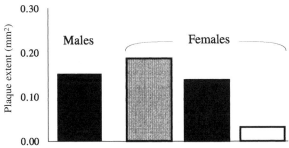

Figure 15.2 Coronary artery atherosclerosis (measured as plaque extent) in males and in females in different reproductive conditions. Among females: gray bars = ovariectomized females; black bars = intact socially subordinate females with poor ovarian function; white bars = intact socially dominant females with good ovarian function. (Based on data from Hamm *et al.* (5), Adams *et al.* (8))

istic pathways relating stress to impaired reproductive function in female primates have been identified, suggesting that the stress–ovarian function impairment hypothesis is plausible from a physiological perspective. Activation of the hypothalamic-pituitary-adrenal axis, endogenous opioid pathways, increased prolactin release, and changes in sensitivity to gonadal steroid hormone feedback have all been proposed to mediate the effects of behavioral stress on the reproductive system (24–30). Intriguingly, women with hypothalamic amenorrhea also have increased hypothalamic-pituitary-adrenal activity similar to that observed in subordinate female cynomolgus monkeys (31). The relationship between poor ovarian function during the premenopausal years and CHD risk is also difficult to ascertain in women due to the double challenge of characterizing ovarian function, and detecting an adequate number of clinical CHD events. However, La Vecchia reported that women with a history of irregular menstrual cycles are at increased risk for CHD (32).

Ovarian hormones (particularly estradiol) are also associated with the *function* of the coronary arteries. In response to neuroendocrine signals, coronary arteries either dilate or constrict to modulate the flow of blood to the heart. Inappropriate coronary artery constriction, or vasospasm, early in life may change flow dynamics, injuring the epithelium and exacerbating atherosclerosis. Coronary vasospasm later in life in the presence of exacerbated atherosclerosis may increase the likelihood of myocardial infarction. In cynomolgus monkeys, the coronary arteries of normal cycling females dilate in

response to acetylcholine infused directly into the coronary artery, whereas those of ovariectomized females constrict. The dilation response can be restored in ovariectomized females by administering estradiol, i.e. estrogen replacement therapy (33,34). The coronary arteries of dominant females with good ovarian function dilate in response to an infusion of acetylcholine, whereas those of subordinate females with poor ovarian function constrict in response to acetylcholine (35). Thus, female primates with poor ovarian function may be at increased CHD risk for two reasons: (1) impaired coronary artery function, and (2) increased atherogenesis.

Ovarian function declines at menopause, particularly the production of estradiol and progesterone. Importantly, clinically detectable events occur most frequently during and after the menopausal decline in ovarian function. Thus, the impact of premenopausal ovarian function on CHD risk may be temporally separate from the clinical manifestation of CHD. However, atherogenesis is a dynamic process that occurs over a lifetime. We hypothesize that atherogenesis during young and middle adulthood may be accelerated among socially stressed women. These women enter the menopausal years with exacerbated atherosclerosis. During the estrogen-deficient menopausal years, exacerbated atherosclerosis, combined with a more atherogenic lipid profile and increased likelihood of coronary vasospasm, result in increased CHD among women who experienced excessive premenopausal social stress.

Social Status, Social Stress, and Depression

Social stress is believed to precipitate depression (36–40) Unfortunately, depressive disorders are prevalent and the rate of occurrence is increasing (41). The results of several studies suggest that low social status is associated with increased risk of depression, although the nature of the relationship is unclear (42,43). In one prospective study in which low social status predicted first onset of major depressive disorder, a lack of social support (social isolation) appeared to mediate this relationship, at least in part (44). Thus, social support may reduce risk of depression following stressful life events (45,46).

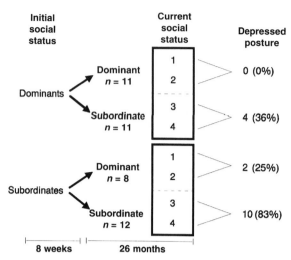

Figure 15.3 The effects of low social status on the prevalence of behavioral depression in female monkeys. (Based on data from Shively *et al.* (47))

The hypothesis that social subordination is stressful, and results in a depressive response in some individuals, was examined in the following experiment. Forty-eight adult female monkeys were fed an atherogenic diet, housed in small social groups, and social status was altered in half of the animals such that half of the subordinates became dominant, and half of the dominants became subordinate (Figure 15.3).

Current subordinates hypersecreted cortisol, were insensitive to negative feedback, and had suppressed reproductive function. Current subordinates received more aggression, engaged in less affiliation, and spent more time alone than dominants. Furthermore, they spent more time fearfully scanning the social environment and displayed more behavioral depression than dominants. Current subordinates with a history of social subordination were preferentially susceptible to a behavioral depression response. The results of this experiment confirm that the stress of social subordination causes hypothalamic-pituitary-adrenal and ovarian dysfunction, and support the hypothesis that chronic, low-intensity social stress may result in depression in susceptible individuals (15,47).

Interim Summary

Low social status in female primates is associated with worsened coronary artery atherosclerosis.

These females are the recipients of hostility/aggression, and they are also relatively socially isolated. Females with low social status are also preferentially susceptible to a depressive response to social stress, particularly if they have a history of social subordination.

Social stress increases the risk of CHD and precipitates bouts of depression in human beings. Low socioeconomic status is associated with increased risk of depression and CHD. The relationship between socioeconomic status and health in human beings is linear; there is no apparent threshold. The upper class has better health than the upper middle class, and so on down the hierarchy. Risk of disease is increased even among relatively low social status employed individuals with adequate health care, nutrition, and shelter. Thus, the health gradient does not appear to be due to poverty, per se (48). Perhaps the reason low social status is associated with increased risk of disease in human beings is because low social status is stressful. Like the monkeys, human primates with low social status have relatively little control over their lives, and low control is a source of chronic stress that could engender physiological responses that are deleterious to health.

REGIONAL ADIPOSITY AND CORONARY ARTERY ATHEROSCLEROSIS IN FEMALES

We examined the relationship between social status, social stress, and central obesity in a series of studies of social group-living cynomolgus monkeys. In all of the experiments discussed below, adult monkeys were fed a moderately atherogenic diet that contained between 0.25 and 0.39 mg cholesterol/calorie and 40% of calories from fat (primarily saturated fat). These monkeys were housed in small social groups of four to six animals of the same gender.

The initial investigation of regional adiposity and coronary artery atherosclerosis was a retrospective necropsy study of 36 adult female cynomolgus monkeys (49). Whole body and regional adiposity were determined using anthropometric measurements. Whole body adiposity did not predict the extent of coronary artery atherosclerosis. However, the relative amount of subcutaneous fat deposited on the trunk (estimated by the ratio of subscapular:triceps skinfold thickness) versus the periphery was associated with coronary artery atherosclerosis extent. Females in the top half of the distribution of subscapular:triceps skinfold ratio had more than three times as much coronary artery atherosclerosis than females in the lower half of the distribution (49).

REGIONAL ADIPOSITY AND METABOLIC ABERRATIONS

Female cynomolgus monkeys with high central fat have higher glucose and insulin concentrations in an intravenous glucose tolerance test than females with relatively low central fat. They also have higher blood pressure and total plasma cholesterol concentrations, and lower HDL cholesterol concentrations compared to low central fat females (50). In women, central obesity has been linked with a metabolic syndrome consisting of impaired glucose tolerance, raised serum triglycerides and low levels of HDL cholesterol (51).

SOCIAL SUBORDINATION AND REGIONAL ADIPOSITY

To determine characteristics of subordinate females which increase their risk of coronary artery atherosclerosis, whole body and regional adiposity were evaluated using anthropometric measurements in 75 adult female cynomolgus monkeys (52,53). Subordinate females were more likely than dominants to be in the top half of the distribution of the subscapular:triceps skinfold ratio. This suggested the possibility of a relationship between stress and patterns of fat distribution that is associated with increased coronary artery atherosclerosis in monkeys and increased risk of coronary heart disease in women. Since that observation, we have attempted to further our understanding of the potential relationship between stress and fat distribution.

SOCIAL STRESS AND REGIONAL ADIPOSITY IN MALES

Since truncal fat patterns are associated with androgenic hormone profiles, it is possible that the androgenic fat distribution pattern observed more frequently in social subordinates is due to ovarian dysfunction. To begin to address this possibility, the relationship between stress and fat distribution patterns was studied in male monkeys. Coronary artery atherosclerosis is exacerbated in male cynomolgus monkeys when their social groups are repeatedly disrupted. Social disruption has been achieved in several experiments by altering the constituency of social groups frequently (e.g. every 4 weeks) for a 2-year period. Generally, the monkeys respond to alterations in group membership by increased aggression and decreased affiliation (54). Thus, repeated social reorganization was used as the stressor in the following study of males.

The monkeys were assigned to treatment groups using a method of stratified randomization that matched the groups for pretreatment plasma cholesterol concentrations. Pretreatment anthropometric measures were used to control for small (non-significant) differences in adiposity that were present prior to treatment. Computed tomography was used to measure intra-abdominal and subcutaneous abdominal fat in forty monkeys and regional skinfold thicknesses were also measured (55). Males that lived in the stress condition produced by repeated social reorganization had significantly higher ratios of intra-abdominal:subcutaneous (IA:SQ) abdominal fat (56).

This experiment provides important evidence supporting the hypothesis that social stress can alter regional fat deposition. The stressor was manipulated by the experimenter rather than resulting from social group living, as in the previous observation of an association between social status and regional fat deposition. These findings also indicate that stress can alter fat distribution patterns independent of ovarian function; however, the mechanism(s) that might relate these two factors remains to be determined.

MECHANISMS MEDIATING THE RELATIONSHIP BETWEEN SOCIAL STRESS AND REGIONAL ADIPOSITY

To identify potential mechanisms through which social stress might alter fat deposition patterns, a study was recently completed in which behavior, the function of the hypothalamic-pituitary-adrenal

Table 15.1 Associations between abdominal fat distribution and behavioral characteristics of female monkeys

	IS:SQ		
	Low	High	P
% time being groomed	12(1.3)	8(1.5)	0.07
% time grooming	13(1.8)	7.5(0.8)	0.03
% time alone vigilant scan	36(2.2)	43(2.8)	0.07
% time alone	45(2.6)	54(3.4)	0.06
% mild aggression—attacker	31(6.3)	13(4.5)	0.05
% mild aggression—victim	12(3.6)	46(9.5)	0.001
% severe aggression—attacker	19(3.5)	17(5.5)	0.75
% severe aggression—victim	11(3.8)	31(9.5)	0.03
Social status (0 = Subordinate, 1 = Dominant)	0.6(0.1)	0.3(0.1)	0.002

IA:SQ, Intra-abdominal to subcutaneous abdominal fat ratio as measured using computed tomography.

axis, and the sympathetic nervous system were characterized in female cynomolgus monkeys. Abdominal fat mass was characterized by computed tomography as previously described (49,55). The monkeys lived in their social groups for $2\frac{1}{2}$ years, and social behavior was recorded throughout this time period. Females above the mean of the ratio of IA:SQ abdominal fat mass were compared to females below the mean.

Females with high IA:SQ abdominal fat ratios spent less time in affiliative social interaction, were more frequently the victims of aggression, and were socially subordinate compared to females with low IA:SQ abdominal fat ratios (Table 15.1).

There was also a modest correlation between behavioral depression and the IA:SQ ratio (Spearman's rho = 0.26, P = 0.05, 1-tailed test), suggesting that females with relatively greater amounts of intra-abdominal fat were more likely to display behavioral depression. Heart rate, a non-invasive indicator of sympathetic nervous system activity, was measured while the animals were in their social groups, using a telemetry system, from 15:00 h to 8:00 h the following day for three consecutive days. Heart rates of these animals are generally lowest at night, increase during the time of day when there is the most activity in their building, and decrease in the afternoon after the activity level in the building declines. Two months following the formation of social groups, there were no differences in high versus low IA:SQ females. However, by 24 months, differences between these groups had emerged. The

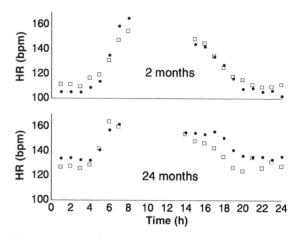

Figure 15.4 Association between abdominal fat distribution and heart rate in female monkeys. (Heart rates were recorded 2 months and 24 months following social group formation.) IA:SQ, Intra-abdominal to subcutaneous abdominal fat ratio as measured using computed tomography; HR, heart rate in beats per minute (bpm). □ Low IA:SQ; ● high IA:SQ

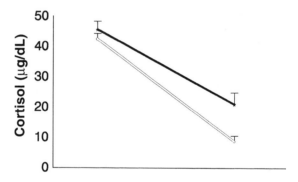

Figure 15.5 Dexamethasone suppression test. Relationship between insensitivity to cortisol negative feedback and abdominal fat distribution. Females with low IA:SQ intra-abdominal to subcutaneous fat reduce cortisol secretion by 79%, whereas those with high IA:SQ abdominal fat reduce cortisol secretion by 54% (<0.05). IA:SQ, intra-abdominal to subcutaneous abdominal fat ratio as measured using computed tomography. White line, low IA:SQ; solid line, high IA:SQ

heart rates of all females were similarly elevated during the day; however, in the afternoon and night, heart rates of the females in the high IA:SQ abdominal fat group were higher than those in the low group ($P = \leq 0.05$; Figure 15.4).

Hypothalamic-pituitary-adrenal (HPA) function was assessed using a dexamethasone suppression test. Suppression of serum cortisol in response to dexamethasone was greater in females in the lower half of the distribution of IA:SQ abdominal fat mass ($P < 0.05$; Figure 15.5). This observation suggests that the central regulatory areas of the HPA axis of females with a relatively low IA:SQ ratio are more sensitive to circulatory cortisol concentrations than those with relatively high IA:SQ. Taken together, these data suggest that females with relatively greater amounts of visceral fat are also characterized by behavioral and physiological attributes indicative of chronic stress. Furthermore, the sympathetic nervous system and the HPA axis may mediate the relationship between social stress and regional adiposity. Our findings in cynomolgus monkeys support the hypothesis proposed by some that stress and a hypersensitive HPA axis are central abnormalities in abdominal obesity of human beings (51).

SUMMARY

In primates, abdominal obesity is associated with low social status, the metabolic syndrome, and increased risk of morbidity and mortality due to depression and cardiovascular disease. Data from studies of monkeys suggest that social stress may be an underlying cause. We hypothesize that the stress of social subordination or social instability causes increased sympathetic nervous and HPA function. The chronic stimulation of these two systems leads to increased blood pressure and heart rate, and imbalances in sex steroid production which result in injury to the artery wall, and deposition of fat in the viscera. Visceral fat depots in turn exacerbate the metabolic effects of stress. Some of these physiological stress responses affect the function of the brain, resulting in depression.

ACKNOWLEDGEMENT

The studies reported here were funded, in part, by grants HL-39789, HL-14164, and HL-40962 from the National Institutes of Health, National Heart, Lung, and Blood Institute, Bethesda, MD.

REFERENCES

1. Brunner EJ, Marmot MG, Nanchahal K, Shipley MJ, Stansfeld SA, Juneja M, Alberti KGMM. Social inequality in coronary risk: central obesity and the metabolic syndrome. Evidence from the Whitehall II study. *Diabetologia* 1997; **40**: 1341–1349.
2. Wingard DL, Suarez L, Barrett-Connor E. The sex differential in mortality from all causes and ischemic heart disease. *Am J Epidemiol* 1983; **117**: 19–26.
3. Vanecek R. Atherosclerosis of the coronary arteries in five towns. *Bull WHO* 1976; **53**: 509–518.
4. Tejada C, Strong JP, Montenegro MR, Restropo C, Solberg LA. Distribution of coronary and aortic atherosclerosis by geographic location, race, and sex. *Lab Invest* 1968; **18**: 509–526.
5. Hamm TE Jr, Kaplan JR, Clarkson TB, Bullock BC. Effects of gender and social behavior on the development of coronary artery atherosclerosis in cynomolgus macaques. *Atherosclerosis* 1983; **48**: 221–233.
6. Jewett DA, Dukelow WR. Cyclicity and gestation length of *Macaca fascicularis. Primates* 1972; **13**: 327–330.
7. Mahoney CJ. A study of the menstrual cycle in *Macaca irus* with special reference to the detection of ovulation. *J Reprod Fertil* 1970; **21**: 153–163.
8. Adams MR, Kaplan JR, Clarkson TB, Koritnik DR. Ovariectomy, social status, and atherosclerosis in cynomolgus monkeys. *Arteriosclerosis* 1985; **5**: 192–200.
9. Kannel WB, Hjortland MC, McNamara PM, Gordon T. Menopause and risk of cardiovascular disease: the Framingham study. *Ann Intern Med* 1976; **85**: 447–452.
10. Adams MR, Kaplan JR, Manuck SR, Koritnik DR, Parks JS, Wolfe MS, Clarkson TB. Inhibition of coronary artery atherosclerosis by 17-beta estradiol in ovariectomized monkeys. *Arteriosclerosis* 1990; **10**: 1051–1057.
11. Bush TL, Barrett-Connor E, Cowan LD, Criqui MH, Wallace RB, Suchindran CM, Tyroler HA, Rifkind BM. Cardiovascular mortality and noncontraceptive use of estrogen in women: results from the Lipid Research Clinics Program Follow-up Study. *Circulation* 1987; **75**: 1102–1109.
12. Shively CA. The evolution of dominance hierarchies in nonhuman primate society. In: Ellyson SL, Dovidio JF (eds) *Power, Dominance, and Nonverbal Behavior.* New York: Springer-Verlag, 1985: 67–88.
13. Shively CA, Kaplan JR, Adams MR. Effects of ovariectomy, social instability and social status on female *Macaca fascicularis* social behavior. *Physiol Behav* 1986; **36**: 1147–1153.
14. Shively CA, Manuck SB, Kaplan JR, Koritnik DR. Oral contraceptive administration, interfemale relationships, and sexual behavior in *Macaca fascicularis. Arch Sex Behav* 1990; **19**: 101–117.
15. Shively CA. Social subordination stress, behavior and central monoaminergic function in female cynomolgus monkeys. *Biol Psychiatry* 1998; **44**: 882–891.
16. Shumaker SA, Hill DR. Gender differences in social support and physical health. *Health Psychol* 1991; **10**: 102–111.
17. Shively CA, Clarkson TB, Kaplan JR. Social deprivation and coronary artery atherosclerosis in female cynomolgus monkeys. *Atherosclerosis* 1989; **77**: 69–76.
18. Watson SL, Shively CA, Kaplan JR, Line SW. Effects of chronic social separation on cardiovascular disease risk factors in female cynomolgus monkeys. *Atherosclerosis* 1998; **137**(2): 259–266.
19. Wilks JW, Hodgen GD, Ross GT. Luteal phase defects in the rhesus monkey: The significance of serum FSH:LH ratios. *J*

Clin Endocrinol Metab 1976; **43**: 1261–1267.

20. Wilks JW, Hodgen GD, Ross GT. Endocrine characteristics of ovulatory and anovulatory menstrual cycles in the rhesus monkey. In: Hafez ESE (ed.) *Human Ovulation*. Amsterdam: Elsevier/North-Holland Biomedical Press, 1979: 205–218.

21. Matteo S. The effect of job stress and job interdependency on menstrual cycle length, regularity and synchrony. *Psychoneuroendocrinology* 1987; **12**: 467–476.

22. Barnea ER, Tal J. Stress-related reproductive failure. *J in Vitro Fertil Embryo Transfer* 1991; **8**: 15–23.

23. Gindoff PR. Menstrual function and its relationship to stress, exercise, and body weight. *Bull N Y Acad Med* 1989; **65**: 774–786.

24. Hayashi KT, Moberg GP. Influence of the hypothalamic-pituitary-adrenal axis on the menstrual cycle and the pituitary responsiveness to estradiol in the female rhesus monkey (*Macaca fascicularis*). *Biol Reprod* 1990; **42**: 260–265.

25. Abbott DH, O'Byrne KT, Sheffield JW, *et al.* Neuroendocrine suppression of LH secretion in subordinate female marmoset monkeys (*Callithrix jacchus*). In: Eley RH (ed.) *Comparative Reproduction in Mammals and Man*. Proceedings of the Conference of the National Center for Research in Reproduction. Nairobi, Institute of Primate Research, National Museums of Kenya, 1989: 63–67.

26. Abbott DH, Saltman W, Schultz-Darken NJ. Hypothalamic switches regulating fertility in primates. Paper presented at the XIVth Congress of the International Society of Primatology, Strasbourg, France, 1992.

27. Gindoff PR, Ferin M. Endogenous opioid peptides modulate the effect of corticotropin-releasing factor on gonadotropin release in the primate. *Endocrinology* 1989; **121**: 837–842.

28. Ferin M. Two instances of impaired GnRH activity in the adult primate: The luteal phase and 'stress'. In: Delemarrevan de Waal HA, *et al.* (eds) *Control of the Onset of Puberty III*. Amsterdam: Elsevier Science Publishers BV, 1989: 265–273.

29. Biller BM, Federoff HJ, Koenig JI, Klibanski A. Abnormal cortisol secretion and responses to corticotropin-releasing hormone in women with hypothalamic amenorrhea. *J Clin Endocrinol Metab* 1990; **70**: 311–317.

30. Cameron JL. Stress and behaviorally induced reproductive dysfunction in primates. *Semin Reprod Endocrinol* 1997; **15**: 37–45.

31. Nappi RE, Petraglia F, Genazzini AD, D'Ambrogio G, Zarta C, Genazzani AR. Hypothalamic amenorrhea: evidence for a central derangement of hypothalamic-pituitary-adrenal cortex axis activity. *Fertil Steril* 1993; **59**: 571–576.

32. La Vecchia C, Decarli A, Franceschi S, Gentile A, Negri E, Parazzini F. Menstrual and reproductive factors and the risk of myocardial infarction in women under fifty-five years of age. *Am J Obstet Gynecol* 1987; **157**: 1108–1112.

33. Williams JK, Adams MR, Klopfenstein HS. Estrogen modulates responses of atherosclerotic coronary arteries. *Circulation* 1990; **81**: 1680–1687.

34. Williams JK, Adams MR, Herrington DM, Clarkson TB. Short-term administration of estrogen and vascular responses of atherosclerotic coronary arteries. *J Am Coll Cardiol* 1992; **20**: 452–457.

35. Williams JK, Shively CA, Clarkson TB. Vascular responses

36. of atherosclerotic coronary arteries among premenopausal female monkeys. *Circulation* 1994; **90**: 983–987.

36. Brown GW, Harris TO. Aetiology of anxiety and depressive disorders in an inner-city population. 1. Early adversity. *Psychol Med* 1993; **23**: 143–154.

37. Brown GW. Life events and affective disorder: Replications and limitations. *Psychosom Med* 1993; **55**: 248–259.

38. Brown GW, Harris TO, Eales MJ. Aetiology of anxiety and depressive disorders in an inner-city population. 2. Comorbidity and adversity. *Psychol Med* 1993; **23**: 155–165.

39. Brown GW, Moran P. Clinical and psychosocial origins of chronic depressive episodes. I: A community survey. *Br J Psychiatry* 1994; **165**: 447–456.

40. Brown GW, Harris TO, Hepworth C. Loss, humiliation and entrapment among women developing depression: a patient and non-patient comparison. *Psychol Med* 1995; **25**: 7–21.

41. Fombonne E. Increased rates of depression: update of epidemiological findings and analytical problems. *Acta Psychiatr Scand* 1994; **90**: 145–156.

42. Murphy JM, Olivier DC, Monson RR, Sobol AM, Federman EB, Leighton AH. Depression and anxiety in relation to social status. *Arch Gen Psychiatry* 1991; **48**: 223–229.

43. Cole DA, Carpentieri S. Social status and the comorbidity of child depression and conduct disorder. *J Consult Clin Psychol* 1990; **58**: 748–757.

44. Bruce ML, Hoff RA. Social and physical health risk factors for first-onset major depressive disorder in a community sample. *Soc Psychiatry Psychiatr Epidemiol* 1994; **29**: 165–171.

45. Aneshensel CS, Stone JD. Stress and depression: A test of the buffering model of social support. *Arch Gen Psychiatry* 1982; **39**: 1392–1396.

46. Serban G. Stress in affective disorders. *Methods Achieve Exp Pathol* 1991; **15**: 200–220.

47. Shively CA, Laber-Laird K, Anton RF. The behavior and physiology of social stress and depression in female cynomolgus monkeys. *Biol Psychiatry* 1997; **41**: 871–882.

48. Marmot MG, Davey Smith G, Stansfeld S, *et al.* Health inequalities among British Civil Servants: The Whitehall II study. *Lancet* 1991; **337**: 1387–1393.

49. Shively CA, Clarkson TB, Miller LC, Weingand KW. Body fat distribution as a risk factor for coronary artery atherosclerosis in female cynomolgus monkeys. *Arteriosclerosis* 1987; **7**: 226–231.

50. Shively CA, Clarkson TB. Body fat distribution and atherosclerosis. In: Howard DF Jr (ed.). *Nonhuman Primate Studies on Diabetes, Carbohydrate Intolerance, and Obesity*. New York: Alan R. Liss, 1988: 43–63.

51. Björntorp P. Body fat distribution, insulin resistance and metabolic diseases. *Nutrition* 1997; **13**: 795–803.

52. Shively CA, Clarkson TB. Regional obesity and coronary artery atherosclerosis in females: a nonhuman primate model. *Acta Med Scand* (Suppl) 1988; **723**: 71–78.

53. Shively CA, Kaplan JR, Clarkson TB. Carotid artery atherosclerosis in cholesterol-fed cynomolgus monkeys: The effects of oral contraceptive treatments, social factors and regional adiposity. *Arteriosclerosis* 1990; **10**: 358–366.

54. Kaplan JR, Manuck SB, Clarkson TB, Lusso FM, Taub DM. Social status, environment, and atherosclerosis in cynomolgus monkeys. *Arteriosclerosis* 1982; **2**: 359–368.

55. Laber-Laird K, Shively CA, Karstaedt N, Bullock BC. Assessment of abdominal fat deposition in female cynomolgus monkeys. *Int J Obes* 1991; **15**: 213–220.

56. Jayo J, Shively CA, Kaplan JR, Manuck SB. Effects of exercise and stress on body fat distribution in male cynomolgus monkeys. *Int J Obes* 1993; **17**: 597–604.

16

Centralization of Body Fat

Per Björntorp
Sahlgrenska University Hospital, Göteborg, Sweden

INTRODUCTION

Centralization of body fat stores has proven to be an index of several serious diseases and their precursor states, indicated by risk factors. Historically this is an observation which originates from anthropologists in the early twentieth century. Kretschmer (1) noticed the difference in disease associations with different body build, mainly from the aspect of his own specialty, which was psychiatry. He observed that the pychnic type frequently suffered from gout, atherosclerotic disease and stroke, and he saw early signs of glucose intolerance as well as abnormal pharmacological reactions of the autonomic nervous system in comparison with, particularly, the leptosomic body build type. Both these types were also different from the aspect of food intake, where the pychnic type increased more readily in body weight. Kretschmer made anthropometric measurements from which the waist-to-hip circumference ratio (WHR) can be calculated. Such calculations show that the pychnic type had a WHR which is well within the risk zone for disease, as recently suggested by the WHO (2). The pychnic type was also more prone to develop depressive symptoms while the leptosomic type often had a schizoid personality.

Jean Vague in Marseille (3) is another pioneer who already 50 years ago saw the differences between gynoid and android obesity and the risk for complications in the latter. Vague was focusing mainly on adipose tissue distribution but also made observations on other diseases than obesity.

All these sharp-sighted clinical observations have been confirmed and extended in modern science with more refined methods, as will be briefly reviewed in this chapter.

Centralization of body fat stores can be measured in a number of ways. The gold standard methods for obtaining absolute masses of various body fat stores are the imaging techniques. These methods are, however, complicated and expensive to use in epidemiological work, where simpler surrogate measurements have to be employed. Such methods include skinfolds, which, however, do not measure intra-abdominal fat masses. Various circumference measurements such as waist circumference or the WHR provide an estimate of internal fat masses. The WHR has probably been somewhat better anchored in prospective studies of disease than the waist circumference, although the latter is slightly easier to measure. The abdominal sagittal diameter seems to provide the most accurate estimation of the important visceral, intra-abdominal fat masses (4).

Utilizing such measurements, it has now become increasingly clear that body fat centralization is a powerful index of prevailing previously established risk factors for disease such as insulin resistance, dyslipidaemia and hypertension, is found with high prevalence in already established disease, and is a powerful independent risk factor for disease in prospective studies. The abnormalities associated with body fat centralization span a wide range of somatic diseases in metabolism and energy intake, such as obesity, cardiovascular and cerebrovascular diseases. Furthermore, respiratory, haematological

International Textbook of Obesity. Edited by Per Björntorp.
© 2001 John Wiley & Sons, Ltd.

and psychiatric diseases as well as cancer show associations with centralization of body fat. This is also the case for personality characteristics, alcohol abuse, socioeconomic and psychosocial handicaps. It is thus apparent that centralization of body fat embraces a large cluster of human life conditions, health and disease.

Only from this wide array of conditions does it seem unlikely that central fat distribution could be a causative factor. It seems more likely that central-ization of body fat is an index of perturbations in profound, central regulation of several vital systems in the body. Such regulations usually have their origin in the hypothalamic–limbic areas of the brain, which regulate vital functions in endocrine, metabolic and haemodynamic systems via neuroen-docrine and autonomic signals to the periphery. This is orchestrated by the central nervous system into appropriate reactions to maintain homeostasis or allostasis. When various factors challenging these counterbalancing mechanisms become too se-vere, homeostasis or allostasis can no longer be maintained, and disease and disease symptoms will appear in the long run.

In this chapter certain new developments within this area will be overviewed. The input into this research emanated originally from the obesity field, where Jean Vague's pioneering work has attracted too little attention. Obesity will, however, only be briefly touched upon here, primarily with emphasis on novel findings. Instead an outlook into other diseases and conditions will be offered. Some, but not all, of these fields are related to obesity, suggest-ing that body fat centralization has a much more fundamental significance for human disease than only in the obesity field.

By approaching various problems in biomedical research with epidemiological techniques on a population basis, it is possible to obtain a wide view on several diseases and their development, provided that a sufficient number of well-selected variables are examined. With this method many conditions can be analysed to search for potential pathogenetic pathways and generate hypotheses for further re-search. Selecting out only one phylogenetic charac-teristic for examination in case control studies limits the focus on the particular selected variable, for example obesity. In our research we have there-fore frequently based observations on epi-demiological studies to obtain a wider outlook on health problems.

OBESITY. THE HYPOTHALAMIC-PITUITARY-ADRENAL (HPA) AXIS

It must now be considered established that central, abdominal obesity is the malignant form of obesity. This condition seems to be associated with various perturbations of the function of the HPA axis. About one-quarter of a male population, selected at random, and all 52 years of age, have signs of an elevated diurnal cortisol secretion, associated with abdominally localized excess of body fat, measured with the sagittal, abdominal diameter, as well as signs of metabolic derangements, characteristic of the metabolic syndrome (5). It seems possible to explain the central fat accumulation as well as the metabolic derangements via effects of cortisol (6,7). The elevated cortisol secretion is seen most clearly when the endogenous activity of the HPA axis is most pronounced, that is before noon (Figure 16.1). During this period reports of perceived stress were also most prevalent (unpublished). This observation is in agreement with results of controlled animal experiments, where chronic stress facilitates this particularly active phase of HPA axis activity (8), and indicates that the men examined were exposed to a stressful environment not only during the day in their ordinary life when their cortisol secretion was measured, but also during a period preceding the examination.

In about 10% of the population the HPA axis displays a depressed activity with less diurnal vari-ation, a 'burn-out' condition (see Figure 16.1). The cortisol secretion is about 75% of controls, and the secretion is again most perturbed during the high activity phase of the HPA axis. This is also in agree-ment with controlled animal experiments of chronic stress (9), and might be the end result of a develop-ment in stages from repeated stress challenges, as in the group of men mentioned above, to eventual burn-out.

In spite of not being elevated, cortisol secretion in this condition is associated with central obesity and its well-known associated risk factors, including hy-pertension and elevated pulse rate. Interestingly, in this group secretions of testosterone and growth hormone are depressed (5), probably a consequence of the challenges on their central regulation by the HPA axis perturbations (10).

Such a burned-out HPA axis has been observed

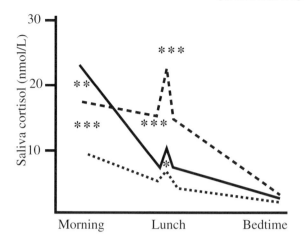

Figure 16.1 Saliva cortisol concentrations in controls (solid line), men with high stress-related cortisol (dashed line), and men with a burn out hypothalamic-pituitary-adrenal axis (dotted line) (from references 5 and 17 and unpublished data). *, $P < 0.05$; **, $P < 0.01$; ***, $P < 0.0001$ (in comparison with controls)

previously in conditions of severe stress such as in war veterans, holocaust victims, chronic pain, and 'vital exhaustion' (9), but it can apparently also be found in the general population. It appears that psychosocial and socioeconomic handicaps as well as alcohol abuse might be involved, but there are most likely other factors involved, yet to be identified, some of which probably have a genetic background (11,12). This condition should have a high priority for further research because of its serious endocrine abnormalities with associated malignant risk factor pattern.

In this condition the pathogenetic factors at play are unlikely to include cortisol secretion, because total cortisol secretion is low. It seems possible that the diminished secretions of sex steroid and growth hormones are involved. Deficiencies in these hormones would be expected to be followed by similar consequences as elevated cortisol, because these hormones counteract and balance the effects of cortisol in both the regulation of visceral fat mass and insulin resistance (6,7).

Another putative pathogenetic pathway might be via elevation of central sympathetic nervous activity, as indicated by the elevations of blood pressure and heart rate in this condition (5). Animal experiments clearly show that when the activity of the HPA axis is insufficient or burned out the sympathetic nervous system is activated in compensation to maintain homeostatic conditions (13). This would

also be expected to be followed by increased mobilization of free fatty acids with hepatic and muscular insulin resistance (14,15) as well as dyslipidaemia and perhaps diminished hepatic clearance of insulin as consequences (16). Free fatty acids are clearly elevated in abdominal obesity (16).

It should be observed at this point that although it seems possible to understand the pathogenetic pathways to centralization of body fat with associated risk factors via elevated cortisol secretion (5), as seen in the group of men with elevated stress-related cortisol secretion, the evidence suggests that the kinetics of diurnal cortisol secretion are at least of equal importance. In the men with elevated stress-related cortisol secretion the increase in diurnal cortisol is limited, about 20% in comparison with controls. The nocturnal cortisol secretion was not measured, and might have been elevated also to add to the total increase in cortisol secretion. It is noteworthy, however, that this group of men had significantly lower cortisol secretion in the earliest measurement after waking up (Figure 16.1). One might speculate that this is a sign of progression towards the low secretion of the group with the burned-out axis.

The burned-out condition is by itself the most powerful evidence suggesting that the perturbed regulation of the HPA axis rather than elevated cortisol secretion might be the crux of the matter in attempts to understand how cortisol secretion is associated with metabolic abnormalities.

The men in the group examined who had a normal HPA axis function with little or no exposure to perceived stress (see Figure 16.1) also had normal secretions of testosterone and growth hormone as well as normal blood pressures and heart rate. This is an apparent picture of normally regulated neuroendocrine and autonomic functions in several axes. Here cortisol secretion was negatively correlated to various risk factors. This means that, for example, absence of body fat centralization was associated with high cortisol, particularly when measured during the physiological stimulation of cortisol by food intake (17). This is an unexpected finding; one would actually have expected the opposite correlation. We have interpreted this to mean that a normally functioning neuroendocrine system as indicated by a high plasticity of the HPA axis, and normally functioning gonadal and growth hormone secretions, is associated with signs of bodily health, a 'mens sana in corpore sano' (18).

Taken together these observations indicate that neuroendocrine regulations are of fundamental importance for somatic health. Regulation of HPA axis activity probably occupies a central role, where cortisol secretion might be considered both as an index of neuroendocrine health or abnormality, with cortisol itself as a trigger of somatic perturbations in some, but not all conditions. These considerations, based on observations, probably explain the complicated results in previous attempts to measure cortisol secretion in obesity.

We have recently finalized a similar population study in women as that reported in men (5,11,17). The situation is different in several important aspects. Hyperandrogeneticity (HA) is a prominent, important abnormality in women related to centralization of body fat. The highest quintile of free testosterone is strongly associated with abdominal obesity and conventional risk factors for cardiovascular disease, stroke and type 2 diabetes mellitus. We have previously shown that HA is a powerful, independent risk factor for these diseases, as well as certain cancers (19), and is therefore probably a major predisposing condition for disease in women. The mechanism of action is likely to be induction of insulin resistance in muscles, which then triggers metabolic disease (20).

The nature of this HA has been examined in the new population study. It seems highly likely that its origin is at least partly adrenal, because steroids secreted mainly by the adrenals such as dihydroepiandrosterone sulphate and cortisol are elevated in parallel. Furthermore, concentrations of free testosterone show associations with features of saliva cortisol concentrations, which have been shown in men to be particularly associated with risk factors, namely low morning cortisol and food-induced cortisol secretion (21). Associations between HA and depressive traits have been found, similar to the associations of cortisol secretion in this condition, previously disclosed in men (22). Further potential background factors are currently being examined.

There are, however, probably also other factors involved. First, the aromatase gene shows polymorphisms in microsatellite areas, associated with elevated androgens and decreased 17β oestradiol, which are the expected consequences of a defect function of the aromatase enzyme, which converts testosterone to 17β oestradiol. A poorly functioning aromatase would therefore be followed by elevated testosterone. This may add to HA.

Furthermore, the androgen receptor gene shows a diminished number of trinucleotide repeats (CAG, glutamine) in the first exon, which might be associated with increased androgen sensitivity.

The polymorphisms found are thus localized to microsatellites with tetra- or trinucleotide repeats in the genes examined. Such abnormalities have introduced a new dimension in the research of genetic abnormalities in polygenic diseases. Monogenic diseases with mutations in exons usually have an all or nothing phylogenetic consequence. The interesting feature with microsatellite polymorphisms is that they often express themselves as quantitative abnormalities of more or less importance (23). For example, we see in the example mentioned above a variation in the expression of HA depending on the number of or lack of nucleotide repeats.

In summary, the currently performed analyses in women suggest that not only adrenal cortisol but also adrenal androgens are associated with central obesity with its risk factors and diseases. Adrenal androgens might well be also elevated in men with central obesity, but would be expected to be followed by minor or no peripheral consequences, because they would add only a minor fraction to testosterone produced in the gonads. The insulin resistance following HA in women is probably the trigger for at least the metabolically related diseases. Additional factors seem to be involved as disease-generating triggers in women with HA, including androgen metabolism and sensitivity.

OBESITY. CORTISOL METABOLISM

Cortisol is subjected to metabolic transformations in the periphery, which are of importance for the impact of cortisol on peripheral target tissues. This area is reviewed in the chapter by Walker and Seckl (Chapter 18), where detailed references can be found, and is only discussed here in relation to the central perturbations of HPA axis activity, reviewed in the preceding section.

There are two main systems regulating cortisol metabolism. One is the 5α reductases which transfer cortisol to tetrahydrocortisone, which is an essentially inactive metabolite excreted in the urine. The other system is the 11β-hydroxysteroid dehydrogenases (HSD), which consist of the HSD1, converting cortisone to cortisol, and the HSD2, converting cortisol to cortisone. In humans cortisone is a much less powerful glucocorticoid than cortisol.

There is evidence for an increased activity in obesity of 5α-reductase and HSD2, which inactivates cortisol. This would be expected to result in less active occupancy of the central glucocorticoid receptors (GR) which regulate cortisol secretion by a negative feedback mechanism (9), and an elevated cortisol secretion would be the expected outcome. In a recent study cortisol measurements have been adjusted for the body mass index (BMI), in an attempt to examine cortisol secretion without the influence of adipose tissue inactivation. This resulted in a visualization of elevated cortisol secretion in obesity (24). Consequently peripheral inactivation of cortisol might explain the elevated cortisol secretion in obesity.

It is, however, apparently not possible to explain why cortisol secretion is particularly elevated in centrally localized obesity, since an elevated cortisol secretion along this mechanism would be expected to be dependent on total mass of adipose tissue irrespective of its localization. Furthermore, if cortisol is rapidly inactivated in the peripheray, this would not be expected to result in peripheral consequences of hypercortisolism, as seen in central obesity.

Local elevations of the HSD1, which has been reported to occur in visceral fat depots, might have local effects but it seems difficult to imagine that a secretion of cortisol from visceral fat would have systemic effects, due to the small mass of this tissue. Cortisol from such elevated secretion would presumably also be inactivated peripherally. It is also difficult to understand the relationships, if any, between mechanisms, working on the regulatory centres of the HPA axis, described in the preceding section, and peripheral metabolism of cortisol. It might be considered that the peripheral enzymes involved in cortisol metabolism are secondarily modified by obesity-related factors such as cotisol itself, insulin and other hormone secretions which are abnormal.

These peripheral conversions of cortisol add to the complexity of this field, but are clearly important for the understanding of the problems involved. Parallel studies of both the central and peripheral mechanisms, regulating the net concentration of circulating glucocorticoids and their interaction with peripheral target tissues, would be needed to understand potential interactions and the resulting outcome.

OBESITY. PERINATAL FACTORS

Perinatal factors are likely to be involved in the problem of centralization of body fat stores. This idea originates from studies by Barker (25), who found that children born small for gestational age frequently develop centralization of body fat and associated metabolic syndrome, 'the small baby syndrome'. Although originally based on statistical observations from populations where intrauterine undernutrition was suspected, this hypothesis has gained considerable support from the results of recent studies.

Subjects with the small baby syndrome and abdominal preponderance of body fat stores have recently been reported to have elevated cortisol secretion (26). This might correspond to the group of men we have studied with elevated stress-related cortisol and centralization of body fat (8,17).

There are experimental studies which indicate potential mechanisms. The HPA axis can be sensitized by intrauterine exposure to immune stress or cytokine exposure or to lipopolysaccharides (27,28), and the handling of newborns has also been shown to be of importance (29). Recent studies have provided further interesting information, probably explaining the effects of prenatal exposure to lipopolysaccharides. These bacterial endotoxins stimulate the secretion of cytokines. Prenatal exposure to interleukin-6, tumour necrosis factor α or dexamethasone, a synthetic glucocorticoid which passes the placental barrier, is followed by permanent sensitization of the HPA axis, leptin-resistant obesity and insulin resistance (30). It seems likely that leptin-resistant obesity is caused by the increased corticosterone secretion from the HPA axis, because a similar condition develops after elevated corticosterone exposure in adult rats (31). This is probably applicable also to humans because it is well known from clinical experience that patients treated with glucocorticoids overeat and become obese. Furthermore, in recent experiments we have been able to show that women taking 25 mg prednisolone daily for a week increase their food intake in spite of elevated leptin concentrations (32).

These interesting developments suggest that centralization of body fat and also the development of obesity might be affected not only by cortisol in adulthood, but also by prenatal factors. Infections during pregnancy might speculatively be involved in such developments.

It is thus apparent that perinatal factors are critical for the development of obesity and centralization of body fat stores with its metabolic associates in adult life. Evidence suggests that this might at least partly be mediated via programming of the regulation of the HPA axis. It will be of interest in the future to find out to what extent 'the small baby syndrome' is involved in the overall prevalence of centralization of body fat and the metabolic syndrome in adult life.

HYPERTENSION

There is now considerable evidence indicating that primary hypertension is frequently associated with centralization of body fat mass (33) and the metabolic syndrome (34,35). From the statistical correspondence between elevated blood pressure and insulin arose the suggestion that elevated blood pressure might be caused by hyperinsulinaemia or its precursor, insulin resistance. This contention is supported by experimental work showing that the central sympathetic nervous system is activated by insulin (36).

New evidence is, however, not in agreement with this chain of events (37). In statistical calculations with blood pressure as the independent variable, HPA axis perturbations take over all statistical power, and blood pressure is no longer dependent on insulin. This suggests that some factor related to HPA axis activity is a major determinant of blood pressure. This is probably the activity of the sympathetic nervous system, which shows signs of parallel activation when the HPA axis is not functioning normally (38). This is a well-described phenomenon with interactions between the central regulation of the HPA axis and the synpathetic nervous system at several levels. In fact, it is difficult to activate one of these axes without interfering with the other, due to this tight coupling of their regulatory centres (10).

It therefore seems likely that the relationship between insulin levels and blood pressure is due to a parallel activation of the HPA axis and the sympathetic nervous system at central levels. It seems likely that the sympathetic nervous system is responsible for blood pressure elevation and the HPA axis for insulin resistance with hyperinsulinaemia following as described above. The HPA axis is presumably also responsible for the centralization of body fat as also discussed above.

In the case of primary hypertension; centralization of body fat stores seems to be a sign of central neuroendocrine disturbances where elevated blood pressure is probably due to a parallel activation of the sympathetic nervous system, also occurring at a central level. It may well be, however, that insulin amplifies this autonomic activation. For further discussion of this problem, see review in Björntorp et al. (35).

MENTAL DEPRESSION

Much to our initial surprise we found in population studies that subjects with traits of depression and anxiety often had centralized fat depots (39). This has also been found in our most recent studies in both men and women (22, and data in preparation). These traits are depressed moods, frequent use of antidepressant drugs and anxiolytics as well as various sleeping difficulties (39–41). This has now also been confirmed from other laboratories (42). As is almost invariably the case, this centralization of body fat is followed by the metabolic syndrome, as well as frequently, by hypertension.

These findings are of interest from at least two aspects. Full-blown melancholic depression is a condition with severe perturbations of several neuroendocrine axes, including activation of the HPA axis with poor suppression of cortisol secretion by dexamethasone, elevated activity of the sympathetic nervous system and inhibition of the hypotalamic-gonadal axis and growth hormone secretion (43). These are exactly the same neuroendocrine perturbations that occur in people with centralization of body fat (see above). Consequently, we believe that depressive traits might be a significant pathogenetic factor which via the neuroendocrine perturbations will lead to body fat centralization and the metabolic syndrome.

Another aspect of interest is that depression is clearly followed by an increased risk for somatic disease and premature mortality, also when suicide is taken into account. Prospective studies have demonstrated that the risk for cardiovascular disease and type 2 diabetes mellitus is clearly increased in subjects with frequent episodes of depression, and the risk power is comparable to that of conventional somatic metabolic risk factors such as dyslipidaemia, insulin resistance and hypertension (44,45). Unfortunately, such risk factors have not been extensively followed in these prospective studies of depression. A very recent study has, however, clearly shown that visceral fat masses are elevated in patients with repeated depressive periods (46).

Taken together this evidence strongly suggests that depressive traits or clinically manifest melancholic depression are associated already at early stages with centralization of body fat masses, and metabolic and circulatory risk factors for prevalent, serious, somatic disease. This probably provides an explanation for the increased somatic morbidity and mortality in depression. The pathogenetic mechanisms are most likely provided by the central multiple neuroendocrine and auto-nomic perturbations, that occur in depression as well as in subjects who present with centralization of body fat. This field has recently been summarized, and the reader is referred to this review for detailed references and further discussion (47).

This has interesting therapeutic implications. Mental depression is improved or cured by modern pharmacological treatment. This is also followed by a correction of the neuroendocrine and autonomic abnormalities. If the proposed chain of pathogenetic events presented above is correct, then metabolic and haemodynamic abnormalities, following the neuroendocrine and autonomic abberations, would also be expected to be improved. Unfortunately, this does not seem to have been systematically followed in psychiatric literature.

We have therefore recently finalized a pilot study with this problem in focus. Men with elevated WHR were treated with an antidepressant inhibiting serotonin reuptake, but without effects on energy balance. This was followed by an apparent normalization of the signs of a perturbed activity of the HPA axis as well as a decreased activity of the sympathetic nervous system, and signs of metabolic correction such as improved glucose tolerance and insulin sensitivity. Interestingly, these men did not show any pathological scores in several depression

scales, and these scores did not change with treatment, perhaps suggesting that metabolic improvements may occur without parallel mental changes (48). In addition, these results suggest that the serotonergic system is involved in neuroeuroendocrine regulation, which is an established phenomenon (10).

ALCOHOL AND SMOKING

There are several reports in the literature that tobacco smoking as well as elevated alcohol consumption is associated with centralization of body fat stores. This is dramatically apparent in the so called pseudo-Cushing syndrome which is due to alcohol abuse. Both tobacco smoking and alcohol intake above a limit of a couple of drinks per day are followed by an activation of the HPA axis, providing a possible link to centralization of body fat stores (49).

PSYCHOSOCIAL AND SOCIOECONOMIC FACTORS

Psychosocial factors have been found to be associated with an elevated WHR in both men and women. The relationships seem stronger in men, with factors such as living alone and divorce. Socioeconomic handicaps are also involved, including poor education, physical type of work, low social class and low income (50,51). This has also recently been observed in the Whitehall studies with strong inverse relationships between socioeconomic status on the one hand and an elevated WHR associated with the metabolic syndrome on the other (52). In a similar treatment of our data we find the same relationships, which are associated with perturbations of the HPA axis. In addition, exposure time for such handicaps seems to worsen the symptoms (53).

It seems likely that exposure to such socioeconomic and psychosocial handicaps provides a background which would frequently expose such individuals to a stressful environment, and activate the stress systems in the lower part of the brain, followed by the neuroendocrine and autonomic cascade of events, eventually leading to central fat accumulation, the metabolic syndrome and disease.

This then might provide an explanation for the social inequality of disease.

PERSONALITY

Accumulating evidence now also suggests that body fat tends to be stored in central depots in certain types of personalities. This includes both normal variants and what has been defined as personality disorders (54,55). Men with an elevated WHR frequently score high on items of 'novelty seeking', and sometimes display antisocial, histrionic and explosive personalities. Personality disorders include schizoid and avoidant, dependent and passive, aggressive characteristics. Men with such personalities might be expected to react to their surroundings in a way that induces stress. Examinations also show that they have high values on various reported stress items such as difficulties in control of not only important things in life but also day to day problems and annoyances, and have a high total score in stress questionnaires. These findings are in concert with the reports of frequent perceived stress periods, associated with perturbed neuroendocrine functions, which supposedly are followed by centralization of body fat (5,17) as discussed in a preceding secretion.

ENDOCRINE DEFICIENCIES

Men with low testosterone, women after menopause and both men and women with growth hormone deficiency without involvement of HPA axis perturbations tend to have abdominal obesity (49). These hormones prevent accumulation of body fat in intra-abdominal depots, and deficiency would then be expected to be followed by enlargement of these depots. The mechanisms whereby this occurs have been largely elucidated, and substitution with the deficient hormone is followed by a specific decrease of visceral fat as well as improvement of the factors included in the metabolic syndrome (6). The prevalence of such conditions seem to be in the order of 10% in the middle-aged male population (56).

CANCER

Cancer is also predicted by increased proportions of the central fat stores. This was first reported in a small number of endometrial carcinomas (57), and has subsequently been reported also for breast carcinoma (58) and confirmed in a larger study of endometrial carcinomas (59). Since these reports seem to suggest that the carcinomas predicted are localized to tissues which are sensitive to sex steroid hormones, one might speculate that the abnormalities of steroid hormone secretion found in abdominal obesity are also involved in this problem. Elevated androgens are closely associated with centralization of fat in women (21,60) as discussed in a preceding section, and probably originate from the adrenals as a consequence of a central drive of the HPA axis. Such abnormalities indicate disturbed secretions of sex steroid hormones which in an unknown way might be associated with these endocrine dependent carcinomas.

GENETIC FACTORS

Genetic factors are clearly involved in the phenomenon of central accumulation of body fat. Such factors could be present locally in the adipose tissues in question, or in the regulatory mechanisms involved in adipose tissue distribution. A major factor in this regard is probably the activity of the HPA axis, which has been shown to be strongly dependent on genetic factors (61).

A first target for examining molecular genetic factors in men with elevated central body fat has been the gene locus of the glucocorticoid receptor (GR), because the men with perturbed diurnal cortisol secretion discussed in the section on obesity often show abnormalities in the suppression of the HPA axis by dexamethasone (5). We then found that a known polymorphism of the GR gene locus, situated in the first intron, was associated with centralization of body fat as well as insulin resistance and, furthermore, an exaggerated stimulated cortisol secretion (62). Furthermore, another polymorphism in the promoter region is associated with elevated basal cortisol secretion (63). There are thus genetic markers for centralization of fat depots in this gene, probably, if functionally significant, acting via regulation of the HPA axis.

In women additional polymorphisms, localized in microsatellites of genes involved in androgen metabolism and sensitivity seem to be involved (21), as discussed in a preceding section.

Other polymorphisms of potential general interest for the syndrome of elevated central fat are those involved in the regulation of the sympathetic nervous system. Such polymorphisms have been found in the beta-2-adrenergic receptor and in the dopamine-2 receptor, both associated with elevated blood pressure. Polymorphisms of the leptin receptor are, however, apparently protective for hypertension in obesity (64–66).

These early findings demonstrate that the syndrome of central fat accumulation is associated with several gene polymorphisms, indicating a complex genetic background of the syndrome.

WHY DOES FAT ACCUMULATE PREDOMINANTLY IN CENTRAL DEPOTS?

The mechanistic, mainly endocrine background to visceral fat accumulation has been reviewed elsewhere (6). One may wonder from a teleological viewpoint why humans in a wide variety of conditions store an excess fraction of body fat in central depots.

These depots are equipped with a very sensitive fat mobilization system, which becomes even more efficient by a dense innervation and a rich blood flow to remove mobilized free fatty acids to the portal circulation, and subsequently after hepatic extraction, to systemic circulation. Accumulation of depot fat in these portally drained depots thus serves as an easily available substrate for important liver and peripheral functions in, for example, muscles. The substrate delivery to the periphery is in the form of both free fatty acids and very low density lipoprotein triglycerides, synthesized in the liver (for review see Björntorp (16). The accumulation of central fat is more pronounced in men than women. Specific localization of fat accumulation seems to have a clear survival value, particularly in men, who were particularly dependent on their muscles for survival in ancient times.

One may also look upon this phenomenon as a reserve depot for periods when the surrounding milieu is threatening, and where much available energy is best stored in easily mobilizable depots, and not, for example, in the gluteo-femoral depot of women, which seems to be constructed for specific child-bearing purposes (6). Such a construction is, however, outdated in current urbanized societies. When this excess is not used for purposes of energy delivery to muscles after longer stressful periods with accumulation of central fat, these depots remain intact as a sign of long-term environmental pressures, which lead to disease by mechanisms involving neuroendocrine and autonomic mechanisms, as discussed above.

GENERAL SUMMARY

This overview has attempted to summarize briefly the multitude of conditions in which central, visceral fat is accumulated in excess. In all these situations there seems to be a neuroendocrine background affecting the HPA as well as other central hormonal axes, often coupled to the autonomic nervous system. This parallel activation is characteristic of an arousal reaction of centres in the lower parts of the brain, constructed for adaptation to surrounding pressures in order to maintain homeostasis or allostasis. The widespread occurrence of elevated central body fat masses suggests by itself that vital, common pathways are activated. The associations between central fat and such diverse conditions as heart disease, stroke, diabetes, obesity, hypertension, cancer, depression, anxiety, endocrine disturbances, personality aberrations, alcohol abuse, socioeconomic and psychosocial handicaps etc., suggest some kind of common pathogenetic denominator. It seems likely that this denominator is a central arousal, induced by factors in a competitive, hectic society. Central fat accumulation may be considered mainly as a conveniently observable indicator of a chronic exposure to such damaging factors, remaining as an outdated survival mechanism. Figure 16.2 illustrates a hypothesis of the putative pathways linking increased central fat mass to diseases and conditions which have been shown to be statistically associated with it.

ACKNOWLEDGEMENT

The studies from the author's laboratory referred to have been performed in collaboration with a large

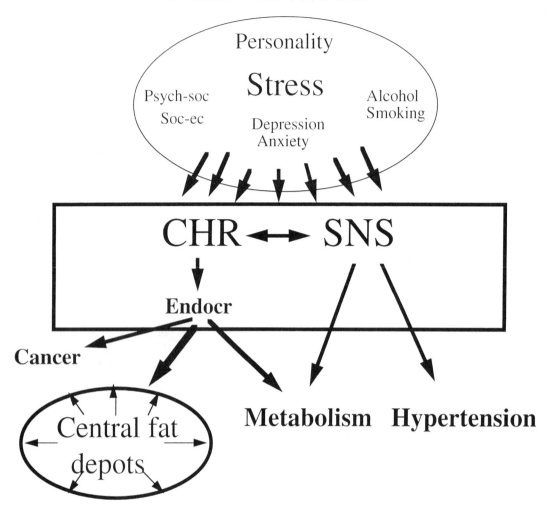

Figure 16.2 Hypothetical explanation to the statistical associations between central fat depot enlargement and a large cluster of different factors. Various stress factors, including psychosocial and socioeconomic handicaps (psycho-soc, soc-ec), depression, anxiety, alcohol and smoking which, dependent on personality characteristics, via corticotrophin-releasing hormone (CRH) and endocrine perturbations, including cortisol, sex steroid and growth hormones (endocr) direct fat to central depots, and constitute risk factors for endocrine type of cancers. In addition, CRH, together with the functionally, tightly connected central sympathetic nervous system (SNS), generates metabolic and haemodynamic (hypertension) risk factors for disease

number of international and Swedish researchers. Their names are found in the reference list.

REFERENCES

1. Kretschmer E. *Physique and Character.* New York: Harcourt, 1936. (Originally published in German 1921.)
2. WHO. *Obesity. Preventing and Managing the Global Epidemic.* Report of a WHO consultation on obesity, Geneva, 3–5 June 1997, WHO/NUT/NCD/98. 1. Geneva: WHO, 1998.
3. Vague J. La différenciation sexuelle facteur déterminant des formes de l'obesite. *Presse Med* 1947; **30**: 339–341.
4. Kvist H, Chowdhury B, Grangård U, Tyle'n U, Sjöström L. Total and visceral adipose tissue volumes derived from measurements with computed tomography in adult men and women: predictive equations. *Am J Clin Nutr* 1988; **48**: 1351–1361.
5. Rosmond R, Dallman MF, Björntorp P. Stress-related cortisol in men: Relationships with abdominal obesity and endocrine, metabolic and hemodynamic abnormalities. *J Clin Endocrinol Metab* 1998; **83**: 1853–1859.
6. Björntorp P. The regulation of adipose tissue distribution in humans. *Int J Obes* 1996; **20**: 291–302.
7. Björntorp P. Neuroendocrine perturbations as a cause of

insulin resistance. *Diabetes/Metabolism Res Rev* 1999; **15**: 1–15.

8. Dallman MF, Akana SF, Scribner KA. Stress, feedback and facilitation in the hypothalamo-pituitary-adrenal axis. *J Neuroendocrinol* 1992; **4**: 516–526.

9. McEwen BS. Protective and damaging effect of stress mediators. *N Engl J Med* 1998; **338**: 171–179.

10. Chrousos GP, Gold PW. The concept of stress and stress system disorders. Overview of physical and behavioral homeostasis. *JAMA* 1992; **267**: 1244–1252.

11. Rosmond R, Lapidus L, Björntorp P. The influence of occupational and social factors on obesity and fat distribution in middle-aged men. *Int J Obes* 1996; **20**: 599–607.

12. Larsson B, Seidell J, Svärdsudd K, Wilhelmsen L. Tibblin G, Björntorp P. Obesity, adipose tissue distribution and health in men—the study of men born in 1913. *Appetite* 1989; **13**: 37–44.

13. Plotsky PM, Cunningham Jr ET, Widmaier EP. Catecholaminergic modulation of corticotropin-releasing factor and adrenocorticotropin secretion. *Endocr Rev* 1989; **19**: 437–458.

14. Randle P, Garland P, Hales N, Newsholme E. The glucose-fatty acid cycle: its role in insulin sensitivity and the metabolic disturbances in diabetes mellitus. *Lancet* 1963; 785–789.

15. Groop LC, Saloranta C, Shank M, Bonadonna RC, Ferrannini E, DeFronzo RA. The role of free fatty acid metabolism in the pathogenesis of insulin resistance in obesity and non-insulin dependent diabetes mellitus. *J Clin Endocrinol Metab* 1971; **72**: 96–107.

16. Björntorp P. 'Portal'adipose tissue as a generator of risk factors for cardiovascular disease and diabetes. *Arteriosclerosis* 1900; **10**: 493–496.

17. Rosmond R, Holm G, Björntorp P. Food-induced secretion in relation to anthropometric, metabolic and hemodynamic variables in men. *Int J Obes* 2000; **24**: 416–422.

18. Chrousos GP, Gold PW. Editorial: A healthy body in a healthy mind—and vice versa—the damaging power of 'uncontrollable' stress. *J Clin Endocrinol Metab* 1998; **83**: 1842–1845.

19. Björntorp P. Abdominal fat distribution and disease: An overview of epidemiological data. *Ann Med* 1992; **24**: 15–18.

20. Björntorp P. Metabolic implications of body fat distribution. *Diabetes Care* 1991; **14**: 1132–1143.

21. Baghaei F, Rosmond R, Eriksson E, Holm G, Björntorp P. Disease predictors and adrogens in women. 2000. Submitted for publication.

22. Rosmond R, Björntorp P. Endocrine and metabolic aberrations in men with abdominal obesity in relation to anxio-depressive infirmity. *Metabolism* 1998; **47**: 1187–1193.

23. Comings DE. Polygenic inheritance and micro/minisatellites. *Mol Psychiatry* 1998; **3**; 21–31.

24. Walker BR, Soderberg S, Lindahl B, Olsson T. Independent effects of obesity and cortisol in predicting cardiovascular risk factors in men and women. *J Intern Med* 2000; **247**: 198–204.

25. Barker DJP. Fetal origins of coronary heart disease. *BMJ* 1995; **311**: 171–174.

26. Phillips DIW, Barker DJP, Fall CHD. Elevated plasma cortisol concentrations; a link between low birthweight and the insulin resistance syndrome? *J Clin Endocrinol Metab* 1998; **83**: 757–760.

27. Reul JMHM, Stec J, Wiegers GJ. Prenatal immune challenge alters the hypothalamic-pituitary axis in adult rats. *J Clin Invest* 1994; **93**: 2600–2607.

28. Nilsson C, Larsson B-M, Jennische E, Eriksson E, Björntorp P, York DA, Holmäng A. Prenatal endotoxin exposure results in leptin resistance, obesity and insulin resistance in adult male rats. 2000. Submitted for publication.

29. Meaney MJ, McCormick CM, Smythe JW, Sharma S. Sex specific effects of prenatal stress on hypothalamic-pituitary-adrenal responses to stress and brain glucocorticoid density in adult rats. *Brain Res* 1995; **84**: 55–61.

30. Dahlberg J, Nilsson C, Jennische E, Hoi-Por Ho, Eriksson E, Niklasson A, Björntorp P, Albertsson-Widkland K, Holmäng A. Prenatal cytokine exposure results in obesity, and sex-specific programming of neuroendocrine axes in adult rats. 2000. *Amer J Physiol*, in press.

31. Zakrzewska KE, Cusin J, Sainsbury A, Rohner-Jeanrenaud F, Jeanrenaud B. Glucocorticoids as counterregulatory hormones of leptin: toward an understanding of leptin resistance. *Diabetes* 1997; **46**: 717–719.

32. Uddén J, Björntorp P, Arner P, Barkeling B, Meurling L, Hill M, Rössner S. Glucocorticoids induce leptin resistance in women. 2000. Submitted for publication.

33. Krotkiewski M, Björntorp P, Sjöström L, Smith U. Impact of obesity on metabolism in men and women. *J Clin Invest* 1983; **72**: 1150–1162.

34. Ferrannini E, Buzzigoli G, Bonadonna R. Insulin resistance in essential hypertension. *N Engl J Med* 1987; **317**: 350–357.

35. Björntorp P, Holm G, Rosmond R, Folkow B. Hypertension and the metabolic syndrome. Closely related central origin? *Blood Press.* 2000; **9**: 71–82.

36. Landsberg L, Young JB. Insulin-mediated glucose metabolism in the relationship between dietary intake and the sympathetic nervous system activity. *Int J Obes* 1985; **9**: 63–68.

37. Rosmond R, Björntorp P. Blood pressure in relation to obesity, insulin and the hypothalamic-pituitary-adrenal axis in Swedish men. *J Hypertens* 1998; **16**: 1721–1726.

38. Ljung T, Holm G, Friberg P, Dallman MF, Mc Ewen BC, Björntorp P. The activity of the hypothalamic-pituitary-adrenal axis and the sympathetic nervous system in men with elevated waist/hip circumference ratio. *Obes Res* 2000; **8**: 487–495.

39. Lapidus L, Bengtsson C, Hällström T, Björntorp P. Obesity, adipose tissue distribution and health in women—results from a population study in Gothenburg, Sweden. *Appetite* 1989; **12**: 25–35.

40. Rosmond R, Björntorp P. Psychiatric ill-health in women and its relationship to obesity and fat distribution. *Obes Res* 1998; **6**: 338–345.

41. Rosmond R, Lapidus L, Mårin P, Björntorp P. Mental distress, obesity and body fat distribution in middle-aged men. *Obes Res* 1996; **4**: 245–252.

42. Wing RR, Matthews KA, Kuller LH, Meilahn EN, Plantinga P. Waist to hip ratio in middle-aged women. Associations with behavioral and psychosocial factors and with changes in cardiovascular risk factors. *Arterioscler Thromb* 1991; **11;** 1250–1257.

43. Gold PW, Chrousos GP. The endocrinology of melancholic and atypical depression: relation to neurocircuitry and so-

matic consequences. *Proc Assoc Am Physicians* 1999; **111**: 22–34.

44. Pratt LA, Ford DE, Crum RM, Arnenian HK, Fallo JJ, Eaton WW. Depression, psychotropic medication, and risk of myocardial infarction. Prospective data from the Baltimore ECA follow-up. *Circulation* 1996; **94**: 3123–3129.

45. Eaton WW, Armenian H, Gallo J, Pratt L, Ford DE. Depression and risk for onset of type II diabetes. A prospective population-based study. *Diabetes Care* 1996; **19**: 1097–1102.

46. Thakore JH, Richards PJ, Reznek RH, Martin A, Dinan TG. Increased intra-abdominal fat mass in patients with major depressive illness as measured by computed tomography. *Biol Psychiatry* 1997; **41**: 1140–1142.

47. Björntorp P. Epidemiology of the relationship between depression and physical illness. In Thakore JH (ed.) *Depression, a Stress-related Disorder: Physical Consequences and Potential Treatment Implications.* Petersfield, UK: Wrightson, 2001, in press.

48. Ljung T, Ahlberg A-C, Holm G, Friberg P, Andersson B, Eriksson E, Björntorp P. Treatment of men with abdominal obesity with a serotonin reuptake inhibitor. A pilot study. 2000; submitted for publication.

49. Björntorp P. Visceral obesity: a 'civilisation syndrome'. *Obes Res* 1993; **1**: 206–222.

50. Rosmond R, Björntorp P. Psychosocial and socioeconomic factors in women and their relationship to obesity and regional fat distribution. *Int J Obes* 1999; **23**: 138–145.

51. Rosmond R, Lapidus L, Björntorp P. The influence of occupational and social factors on obesity and body fat distribution in middle-aged men. *Int J Obes* 1996; **20**: 599–607.

52. Brunner EJ, Marmot MG, Nanchatal K. Social inequality and coronary risk: central obesity and the metabolic syndrome. Evidence from the Whitehall II study. *Diabetaologia* 1997; **40**: 1341–1349.

53. Rosmond R, Björntorp P. Occupational status, cortisol secretory pattern and visceral obesity in middle-aged men. 1999; *Obes Res* 2000; **8**: 445–450.

54. Rosmond R, Eriksson E, Björntorp P. Personality disorders in relation to anthropometric and metabolic factors. *J Endocrinol Invest* 1999; **22**: 279–288.

55. Ahlberg A-C, Ljung T, Rosmond R, McEwen BC, Holm G, Björntorp P, Akesson H-O. Mood disturbance and anthropometric measurements in men. 2000, submitted for publication.

56. Rosmond R, Björntorp P. The interactions between hypothalamic-pituitary-adrenal axis activity, testosterone, insulin-like growth factor I and abdominal obesity with metabolism and blood pressure in men. *Int J Obes Relat Metab Disord* 1998; **22**: 1184–1196.

57. Lapidus L, Helgesson Ö, Merck C, Björntorp P. Adipose tissue distribution and female carcinomas. A 12 year follow-up of the participants in the population study of women in Gothenburg, Sweden. *Int J Obes* 1988; **12**: 361–368.

58. Folsom AR, Kaye SA, Prineas RJ, Potter JD, Gapstur SM, Wallace RB. Increased incidence of carcinoma of the breast associated with abdominal adiposity in postmenopausal women. *Am J Epidemiol* 1990; **131**: 794–803.

59. Schapira DV, Kumar NB, Lyman GH, Cavanagh D, Roberts WS, LaPolla J. Upper-body fat distribution and endometrial cancer risk *JAMA* 1991; **266**: 1808–1811.

60. Peiris AN, Mueller RA, Struve MF, Smith GA, Kissebah AH. Relationship of androgenic activity to splanchnic insulin metabolism and peripheral glucose utilisation in premenopausal women. *J Clin Endocrinol Metab* 1987; **64**: 162–169.

61. Linkowski P, Van Ouderbergen A, Kerkhofs M, Bosson D, Mendlewicz J, Van Cauter E. Twin study of the 24-h cortisol profile: Evidence for genetic control of the human circadian clock. *Am J Physiol* 1993; **264**: E173–181.

62. Rosmond R, Chagnon YC, Holm G, Chagnon M, Pérusse L, Carlsson B, Bouchard C, Björntorp P. A Bcl I restriction fragment length polymorphism of the glucocorticoid receptor gene locus is associated with abdominal obesity, leptin and dysregulation of the hypothalamic-pituitary-adrenal axis. *Obes Res* 2000; **8**: 211–218.

63. Rosmond R, Chagnon YC, Chagnon M, Pérusse L, Bouchard C, Björntorp P. A polymorphism of the 5′-flanking region of the glucocorticoid receptor gene locus is associated with basal cortisol secretion in men. *Metabolism* 2000, in press.

64. Rosmond R, Ukkola U, Chagnon M, Bouchard C, Björntorp P. Polymorphisms of the β2-adrenergic receptor gene (ADRB2) in relation to cardiovascular risk factors in men. 1999, submitted for publication.

65. Rosmond R, Rankinen T, Chagnon M, Pérusse L, Bouchard C, Björntorp P. A polymorphism of the dopmine 2 receptor 2 gene locus is associated with elevated blood pressure and personality disorders in men. *J Clin Endocrinol Metab* 2000; in press.

66. Rosmond R, Chagnon YC, Holm G, Chagnon M, Pérusse L, Lindell K, Carlsson B, Bouchard C, Björntorp P. Hypertension in obesity and the leptin receptor gene locus. *Obes Res* 2000 (in press).

17

Obesity and Hormonal Abnormalities

Renato Pasquali and Valentina Vicennati

Endocrinology, S. Orsola-Malpighi Hospital, Univesity Alma Mater Studiorum, Bologna, Italy

INTRODUCTION

Obesity is associated with multiple alterations in the endocrine system, including abnormal circulating blood hormone concentrations, which can be due to changes in the pattern of their secretion and/or metabolism, altered hormone transport and/or action at the level of target tissues. In recent years a great stimulus in both basic and clinical research has, on one hand, produced a great deal of knowledge on the pathophysiology of obesity, and, on the other, led to the discovery of new hormones, such as leptin (1) and orexins (2).

This chapter reviews the main alterations in the classic endocrine systems, specifically those related to the hypothalamic-pituitary-gonadal (HPG) axis, the growth hormone/insulin-like growth factor 1 (GH/IGF-1) axis, and the hypothalamic-pituitary-adrenal (HPA) axis. The discussion will focus on human endocrinology, and animal studies will be referred to only when relevant to the organization of current knowledge. Several other endocrine systems will not be discussed, and readers are referred to extensive recent reviews in the field (3,4).

The recent discovery of the product of the *ob* gene, leptin, has pointed to the role of adipose tissue as an endocrine organ, capable of interacting with the central nervous system and other peripheral tissues by an integrated network, mainly devoted to the regulation of the energy balance and fuel stores.

The impressive growth of knowledge that has followed the discovery of leptin in 1996 is under continuous investigation. Other chapters of this book review this exciting topic, which will probably radically modify our clinical and therapeutic approach to obesity and related metabolic disorders in the next few years.

THE HPG AXIS IN FEMALES (Table 17.1)

Sex Steroid and Gonadotropin Concentration and Metabolism

An increase in body weight and fat tissue is associated with several abnormalities of sex steroid balance in premenopausal women. They involve both androgens and estrogens and their main transport protein, sex hormone-binding globulin (SHBG). Changes in SHBG, which binds testosterone and dihydrotestosterone (DHT) with high affinity and estrogens with lower affinity, also lead to an alteration of androgen and estrogen delivery to target tissues. The concentrations of SHBG are regulated by a complex of factors, which include estrogens, iodothyronines and growth hormone (GH) as stimulating, and androgens and insulin as inhibiting factors (5). The net balance of this regulation is probably responsible for decreased SHBG con-

International Textbook of Obesity. Edited by Per Björntorp.

Table 17.2   Main alterations of the hypothalamic-pituitary-gonadal axis in obese women

Condition	Alterations
Effect of obesity on sex hormones	Increased SHBG-bound and non SHBG-bound androgen production rate and metabolic clearance rate
	Reduced SHBG synthesis and concentrations
	Increased percentage free testosterone fraction
	Normal gonadotropin secretion
	Increased estrogen production rate
	Altered active/inactive estrogen balance
Impact of central obesity	Worsened androgen imbalance
	Treatment with androgens increases visceral fat in postmenopausal women
Obesity, hyperandrogenism and PCOS	Half PCOS women are overweight or obese
	Obesity may have a pathogenetic role in the development of hyperandrogenism in PCOS
	Obese women with PCOS have a prevalence of visceral fat distribution
	Hyperinsulinemia represents a pathogenetic factor of hyperandrogenism
	The metabolic syndrome is part of the obesity–PCOS association
Effects of weight loss	In simple obesity, improvement of androgen and SHBG imbalance
	In obese women with PCOS reduction of hyperinsulinemia and insulin resistance, hyperandrogenism, and improvement of all clinical features, including fertility rate

PCOS, polycystic ovary syndrome; SHBG, sex hormone-binding globulin.

centrations in obesity, in inverse proportion to the increase in body weight (4,5). Body fat distribution has important effects on SHBG concentrations in obese women. In fact, those with central obesity usually have lower SHBG concentrations in comparison to their age- and weight-matched counterparts with peripheral obesity (6). Insulin seems to play a dominant role in this context. Numerous epidemiological studies have, in fact, demonstrated a significantly negative correlation between insulin and SHBG blood levels, suggesting a cause–effect relationship (7). Moreover, studies *in vitro* have shown that insulin inhibits SHBG hepatic synthesis (8), and suppression (9) or stimulation (10) of insulin secretion *in vivo* has been found to be inversely associated with changes in SHBG concentrations, at least in hyperandrogenic obese women. Not surprisingly, reduced SHBG concentrations are therefore commonly associated with obesity, particularly in the central phenotype, type 2 diabetes, hyperandrogenic states such as polycystic ovary syndrome (PCOS), and cardiovascular atherosclerotic diseases (11), all conditions characterized by hyperinsulinemia and insulin resistance. On the other hand, not all obese women have reduced levels of SHBG, in spite of similar circulating androgen and estrogen concentrations, similar body weight and pattern of fat distribution. It has been suggested, for example, that dietary factors may help to explain these discrepancies. In fact, a significantly negative correla-

tion has been found in premenopausal women between lipid intake and SHBG levels (12). Moreover, experiments performed in men have demonstrated that high lipid intake significantly decreased SHBG concentrations, although contradictory data have been reported by others (see reference 12 for review).

Although the urinary excretion rate of 17-keto-steroids may be higher than normal in obese women (4), the levels of the main androgens are usually high only in obese women with amenorrhea and are normal in those with regular menstrual cycles (12). Gonadotropin secretory dynamics also appear to be normal in eumenorrheic obese women (4). The reduction of SHBG increases the metabolic clearance rate of circulating SHBG-bound steroids, specifically testosterone, DHT and androstane 3, 17β-diol (3A-diol), which is the principal active metabolite of DHT (13). However, this is compensated for by elevated production rates. The metabolism of the androgens not bound to SHBG is also modified by obesity. In fact, both production rates and metabolic clearance rates of dehydroepiandrosterone (DHEA) and androstenedione are equally increased in obesity (14,15), so that no difference in blood concentrations of the hormones is usually found in comparison to normal-weight individuals. Androgen production and metabolism may also show several differences in relation to the pattern of body fat distribution. Kirschner *et al.* (15), for example, found that premenopausal women with central obesity had higher testosterone production rates than those with peripheral obesity, whereas no differences in androstenedione and DHT production rate values were found. Accordingly, metabolic clearance rates of testosterone and DHT were significantly higher in the former than in the latter. The maintenance of normal circulating levels of these hormones in obesity suggests the presence of a servo-mechanism of regulation which adjusts both the production rate and the metabolic clearance rate of these hormones to body size. In women with obesity, the rates of androgen production increase but, due to the appreciable quantity of circulating blood passing through the adipose tissue, androgens may be cleared (metabolized) not only in the liver but also in the fat. In turn, this will result in a reduction in hormone uptake by androgen-sensitive tissues. Although speculative, this hypothesis may explain why most obese women seem to be protected against the biological effects of excessive androgen production, such as hirsutism and menstrual disturbances (13).

Obesity can also be considered a condition of exaggerated estrogen production. It has been demonstrated that the conversion of androgens to estrogen in peripheral tissues is significantly correlated with body weight and the amount of body fat (16). Several other factors can contribute to this condition of 'functional hyperestrogenism' (12). Due to reduced SHBG synthesis and lower circulating SHBG concentrations in obesity, the free estradiol fraction increases, thus increasing exposure of target tissues to this hormone. Moreover, the metabolism of estrogens is altered in obese women. A decreased formation of inactive estradiol metabolites, such as 2-hydroxyestrogens, which are virtually devoid of peripheral estrogen activity, is observed, together with a higher than normal production of estrone sulfate (which represents an important reservoir of active estrogens, particularly estrone), due to the concurrent reduction of its metabolic clearance and increased production rate. The final result of these metabolic derangements on estrogens is an increased ratio of active to inactive estrogens in obese women. In spite of these alterations, blood estrogen concentrations are usually normal or only slightly elevated in both premenopausal and postmenopausal obese women (3,4). This may be related to the fact that enlarged body fat may act as deposits for excess formed estrogen, thus contributing to maintain normal circulating hormone concentrations.

Most sex steroid and SHBG alterations can be improved by reducing body weight (17).

The Impact of Body Fat Distribution

Due to the greater reduction of SHBG concentrations, percentage free testosterone fraction tends to be higher in centrally obese women than in those with peripheral obesity (18). Moreover, there are hardly ever systematic differences in the concentrations of principal C19 androgens between women with central and peripheral obesity, although the former may have higher androstenedione levels than the latter (19). This may be due to the fact that androgen production rates are higher in women with central obesity than in their peripheral counterparts (see above). An inverse correlation exists between waist-to-hip ratio (WHR) (or other indices of body fat distribution) and testosterone or SHBG concentrations, regardless of body fatness and body mass index (BMI) (18). Therefore, a condition of 'relative functional hyperandrogenism' may be present in women with the central obesity phenotype. This may play an important role in the development of visceral fat deposits. Androgen receptors are expressed in the adipose tissue, with a higher density in intra-abdominal than subcutaneous deposits, at least in rats (20). In concert with GH and catecholamines, testosterone activates the lipolytic cascade particularly in the visceral adipocytes, thus favoring increased free fatty acid release (20). These events are suggested as participating in the development of insulin resistance and compensatory hyperinsulinemia, both conditions invariably associated with central obesity. Increased insulin levels can in turn produce an inhibition of SHBG synthesis, which further aggravates the androgen imbalance. Since hyperinsulinemia *per se* appears to play a role in the development of visceral fatness, hyperinsulinemia and 'functional hyperandronism' in the central obesity phenotype may participate in a coordinated fashion to increase visceral fat deposits in obese women. This is further supported by the finding that exogenous androgen administration in obese postmenopausal women has been shown to cause a significant gain in visceral fat (as measured by computed tomography scan) and a relatively greater loss of subcutaneous fat in comparison with placebo (21).

Obesity and Hyperandrogenism in Premenopausal Women: a Link with the PCOS

Approximately half the women with PCOS are overweight or obese (12). This association has aroused a great deal of interest in recent years, particularly since the discovery that PCOS women are often hyperinsulinemic and that the degree of hyperandrogenism may be positively and significantly correlated with that of hyperinsulinemia (10). The association between obesity and hyperandrogenism develops during puberty, and common pathogenetic mechanisms primarily appear to involve a dysregulation of insulin secretion and action and also of the GH/IGF-I system (22). Recently, however, it has been suggested that in obese women with PCOS, higher than normal ovarian secretion of androgens is associated with birthweight and maternal obesity, suggesting that intrauterine factors may play a role in the development of the syndrome later in life (23). Premenopausal women with PCOS are clinically characterized by several signs and symptoms related to hyperandrogenism and hyperinsulinemia, including chronic anovulation, hirsutism and acne. Hyperandrogenism, hyperinsulinemia and insulin resistance and all clinical features tend to be more severe in PCOS women with abdominal body fat distribution (24). Altered lipid profile represents another associated metabolic characteristic.

Pathophysiological aspects of the association between obesity and PCOS have been extensively reviewed in recent years (12,25,26). There may be various mechanisms by which obesity may influence hyperandrogenism in premenopausal women with PCOS. The pivotal role of insulin was first suggested on the basis of the significant positive correlation observed between the degree of hyperandrogenism and that of hyperinsulinemia in women with PCOS (9). *In vitro* studies have subsequently demonstrated that insulin is capable of stimulating androgen secretion by the ovaries, reducing aromatase activity in peripheral tissues and, finally, reducing SHBG synthesis in the liver (9,26,27). *In vivo*, numerous studies have demonstrated that both acute and chronic hyperinsulinemia can stimulate testosterone production and that suppression of insulin levels can conversely decrease androgen concentrations (9,26). The fact

that hyperinsulinemia and insulin resistance are invariably associated with obesity and, particularly, abdominal-visceral obesity, represents the basis for the hypothesis supporting its role in the development of hyperandrogenism in PCOS women. Sufficient data demonstrate that suppression of insulin levels by diet (28,29) or chronic insulin sensitizing agent administration, such as metformin (23), troglitazone (30), or D-*chiro*-inositol (31) can improve not only the hyperandrogenic state but also the degree of hirsutism and the fertility rate. These data obviously add further emphasis to the role of obesity-related hyperinsulinemia as a co-factor responsible for increased androgen production in obese PCOS women.

As reported above, obesity is associated with supranormal estrogen production. Since estrogens exert a positive feedback regulation upon gonadotropin release, increased ovarian androgen production in obese PCOS women could be partly favored by increased luteinizing hormone (LH) secretion secondary to prevailing hyperestrogenemia (32). Obesity, as well as PCOS, is also characterized by increased opioid system activity, and studies *in vitro* and *in vivo* have shown that β-endorphin is able to stimulate insulin secretion. Moreover, the administration of β-endorphin can reduce LH release at the hypophyseal level in normal but not in PCOS women (33). The possibility that increased opioid activity may favor the development of hyperinsulinemia and, in turn, of hyperandrogenism, is further supported by the finding that both acute and chronic administration of opioid antagonists, such as naloxone and naltrexone, suppresses both basal and glucose-stimulated insulin blood concentrations in a small group of obese women with PCOS and acanthosis nigricans (34). Finally, there are theoretical possibilities that diet may play some role in the development of the obesity–PCOS association, although very few studies have addressed this issue. In fact, a higher than usual lipid intake has been described in PCOS women by some authors (35). Mechanisms by which high lipid intake may be responsible for altered androgen balance in susceptible women with obesity and PCOS have been summarized above.

Table 17.2 Main alterations of the hypothalamic-pituitary-gonadal axis in obese men

Condition	Alterations
Effect of obesity on sex hormones	Reduced testosterone (free and total), and C19 steroids
	Reduced SHBG concentrations
	Reduced luteinizing hormone secretion
	Increased estrogen production rate
	Altered aromatase activity (?)
Impact of body fat distribution	Men with hypogonadism have typically enlarged visceral fat depots
	Relationship with waist-to-hip ratio (and other indices of fat distribution) controversial
	Association between androstane 3, 17β-diol glucuronide and visceral fatness
Effects of weight loss	Improved sex hormone imbalance (increase of testosterone)
	SHBG can be restored to normal when near-normal body mass index is achieved
Effect of testosterone therapy	Reduction of visceral fat
	Improvement of all parameters of the metabolic syndrome

SHBG, sex hormone-binding globulin.

Effects of Weight Loss and Reduction of Insulin Concentrations in Obese Hyperandrogenic Women with PCOS

There is long-standing clinical evidence concerning the efficacy of weight reduction upon both the clinical and endocrinological features of obese women presenting PCOS. Reduction of hyperandrogenemia (namely testosterone, androstenedione, and dehydroepiandrosterone sulfate (DHEA-S)) (28,29) appears to be the key factor responsible for these effects. However, weight loss primarily improves insulin sensitivity and reduces hyperinsulinemia, and changes in testosterone and insulin concentrations are significantly correlated, regardless of body weight variations (28,29). Recent studies have suggested that hyperinsulinemia may be responsible for increased activity of the ovarian cytocrome P450c17 system, which has been implicated in ovarian hyperandrogenism in many PCOS women (36). Reduction of insulin concentrations by diet (37), metformin (27), or D-*chiro* inositol (31) has been demonstrated to reduce this enzyme activity and, consequently, ovarian androgen production. Finally, weight loss and/or insulin sensitizers also significantly improved ovulation and fertility rate (28,29,31,37), further supporting the role of hyperinsulinemia in the pathogenesis of hyperandrogenism in women with obesity and PCOS. The effects of dietary-induced weight loss on androgen levels (except SHBG) seem to be peculiar to obese hyperandrogenic women, since they have not been reported in non-PCOS obese women (17).

THE HPG AXIS IN MALES (Table 17.2)

Sex Steroid and Gonadotropin Concentration and Metabolism

Contrary to what occurs in obese women, with increasing body weight testosterone (total and free) blood concentrations progressively decrease in obese men (36). Reduced testosterone levels are associated with a progressive decrease of SHBG concentrations as body weight increases (38). Spermatogenesis and fertility are not affected in the majority of obese men, although they may be reduced in subjects with massive obesity (3). Serum testosterone is also inversely correlated with body weight in men with Kinefelter's syndrome (3), thus supporting the causal relationship between obesity and hypotestosteronemia. Serum levels of other sex steroids have also been examined in obese men. Androstenedione concentrations are usually normal or slightly reduced (39) and are not correlated with the degree of obesity (4). Likewise, concentrations of DHT are usually normal (4). Other C19 steroids, such as DHEA and 3 A-diol and androstenediol (Δ5-diol), may be reduced in obesity (39). As previously reported for women, estrogen production rates are increased in male obesity in proportion to body weight, and blood concentrations of all major estrogens, particularly estrone, may be normal (3,4) or slightly increased (4). Altered estrogen metabolism in obesity presumably reflects the aromatase activity of the adipose tissue, which is responsible for active conversion of androgens into estrogens.

Gonadotropin secretion is also impaired in obesity. In fact, pulsatility studies have shown that obese men have a reduced LH secretory mass per secretory burst without any change in burst number, implying a reduction of total LH secretion from the pituitary, probably due to impaired secretion of the gonadotropin releasing hormone at the hypothalamic level (40). The absence of clinical signs of hypogonadism can be explained by the fact that the testosterone free-fraction represents only 2% of total testosterone, and that obesity predominantly affects circulating bound testosterone, due to the concurrent decreases of SHBG production.

The Impact of Body Fat Distribution

There are contradictory data on the relationship between body fat distribution and T in male obesity. Although some clinical (41) and epidemiological (42) studies found an association between testosterone and WHR values, others in which anthropometry (43) or magnetic resonance (44) were used failed to confirm these results. This suggests that the relationship between sex steroids and WHR may be the result of the shared covariance of WHR and total adiposity, rather than a direct relationship. This is not surprising, since obesity in males is almost always associated with a parallel increase in abdominal and visceral fat, which means that the central distribution of body fat in males depends on the actual presence of obesity. Other studies confirmed that reduction of C19 steroid precursors, such as DHEA, androstenedione, Δ5-diol, is predominantly associated with body fatness rather than with excess visceral fat accumulation (39). Conjugation of steroids with glucuronic acid has been suggested to play a major role in the intracellular levels of unconjugated steroids as well as their biological activity. Recent studies have shown that 3A-diol glucuronide (3A-diol-G) levels are significantly higher in obese men, particularly in those with the visceral phenotype (39). Since glucuronide conjugates have been considered better markers of peripheral androgen metabolism than circulating free steroids, the association between 3A-diol-G and visceral fatness suggests that increased visceral adipose tissue accumulation is a condition in which steroid metabolism is altered (45).

Hypotestosteronemia in male obesity thus appears to be largely justified by the coexistence of peripheral (i.e. reduced SHBG synthesis) and central (i.e. reduced LH secretion) factors. On the other hand, both SHBG and testosterone are significantly and negatively correlated with insulin levels, even after adjusting for BMI and WHR values (43). The inverse relationship with SHBG can be easily explained by the fact that insulin inhibits SHBG synthesis in the liver. A confirmatory role for the insulin effect *in vivo* has been reported, since suppression of insulin concentrations by diazoxide has been found to increase circulating SHBG in both normal-weight and obese individuals (46). The inverse relationship between testosterone and insulin deserves further consideration. In fact, low testosterone levels can be found in streptozotocin-induced diabetic rats (47) and in males with type 1 diabetes (48). In insulin-deficient rats and humans insulin replacement restores testosterone concentrations to normal (47). In obese men, moderate hyperinsulinemia, such as that obtained during a hyperinsulinemic euglycemic clamp, increased testosterone concentrations, whereas suppression of insulin by short-term diazoxide administration produced the opposite phenomenon (49). Taken together, these data support the concept that insulin may have a 'direct' stimulatory effect on testosterone production, similar to that demonstrated in women. Therefore, reduced testosterone levels in obese males appear to result from several complementary factors, including lower gonadotropin secretion and the balanced effects of insulin on SHBG (inhibition) and testosterone (stimulation).

The Effects of Weight Loss and Testosterone Replacement Therapy

Weight reduction by both dietary intervention or surgical procedures can increase testosterone and SHBG concentrations, provided substantial weight loss is achieved (3). When massively obese men return to a near-normal BMI, SHBG concentrations fall within the reference values for normal-weight individuals (50). Although there are no kinetic data on estrogen production following weight loss in obese men, it is likely that estrogen metabolism and peripheral production improve as weight loss increases.

Correction of hypotestosteronemia can also be

Table 17.3 Main alterations of the growth hormone/insulin-like growth factor 1 (GH-IGF-I) axis in obesity

Condition	Alterations
Effect of obesity on GH	Reduced GH levels in proportion to body fat
	Blunted response to any stimuli (including GHRH, GHRP-6 superanalogs, etc.)
	Reduced pituitary GH secretion
	Increased GH metabolic clearance rate
Relationship with body fat distribution	Children and adults with GH deficiency typically have visceral obesity
Effect of obesity on the IGF-I system	IGF-I concentration normal or reduced (particularly in visceral obesity)
	Increased free IGF-I fraction
Effects of weight loss	Improvement of basal and stimulated GH levels (in proportion to body fat loss)
	Possible effects of nutrition on GH secretion
Effect of GH replacement therapy	Reduction of visceral fat, in both GH-deficient (children and adults) patients and in obese individuals

achieved by exogenous testosterone administration. Recent studies have in fact demonstrated that it may have a beneficial effect not only by reducing body fat, particularly visceral fat (51), but also on all major parameters of the metabolic syndrome, by reducing hyperlipidemia and hyperinsulinemia and improving peripheral insulin sensitivity (51). Although much more research is needed in this area, this promising approach appears to have potential therapeutic applications in the near future.

THE GH/IGF-I AXIS (Table 17.3)

Basal GH Levels and Secretion and Dynamic Studies

Basal GH levels are markedly reduced in obesity (52,53). This is particularly due to a significant reduction of GH secretory burst mass in the pituitary (52). The extent of this alteration appears to be inversely proportional to the excess body fat (4). Indirect evidence for this is that in subjects with increased body weight due to enlarged lean body mass, such as body builders, GH output and peripheral concentrations are not reduced and GH response to insulin-induced hypoglycemia is in fact normal. Obese subjects are also characterized by blunted GH secretion to all stimuli of GH release, including GHRH, insulin-induced hypoglycemia, L-dopa, arginine, glucagon, exercise, opioid peptides, clonidine, nicotinic acid, or states such as deep sleep (3,54).

Mechanisms responsible for reduced GH levels in obesity are probably multiple. Studies performed in both rhesus monkeys (55) and humans (53) have shown that GH metabolic clearance rate is increased in obesity, in proportion to body weight. The blunted response to growth hormone releasing hormone (GHRH) rules out the possibility that a hypothalamic GHRH deficit may be responsible for reduced GH in obesity. Short-term fasting increases GH levels in obese subjects regardless of body weight loss (56), thus suggesting that GH deficiency in obesity may be a functional reversible state. Pre-treatment with the cholinergic agonist pyridistigmine (57), which suppresses endogenous somatostatin, improves GH release, indicating that enhanced somatostatinergic tone may be responsible, at least in part, for pretreatment reduced GH levels. However, when eliminating the presumed higher than normal somatostatin tone with pyridostigmine, the GH response in obese individuals after any stimuli is still lower than normal (57). GHRP-6 is a potent synthetic exapeptide which specifically stimulates GH release in a dose–response fashion, by interacting with specific hypophyseal and hypothalamic receptors. GH response to GHRP-6 or other peptides of the same family can be decreased by pretreatment with GHRH antiserum, which indicates a degree of dependency of the GHRP-6 action on GHRH. Recent studies have shown that GH response to GHRP-6 was almost twice that induced by GHRH, regardless of cholinergic stimulation by pyridostigmine, and that the combination of these peptides elicited the largest GH discharge ever seen after any stimulus (54). Therefore, other than increased somatostatinergic tone, impaired GH secretion in obesity appears to be a functional reversible state, due to still undefined altered somatotrophic function. Whether GHRH resistance or other mechanisms acting at the pituitary levels are co-responsible for blunted GH release in obesity remains to be investigated.

Other factors have been implicated in reducing GH levels. Obesity is a condition of altered and supranormal free fatty acid (FFA) production. Increased FFAs are postulated to inhibit basal GH secretion, by mechanisms independent of effects on somatostatinergic tone (3). This is further supported by the fact that FFA inhibition by antilipolytic agents such as acipimox have been demonstrated to potentiate GH responsiveness to GHRH, with or without pyridostigmine pretreatment (58).

Sex steroids, specifically testosterone and estradiol, have positive effects on GH secretion (3) probably by influencing the pulsatile mode of GH release (52). Basal GH secretory bursts, which are reduced in obesity, are positively correlated with estradiol and testosterone concentrations (50), which further indicates a close relationship between sex steroid imbalance and GH secretory dynamics in the obese state.

Serum (IGF-I) Levels

Levels of IGF-I in obesity have been variously reported to be increased, normal, or decreased (3,4). However, although obese children have lower than normal GH levels in basal conditions and after stimulatory testing, they grow normally, which suggests that IGF-I action in the target tissues for growth is indeed adequate for growth and development before, during, and after puberty (3). Interestingly, it has been found that free IGF-I levels are actually increased in obese subjects (59). An increase in free IGF-I levels could be involved in the decline in GH levels with increasing body fat, via feedback inhibition of GH secretion at the pituitary level. Serum IGF-I levels are particularly reduced in subjects with visceral obesity (60) and an inverse relationship has been found with the amounts of visceral fat, independent of total fat mass (61) in a cohort of subjects ranging from normal weight to obesity. Since insulin regulates IGF-I metabolism *via* its stimulatory effects on the synthesis of IGF binding protein 1 (IGF-BP-I), altered IGF-I in obesity, particularly the visceral phenotype, may reflect prevailing hyperinsulinemia in the blood circulation.

Effect of Weight Loss

Weight reduction significantly improves basal and stimulated GH levels, in proportion to the amount of body weight lost (3). However, there are no studies confirming that weight loss can completely restore GH secretion to normal. This is probably due to the fact that it is difficult to regain a normal weight, particularly in subjects with massive obesity. On the other hand, nutrition itself is an important factor regulating GH secretion and metabolism. As mentioned above, short-term fasting can partially restore baseline and stimulated GH concentrations (56). Starvation is associated with increased GH levels. Therefore, in conditions of energy deficit, absolute or relative GH increase appears to represent an adaptive mechanism by which the body provides fuels from lipolytic pathways to support energy balance. Since weight loss in obese patients can be achieved by varying degree of energy restriction, it would be interesting to investigate how much the positive effect of partial weight loss on GH secretion is due to a reduction of body fat and how much to energy restriction *per se*, particularly in carbohydrates.

Effects of GH Administration

GH has a potent lipolytic activity and therefore, suppressed GH levels in obesity can be viewed as an unbalanced lipogenetic condition, which could probably be responsible for the perpetuation of the obese state once established. In fact, obese subjects have elevated insulin levels as a consequence of the insulin resistance state with respect to carbohydrate metabolism, but the adipose tissue remains sensitive to the antilipolytic effects of insulin. Evidence from animal and human studies supports the hypothesis that GH administration in obesity may stimulate lipolytic pathways and can provide a valuable adjunct to diet in inducing weight loss. Ventromedial hypothalamic lesions in rats produce obesity, hyperinsulinemia and decreased GH secretion. When administered to hypophysectomized ventromedial-lesioned rats, GH prevents both hyperphagia and development of obesity (62). Genetically obese Zucker *fa/fa* rats also have decreased GH secretion and GH treatment results in reduced lipid deposition (62). In GH-deficient children, many of whom

Table 17.4 Main alterations of the hypothalamic-pituitary-adrenocortical axis in obesity

Condition	Alterations
Basal ACTH/cortisol in obesity	Increased cortisol metabolic clearance rate
	Increased ACTH pulse frequency
	Normal cortisol axis diurnal rhythm
	Normal 24-hour ACTH/cortisol concentrations
	Reset to lower resilient axis (?)
	Altered cortisol suppression after overnight dexamethasone (?)
Effects of body fat distribution	High glucocorticoid receptor density in the visceral adipose tissue
	Altered cortisol production in the visceral adipose tissue (increased/decreased activity of the 11β-HSD)
	Reduced ACTH pulse amplitude
	Positive relationship between visceral fat and daily urinary free cortisol excretion rate
	Lower suppression to submaximal dexamethasone administration (?)
	relationship with perceived stress-dependent free salivary cortisol levels
	Increased CBG binding capacity in parallel to insulin resistance
Dynamic studies	Increased ACTH/cortisol response to CRH, CRH + AVP, ACTH, acute stress, insulin-induced hypoglycemia (?), meals (?)
	Increased ACTH respone to CRH + AVP (normal-weight individuals: reduced) during mild increase of NE blood levels (reference 94)

ACTH, adrenocorticotropin; CBG, corticosteroid-binding globulin; CRH, corticotropin-releasing hormone; AVP, arginine vasopressin.

are obese, GH administration reduces body fat (63). The same occurs in subjects with adult GH deficiency (64), and in elderly subjects who underwent therapy with GH to increase lean body mass and improve fitness (65). Exogenous GH administration also reduced fat stores, particularly in the visceral depots, in GH-deficient adult subjects (66). These effects can be additive to those dependent on diet restriction, but they may also occur in conditions of eucaloric intake (67). Interestingly, the magnitude of this effect appears to be independent of initial body weight and endogenous GH status (67). One limitation of GH administration is related to the possibility that long-term GH treatment worsens glucose tolerance and insulin resistance, although the contrary has been reported by some studies (66). Perhaps the administration of GH in a manner that stimulates normal physiological secretion rather than pharmacological doses would circumvent or lessen its effects on carbohydrate metabolism in the long term.

of the metabolic syndrome, due to the biological effects of prevailing hypercortisolemia. The main metabolic abnormality of cortisol excess is insulin resistance, which develops by cellular mechanisms that have been largely elucidated (68). Briefly, glucocorticoids inhibit glucose uptake by peripheral tissues, stimulate gluconeogenesis, and cause increased postabsorptive glucose and insulin. In insulin-sensitive tissues, glucocorticoids impair post-receptor insulin function by mechanisms that involve interaction with glucose transporters (68). Treatment of hypercortisolism by pituitary or adrenal surgical procedures can completely reverse these abnormalities.

Subjects with visceral obesity may be characterized by several Cushing-like features, i.e. abdominal striae, buffalo hump, facial plethora, etc., and have associated abnormalities of the metabolic syndrome. Theoretically, these abnormalities may be related, at least in part, to alterations of cortisol metabolism and hyperactivity of the HPA axis.

THE HPA AXIS (Table 17.4)

Similarities Between Visceral Obesity and Cushing's Syndrome

Patients with Cushing's syndrome have typically enlarged visceral fat deposits and show all features

ACTH and Cortisol Concentrations in Basal Conditions

It is well recognized that cortisol metabolism may be increased in obesity. This may be due to the coordinated interference of several factors. First, the concentrations of corticosteroid-binding glubulin (CBG) may be reduced in obesity, although not systematically (3). Moreover, glucocorticoid receptors have been demonstrated in adipose tissue by different techniques, all of which show that they are significantly more dense in visceral than in subcutaneous adipose tissue (69). Finally, adipose tissue can metabolize cortisol to cortisone and vice versa, a reaction that is catalyzed by the 11β-hydroxysteroid dehydrogenase (11β-HSD) enzyme system. Bujalska and coworkers (70) found that the production of cortisol from cortisone in the omental fat taken from normal-weight and obese patients undergoing surgical procedures was significantly higher than in the subcutaneous fat, due to the increased expression of the 11β-HSD isoform type 1 (a low-affinity NADP(H)-dependent dehydrogenase/oxoreductase), this activity being further enhanced by tissue exposure to cortisol and insulin. The increased 'production' of cortisol could ensure a constant exposure of glucocorticoids to omental tissue, therefore playing a potential role in determining differentiation and mass increase of such a tissue, as recently suggested (71) and, in addition, may represent an inappropriate feedback signal at the neuroendocrine levels, able to modify both the basal activity of the HPA axis and its response to stimulatory and/or inhibitory factors. The concept that obesity may be associated with increased activity of the 11β-HSD has been recently supported by human studies which demonstrated an increased ratio of daily urinary cortisol-to-cortisone metabolite secretion in obese subjects, particularly in those with the abdominal phenotype (72), although controversial findings have also been reported (73).

In unselected obese subjects, normal values have been reported for plasma cortisol, plasma unbound cortisol, 24 h mean plasma cortisol, urinary free-cortisol excretion, and circadian rhythms of plasma and urine cortisol (74). On the other hand, a higher than normal 24 h urine free-cortisol excretion has been reported in women with visceral obesity, and a positive correlation with anthropometric parameters of visceral fat distribution was found (75–77), suggesting that cortisol production may increase as the amounts of visceral fat enlarge.

The impact of obesity on adrenocorticotropin (ACTH) and cortisol pulsatile rhythm has been poorly investigated and available data, which predominantly refer to obese men, often yielded conflicting results. Although several studies reported

normal plasma cortisol levels and daily circadian rhythms, others found either lower than normal single samples or lower 24 h integrated cortisol levels in obese men (3). In all these studies, however, ACTH dynamics were not investigated. Studies in obese women are very scarce. Recently, it has been demonstrated that premenopausal women with visceral obesity may have several abnormalities of ACTH (but not cortisol) pulsatile secretion (78), specifically higher than normal ACTH pulse frequency and reduced ACTH pulse amplitude, particularly during the morning, without any significant change in mean basal ACTH blood concentrations. The mechanisms responsible for these alterations are still unclear. Recently it has been demonstrated that a highly significant inverse relationship between rapid fluctuations in plasma leptin and those of ACTH and cortisol exists in normal men, and that obese individuals, in whom higher than normal leptin levels are present, maintain unaltered both leptin diurnal variability and pulsatile secretion (79), with higher pulse height resulting in higher mean daily leptin concentrations in the blood. Therefore one of the central effects of leptin in the central nervous system might be the acute suppression of the HPA axis. Whether increased brain leptin concentrations in obesity may be in some way responsible for altered ACTH pulsatility, particularly in the visceral phenotype, remains, however, to be clarified.

Effects of Meals on ACTH and Cortisol Concentrations

Meals are potent stimulators of adrenocortical function. In fact, food ingestion, particularly at noon, elicits sustained cortisol release regardless of its pulsatile rhythm (80). The increase in cortisol concentrations appears to be higher in women with visceral obesity than in those with subcutaneous obesity and controls (78,81,82). Theoretically, this could reflect an altered responsiveness of the adrenals to ACTH in obesity. Whatever the mechanism of action, these findings suggest that women with visceral obesity are inappropriately exposed to supranormal cortisol levels, which, in turn, may have a negative impact on the regulation of postprandial fuel metabolism and on insulin action in peripheral tissues.

The Activity of the HPA Axis: Dynamic Studies

Studies in obese subjects not selected on the basis of the pattern of body fat distribution have demonstrated that both ACTH and cortisol response to corticotropin-releasing hormone (CRH) was either normal or reduced (74) when compared to normal-weight controls. On the other hand, Weaver and coworkers (83) found that obese women representing a wide spectrum from 'gynoid' to 'android' obesity had significantly higher ACTH response to insulin-induced hypoglycemia with respect to controls, although no significant relationship between fat distribution and hormonal response was reported. Recently, however, several studies have reported data supporting the concept that obese women with visceral body fat distribution may have hyperactivity of the HPA axis (75,76,84). This alteration is characterized by exaggerated ACTH and cortisol response to intravenous administration of CRH alone (76) or combined with arginine vasopressin (AVP) (84), and by higher than normal cortisol response to intravenous ACTH stimulation or acute stress challenge (75,84,85). In addition, visceral obese women also have hyperactivity of the HPA axis to opioid blockade which can be completely reversed by increasing the serotoninergic receptor activation by dexfenfluramine (86). Other studies indicate that obese men also have a higher than normal ACTH (but not cortisol) response to combined CRH/AVP administration and that this alteration may be significantly correlated with the insulin concentrations, regardless of BMI and WHR values (87). In addition, a decrease in the inhibition of cortisol secretion by single low-dose (0.5 mg overnight) dexamethasone administration and an inverse correlation between the decrease of serum cortisol and the WHR has been found by other investigators (88). This supports the concept that increased sensitivity and/or responsiveness by CRH receptors in the brain could be due, at least in part, to the deficient control of CRH receptors by the inhibitory feedback action of glucocorticoids on the system.

The mechanisms responsible for neuroendocrine abnormalities are still unclear and need to be elucidated. First, they could be due to a primary neuroendocrine alteration leading to increased sensitivity to CRH or ACTH-secreting cells or to increased CRH flow towards the pituitary. Another quite convincing theory, however, claims that the HPA hyperactivity may represent part of an altered response to acute and/or chronic stress which can be independent of the mechanisms responsible for feedback regulation (69). Several studies have in fact demonstrated that a similar neuroendocrine adaptation takes place during the reaction behaviour in laboratory animals exposed to various socioenvironmental stressors. For example, Shively and her colleagues (89) exposed cynomolgus macaques to chronic physical and psychological stress, and subsequently showed that the animals developed high visceral fat deposition, which was combined with insulin resistance, hyperinsulinemia and impaired glucose tolerance, adrenal hypertrophy, enhanced cortisol response to ACTH stimulation, altered lipid profiles and incidence of coronary artery atherosclerosis significantly greater than controls. Theoretically, women with visceral obesity may have hyperactivity of the HPA as a consequence of maladaptation to chronic stress exposure. In this model, a key role is represented by the combination of events involving maladaptation to altered coping reaction to chronic stress. In fact, these abnormalities include increased or unbalanced ACTH and cortisol response. Recent data from epidemiological studies by Björntorp's group appear to be consistent with the hypothesis and with the aforementioned animal data. In fact, they found a strong association between symptoms of mental distress (such as anxiety, depression, etc.), smoking habits and alcholic consumption, as well as certain psychosomatic diseases and, finally, low socioeconomic conditions and abdominal obesity in both males and females (90–93). Furthermore, in a large cohort of middle-aged men they recently demonstrated a significant interaction between diurnal cortisol secretion (measured in saliva) related to perceived stress and several anthropometric, endocrine and metabolic variables (82). Moreover, they found that a non-stressed HPA axis was characterized by increased cortisol variance, whereas chronically stressed subjects presented decreased cortisol variance, mostly due to evening nadir elevation, morning zenith decrease and inadequate suppression of morning cortisol by overnight dexamethasone (82). In addition, there are data consistent with a dysregulation of the noradrenergic control of the HPA axis during acute mild stress in subjects with obesity, particularly the abdominal phenotype (94).

All these findings suggest chronic neuroendocrine (at the CRH level?) hyperactivity in stressed individuals and a reset of their HPA axis to a lower resilient state. In addition, they are consistent with aforementioned data from Shively obtained in cynomolgus macaques. On the other hand, much more data are needed to clarify this complex interaction between environmental factors and the pathophysiology of human obesity and related metabolic and cardiovascular comorbidities.

To summarize, there is increasing evidence that the activity of the HPA axis is dysregulated in many obese individuals, particularly those with the visceral phenotype. At least two distinct alterations can be observed. The first, which appears to be central in origin, is characterized by altered ACTH pulsatile secretory dynamic and diurnal chronobiology, and by a hyperesponsiveness of the HPA axis to different neuropeptides and acute stress events and, possibly, to selected dietary factors. The other appears to be located in the periphery, namely the visceral adipose tissue, which is characterized by elevated cortisol traffic and, probably, by supranormal cortisol production. It is also possible that this last alteration may be responsible, at least in part, for inappropriate feedback signals at the neuroendocrine level and altered ACTH secretion.

CONCLUSIONS

This chapter focuses on the main alterations of the HPG axis, the GH/IGF-I axis and the HPA axis in human obesity. Many of these alterations may have a pathogenetic role in the development of excess body fat, particularly visceral fat, and related metabolic abnormalities. Indirect evidence of this is that all obese subjects with GH deficiency, endogenous hypercortisolism and, in males, hypogonadism, have enlarged visceral fat depots. At variance, a prevalence of visceral body fat distribution is typically associated with hyperandrogenism in women with obesity alone and in those with PCOS. This gender dichotomy obviously needs to be further elucidated. Finally, there are preliminary physiopathological and clinical studies suggesting that hormonal replacement treatment may have a potential application in the treatment of obesity, particularly the visceral phenotype.

REFERENCES

1. Bray GA, York DA. Leptin and clinical medicine: a new piece in the puzzle of obesity. *J Clin Endocrinol Metab* 1997; **82**: 2771–2776.
2. Sakurai T, Amemiya A, Ishii M, Matsuzaki I, Chemelli R, Tanaka H, Clay Williams S, Richardson JA, Kozlowski GP, Wilson S, Arch JRS, Buckingham RE, Haynes AC, Carr SA, Annan RS, McNulty DE, Liu WS, Terret JA, Elshourbagy NA, Bergsma DJ, Yanagisawa M. Orexins and orexin receptors: a family of hypothalamic neuropep-tides and G-protein-coupled receptors that regulate feeding behavior. *Cell* 1998; **92**: 573–585.
3. Smith SR. The endocrinology of obesity. *Endocr Metab Clin NA* 1996; **25**: 921–942.
4. Glass AR. Endocrine aspects of obesity. *Med Clin NA* 1989; **73**: 139–160.
5. Von Shoultz B, Carlstrom K. On the regulation of sex-hormone-binding globulin. A challenge of old dogma and outlines of an alternative mechanism. *J Steroid Biochem* 1989; **32**: 327–334.
6. Pasquali R, Casimirri F, Platè L, Capelli M. Characterization of obese women with reduced sex hormone-binding globulin concentrations. *Horm Metabol Res* 1990; **22**: 303–306.
7. Preziosi P, Barrett-Connor E, Papoz L, Roger M, Saint-Paul M, Nahoul K, Simon D. Interrelationship between plasma sex hormone-binding globulin and plasma insulin in healthy adult women: the Telecom study. *J Clin Endocrinol Metab* 1993; **76**: 283–287.
8. Plymate SR, Matej LA, Jones RE, Friedl KE. Inhibition of sex hormone-binding globulin in the human hepatoma (HepG2) cell line by insulin and prolactin. *J Clin Endocrinol Metab* 1988; **67**: 460–464.
9. Nestler JE, Baralascini CO, Matt DW, Steingold KA, Plymate SR, Clore JN, Blackard WG. Suppression of serum insulin diazoxide reduces serum testosterone levels in obese women with polycystic ovary syndrome. *J Clin Endocrinol Metab* 1989; **68**: 1027–1032.
10. Poretsky L. On the paradox of insulin-induced hyperandrogenism in insulin-resistant states. *Endocr Rev* 1991; **12**: 3–13.
11. Björntorp P. The association between obesity, adipose tissue distribution and diseases. *Acta Med Scand* 1988; **723** (Suppl): 121–134.
12. Pasquali R, Casimirri F. The impact of obesity on hyperandrogenism and polycystic ovary in premenopausal women. *Clin Endocrinol (Oxf)* 1993; **39**: 1–16.
13. Samojlik E, Kirschner MA, Silber D, Schneider G, Ertel NH. Elevated production and metabolic clearance rates of androgens in morbidly obese women. *J Clin Endocrinol Metab* 1984; **59**: 949–954.
14. Kurtz BR, Givens JR, Koinindir S, Stevens MD, Karas JG, Bittle JB, Judge D, Kitabki AE. Maintenance of normal circulating levels of Δ4-androstenedione and dehydroepiandrosterone in simple obesity despite increased metabolic clearance rates: evidence for a servo-control mechanism. *J Clin Endocrinol Metab* 1987; **64**: 1261–1267.
15. Kirschner MA, Samojlik E, Drejka M, Szmal E, Schneider G, Ertel N. Androgen-estrogen metabolism in women with

upper body versus lower body obesity. *J Clin Endo-crinol Metab* 1990; **70**: 473–479.

16. Siiteri PK. Extraglandular estrogen formation and serum binding of estradiol: relationship to cancer. *J Endocrinol* 1981; **89**: 119P–129P.

17. Grenman S, Konnemaa T, Iryale K, Kaiola HL, Grouroos M. Sex steroid, gonadotropin, cortisol, and prolactin in healthy, massively obese women: correlation with abdominal fat cell size and effect of weight loss. *J Clin Endocrinol Metab* 1986; **63**: 1257–1261.

18. Evans DJ, Hoffmann RG, Kalkhoff RK, Kissebah AH. Relationship of androgenic activity to body fat topography, fat cell morphology and metabolic aberrations in premenopausal women. *J Clin Endocrinol Metab* 1983; **57**: 304–310.

19. Pasquali R, Casimirri F, Cantobelli S, Morselli-Labate AM, Venturoli S, Paradisi R, Zannarini L. Insulin and androgen relationship with abdominal body fat distribution in women with and without hyperandrogenism. *Horm Res* 1993; **39**: 179–187.

20. Björntorp P. The regulation of adipose tissue distribution in humans. *Int J Obes* 1996; **20**: 291–302.

21. Lovejoy JC, Bray GA, Bourgeois MO, Macchiavelli R, Rood JC, Greeson C, Partington C. Exogenous androgens influence body composition and regional body fat distribution in obese postmenopausal women—A clinical research center study. *J Clin Endocrinol Metab* 1996; **81**: 2198–2203.

22. Apter D, Butzow T, Laughlin GA, Yen SSC. Metabolic features of polycystic ovary syndrome are found in adolescent girls with hyperandrogenism. *J Clin Endocrinol Metab* 1995; **80**: 2966–2973.

23. Cresswell JL, Barker DJP, Osmond C, Egger P, Phillips DIW, Fraser RB. Fetal growth, length of gestation, and polycystic ovaries in adult life. *Lancet* 1997; **350**: 1131–1135.

24. Pasquali R, Casimirri F, Venturoli S, Morselli Labata AM, Reho S, Pezzoli, Paradisi R. Body fat distribution has weight-independent effects on clinical, hormonal, and metabolic features of women with polycystic ovary syndrome. *Metabolism* 1994; **43**: 706–713.

25. Dunaif A. Insulin resistance and the polycystic ovary syndrome: mechanism and implications for pathogenesis. *Endocr Rev* 1997; **18**: 774–800.

26. Poretsky L, Cataldo NA, Rosewaks Z, Giudice LC. The insulin-related ovarian regulatory system in health and disease. *Endocr Rev* 1999; **20**: 1–48.

27. Nestler JE, Jakubowicz DJ. Decreases in ovarian cytochrome P450c17α activity and serum free testosterone after reduction of insulin secretion in polycystic ovary syndrome. *N Engl J Med* 1996; **335**: 617–623.

28. Kiddy DS, Hamilton-Fairley D, Bush A, Short F, Anyaoku V, Reed MJ, Franks S. Improvement in endocrine and ovarian function during dietary treatment of obese women with polycystic ovary syndrome. *Clin Endocrinol (Oxf)* 1992; **36**: 105–111.

29. Pasquali R, Antenucci D, Casimirri F, Venturoli S, Paradisi R, Fabbri R, Balestra V, Melchionda N, Barbara L. Clinical and hormonal characteristics of obese amenorrheic hyperandrogenic women before and after weight loss. *J Clin Endocrinol Metab* 1989; **68**: 173–179.

30. Dunaif A, Scott D, Finegood D, Quantana B, Whitcomb R. The insulin-sensitizing agent, troglitazone, improves metabolic and reproductive abnormalities in the polycystic ovary syndrome. *J Clin Endocrinol Metab* 1996; **81**: 3299–3306.

31. Nestler JE, Jakubowicz DJ, Reamer P, Gunn RD, Allan G. Ovulatory and metabolic effects of D-*chiro* inositol in the polycystic ovary syndrome. *N Engl J Med* 1999; **340**: 1314–1320.

32. Yen SSC. The polycystic ovary syndrome. *Clin Endocrinol (Oxf)* 1980; **12**: 177–208.

33. Reid RL, Yen SSC. β-endorphin stimulates the secretion of insulin and glucagon in humans. *J Clin Endocrinol Metab* 1981; **52**: 592–594.

34. Givens JR, Wiedemann E, Andersen RN, Kitabchi AE. β-endorphin and β-lipotropin plasma levels in hirsute women: correlation with body weight. *J Clin Endocrinol Metab* 1980; **50**: 915–917.

35. Wild RA, Painter PC, Coulson RB, Carruth KB, Ranney GB. Lipoprotein lipid concentrations and cardiovascular risk in women with polycystic ovary syndrome. *J Clin Endocrinol Metab* 1985; **61**: 946–951.

36. Ehrmann DA, Rosenfield RL, Barnes, RB, Brigell DF, Sheikh Z. Detection of functional hyperandrogenism in women with androgen excess. *N Engl J Med* 1992; **327**: 157–162.

37. Yakubowicz DJ, Nestler JE. 17α hydroxyprogesterone response to leuprolide and serum androgens in obese women with and without polycystic ovary syndrome after dietary weight loss. *J Clin Endocrinol Metab* 1997; **82**: 556–560.

38. Zumoff B, Strain G, Miller LK, Rosner W, Senie R, Seres D, Rosenfield RS. Plasma free and non-sex-hormone-binding-globulin-bound testosterone are decreased in obese men in proportion to their degree of obesity. *J Clin Endo-crinol Metab* 1990; **71**: 929–931.

39. Tchernoff A, Després J-P, Bélanger A, Dupont A, Prud'homme D, Moorjani S, Lupien PJ, Labrie F. Reduced testosterone and adrenal C_{19} steroid levels in obese women. *Metabolism* 1995; **44**: 513–519.

40. Vermeulen A, Kaufman JM, Deslypere JP, Thomas G. Attenuated luteinizing hormone (LH) pulse amplitude but normal LH pulse frequency, and its relation to plasma androgens in hypogonadism of obese men. *J Clin Endo-crinol Metab* 1993; **76**: 1140–1146.

41. Seidell JC, Björntorp P, Sjöström L, Kvist H, Sannerstet R. Visceral fat accumulation in men is positively associated with insulin, glucose, and C-peptide levels, but negatively with testosterone levels. *Metabolism* 1990; **39**: 897–901.

42. Khaw KT, Barret-Connor E. Lower endogenous androgens predict central adiposity in men. *Ann Epidemiol* 1992; **2**: 675–682.

43. Pasquali R, Casimirri F, Cantobelli S, Melchionda N, Morselli Labate AM, Fabbri R, Capelli M, Bortoluzzi L. Effect obesity and body fat distribution on sex hormones and insulin in men. *Metabolism* 1991; **40**: 101–104.

44. Leenen R, van der Koy K, Seidell JC, Deurenberg P, Kopperschaar HPF. Visceral fat accumulation in relation to sex hormones in obese men and women undergoing weight loss therapy. *J Clin Endocrinol Metab* 1994; **78**: 1515–1520.

45. Tchernoff A, Labrie F, Bélanger A, Prud'homme D, Bouchard C, Tremblay A, Nadeau A, Després JP. Androstane-3alpha, 17β-Diol glucuronide as a steroid correlate of visceral obesity in men. *J Clin Endocrinol Metab* 1997; **82**: 1528–1534.

46. Pasquali R, Casimirri F, De Iasio R, Mesini P, Boschi S,

Chierici R, Flamia R, Biscott M, Vicennati V. Insulin regulates testosterone and sex hormone-binding globulin concentrations in adult normal weight and obese men. *J Clin Endocrinol Metab* 1995; **80**: 654–658.

47. Lopez Blanco F, Fanjiul LF, Ruiz de Galarreta CM. The effect of insulin and lutenizing hormone treatment of serum concentrations of testosterone and dihydrotestosterone and testicular 3β-hydroxysteroid-dehydrogenase activity in intact and hypophysectomized rats. *Endocrinology* 1989; **109**: 1248–1253.

48. Fushimi H, Horie H, Inoue T. Low testosterone levels in diabetic men and animals: a possible role in testicular impotence. *Diab Res Clin Pract* 1989; **6**: 297–301.

49. Pasquali R, Macor C, Vicennati C, Novo F, De Iasio R, Mesini P, Boschi S, Casimirri F, Vettor R. Effects of acute hyperinsulinemia on testosterone serum concentrations in adult obese and normal-weight men. *Metabolism* 1997; **46**: 526–529.

50. Pasquali R, Vicennati V, Scopinaro N, Marinari G, Flamia R, Casimirri F, Gagliari L. Achievement of near-normal body weight as the prerequisite to normalize sex hormone-binding globulin concentrations in massively obese men. *Int J Obes* 1997; **21**: 1–5.

51. Marin P, Holmang S, Jonsson L, Sjöström L, Kvist H, Holm G, Lindstedt G, Björntorp P. The effects of testosterone treatment on body composition and metabolism in middle-aged obese men. *Int J Obes* 1992; **16**: 991–997.

52. Veldhuis JD, Iranmanesh A, Ho KKY, Waters MJ, Johnson ML, Lizarralde G. Dual defects in pulsatile growth hormone secretion and clearance subserve the hyposomatotropinism of obesity in man. *J Clin Endocrinol Metab* 1991; **72**: 51–59.

53. Kopelman PG. Neuroendocrine function in obesity. *Clin Endocrinol (Oxf)* 1988; **28**: 675–689.

54. Cordido F, Casanueva FF, Dieguez C. Cholinergic receptor activation by pyridostigmine restores growth hormone (GH) responsiveness to GH-releasing hormone administration in obese subjects. *J Clin Endocrinol Metab* 1989; **68**: 290–293.

55. Dubey AK, Hanukoglu A, Hamsen BC, Kowarski AA. Metabolic clearance rates of synthetic human growth hormone in lean and obese male rhesus monkeys. *J Clin Endocrinol Metab* 1988; **67**: 1064–1067.

56. Williams T, Berelowitz M, Joffe J, Thorner MO, Rivier J, Vale W, Frohman LA. Impaired growth hormone responses to growth-hormone releasing factor in obesity. A pituitary defect reversed with weight reduction. *N Engl J Med* 1984; **311**: 1403–1407.

57. Cordido F, Penalva A, Dieguez C, Casanueva FF. Massive growth hormone (GH) discharge in obese subjects after combined administration of GH-releasing hormone and GHRP-6: Evidence for a marked somatotroph secretory capability in obesity. *J Clin Endocrinol Metab* 1993; **76**: 819–823.

58. Lee EJ, Nam SY, Kim KR, Lee HC, Cho JH, Nam MS, Song YD, Lim SK, Huh KB. Acipimox potentiates growth hormone (GH) response to GH-releasing hormone with or without pyridostigmine by lowering serum free fatty acid in normal and obese subjects. *J Clin Endocrinol Metab* 1995; **80**: 2495–2498.

59. Frystyk J, Vestbo E, Skjaerbaek C, Mogensen CE, Ørskov H. Free insulin-like growth factors in human obesity. *Metabolism* 1995; **44** (Suppl) 37–44.

60. Rasmussen MH, Frystyk J, Andersen T, Breum L, Christian-

sen JS, Hilsted J. The impact of obesity, fat distribution and energy restriction on insulin like growth-factor-1 (IGF-1) IGF-binding protein-3, insulin and growth hormone. *Metabolism* 1994; **43**: 315–319.

61. Rasmussen MH, Hvidberg A, Juul A, Main KM, Gotfredsen A, Skakkebæ NE, Hilsted J. Massive weight loss restores 24-hour growth hormone release profiles and serum insulin-like growth factor-1 levels in obese subjects (published erratum appears in *J Clin Endocrinol Metab* 1995; **80**: 2446) *J Clin Endocrinol Metab* 1995; **80**: 1407–1415.

62. Williams T, Frohman LA. Potential therapeutic implications for growth hormone and growth-hormone releasing hormone in conditions other than growth retardation. *Pharmacotherapy* 1986; **6**: 311–318.

63. Rosembaum M, Gertner JM, Leibel R. Effects of systemic growth hormone (GH) administration on regional adipose tissue distribution and metabolism in GH-deficient children. *J Clin Endocrinol Metab* 1989; **69**: 1274–1281.

64. Solomon F, Cenco RC, Herp R, Sonksen PH. The effects of treatment with recombinant human GH on body composition and metabolism in adults with GH deficiency. *N Engl J Med* 1989; **321**: 1797–1803.

65. Rudman D, Feller AG, Nagrai HS, Gergans GA, Lalitha PA, Goldberg AF, Schlenker RA, Cohn L, Rudman IW, Mattson DE. Effects of human growth hormone in men over 60 years old. *N Engl J Med* 1990; **323**: 1–6.

66. Hwu CM, Kwok CF, Lai TY, Shih KC, Lee TS, Hsiao LC, Lee SH, Fang VS, Ho LT. Growth hormone (GH) replacement reduces total body fat and normalizes insulin sensitivity in GH-deficient adults: a report of one-year clinical experience. *J Clin Endocrinol Metab* 1997; **82**: 3285–3292.

67. Skaggs SR, Crist DM. Exogenous human growth hormone reduces body fat in obese women. *Horm Res* 1991; **35**: 19–24.

68. McMahon M, Gerich J, Rizza R. Effects of glucocorticoids on carbohydrate metabolism. *Diab Metab Rev* 1988; **4**: 17–30.

69. Björntorp P. Visceral obesity: a 'Civilization syndrome'. *Obes Res* 1993; **1**: 206–222.

70. Bujalska IJ, Kumar S, Stewart PM. Does central obesity reflect 'Cushing's disease of the omentum'? *Lancet* 1997; **349**: 1210–1213.

71. Bujalska IJ, Kumar S, Hewison M, Stewart PM. Differentiation of adipose stromal cells: the roles of glucorticoids and 11β-hydroxysteroid dehydrogenase. *Endocrinology* 1999; **140**: 3188–3196.

72. Andrew R, Phillips DIW, Walker BR. Obesity and gender influence cortisol secretion and metabolism in man. *J Clin Endocrinol Metab* 1998; **83**: 1806–1809.

73. Stewart PM, Boulton A, Kumar S, Clark PMS, Shachleton CHL. Cortisol metabolism in human obesity: impaired cortisone–cortisol conversion in subjects with central adiposity. *J Clin Endocrinol Metab* 1999; **84**: 1022–1027.

74. Chalew S, Nagel H, Shore S. The hypothalamic-pituitary-adrenal axis in obesity *Obes Res* 1995; **3**: 371–382.

75. Marin P, Darin N, Anemiya T, Anderson B, Jern S, Björntorp P. Cortisol secretion in relation to body fat distribution in obese premenopausal women. *Metabolism* 1992; **41**: 882–886.

76. Pasquali R, Cantobelli S, Casimirri F, Capelli M, Bortoluzzi F, Flamia R, Morselli-Labate AM, Barbara L. The hypothalamic-pituitary-adrenal axis in obese women with dif-

ferent patterns of body fat distribution. *J Clin Endo-crinol Metab* 1993; **77**: 341–346.

77. Duclos M, Corcuff J-B, Etcheverry N, Rushedi M, Tabarin A, Roger P. Abdominal obesity increases overnight cortisol excretion. *J Endocrinol Invest* 1999; **22**: 465–471.

78. Pasquali R, Biscotti M, Spinucci G, Vicennati V, Genazzani AD, Sgarbi L, Casimirri F. Pulsatile rhythm of ACTH and cortisol in premenopausal women: effect of obesity and body fat distribution. *Clin Endocrinol (Oxf)* 1998; **48**: 603–612.

79. Licinio J, Mantzoros C, Negrao AB, Cizza G, Wong ML, Bongiorno PB, Chrousos GP, Karp B, Allen C, Flier JS, Gold PW. Human leptin levels are pulsatile and inversely related to pituitary-adrenal function. *Nat Med* 1997; **3**: 575–579.

80. Quigley ME, Yen SSC. A mid-day surge in cortisol levels. *J Clin Endocrinol Metab* 1979; **49**: 945–947.

81. Korbonits M, Trainer PJ, Nelson ML, Howse I, Kopelman PG, Besser GM, Grossman AB, Svec F. Differential stimulation of cortisol and dehydroepiandrosterone levels by food in obese and normal subjects: relation to body fat distribution. *Clin Endocrinol (Oxf)* 1996; **45**: 699–706.

82. Rosmond R, Dallman MF, Björntorp P. Stress-related cortisol secretion in men: relationships with abdominal obesity and endocrine, metabolic and hemodynic abnormalities. *J Clin Endocrinol Metab* 1998; **83**: 1853–1859.

83. Weaver JU, Kopelman PG, McLoughlin L, Forsling MI, Grossman A. Hyperactivity of the hypothalamic-pituitary-adrenal axis in obesity: a study of ACTH, AVP, β-lipotropin and cortisol responses to insulin-induced hypoglycemia. *Clin Endocrinol (Oxf)* 1993; **39**: 345–350.

84. Pasquali R, Anconetani B, Chattat, Biscotti M, Spinucci G, Casimirri F, Vicennati V, Carcello A, Morselli-Labate AM. Hypothalamic-pituitary-adrenal axis activity and its relationship to the autonomic nervous system in women with visceral and subcutaneous obesity: effects of cortico-tropin-releasing factor/arginine-vasopressin test and of stress. *Metabolism* 1996; **45**: 351–356.

85. Moyer AE, Rodin J, Grilo CM, Cummings N, Larson LM, Rebuffé-Scrive M. Stress-induced cortisol response and fat distribution in women. *Obes Res* 1994; **2**: 255–262.

86. Boushaki FZ, Rasio E, Serri O. Hypothalamic-pituitary-adrenal axis in abdominal obesity: effects of dexfenfluramine. *Clin Endocrinol (Oxf)* 1997; **46**: 461–466.

87. Pasquali R, Gagliardi L, Vicennati V, Gambineri A, Colitta D, Ceroni L, Casimirri F. ACTH and cortisol responses to combined corticotropin releasing hormone-arginine vasopressin stimulation in obese males and its relationship to body weight, fat distribution and parameters of the metabolic syndrome. *Int J Obes* 1999; **23**: 419–424.

88. Ljung T, Anderson B, Bengtsson BA, Björntorp P, Marin P. Inhibition of cortisol secretion by dexamethasone in relation to body fat distribution: a dose–response study. *Obes Res* 1997; **4**: 277–282.

89. Shively C, Clarkson T. Regional obesity and coronary atherosclerosis in females: a non-human primate model. *Acta Med Scand* 1979; **723** (Suppl): 71–78.

90. Lapidus L, Bengtson C, Hallstrom T, Björntorp P. Obesity, adipose tissue distribution and health in women from a population study in Götenborg, Sweden. *Appetite* 1989; **12**: 25–35.

91. Rosmond R, Björntorp P. Endocrine and metabolic aberrations in men with abdominal obesity in relation to anxio-depressive infirmity. *Metabolism* 1998; **47**: 1187–1193.

92. Rosmond R, Lapidus L, Björntorp P. The influence of occupational and social factors on obesity and body fat distribution in middle-aged men. *Int J Obes* 1996; **20**: 599–607.

93. Rosmond R, Lapidus L, Marin P, Björntorp P. Mental distress, obesity and body fat distribution in middle-aged men. *Obes Res* 1996; **4**: 245–252.

94. Pasquali R, Vicennati V, Calzoni F, Gnudi U, Gambineri A, Ceroni L, Coltelli P, Menozzi R, Sinisi R, Del Rio G. α2-adrenoreceptor regulation of the hypothalamic-pituitary-adrenocortical axis in obesity. *Clin Endocrinol* 2000; **52**: 413–421.

18

Cortisol Metabolism

Brian R. Walker and Jonathan R. Seckl

Western General Hospital, Edinburgh, UK

INTRODUCTION

Cortisol is the principal glucocorticoid hormone in humans, contributing to homeostatic regulation of basal metabolism and salt and water balance, and modulating the response to stress. Normal adult human adrenal glands secrete around 5–15 mg per day of cortisol. Only a small fraction is excreted as free cortisol in urine, saliva or bile. The rest is cleared by several metabolic pathways before conjugation and urinary excretion. In the past the enzymes responsible for this metabolism of cortisol received little interest, and indeed were considered to be more important for their other activities, including metabolism of exogenous xenobiotics. However, within the last 15 years, major research programmes have developed around these enzymes following recognition that peripheral metabolism of steroids is not only a means of clearing hormone from the circulation but also plays a key role in determining local responses to hormone. By reversible interconversion with inactive metabolites, the highest intracellular cortisol concentrations can be targeted to specific tissues. This, together with modulation of cortisol secretion by the hypothalamic-pituitary-adrenal axis and modulation of corticosteroid receptor expression and signalling, provides a complex system of regulating glucocorticoid action in a tissue-specific manner (Figure 18.1). In addition, there is interplay between these different determinants of cortisol action since, for example, the rate of metabolic clearance of cortisol by peripheral enzymes influences circulating levels, and thereby affects feedback control of the hypothalamic-pituitary-adrenal axis.

Excessive cortisol secretion in Cushing's syndrome is one of the classical causes of secondary obesity. Effects of excess cortisol on adipose tissue are complex, since central (i.e. visceral, abdominal, facial, and nape of neck) fat deposition is increased, while peripheral fat is reduced. This may result from opposing effects of glucocorticoids which on the one hand increase lipolysis and downregulate lipoprotein lipase—thereby liberating free fatty acids from peripheral fat—but on the other hand stimulate pre-adipocyte differentiation and enhance substrate flux in favour of gluconeogenesis and free fatty acid supply to central fat [1,2]. Tissue specificity of glucocorticoid action on fat may be explained by regional differences in both glucocorticoid receptor expression [3] and pre-receptor metabolism of cortisol by 11β-hydroxysteroid dehydrogenase type 1 [4]. Probably of equal importance in glucocorticoid-induced obesity is central stimulation of appetite, mediated by complex interactions between hypothalamic responses to glucocorticoids, leptin and neuropeptide Y [5].

Against this background, the importance of glucocorticoids in obesity has been investigated in animal models and in humans. Early studies focused on glucocorticoid secretion and circulating levels. Recent studies demonstrated altered peripheral metabolism of cortisol in obesity which may have important effects on tissue response to glucocorticoids. In this chapter, we review current knowledge of enzymes which metabolize cortisol,

International Textbook of Obesity. Edited by Per Björntorp.

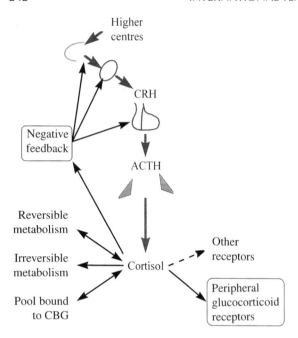

Figure 18.1 Determinants of cortisol activity. The cartoon shows the multiple steps—from the cerebral cortex through hippocampus, hypothalamus, anterior pituitary and adrenal cortex—which regulate cortisol secretion. In addition, it shows that the peripheral response to a given amount of secreted cortisol is determined by the balance between peripheral cortisol clearance, sequestration—in corticosteroid-binding globulin (CBG) or reversibly inactivated steroid (cortisone)—and interaction with corticosteroid receptors. Other factors then influence the effect of receptor activation (see Figure 18.5). CRH, corticotrophin-releasing hormone; ACTH, adrenocorticotrophin

with an emphasis on the 11β-hydroxysteroid dehydrogenases, for which there is strongest evidence of an influence on responses of tissues to glucocorticoids. We also discuss the consequences of deranged activity of these enzymes, and the recent evidence that this is important in subjects with idiopathic obesity. Finally, we discuss the opportunities for therapeutic manipulation of cortisol activity and its relevance to obesity.

PHYSIOLOGY OF CORTISOL METABOLISM

Pathways of Cortisol Metabolism

The principal metabolites of cortisol are shown in Figure 18.2. The enzymes directly metabolizing cor-

tisol include the A-ring reductases (5α- and 5β-reductases), 6β-hydroxylase, 20-reductase, and 11β-hydroxysteroid dehydrogenases. In rats and mice, which lack 17-hydroxylase in their adrenal cortex, the principal glucocorticoid is corticosterone, which is subject to analogous metabolism.

11β-Hydroxysteroid Dehydrogenases (11β-HSDs)

These enzymes catalyse the interconversion of cortisol (or corticosterone) with its inactive metabolite cortisone (or 11-dehydrocorticosterone) (6). Two isozymes have been cloned (7–10) and their characteristics are shown in Table 18.1.

11β-HSD type 2 is a high affinity (low nM Km for cortisol), NAD-dependent dehydrogenase which rapidly converts cortisol to cortisone. Although expressed in many tissues during fetal life (11–14) including the placenta (10,15,16), in adults it is expressed principally in tissues where aldosterone induces its classical effects on sodium excretion, including distal nephron, sweat glands, salivary glands and colonic mucosa (17,18). There is some expression in other epithelial cells, e.g. in lung (19,20) and endothelium (21,22), and in some reports in stromal tissue in lymph nodes (23).

11β-HSD1 is a lower affinity, NADPH-dependent enzyme. Although it converts cortisol to cortisone when removed from its intracellular environment, and for several years it was thought to be responsible for inactivation of cortisol in the kidney (24), in most if not all intact cells and organs this enzyme is a predominant reductase, reactivating inert cortisone into cortisol (4,25–29). This preponderant reductive direction *in vivo* appears to be more due to the intracellular 'context' of 11β-HSD1 in the inner leaflet of the endoplasmic reticulum than to any structural feature, such as glycosylation (30), although the mechanisms determining directionality of the reaction have not been confirmed as yet. 11β-HSD1 is present in kidneys of rats and some other species, but there is negligible 11β-HSD1 expression in adult human kidney (31). However, the 11β-HSD1 isozyme is widely expressed in other tissues (32), including liver, adipose tissue (4,33), lung (34), skeletal muscle, vascular smooth muscle (35,36), anterior pituitary gland, brain (37–39) and adrenal cortex (40).

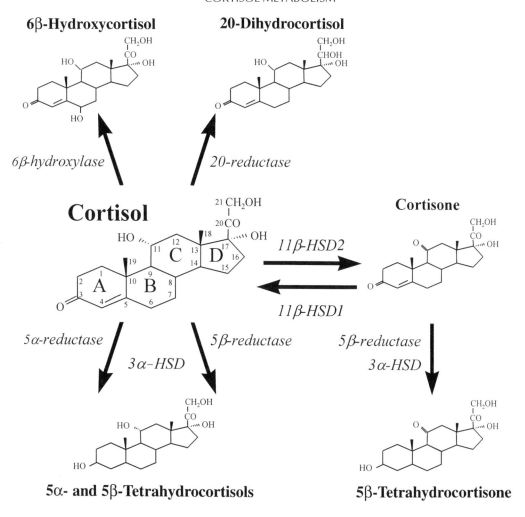

Figure 18.2 Principal routes of metabolism of cortisol. The conversion to tetrahydrocortisols and tetrahydrocortisone is by two steps. HSD, hydroxysteroid dehydrogenase

A-Ring Reductases

5α- and 5β-reductases catalyse the reduction of the 4,5 double bond in the A-ring (Figure 18.2) to generate 5α- or 5β-dihydrocortisol. These dihydro-metabolites are then subject to rapid metabolism in the liver by 3α-hydroxysteroid dehydrogenase. The latter reaction is not rate-limiting and the majority of cortisol metabolites are excreted as 5α- or 5β-tetrahydrocortisols. 5α-tetrahydrocortisol is also known as allo-tetrahydrocortisol. These reactions are not significantly reversible. 5β-reductase is expressed mainly in liver, where it also plays a major

role in bile acid metabolism (41). 5α-reductase activity is catalysed by two isozymes from different genes (Table 18.2) (42). 5α-reductase type 1 is expressed in liver, non-genital skin, brain and to a lesser extent in stromal cells of adipose tissue (43). In addition to metabolizing cortisol, it also converts testosterone to the more potent androgen receptor agonist 5α-dihydrotestosterone. 5α-reductase type 2 is expressed in human liver, specific areas of the developing central nervous system (CNS) involved in reproductive behaviour, prostate and genital skin. In the latter tissues it is essential to enhance local androgen receptor activation and development of the

Table 18.1 Characteristics of 11β-hydroxysteroid dehydrogenases

	11β-HSD1	Homology	11β-HSD2
Protein	34 kDa	20%	40 kDa
	287–292 amino acids		405–427 amino acids
Gene	> 20 kb cDNA ~ 1200 bp	21%	5.3 kb cDNA ~ 1900 bp
	Chromosome 1		Chromosome 16
	6 exons		5 exons
Cofactor affinity	NADP(H)		NAD
Substrate affinity			
Corticosterone	$1.8\,\mu M$		5 nM
Cortisol	$17\,\mu M$		50 nM
11-dehydrocortisone	~ 120 nM		Negligible
Dexamethasone	negligible		500 nM
Favoured reaction	Reductase		Dehydrogenase
Sites expressed	Liver		Distal nephron
	Adipose tissue		Colonic mucosa
	Skeletal muscle		Salivary gland
	Lung		Sweat gland
	Brain		Lung
	Pituitary		Lymph node
	Vascular smooth muscle		Vascular endothelium
	Adrenal cortex		Placenta
	Ovary		Extensive fetal tissues (to
	Testis (some species)		midgestation only)

Table 18.2 Characteristics of 5α-reductases

	5α-Reductase type 1	Homology	5α-Reductase type 2
Protein	23 kDa	50%	21 kDa
	259 amino acids		254 amino acids
Gene	cDNA 2100 bp		cDNA 2437 bp
	Chromosome 5		Chromosome 2
Cofactor affinity	NADPH		NADPH
Substrate affinity			
Testosterone	$1.7\,\mu M$		$0.2\,\mu M$
Cortisol	$18.9\,\mu M$		$11.1\,\mu M$
Favoured reaction	Reductase		Reductase
Sites expressed	Liver		Prostate
	Adipose stromal cells		External genitalia
	Non-genital skin		Genital skin
	Brain		Liver (human)

male phenotype and secondary sexual characteristics (44). Its contribution to metabolism of cortisol is uncertain.

Metabolism to Polar Steroids

The cytochrome p450 microsomal enzyme 6β-hydroxylase and 20-reductase (20α- and 20β-HSDs) are mainly expressed in the liver (45–48). The former is upregulated by glucocorticoids. These pathways account for only a small fraction (< 10%) of cortisol metabolites but may be more important in the metabolism of synthetic glucocorticoids (see below). 20α- and 20β-HSDs also catalyse further reduction of tetrahydrocorticoids to cortols and cortolones. Finally, p450scc and 21-oxidase catalyse the terminal oxidation steps to 11-hydroxy-etiocholanolone and cortolic/cortolonic acids, respectively.

Sites of Cortisol Metabolism

Inactivation of Cortisol

The most active metabolism of cortisol occurs in liver and kidney. It is hard to quantify the contribution of other sites but 11β-HSD2 expressed at lower levels in large organs such as lung, skin and (perhaps) vasculature may be important, as may 5α-reductase expressed in adipose stromal cells and skin.

Estimates of hepatic clearance of cortisol are not available in humans because of the difficulty of obtaining portal venous samples and measuring hepatic blood flow. Experiments in animals in isolated perfused livers (49) suggest that the majority of cortisol is inactivated, principally to A-ring reduced metabolites, on single pass through the liver. However, this is offset by reactivation of cortisone into cortisol by hepatic 11β-HSD1 (26), so that the overall gradient of cortisol across the liver may be quite small.

In humans, around 10% of cortisol is extracted on single pass through each kidney (50). A minority is filtered in the glomerulus and excreted as urinary free cortisol, but most is inactivated to cortisone by 11β-HSD2 in the distal nephron. This has been confirmed by observations that nephrectomized patients have very low circulating cortisone levels (51), and by measurement of arteriovenous differences in 11α-^{3}H-cortisol from which the ^{3}H label is cleaved irreversibly by 11β-HSD2 (Figure 18.3) (50).

Reactivation of Cortisol

The half-life of cortisol in the circulation is about 90 minutes. However, the half-life of 11α^{3}H-cortisol, from which the ^{3}H is removed by 11β-HSD type 2, is about 40 minutes. This discrepancy suggests that there is significant reversible 'shuttling' between cortisol and its 11-oxidized metabolite. The only major metabolic pathway of cortisol which is reversible (Figure 18.2) is its interconversion with cortisone. There is a large pool of cortisone in plasma available for reactivation and widespread expression of the 11β-HSD1 enzyme for which cortisone is the principal substrate. Plasma levels of cortisol (∼ 500 nM peak in the morning and ∼ 100 nM trough in the evening) are higher than those of cortisone (∼ 70 nM), but, unlike cortisol, cortisone is not highly protein bound and is not subject to

marked diurnal variation (26). So, especially in the evening, free cortisone concentrations in plasma exceed those of cortisol. This cortisone is derived both from generation by 11β-HSD2 in kidney, and from adrenocortical secretion. 11β-HSDs are expressed in the adrenal gland (40,52–54) and cortisone is elevated in plasma from the adrenal vein (26,55).

The capacity to reactivate cortisone to cortisol was the basis for the first therapeutic use of glucocorticoids, which relied upon administration of cortisone acetate. After oral administration, relatively little cortisone is detected in peripheral plasma (Figure 18.4) consistent with extensive first pass metabolism in the liver. Indeed, efficient reductase activity of 11β-HSD1 has been confirmed in isolated perfused liver in vitro (49), and by arteriovenous sampling in vivo (26). In addition, however, endogenous cortisone in the systemic circulation may be reactivated to cortisol by 11β-HSD1 in many other sites (Table 18.1). Thus, elevated ratios of cortisol/cortisone relative to circulating ratios have been detected in lung (bronchoalveolar lavage fluid) (56), and subcutaneous adipose tissue (arteriovenous sampling) (57). The absolute rate at which cortisol is generated by this peripheral reactivation has not been compared with the rate of adrenocortical de novo synthesis and secretion, since use of suitable tracer steroids has yet to be reported.

Impact of Cortisol Metabolism on Tissue Response

The effects of corticosteroids are mediated by intracellular receptors which function as transcription factors inducing and repressing the expression of a host of target genes. Many such transcriptional effects are mediated by direct contact of the receptors with target gene DNA via 'glucocorticoid response elements' in their 5' promoter regions (Figure 18.5), others occur via actions upon other DNA-bound transcription factors, such as AP1, NFkB and CREB. The corticosteroid receptors are members of the steroid/thyroid intracellular receptor superfamily (Table 18.3) which are widely expressed. Almost without exception, the access of ligands to receptors in this family is modulated by 'pre-receptor' metabolism, and tissue-specific

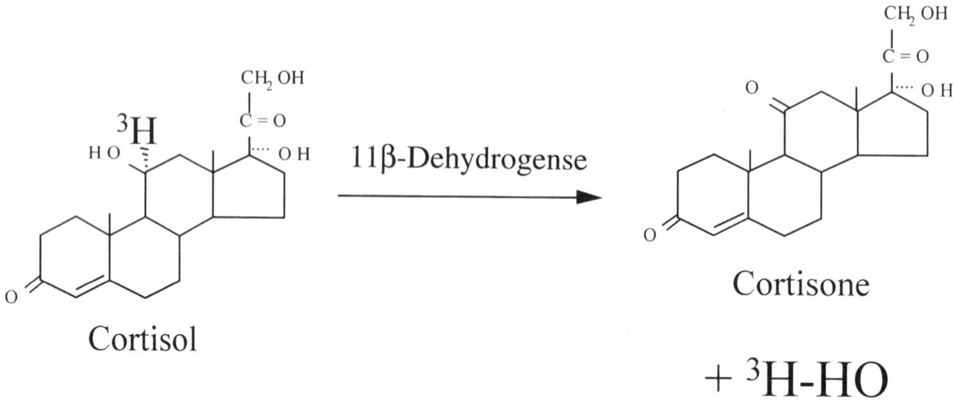

Figure 18.3   Use of 11α-^{3}H-cortisol as a tracer to measure 11β-HSD2 activity *in vivo*. 11β-dehydrogenase activity is assessed from the rate of accumulation of ^{3}H-HO

Table 18.3   Examples of members of the steroid/thyroid intracellular receptor superfamily and the enzymes which modulate access of ligands

Receptor	Principal ligand	Enzyme modulating ligand concentration
Glucocorticoid receptor	Cortisol	11β-HSD1
Mineralocorticoid receptor	Aldosterone	
	Cortisol	11β-HSD2
Oestrogen receptor(s)	Oestradiol	17β-HSD
		Aromatase
Androgen receptor	Dihydrotestosterone	5α-reductase type 2
Thyroid hormone receptor	Triiodothyronine	5′-monodeiodinase

responsiveness is modulated by a combination of local control of receptor expression, pre-receptor enzyme expression, and availability of key transcription factors (58). Relatively recent research has established that pre-receptor metabolism of glucocorticoids is also an important determinant of tissue-specific responses. There is strong evidence for such a role for 11β-HSD enzymes; the potential for other cortisol metabolizing enzymes to modulate local corticosteroid receptor activation has yet to be addressed.

Mineralocorticoid Receptor Activation

Although corticosteroid receptors were initially classified according to their *in vivo* binding characteristics as 'mineralocorticoid' (type I) or 'glucocorticoid' (type II) receptors, when the mineralocorticoid receptor was cloned and expressed it was found to have remarkable sequence homology with the glucocorticoid receptor and to bind cortisol and aldosterone with equal affinity (59). Moreover, in

vivo the mineralocorticoid receptor was shown to bind glucocorticoids in some tissues (e.g. hippocampus) but not in others (e.g. distal nephron) (60), despite glucocorticoid concentrations in plasma being two to three orders of magnitude higher than concentrations of mineralocorticoids. This paradox has been explained on the basis of the tissue-specific expression of 11β-HSD2 (24,61).

There are circumstances in which activity of 11β-HSD2 is impaired, including congenital mutations in the 11β-HSD2 gene (62), pharmacological inhibition of the enzyme (e.g. with liquorice derivatives such as glycyrrhetinic acid or carbenoxolone) (63,64), or transgenic disruption of the gene in mice (65). In these circumstances, glucocorticoids gain inappropriate access to mineralocorticoid receptors (24,61), resulting in profound sodium retention and potassium wasting, with hypertension and hypokalaemic alkalosis. This occurs despite low concentrations of aldosterone, and has been termed the syndrome of 'apparent' mineralocorticoid excess (66). Diagnosis of this syndrome is discussed further

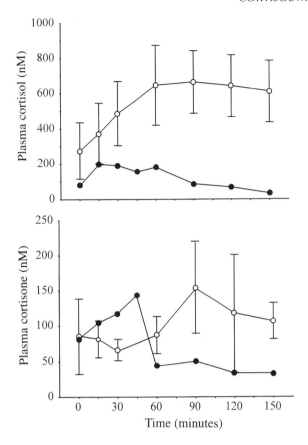

Figure 18.4 Plasma cortisol and cortisone following oral administration of cortisone in humans. Data are from 10 healthy women (open symbols) who received dexamethasone 250 μg orally at 2300 h then cortisone 25 mg by mouth at 0830 h. Plasma cortisol and cortisone were measured at the intervals shown after cortisone. Note the inconsistent and relatively small rise in plasma cortisone by contrast with the substantial rise in cortisol. This is consistent with avid 11β-HSD1 conversion of cortisone to cortisol on first pass metabolism through the liver. Data are also shown for a 36-year-old female patient (solid symbols) with probable congenital 11β-HSD1 deficiency. Note the very poor generation of cortisol and early peak of cortisone. Adapted from Jamieson *et al.* (93)

below. Thus, 11β-HSD2 activity is important in preventing glucocorticoids from gaining access to mineralocorticoid receptors. This mechanism explains the selectivity of mineralocorticoid receptors for aldosterone in sites where 11β-HSD2 is active, including distal nephron, sweat glands, salivary glands and colonic mucosa. In sites where 11β-HSD2 is not expressed, such as hippocampus, glucocorticoids readily gain access to mineralocorticoid receptors *in vivo*.

Glucocorticoid Receptor Activation

More recent studies have addressed the possibility that pre-receptor reactivation of cortisol from cortisone by 11β-HSD1 may also regulate intracellular receptor activation. As above, 11β-HSD1 is expressed in sites which are not classical targets for aldosterone, but which are important sites where glucocorticoids modulate carbohydrate and lipid metabolism, including liver and adipose tissue. Surprisingly, the affinity of glucocorticoid receptors for cortisol is 10–40-fold lower than that of mineralocorticoid receptors (59). Reactivation of cortisone to cortisol may therefore be an important mechanism for maintaining adequate exposure of glucocorticoid receptors to their endogenous ligand in key target sites, especially during the trough of circulating cortisol levels at night.

In Liver

In support of this hypothesis, pharmacological inhibition of 11β-HSD1 reductase activity with carbenoxolone in humans (67) or oestrogen administration in male rats (68), or transgenic disruption of the 11β-HSD1 gene in mice (69), results in altered carbohydrate metabolism consistent with impaired activation of hepatic glucocorticoid receptors (Figure 18.6). These receptors have numerous interactions with insulin in regulating hepatic glucose metabolism (1), including upregulation of the rate-limiting enzyme in gluconeogenesis, phosphenolpyruvate carboxykinase (PEPCK). Impaired 11β-HSD1 activity is characterized by impaired PEPCK expression and/or activity, either at baseline or in response to the stimulus of fasting (Figure 18.6). Similarly, induction of another hepatic glucocorticoid-regulated gene product, glucose-6-phosphatase, is also deficient in 11β-HSD1 null mice (69).

In Adipose Tissue

A key question is whether 11β-HSD1 influences glucocorticoid receptor activation in other sites as well as in liver. The 11β-HSD inhibitor carbenoxolone enhances insulin sensitivity in healthy humans (Figure 18.6) (67). This could not be attributed to altered uptake of glucose in skeletal muscle, as measured by forearm arteriovenous glucose uptake, so it must result from enhanced sup-

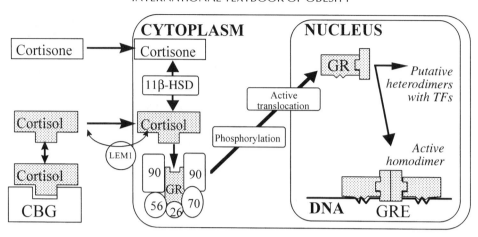

Figure 18.5 Regulation of gene transcription by corticosteroid receptors 11β-HSD, 11β-hydroxysteroid dehydrogenases; GR, glucocorticoid receptor; ⎰⎱, zinc fingers, which bind to DNA; 90, 70, 56, and 26 indicate heatshock proteins of these molecular weights, in kDa, which dissociate from the activated receptor; TF, transcription factor, e.g. AP-1; GRE, glucocorticoid response element, typically a palindromic sequence to which the receptors bind; LEM1, a yeast transmembrane transporter; CBG, corticosteroid-binding globulin

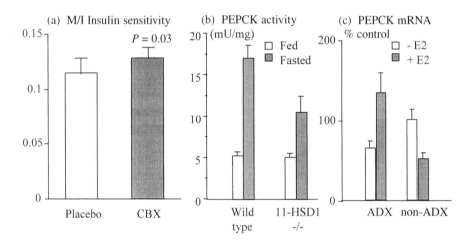

Figure 18.6 Evidence that 11β-HSD1 influences insulin sensitivity in humans, mice and rats. (a) Comparison of results of euglycaemic hyperinsulinaemic clamps in healthy men receiving placebo or the 11β-HSD inhibitor carbenoxolone (CBX, 100 mg by mouth 8-hourly for 7 days) in a randomized double-blind cross-over study. Carbenoxolone increased insulin sensitivity by 11.3%. Insulin sensitivity is represented by M/I, which is the rate of glucose infusion during hyperglycaemia (M value) divided by prevailing insulin concentration. Adapted from Walker et al. (67).
(b) Comparison of hepatic phosphoenolpyruvate carboxykinase (PEPCK) activity in wild-type mice and 11β-HSD1 knockout mice under fasted and fed conditions. Although basal activity is not different, 11β-HSD1 knockout mice have less induction of gluconeogenic enzymes when fasted. Adapted from Kotelevtsev et al. (69).
(c) Comparison of the effect of oestradiol (E2) administration on hepatic PEPCK mRNA measured by Northern blot in rats with and without corticosterone. In the absence of corticosterone, oestradiol increases expression of gluconeogenic enzymes. However, in the presence of corticosterone, oestradiol (which potently represses 11β-HSD1 expression and activity in these circumstances) lowers PEPCK mRNA levels. ADX, adrenalectomy. Adapted from Jamieson et al. (68)

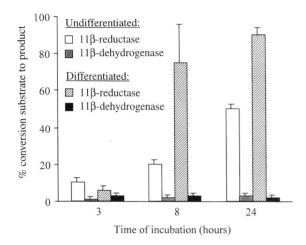

Figure 18.7 11β-HSD activity in 3T3 adipocyte cell line. 11β-HSD activities were measured in the human adipocyte-derived 3T3 cell line, both in cells with the undifferentiated pre-adipocyte phenotype and in cells differentiated to adipocyte phenotype with insulin/cortisol. In both states, 11β-reductase activity (reactivation of cortisone to cortisol) is very much greater than 11β-dehydrogenase activity (inactivation of cortisol to cortisone). Adapted from Napolitano *et al.* (33)

pression of hepatic gluconeogenesis and/or enhanced uptake of glucose in adipose tissue. Experiments to differentiate these possibilities have yet to be reported. The identification of 11β-HSD1 conversion of cortisone to cortisol in adipose stromal cells in primary culture (4), and equivalent activity in a cultured adipocyte cell line (Figure 18.7) (33), has received particularly close attention. Inhibition of this enzyme prevents reactivation of cortisone and glucocorticoid regulation of aromatase expression (70). In human tissue culture this activity is higher in cells obtained from omental fat than subcutaneous fat (4). It has been hypothesized that local regeneration of cortisol in adipose tissue explains the characteristic visceral distribution of fat in Cushing's syndrome, and may explain central adiposity in other circumstances, including growth hormone deficiency (71). In rats, there is no such regional difference in 11β-HSD1 activity in fat (72), but perhaps this explains why rats do not develop glucocorticoid-dependent visceral obesity.

In Brain and Pituitary: Control of Appetite and Hypothalamic-Pituitary-Adrenal Axis

Glucocorticoid receptors are expressed widely in most neurons and glia (73). In contrast, mineralocorticoid receptors are expressed at high levels only in neurons of the hippocampus, septum and a few nuclei of the brainstem. At both receptors, glucocorticoids are involved in altering target gene expression, thereby affecting cellular metabolism and electrophysiological properties, and hence mood, memory and neuroendocrine parameters, as well as cell division, maturation, structure and survival. Indeed glucocorticoids have well-documented effects upon their own release pathways, acting in negative feedback control upon the stimulatory hypothalamic-pituitary-adrenal (HPA) axis. Such feedback occurs at both pituitary and brain levels, most notably in the paraventricular nucleus of the hypothalamus (PVN) and in key supra-hypothalamic sites including the hippocampus (74). This feedback is mediated by glucocorticoid receptors, but there may also be a contribution, especially at low cortisol concentrations, from mineralocorticoid receptors (75).

Adrenal insufficiency and glucocorticoid replacement therapy are associated with alterations in appetite and food intake in humans and in animal models. The mechanisms are rather poorly defined, and may include both glucocorticoid and mineralocorticoid receptor effects. The critical neurons are probably located primarily in specific regions of the hypothalamus, notably the PVN and arcuate nucleus (76). In particular, glucocorticoids appear essential for the increased appetite associated with food (protein) deprivation (77). Glucocorticoid receptors are perhaps more selectively involved in carbohydrate appetite control, at least in rodents, whereas mineralocorticoid receptors have been more implicated in fat appetite (78,79). However, such mechanistic studies have been weakened by the predominant use of peripherally administered steroids which may exert varied and indirect effects upon the CNS.

11β-HSD1 is expressed in neurons of the hippocampus, hypothalamus (including the parvocellular part of the PVN where corticotrophin-releasing hormone (CRH) is synthesized) and anterior pituitary (37–39). Within hippocampal cells, at least, 11β-HSD1 functions as a predominant 11β-reductase *in vitro* (29). Indeed, this glucocorticoid regenerating enzyme appears important in amplifying the deleterious effects of elevated glucocorticoid levels upon neuronal survival in culture. Moreover, 11β-HSD1 null mice show elevated basal levels of glucocorticoids, implying reduced effective glucocorticoid feedback control of the HPA axis (69).

That this occurs in the face of modestly elevated basal plasma glucocorticoid levels suggests that intracellular regeneration of active 11-hydroxy steroids is an important source of the total glucocorticoid signal in the brain as well as in peripheral tissues.

11β-HSD2 has a more restricted distribution than 11β-HSD1 in adult brain. The absence of 11β-HSD2 dehydrogenase activity explains why both glucocorticoid and mineralocorticoid receptors bind cortisol and corticosterone in hippocampus *in vivo* (80). However, 11β-HSD2 is expressed in a limited population of cells in the ventromedial nucleus of the hypothalamus in adult rats (81,82). The dehydrogenase isozyme is also expressed in the central nucleus of the amygdala (81,82), where it is appropriately located to facilitate the specific central actions of aldosterone, but not corticosterone, upon salt appetite (83,84).

The role, if any, in regulation of central appetite of the 11β-HSD enzymes (85), or of other key players in corticosteroid metabolism, such as 5α-reductase, remains unexplored, but could be addressed with the recent construction of 5α-reductase type 1 (86), 11β-HSD1 (69), and 11β-HSD2 (65) knockout mice. Brain-selective, enzyme deficient mice would help to specify the exact locus of any effects seen.

In Other Sites: Further Local and Systemic Modulation of Cortisol Availability

11β-HSDs may also be important in a host of other sites, including in lymphoid tissue where they may modulate cell-mediated immunity (87,88), and in blood vessels where they may modulate glucocorticoid-induced vasoconstriction (89–91).

The fact that tissue-specific differences in cortisol metabolism are important in determining local intracellular corticosteroid receptor activation does not lessen the importance of regulation of circulating cortisol concentrations by the HPA axis (Figure 18.1). Clearly, circulating levels of cortisol—and cortisone—remain important determinants of intracellular cortisol concentrations. There are two ways in which peripheral cortisol metabolism influences feedback regulation of the HPA axis: by influencing local glucocorticoid concentrations in sites where feedback occurs (see above); and by influencing circulating glucocorticoid concentrations.

The metabolic clearance rate for cortisol could play a key role in determining plasma levels of cortisol and resulting feedback regulation of the HPA axis. In circumstances of impaired peripheral inactivation of cortisol (e.g. 11β-HSD2 deficiency (66)), total cortisol production rate falls in order to maintain normal plasma cortisol levels. In circumstances of enhanced cortisol clearance, e.g. 11β-HSD1 deficiency with impaired regeneration of cortisol (92,93), plasma cortisol tends to fall but this is corrected by enhanced ACTH-dependent cortisol secretion. A consequence of this effect is increased secretion of other ACTH-dependent steroids, including adrenal androgens, so that these very rare patients present with hirsutism and menstrual irregularity, as described below. Alterations in other metabolic pathways, e.g. A-ring reductases, is predicted to influence cortisol clearance and negative feedback regulation of the hypothalamic-pituitary-adrenal axis but this has not been subject to experimentation.

Regulation of Cortisol Metabolism

Given the importance of peripheral metabolism in determining tissue-specific differences in response to corticosteroids one would expect exquisite regulation of these enzymes. This may in turn give clues to their dysregulation in obesity.

11β-HSD2 appears to be constitutive, required at all times in the adult to protect mineralocorticoid receptors from inappropriate activation by glucocorticoids. However, during embryonic development, this isozyme is expressed much more widely (12,13,94,95). High fetal tissue expression of 11β-HSD2 is dramatically lost in most organs at the end of midgestation in rodents and humans, presumably allowing tissue exposure to glucocorticoids to occur. The signals for these dramatic and acute changes in 11β-HSD2 expression remain to be elucidated.

11β-HSD1 gene expression and/or activity in adulthood is regulated by a number of factors (Table 18.4). These include factors which are potentially important mediators of the insulin resistance and dyslipidaemia of obesity such as growth hormone, insulin, tumour necrosis factor-α (TNFα), and interleukin-6 (IL-6), as well as glucocorticoids themselves. These effects may be mediated in large

Table 18.4 Regulation of 11β-HSDs

	11β-HSD1	11β-HSD2
Upregulation	Glucocorticoids (183–188) Thyroxine (192–196) IL-5, IL-6, TNFα, IL-1 (198,199)	Oestradiol (189–191) Retinoic acid (197) Dehydroepiandrosterone (200)
Downregulation	Insulin (28,184,188) Oestradiol (172,189,202) Growth hormone (172,175,188) Stress (203,204)	ACTH (26,53,201) Progesterone (191) Growth hormone (174) Nitric oxide (205)

IL, interleukin; TNFα, tumour necrosis factor α.

part by the C/EBP family of transcription factors, for which there are multiple functional binding sites in the 5' region of the 11β-HSD1 gene (96,97).

5β-Reductase activity is lower in female than male rat livers (98) but it is upregulated by oestrogen (99). 5α-Reductase type 1, the principal isozyme in human liver and fat (43), is usually thought to be 'constitutive' and not regulated hormonally (100,101), but there is some evidence that this isozyme is downregulated by androgens (102,103) more so than by oestrogen (104) so that its activity is higher in female liver (105) and adrenal (106). The type 1 isozyme is not regulated by growth hormone (105,107). 5α-Reductase type 2 is expressed mainly in the prostate, but also in liver, where it is upregulated by androgens (42), oestrogens (108) and growth hormone (107).

In addition to regulation of expression of enzymes metabolizing cortisol, the activity of these enzymes has been suggested to be influenced by the prevailing concentrations of a large number of endogenous competitive inhibitors, largely other steroids, sterols and their derived bile acids (Table 18.5). Although present at sufficiently high concentrations to be detected in extracts of urine (109), the relevance of these inhibitors *in vivo* remains uncertain (110–114).

Metabolism of Synthetic Corticosteroids

Modifications of steroid structures has long been recognized to affect their affinity for corticosteroid receptors. In addition, their affinity for metabolizing enzymes may be altered. Thus, 9α-fluorocortisol (also known as fludrocortisone) has preserved affinity for mineralocorticoid and glucocorticoid receptors, but the steroid is no longer inactivated by 11β-HSD2 in the distal nephron (115) and is therefore a potent mineralocorticoid. By contrast, prednisolone differs from cortisol in having a 1,2 double bond in the A-ring which increases affinity for glucocorticoid receptors but retains metabolism by 11β-HSDs (116). Dexamethasone and beclomethasone have a combination of these modifications (9α-fluoro, 16α-methyl and 9α-choloro, 16β-methyl, respectively) which increase affinity for glucocorticoid receptors and lower affinity for mineralocorticoid receptors. Interestingly, the 9α-fluoro modification in dexamethasone appears to dictate metabolism by 11β-HSD1 that is exclusively reductive, even with semi-purified enzyme which will act as an effective 11β-dehydrogenase for cortisol and corticosterone (117). This interaction between substrate and 11β-HSD1 is unique, since other substrates are metabolized

Table 18.5 Inhibitors of 11β-HSDs

Endogenous	Exogenous	Unidentified
11-OH-progesterone (206–208)	Glycyrrhetinic acid (63,155,209)	'GALFs' (109,110,112,210–213)
3α,5β-Tetrahydroprogesterone (214)	Glycyrrhizic acid	ACTH-dependent inhibitors (26)
3α,5β-Tetrahydro-11-deoxy-corticosterone	Carbenoxolone (64)	
11-Epicortisol	CHAPS (215)	
Chenodeoxycholic acid	Ketoconazole	
Cholic acid (216,217)	Saiboku-To (218,219)	
	Gossypol (220,221)	
	Metyrapone (222–224)	
	11-Epiprednisolone	
	Frusemide (225–227)	
	Bioflavinoids (228,229)	

Table 18.6 Biochemical features of deranged 11β-HSD activity

	Apparent mineralocorticoid excess type 1	Apparent mineralocorticoid excess type 2	Apparent cortisone reductase deficiency	Liquorice administration	Carbenoxolone administration
11β-dehydrogenase					
Half life of (11α³H)-cortisol	↑	↑	No data	↑	↑
11β-reductase:					
Conversion of oral cortisone to cortisol	→	↓	↓	→	↓
Urinary cortisol metabolites:					
(5β- +5α-THF)/THE ratio	↑	→	↓	↑	→
5α-/5β-THF ratio	↑	→	↓	↑	→
Cortisol/Cortisone ratio	↑	↑	→	↑	↑
Total cortisol metabolites	↓	↓	↑	↓	↓

THF, tetrahydrocortisol; THE, tetrahydrocortisone.

equally in 11β-reductase and 11β-dehydrogenase directions when the 11β-HSD1 enzyme is semi-purified. Conversely, 11β-HSD2 metabolizes dexamethasone in both directions despite only being able to oxidize cortisol to cortisone and not vice versa (118,119). Perhaps as a result of such attenuated metabolism by the pathways in Figure 18.1, synthetic glucocorticoids are then preferentially metabolized by other enzymes, particularly 6β-hydroxylase.

PATHOLOGY OF CORTISOL METABOLISM

Much of what we have learnt of the physiology of cortisol metabolism has been inferred from observations of the consequences of pathology. In this section, we review these pathological clinical syndromes and experimental models.

Measurement of Cortisol Metabolism in Humans

The established technique for assessing different routes of cortisol metabolism in humans is to measure the principal metabolites of cortisol in urine, using gas chromatography–mass spectrometry (GCMS) (120,121). Examples of major enzyme defects and associated changes in ratios of metabolites are given below. However, these ratios must be interpreted with caution, since they reflect only relative excretion and not flux or turnover through different metabolic pathways. For example, the ratio of the principal metabolites of cortisol/cortisone, i.e. (5α- + 5β- tetrahydrocortisol)/(5β-tetrahydrocortisone), is elevated if 11β-HSD2 is congenitally deficient (66) or inhibited by liquorice (63). However, in theory this could also result from a primary increase in 11β-HSD1 activity. Moreover, dramatic changes in 11β-HSD activity may occur in a tissue-specific manner, but be balanced so that there is no net change in cortisol/cortisone metabolite ratio. An example is that carbenoxolone inhibits both 11β-HSD1 and 11β-HSD2 and, despite marked cortisol excess in kidney and deficiency in liver, there is no *net* change in urinary cortisol/cortisone metabolite ratio (64). Nevertheless, all syndromes in which renal 11β-HSD2 is deficient, including carbenoxolone administration, appear to be associated with increased urinary free cortisol/cortisone ratio (122,123), since this reflects specifically intrarenal cortisol and cortisone concentrations without 'adjustment' by 11β-HSD1 elsewhere (Table 18.6) (Figure 18.8).

Primary changes in A-ring reductases are predicted to change the ratio of cortisol/cortisone metabolites too. It was suggested that A-ring reductase activity could be inferred from an 'A-ring reductase quotient' (i.e. free urinary cortisol/tetrahydrocortisol) (124) but this is not valid if the urinary free cortisol concentration is also altered, e.g. increased because of impaired intrarenal cortisol inactivation by 11β-HSD2 (125). Confusion over the interpretation of urinary metabolite ratios has therefore been an important limitation to the inves-

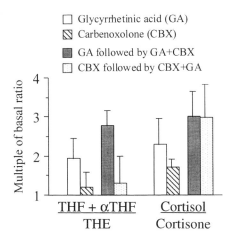

□ Glycyrrhetinic acid (GA)
▨ Carbenoxolone (CBX)
▩ GA followed by GA+CBX
□ CBX followed by CBX+GA

Figure 18.8 Sensitivity of urinary cortisol metabolite ratios to inhibition of 11β-HSD. Data are from six healthy men treated for 2 days with carbenoxolone followed by 2 days with glycyrrhetinic acid plus carbenoxolone, or 2 days with glycyrrhetinic acid followed by 2 days with glycyrrhetinic acid plus carbenoxolone. Urinary cortisol metabolites were measured by gas chromatography–mass spectrometry (GCMS) in 24 h urine samples. The ratio of A-ring reduced metabolites of cortisol/cortisone (i.e. tetrahydrocortisols/tetrahydrocortisone; THFs/THE) was elevated following glycyrrhetinic acid but not carbenoxolone. This ratio reflects the balance between 11β-HSD1 and 11β-HSD2 activities; glycyrrhetinic acid inhibits only 11β-HSD2 while carbenoxolone inhibits 11β-HSD1. In contrast, the ratio of urinary cortisol/cortisone is elevated with all manipulations. This ratio reflects intrarenal cortisol/cortisone ratio which is determined by 11β-HSD2 and not 11β-HSD1. Adapted from Best and Walker (123)

tigation of cortisol metabolism in clinical research (126).

Additional methods to assess specific enzymes include dynamic assessments and tissue-specific sampling. $11\alpha^3$H-Cortisol (Figure 18.3) is cleaved by 11β-dehydrogenase (probably exclusively 11β-HSD2 in humans) to unlabelled cortisone and ^{3}H-H_2O, and can therefore distinguish impaired dehydrogenase from enhanced reductase (50,63,64,127,128). However, the use of radioisotopes in human research is increasingly difficult to justify on ethical grounds. An alternative approach using stable isotope labelling with deuterium has been reported (129) and shows promise. Alternatively, to measure 11β-HSD1, cortisone can be administered orally and the rate of cortisol appearance in peripheral plasma taken to indicate first pass hepatic metabolism by 11β-HSD1 (Figure 18.4) (64,93,130,131). However, this is potentially confounded by the rate of clearance of cortisol from peripheral plasma, and frequent sampling has not always been employed to allow estimates of rate of appearance. A simple estimate of peak plasma cortisol obtained may not be such a specific index of 11β-HSD1.

Tissue-specific sampling requires measurements in venous effluent from the site of interest or from fluid in equilibrium with interstitial fluid at that site. This has been achieved with difficulty for human liver (26), lung (56), and abdominal subcutaneous fat (57). However, the high variability of these measurements may obscure important differences. These techniques would be enhanced by including tracer cortisol or cortisone and examining rates of conversion rather than just cortisol/cortisone ratios.

With these limitations in mind, it has still been possible to define several syndromes on the basis of biochemical measurements, several of which have since been explained by molecular defects.

Congenital Syndromes in Humans

11β-HSD2 Deficiency: 'Apparent Mineralocorticoid Excess Syndrome'

This autosomal recessive disorder is rare, with fewer than 50 cases reported worldwide since 1974 (132,133). It usually presents in childhood with hypokalaemia (polyuria, myopathy), severe hypertension, and complications including stroke and cardiac arrest. Investigation reveals low plasma renin activity, low plasma aldosterone (and low levels of other mineralocorticoids including 11-deoxycorticosterone), and hypokalaemic alkalosis which improves with mineralocorticoid receptor antagonists (spironolactone) or post-receptor sodium channel antagonists (amiloride). In the absence of a measurable mineralocorticoid in serum of these patients the cause remained obscure for some years, hence the term 'apparent' mineralocorticoid excess. It was then recognized that, although plasma cortisol concentrations are normal, the condition improves following suppression of cortisol with dexamethasone, while additional administration of cortisol induces profound mineralocorticoid excess (134,135). Moreover, analysis of urinary metabolites of cortisol reveals an elevated ratio of the metabolites of cortisol versus those of cortisone, and the half-life of $11\alpha^3$H-cortisol (Figure 18.3) is dramatically prolonged, consistent with 11β-dehydrogenase deficiency. Total cortisol metabolite excretion is reduced (consistent with a compensatory fall in cortisol production rate) but urinary free cortisol concentrations are elevated (consistent with impaired intrarenal cortisol metabolism).

Following cloning of human 11β-HSD2 in 1994, a series of mutations in the 11β-HSD2 gene have been reported. Patients with the syndrome of apparent mineralocorticoid excess are more commonly homozygotes than compound heterozygotes for such mutations (62), suggesting that there is a low prevalence of heterozygous inactivating mutations in the population and most cases arise from consanguinity. Heterozygotes in these families may have more subtle abnormalities of cortisol metabolism and milder hypertension (135,136), but their blood pressure has been easily controlled by conventional means, indicating that there is considerable redundancy or excess capacity in 11β-HSD2 activity in human kidney. Intriguingly, polymorphisms of a microsatellite in the 11β-HSD2 gene on chromosome 16p have recently been associated with variations in 11β-HSD activity and with the individual blood pressure response to salt loading (137).

An additional feature of this syndrome has emerged quite recently. 11β-HSD2 is present in placenta (10,11), where it is thought to protect the fetus from inappropriate exposure to maternal cortisol (138). Excessive glucocorticoid exposure of the fetus results in growth retardation. In retrospective studies, birthweight has been found to be low in patients with 11β-HSD2 deficiency (133,139). In some (140), but not all (14,141), studies there is an inverse relationship between placental 11β-HSD activity and birthweight in otherwise healthy individuals. Extensive epidemiological studies have linked low birthweight with subsequent adverse risk factors for cardiovascular disease, including hypertension and insulin resistance (142). Prenatal treatment of rats with either dexamethasone, which is a poor 11β-HSD2 substrate and so directly accesses the fetus, or carbenoxolone which inhibits 11β-HSD, lowers birthweight and programs permanent hypertension and hyperglycemia in the adult offspring (143–145). However, while the hypertension and insulin resistance in low birthweight babies may be amplified by subsequent obesity (146), current data do not suggest that obesity itself is programmed by these early

determinants of metabolic and cardiovascular development.

11β-HSD1 Deficiency: 'Apparent Cortisone Reductase Deficiency'

This syndrome has been reported in just four patients (92,93,147,148). All are female and presented with hirsutism and menstrual irregularity. Investigation reveals mild ACTH-dependent adrenal androgen excess. Urinary cortisol metabolites are strikingly abnormal, with markedly elevated cortisone metabolite excretion and elevated total cortisol metabolite excretion. Urinary free cortisol/cortisone ratio is normal. The conversion of cortisone, administered orally, into cortisol in peripheral plasma was markedly impaired in one affected patient, and unlike healthy volunteers a peak of cortisone was also detected in peripheral plasma (Figure 18.4).

Although all of these features are consistent with 11β-HSD1 deficiency, no mutation in the 11β-HSD1 gene exons or exon/intron boundaries has yet been reported (93,149). It remains possible that an alternative abnormality of cortisol metabolism, such as 5β-reductase deficiency, might be responsible for shifting the excretion of cortisol metabolites in favour of cortisone; hence the term 'apparent' cortisone reductase deficiency.

Given the proposed role of 11β-HSD1 to maintain local cortisol concentrations in adipose tissue (4), one might expect these patients to be thin with lipoatrophy. In fact, this appears not to occur; indeed, at least one of these patients is obese.

Combined 11β-HSD1 and 11β-HSD2 Deficiency

A small series of patients with a so-called syndrome of apparent mineralocorticoid excess 'type 2' have been described (128). In these four patients, cortisol-dependent mineralocorticoid excess has been documented, and impaired 11β-dehydrogenase activity has been confirmed by measurement of $11\alpha^{3}$H-cortisol half-life and urinary free cortisol/cortisone ratio. However, overall cortisol/cortisone metabolite ratios are not deranged and the conversion of oral cortisone into cortisol in peripheral plasma is impaired. This suggests that there is a combination of 11β-HSD1 and 11β-HSD2 deficiency, as occurs after carbenoxolone administra-

Table 18.7 Features of transgenic deletion of 11β-HSDs

11β-HSD1 −/−	11β-HSD2 −/−
Lower blood glucose after overfeeding with obesity	Severe hypertension
Lower blood glucose after stress	Hypokalaemia
Impaired activation of gluconeogenesis (PEPCK) on fasting	Renal structural abnormalities
Hypercorticosteronaemia	Increased risk of early postnatal death
Altered neonatal lung maturation	

tion (see below). The molecular defect remains to be elucidated. A non-coding mutation in 11β-HSD2 has been preliminarily reported in these patients (150), but whether this accounts for the syndrome remains unclear since it does not explain their impaired 11β-HSD1 activity.

Interestingly, these patients all come from the Mediterranean island of Sardinia, where there is an association between hypertension and elevated ratios of cortisol/cortisone metabolites (151), and a high prevalence of the polymorphisms in the 11β-HSD2 gene which have been associated with salt-sensitive hypertension (137).

A-Ring Reductase Deficiencies

The congenital syndrome of 5α-reductase type 2 deficiency results in impaired generation of dihydrotestosterone in key androgen target tissues (44). While testosterone levels are relatively low before puberty, this results in feminization of males including ambiguous genitalia. However, after puberty higher circulating testosterone levels overcome the defect and males develop full secondary sexual characteristics, so that males reared as girls may be re-assigned as men. The consequences of this enzyme defect on cortisol metabolism have, however, not been studied.

Congenital syndromes of 5α-reductase type 1 or 5β-reductase deficiency have not been described.

Interactions Between A-ring Reductases and 11β-HSDs

A paradox in syndromes of 11β-HSD deficiency is that there are also changes in the relative excretion of 5α-tetrahydrocortisol and 5β-tetrahydrocortisol. These remain poorly understood. Following liquorice or carbenoxolone administration, the relative excretion of 5β-tetrahydrocortisol falls (63,64), which could be explained by inhibition of 5β-reductase by these compounds (152). However, the same

relative fall in 5β-reduced cortisol metabolites occurs in congenital 11β-HSD2 deficiency. No obvious artefact of measurement (see above) can explain this. It suggests that there is a more complex interplay between the different pathways of cortisol metabolism than we currently understand.

Animal Models

Transgenic knockout mice have been generated for several of these key glucocorticoid metabolizing enzymes.

11β-HSD2 Knockout Mice

These animals faithfully reproduce the phenotype of the syndrome of apparent mineralocorticoid excess (AME) in humans, with hypertension and hypokalaemia which can be ameliorated by dexamethasone or spironolactone treatment and exacerbated by physiological doses of corticosterone (Table 18.7) (65). Interestingly, they also exhibit structural abnormalities in kidney from infancy (distal tubular hyperplasia and hypertrophy) which do not appear to reverse with spironolactone, suggesting a possible basis for the difficulties in treating established hypertension in AME merely with cortisol suppression or anti-mineralocorticoids.

11β-HSD1 Knockout Mice

The generation of these mice has confirmed the importance of 11β-HSD1 in modulating glucocorticoid action in several target tissues (69). They show a complete inability to convert 11-dehydrocorticosterone (the equivalent of cortisone in humans) to corticosterone (equivalent to cortisol), indicating that 11β-HSD1 is the only major 11β-reductase enzyme, at least in mice. This defect affects multiple tissues, and the following evidence has been obtained that it results in attenuated glucocorticoid action in liver, brain and possibly peripheral fat.

In the liver, PEPCK, the rate-limiting enzyme in gluconeogenesis which is downregulated by insulin and upregulated by glucocorticoids, shows an impaired induction in response to fasting in 11β-HSD $-/-$ animals (Figure 18.6c). This is consistent with the interpretation of pharmacological experiments (see above) that 11β-HSD1 maintains intrahepatic glucocorticoid receptor activation.

When 11β-HSD1 $-/-$ animals are fed a high-fat cafeteria diet, they gain less weight and have lower plasma glucose levels than wild-type controls. The latter is consistent with effects on the hepatic gluconeogenic response to insulin, but the former may be explained by additional central effects of 11β-HSD1 on regulation of energy expenditure and/or an influence of 11β-HSD1 on adipocyte metabolism. Appetite and energy expenditure have yet to be examined. Interestingly, however, body fat distribution in animals on normal chow is not obviously different from wild type.

11β-HSD1 $-/-$ mice are also hyper-corticosteronaemic, consistent with a defect in negative feedback regulation of the hypothalamic-pituitary-adrenal axis.

5α-Reductase Knockout Mice

Mice with transgenic deletion of both isozymes of 5α-reductase have been reported (86,153). The 5α-reductase type 2 knockout, surprisingly, has no abnormality of prostate or genital development but in rodents 5α-reductase type 1 is co-expressed and could compensate. The 5α-reductase type 1 knockout also has no major phenotypic abnormality, except an increased risk of *in utero* death attributed to diversion of androgens to oestrogens instead of 5α-dihydrotestosterone (86). However, glucocorticoid metabolism and action has not been reported in these animals.

Pharmacological Manipulation

Liquorice and its Derivatives

Extracts from the liquorice root have been used as confectionery and in therapy for dyspepsia for dec-

ades (154). Some people habitually consume excessive quantities of liquorice, although whether there is a liquorice withdrawal syndrome—suggesting that the material is truly 'addictive'—has not been established. The active constituents of liquorice include glycyrrhizic acid and its metabolite glycyrrhetinic acid (Figure 18.9). A related hemisuccinate, carbenoxolone, remains a licensed medication for dyspepsia in UK.

A long-recognized side effect of liquorice ingestion is sodium retention, leading to hypertension and even heart failure. This is accompanied by hypokalaemia and suppression of plasma renin activity and aldosterone and was at one time attributed to direct activation of mineralocorticoid receptors by liquorice. However, these side effects are dependent upon the presence of cortisol. Stewart and Edwards showed that liquorice derivatives, particularly glycyrrhetinic acid, inhibit 11β-HSDs and enhance binding of glucocorticoids to mineralocorticoid receptors (24,61,63,155). Liquorice administration therefore reproduces the syndrome of apparent mineralocorticoid excess, including elevated ratios of cortisol/cortisone and of their metabolites in urine and prolonged half-life of $11\alpha^3$H-cortisol (Table 18.6).

Further studies showed that carbenoxolone also induces cortisol-dependent mineralocorticoid excess and inhibits 11β-HSD *in vitro* (64). However, there were several differences between the effects of carbenoxolone and liquorice/glycyrrhetinic acid in humans (Table 18.6). While carbenoxolone increases urinary free cortisol/cortisone and prolongs the half-life of $11\alpha^3$H-cortisol, it does not alter ratios of A-ring reduced urinary metabolites of cortisol versus cortisone (Figure 18.8). This paradox is explained by the observation that carbenoxolone, but not liquorice, inhibits the conversion of cortisone to cortisol by 11β-HSD1 in liver (64,156). Thus, inhibition of 11β-HSD2 in kidney is balanced by inhibition of 11β-HSD1 in liver and there is no change in overall equilibrium between cortisol and cortisone despite marked changes in intrarenal and intrahepatic cortisol concentrations (125). This is an important observation to bear in mind when interpreting urinary cortisol metabolite results in other clinical syndromes (see above). As a result, carbenoxolone produces additional clinical effects, including enhancing insulin sensitivity (Figure 18.4) (67). The reasons for this discrepancy are not clear, since carbenoxolone and glycyrrhetinic acid have

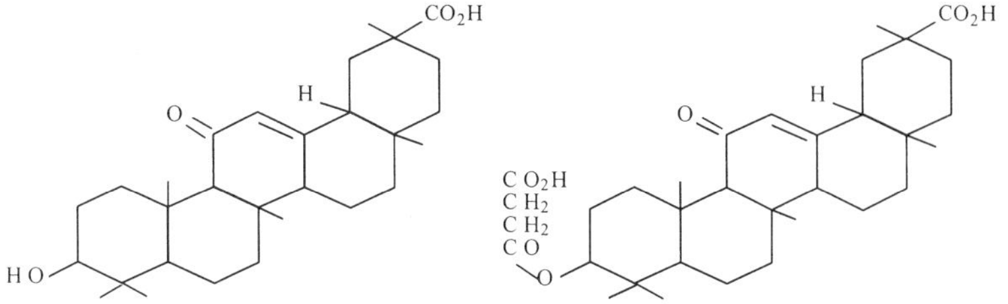

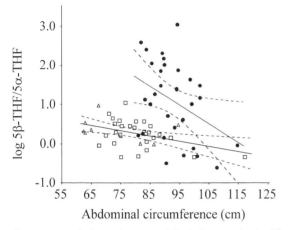

Glycyrrhetinic acid   Carbenoxolone

Figure 18.9 11β-HSD inhibitors. Glycyrrhetinic acid is the principal active constituent of liquorice. Carbenoxolone is a synthetic hemisuccinate derivative

Figure 18.10 A-ring reductase activity in human obesity. The ratio 5β-/5α-tetrahydrocortisol reflects relative activities of 5α- and 5β-reductases. This study of 68 healthy men (filled symbols) and postmenopausal women (open symbols; triangles indicate those receiving oestrogen replacement therapy) aged 47–53 years from a cross-sectional cohort study revealed higher excretion of 5α-tetrahydrocortisol in subjects with central obesity. Adapted from Andrew *et al.* (163)

similar affinities for both 11β-HSD isozymes *in vitro*. It probably relates to pharmacokinetic factors, perhaps because carbenoxolone is water soluble whereas glycyrrhetinic acid is lipid soluble and hydrophobic.

The effects of liquorice derivatives are not selective for 11β-HSD enzymes. These compounds also inhibit enzymes metabolizing prostaglandins (157). In addition, they inhibit 5β-reductase *in vitro* (see below) (152).

5α-Reductase Inhibitors

Arguably the most successful example of therapeutic manipulation of pre-receptor ligand metabolism to date is the use of finasteride to inhibit

5α-reductase type 2. This is used in the treatment of benign prostatic hyperplasia and in prostatic carcinoma. It has a weak effect to reduce androgen receptor activation in skin and may be useful in the treatment of hirsutism and male-pattern baldness. Finasteride is relatively, but not completely, specific for the human type 2 5α-reductase isozyme. It has also been shown to alter cortisol metabolism in one small study (158), although the impact on glucocorticoid receptor activation was not assessed.

Selective 5α-reductase type 1 inhibitors exist (159), but have not been employed therapeutically.

ALTERED CORTISOL METABOLISM IN OBESITY

Cortisol Metabolism in Primary Obesity

Relatively small case-control studies, almost exclusively in women, showed that obesity, particularly of predominantly abdominal distribution, is associated with increased urinary free cortisol excretion (160–162). However, as detailed above, urinary free cortisol forms a very small fraction of total cortisol metabolite excretion. More convincingly, recent large studies confirm that total cortisol production rate is somewhat enhanced in obesity in men as well as women (131,163,164). This is further supported by evidence of enhanced responsiveness of the hypothalamic-pituitary-adrenal axis to ACTH and CRH (161,165). However, in obesity plasma cortisol levels are not consistently elevated. Indeed, peak plasma cortisol levels in the morning are low (166–169). The combination of increased secretion with low morning plasma levels suggests either that diurnal variation of cortisol secretion is disrupted, or that peripheral metabolism of cortisol is enhanced.

Previous studies using radioisotope tracers showed that metabolic clearance rate for cortisol is indeed enhanced in obesity (170). Very recent studies have identified which specific pathways of cortisol metabolism are involved. In a study of 68 men and women, we reported elevated ratios of cortisol/cortisone metabolites in obese men and elevated excretion of 5α-reduced metabolites in obese men and women (Figure 18.10) (163). Our finding of enhanced 5α-reduced metabolites in obesity has been confirmed in a further independent study of nearly 500 men and women (164) and in our own unpublished observations in an additional 300 subjects. It is likely that the same change explains the observation of increased 5α-reduced cortisol metabolites in polycystic ovary syndrome (171). We have also observed increased hepatic 5α-reductase type 1 activity in liver of leptin-resistant, obese Zucker rats (72).

However, cortisol/cortisone metabolite ratios have proved less consistent in further studies. Stewart and colleagues (131) studied 36 men and women and reported that the obese group ($n = 12$) had impaired conversion of oral cortisone to cortisol in peripheral plasma—suggesting impaired hepatic 11β-reductase activity (Figure 18.4). This was associated with lower ratios of cortisol/cortisone metabolites, and relatively impaired inactivation of cortisol by 5α-reductase (Figure 18.2). By contrast, Katz *et al.* examined arteriovenous differences in cortisol/cortisone ratio across subcutaneous abdominal fat and found a trend towards increased 11β-HSD1 activity in obesity (57). A likely explanation for these discrepancies is that there are tissue-specific differences in the activity of 11β-HSD type 1 in obesity (72), with impaired conversion of cortisone to cortisol in liver but normal or enhanced conversion in adipose tissue and perhaps other sites. The sum may frequently be no overall change in urinary metabolites. Indeed, we have evidence in favour of such tissue-specific changes in 11β-HSD1 activity from leptin-resistant obese Zucker rats (72).

We have therefore proposed that in obesity enhanced cortisol clearance by 5α-reductase may lower plasma cortisol levels, thereby reducing negative feedback and providing a key stimulus to the hypothalamic-pituitary-adrenal axis. Such enhanced cortisol clearance will be exacerbated by impaired regeneration of cortisol from cortisone by reduced 11β-HSD1 in liver. However, this results in an elevated pool of cortisol metabolites, including cortisone, available for potential reactivation. In tissues where 11β-HSD1 activity is maintained or even enhanced (e.g. adipose tissue), the local cortisol levels may be elevated in the face of overall increased metabolic clearance rate (Figure 18.11).

At present we can only speculate on the mechanism of altered cortisol metabolism in obesity. The regulation of relevant enzymes by hormones which are disturbed in obesity is clearly relevant (Table 18.4), but none of these have yet been manipulated in obese subjects to assess reversibility of the dysregulation of cortisol metabolism.

Cortisol Metabolism and Growth Hormone Deficiency

Adult growth hormone deficiency is associated with a syndrome which includes lethargy, dyslipidaemia and central obesity. The mechanisms whereby growth hormone and insulin-like growth factor 1 (IGF-1) influence body fat distribution are poorly characterized, and may be mediated indirectly by changes in glucocorticoid receptor activation. In growth-hormone deficient rats, female pattern (continuous administration) growth hormone replacement potently downregulates hepatic 11β-HSD1 expression (172). By contrast, male pattern (pulsatile) growth hormone does not affect enzyme activity. Similar effects of growth hormone and IGF-1 have been reported in human adipose stromal cells in primary culture. In humans, evidence is restricted to interpretation of urinary cortisol metabolites, and studies in hypopituitary patients are confounded by the effect of oral cortisol replacement therapy. However, it appears that continuous (daily subcutaneous injection) growth hormone replacement inhibits 11β-HSD1 on the basis that cortisol/cortisone metabolite ratios are lower and urinary free cortisol/cortisone ratios either unchanged or elevated (173–175). Thus, growth hormone deficiency may well be associated with enhanced adipose 11β-HSD1 and higher intra-adipose cortisol concentrations. It is an intriguing speculation that many of the benefits of growth hormone replacement in adult hypopituitary patients—reduced central adiposity, normalization of dyslipidaemia, and

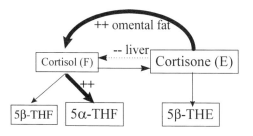

Figure 18.11 A model of consequences of tissue-specific changes in cortisol metabolism in obesity

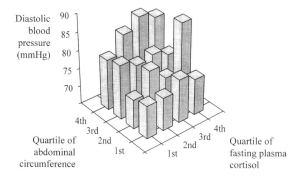

Figure 18.12 Interaction of increasing plasma cortisol and obesity in predicting blood pressure. Data are from 226 otherwise healthy men and women from the MONICA cross-sectional cohort study in northern Sweden. Obesity in this population is associated with lower 0900 h plasma cortisol concentrations, but both obesity and higher plasma cortisol are independently associated with higher blood pressure. This emphasizes that the mechanisms underlying elevated cortisol concentrations in hypertension are likely to be different from those in obesity, and it is those obese subjects who fail to show a characteristic fall in plasma cortisol levels who may be subject to the greatest metabolic complications. Adapted from Walker et al. (167)

enhanced insulin sensitivity—might perhaps be achieved at no cost by lowering the replacement dose of oral hydrocortisone!

Interactions Between Cortisol, Obesity and Other Cardiovascular Risk Factors

Cushing's syndrome is characterized not only by central obesity, but also by hypertension, dyslipidaemia, insulin resistance, and glucose intolerance. This cluster of clinical features bears remarkably similarity to the cluster which occurs in the metabolic syndrome (Reaven's syndrome X; the insulin resistance syndrome). It is possible that a more subtle increase in cortisol action explains the association between these features of the metabolic syndrome and obesity.

In case-control and cross-sectional studies, high blood pressure is associated with elevated cortisol concentrations (in blood, saliva or urine) (164,168,176–179), impaired peripheral inactivation of cortisol by 11β-HSD2 (127,151), and enhanced tissue sensitivity to glucocorticoids as measured by the intensity of dermal vasoconstriction following topical application of beclomethasone (179,180). Similarly, insulin resistance and glucose intolerance are associated with higher circulating cortisol levels (169) and increased dermal vasoconstrictor sensitivity to beclomethasone (179,180). Higher morning plasma cortisol concentrations and increased responsiveness to ACTH also occur in adults with the additional cardiovascular risk factor of low birthweight (169,181). However, all of these associations between cortisol activity and hypertension/insulin resistance are independent of obesity. Obesity is associated with lower (not higher) plasma cortisol, no change in 11β-HSD2 (rather, alterations in 11β-HSD1; see above), and no difference in dermal responses to glucocorticoids.

From these observational studies it is not possible to dissect causality but they do not favour a proposed unifying hypothesis (182) which ascribes the associations between obesity and other features of the metabolic syndrome X to enhanced cortisol secretion. Rather, there may be a primary increase in hypothalamic-pituitary-adrenal axis activity and tissue sensitivity to glucocorticoids in subjects with hypertension/insulin resistance which does not directly predispose to obesity. However, if these individuals become obese, then perhaps acquired changes in 5α-reductase and 11β-HSD1 activities result in higher local glucocorticoid concentrations and amplification of hypertension and insulin resistance. In support of this concept of 'amplification' by obesity, the highest blood pressure in cross-sectional studies occurs amongst relatively rare individuals who are most obese but who have the highest morning plasma cortisol (167,169) (Figure 18.12).

Therapeutic Opportunities

No matter whether the changes in cortisol metabolism are primary or secondary to obesity and/or its associated neurohumoral disturbances, their influence on the hypothalamic-pituitary-adrenal axis and glucocorticoid receptor activation may be a key step in the cascade leading to adverse metabolic consequences of obesity. Therefore, therapeutic intervention to reverse the tissue-specific alterations in cortisol metabolism in obesity may be extremely useful. The results of experiments with 11β-HSD1 and 5α-reductase inhibitors in obesity are awaited with interest.

CONCLUSIONS

This chapter presents evidence that variations in cortisol metabolism play a key role in modulating cortisol secretion and action. There is a clear hypothesis that these mechanisms are important in obesity, but the limitations of current methodology for assessing cortisol metabolism *in vivo* in humans mean that current data remain preliminary. Nevertheless, the results suggest that there are tissue-specific changes in cortisol metabolism in obesity which predict enhanced glucocorticoid action in adipose tissue but not liver. We suggest that these changes are secondary to the obesity but nonetheless may amplify the link between elevated cortisol activity and hypertension or insulin resistance which we have observed in other studies. This area is likely to be the focus of important research in the next few years, when we will learn whether therapeutic manipulation of cortisol metabolism is to become a successful novel approach to limiting the metabolic consequences of obesity.

ACKNOWLEDGEMENTS

Our studies are supported by major grants from the British Heart Foundation and Wellcome Trust. We are grateful to Dr Ruth Andrew for assistance with preparation of material for this chapter.

REFERENCES

1. Andrews RC, Walker BR. Glucocorticoids and insulin resistance: old hormones, new targets. *Clin Sci* 1999; **96**: 513–523.
2. Samra JS, Clark ML, Humphreys SM, MacDonald IA, Bannister PA, Frayn, KN. Effects of physiological hypercortisolemia on the regulation of lipolysis in subcutaneous adipose tissue. *J Clin Endocrinol & Metabol* 1998; **83**: 626–631.
3. Bronnegard M, Arner P, Hellstrom L. Glucocorticoid receptor messenger ribonucleic acid in different regions of human adipose tissue. *Endocrinology* 1990; **127**: 1689–1696.
4. Bujalska IJ, Kumar S, Stewart PM. Does central obesity reflect 'Cushing's disease of the omentum'? *Lancet* 1997; **349**: 1210–1213.
5. Bjorntorp P, Holm G, Rosmond R. Hypothalamic arousal, insulin resistance and type 2 diabetes mellitus. *Diabet Med* 1999; **16**: 373–381.
6. Monder C, White PC. 11β-Hydroxysteroid dehydrogenase. *Vitam Horm* 1993; **47**: 187–271.
7. Agarwal AK, Monder C, Eckstein B, White PC. Cloning and expression of rat cDNA encoding corticosteroid 11β-dehydrogenase. *J Biol Chem* 1989; **264**: 18939–18943.
8. Agarwal AK, Mune T, Monder C, White PC. NAD$^+$-dependent isoform of 11β-hydroxysteroid dehydrogenase. Cloning and characterisation of cDNA from sheep kidney. *J Biol Chem* 1994; **269**: 25959–25962.
9. Albiston AL, Obeyesekere VR, Smith RE, Krozowski ZS. Cloning and tissue distribution of the human 11β-hydroxysteroid dehydrogenase type 2 enzyme. *Mol Cell Endocrinol* 1994; **105**: R11–R17.
10. Brown RW, Chapman KE, Koteletsev Y, Yau JL, Lindsay RS, Brett LP, Leckie CM, Murad P, Lyons V, Mullins JJ, Edwards CRW, Seckl JR. Cloning and production of antisera to human placental 11β-hydroxysteroid dehydrogenase type 2. *Biochem J* 1996; **313**: 1007–1017.
11. Murphy BEP, Branchaud CTL. Fetal metabolism of cortisol. *Curr Top Exp Endocrinol* 1983; **5**: 197–229.
12. Brown RW, Diaz R, Robson AC, Kotelevtsev YV, Mullins JJ, Kaufman MH, Seckl JR. The ontogeny of 11beta-hydroxysteroid dehydrogenase type 2 and mineralocorticoid receptor gene expression reveal intricate control of glucocorticoid action in development. *Endocrinology* 1996; **137**: 794–797.
13. Stewart PM, Murry BA, Mason JI. Type 2 11β-hydroxysteroid dehydrogenase in human fetal tissues. *J Clin Endocrinol Metab* 1994; **78**: 1529–1532.
14. Stewart PM, Rogerson FM, Mason JI. Type 2 11β-hydroxysteroid dehydrogenase messenger RNA and activity in human placenta and fetal membranes: its relationship to birth weight and putative role in fetal steroidogenesis. *J Clin Endocrinol Metab* 1995; **80**: 885–890.
15. Brown RW, Chapman KE, Murad P, Edwards CW, Seckl JR. Purification of 11beta-hydroxysteroid dehydrogenase type 2 from human placenta utilizing a novel affinity labelling technique. *Biochem J* 1996; **313**: 997–1005.
16. Waddell BJ, Benediktsson R, Brown RW, Seckl JR. Tissue-specific messenger ribonucleic acid expression of 11beta-hydroxysteroid dehydrogenase types 1 and 2 and the glucocorticoid receptor within rat placenta suggests exquisite local control of glucocorticoid action. *Endocrinology* 1998; **139**: 1517–1523.
17. Smith RE, Maguire JA, Stein-Oakley AN, Sasano H, Takahashi K, Fukushima K, Krozowski ZS. Localization of 11beta-hydroxysteroid dehydrogenase type II in human epithelial tissues. *J Clin Endocrinol Metab* 1996; **81**: 3244–3248.
18. Hirasawa G, Sasano H, Takahashi K-I, Fukushima K,

Suzuki T, Hiwatashi, Toyota T, Krozowski ZS, Nagura H. Colocalization of 11beta-hydroxysteroid dehydrogenase type II and mineralocorticoid receptor in human epithelia. *J Clin Endocrinol Metab* 1997; **82**: 3859–3863.

19. Suzuki T, Sasano H, Suzuki S, Hirasawa G, Takeyama J, Muramatsu Y, Date F, Nagura H, Krozowski ZS. 11beta-Hydroxysteroid dehydrogenase type 2 in human lung: Possible regulator of mineralocorticoid action. *J Clin Endocrinol Metab* 1998; **83**: 4022–4025.

20. Page N, Warriar N, Govindan MV. 11beta-Hydroxysteroid dehydrogenase activity in human lung cells and transcription regulation by glucocorticoid. *Am J Physiol (Lung Cellular and Molecular Physiology)* 1994; **267**: L464–L474.

21. Brem AS, Bina RB, King TC, Morris DJ. Localization of 2 11beta-OH steroid dehydrogenase isoforms in aortic endothelial cells. *Hypertension* 1998; **31**: 459–462.

22. Hatakeyama H, Inaba S, Miyamori I. 11beta-Hydroxysteroid dehydrogenase in cultured human vascular cells: Possible role in the development of hypertension. *Hypertension* 1999; **33**: 1179–1184.

23. Hennebold JD, Ryu S-Y, Mu H-H, Galbraith A, Daynes RA. 11—Hydroxysteroid dehydrogenase modulation of glucocorticoid activities in lymphoid organs. *Am J Physiol* 1996; **270**: R1296–R1306.

24. Edwards CRW, Stewart PM, Burt D, Brett L, McIntyre MA, Sutanto WS, DeKloet ER, Monder C. Localisation of 11β-hydroxysteroid dehydrogenase—tissue specific protector of the mineralocorticoid receptor. *Lancet* 1988; **ii**: 986–989.

25. Agarwal AK, Tusie-Luna M-T, Monder C, White PC. Expression of 11β-hydroxysteroid dehydrogenase using recombinant vaccinia virus. *Mol Endocrinol* 1990; **4**: 1827–1832.

26. Walker BR, Campbell JC, Fraser R, Stewart PM, Edwards CRW. Mineralocorticoid excess and inhibition of 11β-hydroxysteroid dehydrogenase in patients with ectopic ACTH syndrome. *Clin Endocrinol (Oxf)* 1992; **27**: 483–492.

27. Low SC, Chapman KE, Edwards CRW, Seckl JR. 'Liver-type' 11β-hydroxysteroid dehydrogenase cDNA encodes reductase but not dehydrogenase activity in intact mammalian COS-7 cells. *J Mol Endocrinol* 1994; **13**: 167–174.

28. Jamieson PM, Chapman KE, Edwards CRW, Seckl JR. 11β-Hydroxysteroid dehydrogenase is an exclusive 11β-reductase in primary cultures of rat hepatocytes: effect of physicochemical and hormonal manipulations. *Endocrinology* 1995; **136**: 4754–4761.

29. Rajan V, Edwards CRW, Seckl JR. 11β-Hydroxysteroid dehydrogenase in cultured hippocampal cells reactivates inert 11-dehydrocorticosterone, potentiating neurotoxicity. *J Neurosci* 1996; **16**: 65–70.

30. Agarwal AK, Mune T, Monder C, White PC. 1995 Mutations in putative glycosylation sites of rat 11beta-hydroxysteroid dehydrogenase affect enzymatic activity. *Biochim Biophys Acta (Protein Structure and Molecular Enzymology)* **1248**: 70–74.

31. Stewart PM, Murry BA, Mason JI. Human kidney 11β-hydroxysteroid dehydrogenase is a high affinity nicotinamide adenine dinucleotide-dependent enzyme and differs from the cloned type 1 isoform. *J Clin Endocrinol Metab* 1994; **79**: 480–484.

32. Ricketts ML, Verhaeg JM, Bujalska I, Howie AJ, Rainey WE, Stewart PM. Immunohistochemical localization of type 1 11beta-hydroxysteroid dehydrogenase in human tissues. *J Clin Endocrinol Metab* 1998; **83**: 1325–1335.

33. Napolitano A, Voice MW, Edwards CW, Seckl JR, Chapman KE. 11beta-Hydroxysteroid dehydrogenase 1 in adipocytes: Expression is differentiation-dependent and hormonally regulated. *J Steroid Biochem Mol Biol* 1998; **64**: 251–260.

34. Hundertmark S, Ragosch V, Schein B, Buhler H, Fromm M, Lorenz U, Weitzel HK. 11-Beta-hydroxysteroid dehydrogenase of rat lung: Enzyme kinetic, oxidase–reductase ratio, electrolyte and trace element dependence. *Enzyme Protein* 1993; **47**: 83–91.

35. Walker BR, Yau JL, Brett LP, Seckl JR, Monder C, Williams BC, Edwards CRW. 11β-Hydroxysteroid dehydrogenase in vascular smooth muscle and heart: implications for cardiovascular responses to glucocorticoids. *Endocrinology* 1991; **129**: 3305–3312.

36. Brem AS, Bina RB, King T, Morris DJ. Bidirectional activity of 11β-hydroxysteroid dehydrogenase in vascular smooth muscle cells. *Steroids* 1995; **60**: 406–410.

37. Moisan M-P, Seckl JR, Edwards CRW. 11β-Hydroxysteroid dehydrogenase bioactivity and messenger RNA expression in rat forebrain: localization in hypothalamus, hippocampus and cortex. *Endocrinology* 1990; **127**: 1450–1455.

38. Moisan M-P, Seckl JR, Monder C, Agarwal AK, White PC, Edwards CRW. 11β-Hydroxysteroid dehydrogenase mRNA expression, bioactivity and immunoreactivity in rat cerebellum. *Neuroendocrinology* 1990; **2**: 853–858.

39. Sakai RR, Lakshmi V, Monder C, McEwen BS. Immunocytochemical localization of 11beta-hydroxysteroid dehydrogenase in hippocampus and other brain regions of the rat. *J Neuroendocrinol* 1992; **4**: 101–106.

40. Shimojo M, Whorwood CB, Stewart PM. 11beta-Hydroxysteroid dehydrogenase in the rat adrenal. *J Mol Endocrinol* 1996; **17**: 121–130.

41. Kondo K-H, Kai M-H, Setoguchi Y, Eggertsen G, Sjoblom P, Setoguchi T, Okuda K-I, Bjorkhem I. Cloning and expression of cDNA of human delta4-3-oxosteroid 5beta-reductase and substrate specificity of the expressed enzyme. *Eur J Biochem* 1994; **219**: 357–363.

42. Jenkins EP, Andersson S, Imperato-McGinley J, Wilson JD, Russell DW. Genetic and pharmacological evidence for more than one human steroid 5alpha-reductase. *J Clin Invest* 1992; **89**: 293–300.

43. Killinger DW, Perel E, Daniilescu D, Kharlip L, Lindsay WN. Influence of adipose tissue distribution on the biological activity of androgens. *Ann N Y Acad Sci* 1990; **595**: 199–211.

44. Russell DW, Wilson JD. Steroid 5α-reductase: two genes/two enzymes. *Ann Rev Biochem* 1994; **63**: 25–61.

45. Morris DJ, Latif SA, Rokaw MD, Watlington CO, Johnson JP. A second enzyme protecting mineralocorticoid receptors from glucocorticoid occupancy. *Am J Physiol* 1998; **274**: C1245–C1252.

46. Waxman DJ, Attisano C, Guengerich FP, Lapenson DP. Human liver microsomal steroid metabolism: Identification of the major microsomal steroid hormone 6beta-hydroxylase cytochrome P-450 enzyme. *Arch Biochem Biophys* 1988; **263**: 424–436.

47. Abel SM, Back DJ, Maggs JL, Park BK. Cortisol metabolism in vitro—II. Species difference. *J Steroid Biochem Mol Biol* 1993; **45**: 445–453.

48. Abel SM, Back DJ. Cortisol metabolism in vitro—III. Inhibition of microsomal 6beta- hydroxylase and cytosolic 4-ene-reductas. *J Steroid Biochem Mol Biol* 1993; **46**: 827–832.

49. Bush IE. 11β-hydroxysteroid dehydrogenase: contrast between studies in vivo and studies in vitro. *Adv Biosci* 1969; **3**: 23–39.

50. Hellman L, Nakada F, Zumoff B, Fukushima D, Bradlow HL, Gallacher TF. Renal capture and oxidation of cortisol in man. *J Clin Endocrinol* 1971; **33**: 52–62.

51. Whitworth JA, Stewart PM, Burt D, Atherden SM, Edwards CRW. The kidney is the major site of cortisone production in man. *Clin Endocrinol (Oxf)* 1989; **31**: 355–361.

52. Yang K, Matthews SG. Cellular localization of 11beta-hydroxysteroid dehydrogenase 2 gene expression in the ovine adrenal glan. *Mol Cell Endocrinol* 1995; **111**: R19–R23.

53. Mazzocchi G, Rossi GP, Neri G, Malendowicz LK, Albertin G, Nussdorfer, GG. 11beta-Hydroxysteroid dehydrogenase expression and activity in the human adrenal cortex. *FASEB J* 1998; **12**: 1533–1539.

54. Musajo F, Neri G, Tortorella C, Mazzocchi G, Nussdorfer GG. Intra-adrenal 11beta-hydroxysteroid dehydrogen-ase plays a role in the regulation of corticosteroid secretion: An in vitro study in the rat. *Life Sci* 1996; **59**: 1401–1406.

55. Dazord A, Saez J, Bertrand J. Metabolic clearance rates and interconversion of cortisol and cortisone. *J Clin Endocrinol Metab* 1972; **35**: 24–34.

56. Hubbard WC, Bickel C, Schleimer RP. Simultaneous quantitation of endogenous levels of cortisone and cortisol in human nasal and bornchoalveolar lavage fluids and plasma via gas chromatography-negative ion chemical ionization spectrometry. *Ann Biochem* 1994; **221**: 109–117.

57. Katz JR, Mohamed-Ali V, Wood PJ, Yudkin JS, Coppack SW. An in vivo study of the cortisol-cortisone shuttle in subcutaneous abdominal adipose tissue. *Clin Endocrinol* 1999; **50**: 63–68.

58. Stewart PM, Sheppard MC. Novel aspects of hormone action: intracellular ligand supply and its control by a series of tissue specific enzymes. *Mol Cell Endocrinol* 1992; **83**: C13–18.

59. Arriza JL, Weinberger C, Cerelli G. Cloning of human mineralocorticoid receptor complementary DNA; structural and functional kinship with the glucocorticoid receptor. *Science* 1987; **237**: 268–275.

60. Sheppard K, Funder JW. Mineralocorticoid specificity of renal type 1 receptors; in vivo binding studies. *Am J Physiol* 1987; **252**: E224–E229.

61. Funder JW, Pearce PT, Smith R, Smith AI. Mineralocorticoid action: target tissue specificity is enzyme, not receptor, mediated. *Science* 1988; **242**: 583–585.

62. Wilson RC, Harbison MD, Krozowski ZS, Funder JW, Shackleton CHL, Hanauske-Abel HM, Wei J-Q, Hertecant J, Moran A, Neiberger RE, Balfe JW, Fattah A, Daneman D, Licholai T, New MI. Several homozygous mutations in the gene for 11β-hydroxysteroid dehydrogenase type 2 in patients with apparent mineralocorticoid excess. *J Clin Endocrinol Metab* 1995; **80**: 3145–3150.

63. Stewart PM, Valentino R, Wallace AM, Burt D, Shackleton CHL, Edwards CRW. Mineralocorticoid activity of liquorice: 11β-hydroxysteroid dehydrogenase deficiency comes of age. *Lancet* 1987; **ii**: 821–824.

64. Stewart PM, Wallace AM, Atherden SM, Shearing CH, Edwards CRW. Mineralocorticoid activity of carbenoxolone: contrasting effects of carbenoxolone and liquorice on 11β-hydroxysteroid dehydrogenase activity in man. *Clin Sci* 1990; **78**: 49–54.

65. Kotelevtsev YV, Brown RW, Fleming S, Edwards CRW, Seckl JR, Mullins JJ. Hypertension in mice caused by inactivation of 11β-hydroxysteroid dehydrogenase type 2. *J Clin Invest* 1999; **103**: 683–689.

66. Ulick S, Levine LS, Gunczler P, Zanconato G, Ramirez LC, Rauh W, Rosler A, Bradlow HL, New MI. A syndrome of apparent mineralocorticoid excess associated with defects in the peripheral metabolism of cortisol. *J Clin Endocrinol Metab* 1979; **49**: 757–764.

67. Walker BR, Connacher AA, Lindsay RM, Webb DJ, Edwards CRW. Carbenoxolone increases hepatic insulin sensitivity in man: a novel role for 11-oxosteroid reductase in enhancing glucocorticoid receptor activation. *J Clin Endocrinol Metab* 1995 80: 3155–3159.

68. Jamieson PM, Nyirenda MJ, Walker BR, Chapman KE, Seckl JR. Interactions between oestradiol and glucocorticoid regulatory effects on liver-specific glucocorticoid-inducible genes: possible evidence for a role of hepatic 11β-hydroxysteroid dehydrogenase type 1. *J Endocrinol* 1998; **160**: 103–109.

69. Kotelevtsev YV, Holmes MC, Burchell A, Houston PM, Scholl D, Jamieson PM, Best R, Brown RW, Edwards CRW, Seckl JR, Mullins JJ. 11β-Hydroxysteroid dehydrogenase type 1 knockout mice show attenuated glucocorticoid inducible responses and resist hyperglycaemia on obesity and stress. *Proc Natl Acad Sci USA* 1997; **94**: 14924–14929.

70. Yang K, Khalil MW, Strutt BJ, Killinger DW. 11beta-Hydroxysteroid dehydrogenase 1 activity and gene expression in human adipose stromal cells: Effect on aromatase activity. *J Steroid Biochem Mol Biol* 1997; **60**: 247–253.

71. Weaver JU, Thaventhiran L, Noonan K, Burrin JM, Taylor NF, Norman MR, Monson JP. The effect of growth hormone replacement on cortisol metabolism and glucocorticoid sensitivity in hypopituitary adults. *Clin Endocrinol (Oxf)* 1994; **41**: 639–648.

72. Livingstone DEW, Jones GC, Smith K, Andrew R, Kenyon CJ, Walker BR. Understanding the role of glucocorticoids in obesity: tissue-specific alterations of corticosterone metabolism in obese Zucker rats. *Endocrinology* 2000; **141**: 560–563.

73. de Kloet ER. Brain corticosteroid receptor balance and homeostatic control. *Front Neuroendocrinol* 1991; **12**: 95–164.

74. Jacobson L, Sapolsky R. The role of the hippocampus in feedback regulation of the hypothalamic-pituitary-adrenocortical axis. *Endocr Rev* 1991; **12**: 118–134.

75. Bradbury MJ, Akana SF, Dallman MF. Roles of type I and II corticosteroid receptors in regulation of basal activity in the hypothalamo-pituitary-adrenal axis during the diurnal trough and the peak: Evidence for a nonadditive effect of combined receptor occupation. *Endocrinology* 1994; **134**:

1286–1296.

76. Tempel DL, Leibowitz SF. Adrenal steroid receptors: Interactions with brain neuropeptide systems in relation to nutrient intake and metabolism. *J Neuroendocrinol* 1994; **6**: 479–501.

77. Jacobson L. Glucocorticoid replacement, but not corticotropin-releasing hormone deficiency, prevents adrenalectomy-induced anorexia in mice. *Endocrinology* 1999; **140**: 310–317.

78. Devenport L, Knehans A, Thomas T, Sundstrom A. Macronutrient intake and utilization by rats: Interactions with type I adrenocorticoid receptor stimulation. *Am J Physiol* 1991; **260**: R73–R81.

79. Tempel DL, Leibowitz SF. PVN steroid implants: Effect on feeding patterns and macronutrient selection. *Brain Res Bull* 1989; **23**: 553–560.

80. McEwen BS, de Kloet ER, Rostene W. Adrenal steroid receptors and actions in the nervous system. *Physiol Rev* 1986; **66**: 1121–1188.

81. Robson AC, Leckie CM, Seckl JR, Holmes MC. 11beta-Hydroxysteroid dehydrogenase type 2 in the postnatal and adult rat brain. *Mol Brain Res* 1998; **61**: 1–10.

82. Roland BL, Li KZ, Funder JW. Hybridization histochemical localization of 11beta-hydroxysteroid dehydrogenase type 2 in rat brain. *Endocrinology* 1995; **136**: 4697–4700.

83. McEwen BS, Lambdin LT, Rainbow TC, De Nicola AF. Aldosterone effects on salt appetite in adrenalectomized rats. *Neuroendocrinology* 1986; **43**: 38–43.

84. Sakai RR, Nicolaidis S, Epstein AN. Salt appetite is suppressed by interference with angiotensin II and aldosterone. *Am J Physiol* 1986; **251**: R762–R768.

85. Seckl JR. 11beta-Hydroxysteroid dehydrogenase in the brain: A novel regulator of glucocorticoid action? *Front Neuroendocrinol* 1997; **18**: 49–99.

86. Mahendroo MS, Cala KM, Landrum CP, Russell DW. Fetal death in mice lacking 5alpha-reductase type 1 caused by estrogen excess. *Mol Endocrinol* 1997; **11**: 917–927.

87. Hennebold JD, Mu H-H, Poynter ME, Chen X-P, Daynes RA. Active catabolism of glucocorticoids by 11beta-hydroxysteroid dehydrogenase in vivo is a necessary requirement for natural resistance to infection with Listeria monocytogenes. *Int Immunol* 1997; **9**: 105–115.

88. Hennebold JD, Daynes RA. Inhibition of skin 11beta-hydroxysteroid dehydrogenase activity in vivo potentiates the anti-inflammatory actions of glucocorticoids. *Arch Dermatol Res* 1998; **290**: 413–419.

89. Teelucksingh S, Mackie ADR, Burt D, McIntyre MA, Brett L, Edwards CRW. Potentiation of hydrocortisone activity in skin by glycyrrhetinic acid. *Lancet* 1990; **335**: 1060–1063.

90. Walker BR, Connacher AA, Webb DJ, Edwards CRW. Glucocorticoids and blood pressure: a role for the cortisol/cortisone shuttle in the control of vascular tone in man. *Clin Sci* 1992; **83**: 171–178.

91. Walker BR, Sang KS, Williams BC, Edwards CRW. Direct and indirect effects of carbenoxolone on responses to glucocorticoids and noradrenaline in rat aorta. *J Hypertens* 1994; **12**: 33–39.

92. Phillipou G, Palermo M, Shackleton CHL. Apparent cortisone reductase deficiency; a unique form of hypercortisolism. *J Clin Endocrinol Metab* 1996; **81**: 3855–3860.

93. Jamieson A, Wallace AM, Walker BR, Andrew R, Fraser R, White PC, Connell JMC. Apparent cortisone reductase deficiency: a functional defect in 11β-hydroxysteroid dehydrogenase type 1. *J Clin Endocrinol Metab* 1999; **84**: 3570–3574.

94. Murphy BEP. Ontogeny of cortisol-cortisone interconversion in human tissues; a role for cortisone in human fetal development. *J Steroid Biochem* 1981; **14**: 811–817.

95. Condon J, Gosden C, Gardener D, Nickson P, Hewison M, Howie AJ, Stewart PM. Expression of type 2 11beta-hydroxysteroid dehydrogenase and corticosteroid hormone receptors in early human fetal life. *J Clin Endocrinol Metab* 1998; **83**: 4490–4497.

96. Williams LS, Lyons V, Wallace R, Seckl JR, Chapman KE. CCAAT/enhancer binding protein positively regulates the rat 11beta-hydroxysteroid dehydrogenase type 1 promoter in liver cells. *Biochem Soc Trans* 1997; **25**: 235S.

97. Voice MW, Seckl JR, Chapman KE. The sequence of 5′ flanking DNA from the mouse 11beta- hydroxysteroid dehydrogenase type 1 gene and analysis of putative transcription factor binding sites. *Gene* 1996; **181**: 233–235.

98. Mode A, Rafter I. The sexually differentiated Delta4-3-ketosteroid 5beta-reductase of rat liver. Purification, characterization, and quantitation. *J Biol Chem* 1985; **260**: 7137–7141.

99. Tsuji M, Terada N, Yabumoto H. Hormonal regulation of activities of 4-ene-5beta and 5alpha-reductases and 17beta-ol-dehydrogenase in immature golden hamster ovary. *J Steroid Biochem* 1983; **18**: 777–781.

100. Melcangi RC, Poletti A, Cavarretta I, Celotti F, Colciago A, Magnaghi, Motta M, Negri-Cesi P, Martini L. The 5alpha-reductase in the central nervous system: Expression and modes of control. *J Steroid Biochem Mol Biol* 1998; **65**: 295–299.

101. Berman DM, Tian H, Russell DW. Expression and regulation of steroid 5alpha-reductase in the urogenital tract of the fetal rat. *Mol Endocrinol* 1995; **9**: 1561–1570.

102. Yokoi H, Tsuruo Y, Miyamoto T, Ishimura K. Steroid 5alpha-reductase type 1 immunolocalized in the adrenal gland of normal, gonadectomized, and sex hormone-supplemented rats. *Histochemistry* 1998; **109**: 127–134.

103. Eicheler W, Seitz J, Steinhoff M, Forssmann WG, Adermann K, Aumuller. Distribution of rat hepatic steroid 5alpha-reductase 1 as shown by immunohistochemistry. *Exp Clin Endocrinol Diabetes* 1995; **103**: 105–112.

104. Zyirek M, Flood C, Longcope C. 5alpha-Reductase activity in rat adipose tissue. *Proc Soc Exp Biol Med* 1987; **186**: 134–138.

105. Bullock P, Gemzik B, Johnson D, Thomas P, Parkinson A. Evidence from dwarf rats that growth hormone may not regulate the sexual differentiation of liver cytochrome P450 enzymes and steroid 5alpha-reductase. *Proc Nat Acad Sci USA* 1991; **88**: 5227–5231.

106. Lephart ED, Simpson ER, Trzeciak WH. Rat adrenal 5alpha-reductase mRNA content and enzyme activity are sex hormone dependent. *J Mol Endocrinol* 1991; **6**: 163–170.

107. Reiter E, Kecha O, Hennuy B, Lardinois S, Klug M, Bruyninx M, Closset J, Hennen G. Growth hormone directly affects the function of the different lobes of the rat prostate. *Endocrinology* 1995; **136**: 3338–3345.

108. Suzuki K, Takezawa Y, Suzuki T, Honma S, Yamanaka H. Synergistic effects of estrogen with androgen on the pros-

tate—Effects of estrogen on the prostate of androgen-administered rats and 5-alpha-reductase activity. *Prostate* 1994; **25**: 169–176.

109. Morris DJ, Semafuko WEB, Latif SA, Vogel B, Grimes C, Sheff MF. Detection of glycyrrhetinic acid-like factors (GALFs) in human urine. *Hypertension* 1992; **20**: 356–360.

110. Walker BR, Aggarwal I, Stewart PM, Padfield PL, Edwards CRW. Endogenous inhibitors of 11β-hydroxysteroid dehydrogenase in hypertension. *J Clin Endocrinol Metab* 1995; **80**: 529–533.

111. Walker BR, Williamson PM, Brown MA, Honour JW, Edwards CRW, Whitworth JA. 11β-hydroxysteroid dehydrogenase and its inhibitors in hypertensive pregnancy *Hypertension* 1995; **25**: 626–630.

112. Takeda Y, Miyamori I, Iki K, Inaba S, Furukawa K, Hatakeyama H, Yoneda T, Takeda R. Endogenous renal 11β-hydroxysteroid dehydrogenase inhibitory factors in patients with low-renin essential hypertension. *Hypertension* 1996; **27**: 197–201.

113. Morris DJ, Lo YH, Lichtfield WR, Williams GH. Impact of dietary Na+ on glycyrrhetinic acid-like factors (kidney 11beta- (HSD2)-GALFs) in human essential hypertension. *Hypertension* 1998; **31**: 469–472.

114. Lo YH, Sheff MF, Latif SA, Ribiero C, Silver H, Brem AS, Morris DJ. Kidney 11β-HSD2 is inhibited by glycyrrhetinic acid-like factors in human urine. *Hypertension* 1997; **29**: 500–505.

115. Oelkers W, Buchen S, Diederich S, Krain J, Muhme S, Schoneshofer M. Impaired renal 11β-oxidation of 9alpha-fluorocortisol: an explanation for its mineralocorticoid potency. *J Clin Endocrinol Metab* 1994; **78**: 928–932.

116. Conti M, Frey FJ, Escher G, Marone C, Frey BM. Renal handling of prednisolone/prednisone: Effect of steroid dose and 11beta-hydroxysteroid dehydrogenase. *Nephrol, Dial, Transplant* 1994; **9**: 1622–1628.

117. Best R, Nelson SM, Walker BR. Dexamethasone and 11-dehydrodexamethasone as tools to investigate the isozymes of 11β-hydroxysteroid dehydrogenase *in vitro* and *in vivo*. *J Endocrinol* 1997; **153**: 41–48.

118. Diederich S, Hanke B, Burkhardt P, Muller M, Schoneshofer M, Bahr V, Oelkers W. Metabolism of synthetic corticosteroids by 11beta-hydroxysteroid- dehydrogenases in man. *Steroids* 1998; **63**: 271–277.

119. Li KZ, Obeyesekere VR, Krozowski ZS, Ferrari P. Oxoreductase and dehydrogenase activities of the human and rat 11beta- hydroxysteroid dehydrogenase type 2 enzyme. *Endocrinology* 1997; **138**: 2948–2952.

120. Honour JW. Steroid profiling. *Ann Clin Biochem* 1997; **34**: 32–44.

121. Shackleton CL. Mass spectrometry in the diagnosis of steroid-related disorders and in hypertension research. *J Steroid Biochem Mol Biol* 1993; **45**: 127–140.

122. Palermo M, Shackleton CHL, Mantero F, Stewart PM. Urinary free cortisone and the assessment of 11beta- hydroxysteroid dehydrogenase activity in man. *Clin Endocrinol* 1996; **45**: 605–611.

123. Best R, Walker BR. Additional value of measurement of urinary cortisone and unconjugated cortisol metabolites in assessing the activity of 11β-hydroxysteroid dehydrogenase *in vivo*. *Clin Endocrinol (Oxf)* 1997 47: 231–236.

124. Ulick S, Tedde R, Wang JZ. Defective ring A reduction of cortisol as the major metabolic error in the syndrome of apparent mineralocorticoid excess. *J Clin Endocrinol Metab* 1992; **74**: 593–599.

125. Edwards CRW, Walker BR. Cortisol and hypertension: what was not so apparent about 'apparent mineralocorticoid excess'. *J Lab Clin Med* 1993; **122**: 632–635.

126. Walker BR. How will we know if 11β-hydroxysteroid dehydrogenases are important in common diseases? *Clin Endocrinol* 2000; **52**: 401–402.

127. Walker BR, Stewart PM, Shackleton CHL, Padfield PL, Edwards CRW. Deficient inactivation of cortisol by 11β-hydroxysteroid dehydrogenase in essential hypertension. *Clin Endocrinol (Oxf)* 1993; **39**: 221–227.

128. Mantero F, Tedde R, Opocher G, Fulgheri PD, Arnaldi G, Ulick S. Apparent mineralocorticoid excess type II. *Steroids* 1994; **59**: 80–83.

129. Linberg L, Wang JZ, Arison BH, Ulick S. Synthesis of a deuterium-labeled cortisol for the study of its rate of 11β-hydroxy dehydrogenation in man. *J Steroid Biochem Mol Biol* 1991; **38**: 351–357.

130. Finken MJJ, Andrews RC, Andrew R, Walker BR. Cortisol metabolism in healthy young adults: sexual dimorphism in activities of A-ring reductase but not 11-hydroxysteroid dehydrogenases. *J Clin Endocrinol Metab* 1999; **84**: 3316–3321.

131. Stewart PM, Boulton A, Kumar S, Clark PMS, Shackleton CHL. Cortisol metabolism in human obesity: impaired cortisone—cortisol conversion in subjects with central adiposity. *J Clin Endocrinol Metab* 1999; **84**: 1022–1027.

132. Shackleton CHL, Stewart PM: The hypertension of apparent mineralocorticoid excess syndrome. In: Biglieri EG, Melby JC (eds) *Endocrine Hypertension*. New York: Raven Press, 1990: 155–173.

133. Dave-Sharma S, Wilson RC, Harbison MD, Newfield R, Azar MR, Krozowski, ZS, Funder JW, Shackleton CL, Bradlow HL, Wei J-Q, Hertecant J, Moran A, Neiberger RE, Balfe JW, Fattah A, Daneman D, Akkurt HI, DE, Santis C, New MI. Examination of genotype and phenotype relationships in 14 patients with apparent mineralocorticoid excess. *J Clin Endocrinol Metab* 1998; **83**: 2244–2254.

134. Oberfield SE, Levine LS, Carey RM, Greig F, Ulick S, New MI. Metabolic and blood pressure responses to hydrocortisone in the syndrome of apparent mineralocorticoid excess. *J Clin Endocrinol Metab* 1983; **56**: 332–339.

135. Stewart PM, Corrie JET, Shackleton CHL, Edwards CRW. Syndrome of apparent mineralocorticoid excess: a defect in the cortisol-cortisone shuttle. *J Clin Invest* 1988; **82**: 340–349.

136. Li A, Li KZ, Marui S, Krozowski ZS, Batista MC, Whorwood CB, Arnhold IP, Shackleton CL, Mendonca BB, Stewart PM. Apparent mineralocorticoid excess in a Brazilian kindred: Hypertension in the heterozygote state. *J Hypertens* 1997; **15**: 1397–1402.

137. Lovati E, Ferrari P, Dick B, Jostarndt K, Frey BM, Frey FJ, Schorr U, Sharma AM. Molecular basis of human salt sensitivity: the role of the 11β-hydroxysteroid dehydrogenase type 2. *J Clin Endocrinol Metab* 1999; **84**: 3745–3749.

138. Edwards CRW, Benediktsson R, Lindsay RS, Seckl JR. Dysfunction of placental glucocorticoid barrier: link be-

tween fetal environment and adult hypertension? *Lancet* 1993; **341**: 355–357.

139. Kitanaka S, Tanae A, Hibi I. Apparent mineralocorticoid excess due to 11beta-hydroxysteroid dehydrogenase deficiency: A possible cause of intrauterine growth retardation. *Clin Endocrinol* 1996; **44**: 353–359.

140. Benediktsson R, Calder AA, Edwards CRW, Seckl JR. Placental 11β-hydroxysteroid dehydrogenase: a key regulator of fetal glucocorticoid exposure. *Clin Endo-crinol* 1997; **46**: 161–166.

141. Rogerson FM, Kayes KM, White PC. Variation in placental type 2 11beta-hydroxysteroid dehydrogenase activity is not related to birth weight or placental weight. *Mol Cell Endocrinol* 1997; **128**: 103–109.

142. Barker DJP. Fetal origins of coronary heart disease. *Br Med J* 1995; **311**: 171–174.

143. Benediktsson R, Lindsay RS, Noble J, Seckl JR, Edwards CRW. Glucocorticoid exposure in utero: new model for adult hypertension. *Lancet* 1993; **341**: 339–341.

144. Lindsay RS, Lindsay RM, Waddell BJ, Seckl JR. Prenatal glucocorticoid exposure leads to offspring hyperglycaemia in the rat: studies with the 11β-hydroxysteroid dehydrogenase inhibitor carbenoxolone. *Diabetologia* 1996; **39**: 1299–1305.

145. Lindsay RS, Lindsay RM, Edwards CRW, Seckl JR. Inhibition of 11β-hydroxysteroid dehydrogenase in pregnant rats and the programming of blood pressure in the offspring. *Hypertension* 1996; **27**: 1200–1204.

146. Leon DA, Koupilova I, Lithell HO, Berglund L, Mohsen R, Vagero D, Lithell UB, McKeigue PM. Failure to realise growth potential in utero and adult obesity in relation to blood pressure in 50 year old Swedish men. *Br Med J* 1996; **312**: 401–406.

147. Phillipou G, Higgins BA. A new defect in the peripheral conversion of cortisone to cortisol. *J Steroid Biochem* 1985; **22**: 435–436.

148. Taylor NF, Bartlett WA, Dawson DJ, Enoch BA. Cortisone reductase deficiency: evidence for a new inborn error in metabolism of adrenal steroids. *J Endocrinol* 1984; **102** (Suppl): 90 (Abstract).

149. Nikkila H, Tannin GM, New MI, Taylor NF, Kalaitzoglou G, Monder C, White PC. Defects in the HSD11 gene encoding 11β-hydroxysteroid dehydrogenase are not found in patients with apparent mineralocorticoid excess or 11-oxoreductase deficiency. *J Clin Endocrinol Metab* 1993; **77**: 687–691.

150. Li A, Tedde R, Palermo M, Shackleton CL, Stewart PM. Molecular basis for hypertension in the type II variant of apparent mineralocorticoid excess. *American Journal of Human Genetics* 1998; **63**: 370–379.

151. Soro A, Ingram MC, Tonolo G, Glorioso N, Fraser R. Evidence of coexisting changes in 11β-hydroxysteroid dehydrogenase and 5β-reductase activity in patients with untreated essential hypertension. *Hypertension* 1995; **25**: 67–70.

152. Latif SA, Conca TJ, Morris DJ. The effects of the liquorice derivative, glycyrrhetinic acid, on hepatic 3alpha- and 3β-hydroxysteroid dehydrogenases and 5alpha- and 5β-reductase pathways of metabolism of aldosterone in male rats. *Steroids* 1990; **55**: 52–58.

153. Mala S, Mahendroo MS, Russell DW. Endocrine roles of steroid 5α-reductase isozymes. *Proc Endocr Soc* 1998; **80**: OR50-1 (Abstract).

154. Davis EA, Morris DJ. Medicinal uses of licorice through the millenia: the good and plenty of it. *Mol Cell Endocrinol* 1991; **78**: 1–6.

155. Monder C, Stewart PM, Lakshmi V, Valentino R, Burt D, Edwards CRW. Licorice inhibits corticosteroid 11β-dehydrogenase of rat kidney and liver: in vivo and in vitro studies. *Endocrinology* 1989; **125**: 1046–1053.

156. Walker BR, Edwards CRW. Licorice-induced hypertension and syndromes of apparent mineralocorticoid excess. *Endocrinol Metab Clin N Am* 1994; **23**(2): 359–377.

157. Teelucksingh S, Benediktsson R, Lindsay RS, Burt D, Seckl JR, Edwards CRW, Nan CL, Kelly R. Liquorice. *Lancet* 1991; **337**: 1549.

158. Imperato-McGinley J, Shackleton C, Orlic S, Stoner E. C19 and C21 5beta/5alpha metabolite ratios in subjects treated with the 5alpha-reductase inhibitor finasteride: Comparison of male pseudohermaphrodites with inherited 5alpha-reductase deficiency. *J Clin Endocrinol Metab* 1990; **70**: 777–782.

159. Hirsch KS, Jones CD, Audia JE, Andersson S, McQuaid L, Stamm NB, Neubauer BL, Pennington P, Toomey RE, Russell DW. LY191704: A selective, nonsteroidal inhibitor of human steroid 5alpha- reductase type. *Proc Nat Acad Sci USA* 1993; **90**: 5277–5281.

160. Strain GW, Zumoff B, Strain JJ. Cortisol production in obesity. *Metabolism* 1980; **29**: 980–985.

161. Marin P, Darin M, Amemiya T, Andersson B, Jern S, Bjorntorp P. Cortisol secretion in relation to body fat distribution in obese premenopausal women. *Metabolism* 1992; **41**: 882–886.

162. Pasquali R, Cantobelli S, Casimirri F, Capelli M, Bortoluzzi L, Flamia R, Labate AMM, Barabara L. The hypothalamic-pituitary-adrenal axis in obese women with different patterns of body fat distribution. *J Clin Endocrinol Metab* 1993; **77**: 341–346.

163. Andrew R, Phillips DIW, Walker BR. Obesity and gender influence cortisol secretion and metabolism in man. *J Clin Endocrinol Metab* 1998; **83**: 1806–1809.

164. Fraser R, Ingram MC, Anderson NH, Morrison C, Davies E, Connell JMC. Cortisol effects on body mass, blood pressure, and cholesterol in the general population. *Hypertension* 1999; **33**: 1364–1368.

165. Hautanen A, Adlercreutz H. Altered adrenocorticotropin and cortisol secretion in abdominal obesity: implications for the insulin resistance syndrome. *J Intern Med* 1993; **234**: 461–469.

166. Ljung T, Andersson B, Bengtsson B, Bjorntorp P, Marin P. Inhibition of cortisol secretion by dexamethasone in relation to body fat distribution: a dose-response study. *Obes Res* 1996; **4**: 277–282.

167. Walker BR, Soderberg S, Lindahl B, Olsson T. Independent effects of obesity and cortisol in predicting cardiovascular risk factors in men and women. *J Intern Med* 2000; **247**: 198–204.

168. Rosmond R, Dallman MF, Bjorntorp P. Stress-related cortisol secretion in men: relationships with abdominal obesity and endocrine, metabolic and haemodynamic abnormalities. *J Clin Endocrinol Metab* 1998; **83**: 1853–1859.

169. Phillips DIW, Barker DJP, Fall CHD, Whorwood CB,

Seckl JR, Wood PJ, Walker BR. Elevated plasma cortisol concentrations: an explanation for the relationship between low birthweight and adult cardiovascular risk factors. *J Clin Endocrinol Metab* 1998; **83**: 757–760.

170. Strain GW, Zumoff B, Kream J, Strain JJ, Levin J, Fukushima D. Sex difference in the influence of obesity on the 24 hr mean plasma concentration of cortisol. *Metabolism* 1982; **31**: 209–212.

171. Stewart PM, Shackleton CHL, Beastall GH, Edwards CRW. 5alpha-reductase activity in polycystic ovarian syndrome. *Lancet* 1990; **335**: 431–433.

172. Low SC, Chapman KE, Edwards CRW, Wells T, Robinson ICAF, Seckl JR. Sexual dimorphism of hepatic 11β-hydroxysteroid dehydrogenase in the rat: the role of growth hormone patterns. *J Endocrinol* 1994; **143**: 541–548.

173. Weaver JU, Monson JP, Noonan K, Price C, Edwards A, Evans KA, James I, Cunningham J. The effect of low dose recombinant human growth hormone replacement on indices of bone remodelling and bone mineral density in hypopituitary growth hormone-deficient adults. *Endocrinol Metab* 1996; **3**: 55–61.

174. Walker BR, Andrew R, MacLeod KM, Padfield PL. Growth hormone replacement inhibits renal and hepatic 11β-hydroxysteroid dehydrogenases in ACTH-deficient patients. *Clin Endocrinol* 1998; **49**: 257–263.

175. Gelding SV, Taylor NF, Wood PJ, Noonan K, Weaver JU, Wood DF, Monson, JP. The effect of growth hormone replacement therapy on cortisol–cortisone interconversion in hypopituitary adults: Evidence for growth hormone modulation of extrarenal 11beta-hydroxysteroid dehydrogenase activity. *Clin Endocrinol* 1998; **48**: 153–162.

176. Watt GCM, Harrap SB, Foy CJW, Holton DW, Edwards HV, Davidson HR, Connor JM, Lever AF, Fraser R. Abnormalities of glucocorticoid metabolism and the renin-angiotensin system: a four corners approach to the identification of genetic determinants of blood pressure. *J Hypertens* 1992; **10**: 473–482.

177. Filipovsky J, Ducimetiere P, Eschwege E, Richard JL, Rosselin G, Claude JR. The relationship of blood pressure with glucose, insulin, heart rate, free fatty acids and plasma cortisol levels according to degree of obesity in middle-aged men. *J Hypertens* 1996; **14**: 229–235.

178. Stolk RP, Lamberts SWJ, de Jong FH, Pols HAP, Grobbee DE. Gender differences in the associations between cortisol and insulin sensitivity in healthy subjects. *J Endocrinol* 1996; **149**: 313–318.

179. Walker BR, Phillips DIW, Noon JP, Panarelli M, Best R, Edwards HE, Holton DW, Seckl JR, Webb DJ, Watt GCM. Increased glucocorticoid activity in men with cardiovascular risk factors. *Hypertension* 1998; **31**: 891–895.

180. Walker BR, Best R, Shackleton CHL, Padfield PL, Edwards CRW. Increased vasoconstrictor sensitivity to glucocorticoids in essential hypertension. *Hypertension* 1996; **27**: 190–196.

181. Reynolds RM, Bendall HE, Walker BR, Wood PJ, Phillips DIW, Whorwood CB. Hyper-activity of the hypothalamic-pituitary-adrenal axis may mediate the link between impaired fetal growth and the insulin resistance syndrome. *J Endocrinol* 1998; **159**: OC5 (Abstract).

182. Thornton JE, Cheung CC, Clifton DK, Steiner RA. Regulation of hypothalamic proopiomelanocortin mRNA by leptin in ob/ob mice. *Endocrinology* 1997; **138**: 5063–5066.

183. Lugg MA, Nicholas TE. The effect of dexamethasone on the activity of 11β-hydroxysteroid dehydrogenase in the foetal rabbit lung during the final stage of gestation. *J Pharm Pharmacol* 1978; **30**: 587–589.

184. Hammami MM, Siiteri PK. Regulation of 11β-hydroxysteroid dehydrogenase activity in human skin fibroblasts: enzymatic modulation of glucocorticoid action. *J Clin Endocrinol Metab* 1991; **73**: 326–334.

185. Walker BR, Williams BC, Edwards CRW. Regulation of 11β-hydroxysteroid dehydrogenase activity by the hypothalamic-pituitary-adrenal axis in the rat. *J Endo-crinol* 1994; **141**: 467–472.

186. Low SC, Moisan M-P, Edwards CRW, Seckl JR. Glucocorticoids regulate 11β-hydroxysteroid dehydrogenase activity and gene expression in vivo in the rat. *J Neuroendocrinol* 1994; **6**: 285–290.

187. Idrus RH, Mohammad NB, Morat PB, Saim A, Abdul KK. Differential effect of adrenocorticosteroids on 11beta-hydroxysteroid dehydrogenase bioactivity at the anterior pituitary and hypothalamus in rats. *Steroids* 1996; **61**: 448–452.

188. Liu YJ, Nakagawa Y, Nasuda K, Saegusa H, Igarashi Y. Effect of growth hormone, insulin and dexamethasone on 11beta- hydroxysteroid dehydrogenase activity on a primary culture of rat hepatocytes. *Life Sci* 1996; **59**: 227–234.

189. Smith RE, Funder JW. Renal 11β-hydroxysteroid dehydrogenase activity: effects of age, sex and altered hormonal status. *J Steroid Biochem Mol Biol* 1991; **38**: 265–267.

190. Pepe GJ, Davies WA, Dong K-W, Luo H, Albrecht ED. Cloning of the 11beta-hydroxysteroid dehydrogenase (11beta-HSD)-2 gene in the baboon: Effects of estradiol on promoter activity of 11beta-HSD-1 and -2 in placental JEG-3 cells. *Biochim Biophys Acta (Gene Structure and Expression)* 1999; **1444**: 101–110.

191. Sun K, Yang K, Challis JG. Regulation of 11beta-hydroxysteroid dehydrogenase type 2 by progesterone, estrogen, and the cyclic adenosine 5′-monophosphate pathway in cultured human placental and chorionic trophoblasts. *Biol Reprod* 1998; **58**: 1379–1384.

192. Zumoff B, Bradlow HL, Levin J, Fukushima DK. Influence of thyroid function on the in vivo cortisol-cortisone equilibrium in man. *J Steroid Biochem* 1983; **18**: 437–440.

193. Ichikawa Y, Yoshida K, Kawagoe M, Saito E, Abe Y, Arikawa K, Homma M. Altered equilibrium between cortisol and cortisone in plasma in thyroid dysfunction and inflammatory diseases. *Metabolism* 1977; **26**: 989–997.

194. Hellman L, Bradlow HL, Zumoff B, Gallagher TF. The influence of thyroid hormone on hydrocortisone production and metabolism. *J Clin Endocrinol Metab* 1961; **21**: 1231–1247.

195. Whorwood CB, Sheppard MC, Stewart PM. Tissue specific effects of thyroid hormone on 11β-hydroxysteroid dehydrogenase gene expression. *J Steroid Biochem Mol Biol* 1993; **46**: 539–547.

196. Koerner DR, Hellman L. Effect of thyroxine administration on the 11β-hydroxysteroid dehydrogenases in rat liver and kidney. *Endocrinology* 1964; **75**: 592–601.

197. Tremblay J, Hardy DB, Pereira LE, Yang K. Retinoic acid stimulates the expression of 11beta-hydroxysteroid dehydrogenase type 2 in human choriocarcinoma JEG-3 cells.

Biol Reprod 1999; **60**: 541–545.

198. Evagelatou M, Peterson SL, Cooke BA. Leukocytes modulate 11beta-hydroxysteroid dehydrogenase (11beta-HSD) activity in human granulosa-lutein cell cultures. *Mol Cell Endocrinol* 1997; **133**: 81–88.

199. Escher G, Galli I, Vishwanath BS, Frey BM, Frey FJ. Tumor necrosis factor alpha and interleukin 1beta enhance the cortisone/cortisol shuttle. *J Exp Med* 1997; **186**: 189–198.

200. Homma M, Onodera T, Hirabatake M, Oka K, Kanazawa M, Miwa T, Hayashi. Activation of 11beta-hydroxysteroid dehydrogenase by dehydroepiandrosterone sulphate as an anti-hypertensive agent in spontaneously hypertensive rats. *J Pharm Pharmacol* 1998; **50**: 1139–1145.

201. Diederich S, Quinkler M, Miller K, Heilmann P, Schoneshofer M, Oelkers W. Human kidney 11beta-hydroxysteroid dehydrogenase: Regulation by adreno-corticotropin. *Eur J Endocrinol* 1996; **134**: 301–307.

202. Low SC, Assaad SN, Rajan V, Chapman KE, Edwards CRW, Seckl JR. Regulation of 11β-hydroxysteroid dehydrogenase by sex steroids in vivo: further evidence for the existence of a second dehydrogenase in rat kidney. *J Endocrinol* 1993; **139**: 27–35.

203. Jamieson PM, Fuchs E, Flugge G, Seckl JR. Attenuation of hippocampal 11beta-hydroxysteroid dehydrogenase type 1 by chronic psychosocial stress in the tree shrew. *Stress* 1997; **2**(2): 123–132.

204. Jellinck PH, Dhabhar FS, Sakai RR, McEwan BS. Long-term corticosteroid treatment but not chronic stress affects 11β-hydroxysteroid dehydrogenase type 1 activity in rat brain and peripheral tissues. *J Steroid Biochem Mol Biol* 1997; **60**: 319–323.

205. Sun K, Yang K, Challis JG. Differential regulation of 11 beta-hydroxysteroid dehydrogenase type 1 and 2 by nitric oxide in cultured human placental trophoblast and chorionic cell preparation. *Endocrinology* 1997; **138**: 4912–4920.

206. Souness GW, Latif SA, Laurenzo JL, Morris DJ. 11alpha- and 11beta-hydroxyprogesterone, potent inhibitors of 11beta-hydroxysteroid dehydrogenase (isoforms 1 and 2), confer marked mineralocorticoid activity on corticosterone in the ADX rat. *Endocrinology* 1995; **136**: 1809–1812.

207. Brem AS, Bina RB, King T, Morris DJ. 11betaOH-progesterone affects vascular glucocorticoid metabolism and contractile response. *Hypertension* 1997; **30**: 449–454.

208. Morita H, Zhou M, Foecking MF, Gomez-Sanchez EP, Cozza EN, Gomez, Sanchez CE. 11beta-Hydroxysteroid dehydrogenase type 2 complementary deoxyribonucleic acid stably transfected into Chinese hamster ovary cells: Specific inhibition by 11alpha-hydroxyprogesterone. *Endocrinology* 1996; **137**: 2308–2314.

209. Kato H, Kanaoka M, Yano S, Kobayashi M. 3-mono-glucuronyl-glycyrrhetinic acid is a major metabolite that causes licorice-induced pseudoaldosteronism. *J Clin Endocrinol Metab* 1995; **80**: 1929–1933.

210. Latif SA, Hartman LR, Souness GW, Morris DJ. Possible endogenous regulators of steroid inactivating enzymes and glucocorticoid-induced Na + retention. *Steroids* 1994; **59**: 352–356.

211. Semafuko WEB, Sheff MF, Grimes CA, Latif SA, Sadaniantz A, Levinson P, Morris DJ. Inhibitors of 11β-hydroxysteroid dehydrogenase and 5β-steroid reductase in urine from patients with congestive heart failure. *Ann Clin Lab Sci* 1993; **23**: 456–461.

212. Walker BR, Williamson PM, Brown MA, Honour JW, Edwards CRW, Whitworth JA. 11β-Hydroxysteroid dehydrogenase and its inhibitors in hypertensive pregnancy. *Hypertension* 1995; **25**: 626–630.

213. Roseboom TJ, Van der Meulen JP, Ravelli AJ, Van Montfrans GA, Osmond C, Barker DP, Bleker OP. Blood pressure in adults after prenatal exposure to famine. *J Hypertens* 1999; **17**: 325–330.

214. Latif SA, Sheff MF, Ribeiro CE, Morris DJ. Selective inhibition of sheep kidney 11beta-hydroxysteroid dehydrogenase isoform 2 activity by 5alpha-reduced (but not 5beta) derivatives of adrenocorticosteroids. *Steroids* 1997; **62**: 230–237.

215. Buhler H, Perschel FH, Hierholzer K. Inhibition of rat renal 11β-hydroxysteroid dehydrogenase by steroidal compounds and triterpenoids; structure/function relationship. *Biochim Biophys Act* 1991; **1075**: 206–212.

216. Perschel FH, Buhler H, Hierholzer K. Bile acids and their amidates inhibit 11β-hydroxysteroid dehydrogenase obtained from rat kidney. *Pflug Arch* 1991; **418**: 538–543.

217. Escher G, Nawrocki A, Staub T, Vishwanath BS, Frey BM, Reichen J, Frey FJ. Down-regulation of hepatic and renal 11beta-hydroxysteroid dehydrogenase in rats with liver cirrhosis. *Gastroenterology* 1998; **114**: 175–184.

218. Homma M, Oka K, Niitsuma T, Itoh H. A novel 11β-hydroxysteroid dehydrogenase inhibitor contained in Saiboku-To, a herbal remedy for steroid-dependent bronchial asthma. *J Pharm Pharmacol* 1994; **46**: 305–309.

219. Homma M, Oka K, Ikeshima K, Takahashi N, Niitsuma T, Fukuda T, Itoh H. Different effects of traditional Chinese medicines containing similar herbal constituents on prednisolone pharmacokinetics. *J Pharm Pharmacol* 1995; **47**: 687–692.

220. Song D, Lorenzo B, Reidenberg MM. Inhibition of 11β-hydroxysteroid dehydrogenase by gossypol and bioflavonoids. *J Lab Clin Med* 1992; **120**: 792–797.

221. Wang M-S, Lorenzo JB, Reidenberg MM. NAD- and NADP-dependent 11beta-hydroxysteroid dehydrogen-ase isoforms in guinea pig kidney with gossypol inhibition. *Acta Pharmacol Sinica* 1997; **18**: 481–485.

222. Raven PW, Checkley SA, Taylor NF. Extraadrenal effects of metyrapone include inhibition of the 11-oxoreductase activity of 11beta-hydroxysteroid dehydrogenase: a model for 11-HSD I deficiency. *Clin Endocrinol (Oxf)* 1995; **43**: 637–644.

223. Thomson LM, Raven PW, Smith KE, Hinson JP. Effects of metyrapone on hepatic cortisone–cortisol conversion in the rat. *Endocr Res* 1998; **24**: 607–611.

224. Sampath-Kumar R, Yu M, Khalil MW, Yang K. Metyrapone is a competitive inhibitor of 11beta-hydroxysteroid dehydrogenase type 1 reductase. *J Steroid Biochem Mol Biol* 1997; **62**: 195–199.

225. Fuster D, Escher G, Vogt B, Ackermann D, Dick B, Frey BM, Frey FJ. Furosemide inhibits 11beta-hydroxysteroid dehydrogenase type 2. *Endocrinology* 1998; **139**: 3849–3854.

226. Escher G, Meyer KV, Vishwanath BS, Frey BM, Frey FJ. Furosemide inhibits 11beta-hydroxysteroid dehydrogenase in vitro and in vivo. *Endocrinology* 1995; **136**: 1759–1765.

227. Yin DZ, Lorenzo B, Reidenberg MM. Inhibition of 11beta-hydroxysteroid dehydrogenase obtained from guinea pig kidney by furosemide, naringenin and some other compound. *J Steroid Biochem Mol Biol* 1994; **49**: 81–85.

228. Zhang Y-D, Wang M-S. Inhibition of 11beta-hydroxy-steroid dehydrogenase obtained from guinea pig kidney by some bioflavonoids and triterpenoids. *Acta Pharmacol Sinica* 1997; **18**: 240–244.

229. Lee YS, Lorenzo BJ, Koufis T, Reidenberg MM. Grapefruit juice and its flavonoids inhibit 11beta-hydroxysteroid dehydrogenase. *Clin Pharmacol Ther* 1996; **59**: 62–71.

19

Drug-induced Obesity

Leif Breum[1] and Madelyn H. Fernstrom[2]

[1]Køge Hospital, Køge, Denmark and [2]University of Pittsburgh School of Medicine, Pittsburgh, Pennsylvania, USA

INTRODUCTION

Weight gain is a common, but often overlooked side effect to many widely used drugs. In susceptible individuals the weight gain may result in clinically significant obesity and associated comorbidities. Both tricyclic antidepressant medications and antipsychotic compounds are those prominently cited for producing persistent and problematic body weight gain in many treated patients and have a serious impact on medication compliance to an otherwise beneficial treatment. Furthermore, weight gain is often seen as an improvement of the psychiatric disease and therefore not recognized before the initial body weight is exceeded by several kilos. The mechanisms behind the weight gain are poorly understood. Many of these drugs interfere with central appetite-regulating neurotransmitters and may also produce sedative and anticholinergic effects, ultimately contributing to changes in energy expenditure. The incidence of weight gain during acute and chronic treatment with different classes of frequently prescribed drugs will be reviewed (Table 19.1), as will the possible mechanisms by which such drugs alter energy intake and expenditure, contributing to drug-induced weight gain (Table 19.2). Newer, effective medication classes, without the side effect of weight gain will also be discussed.

ANTIDEPRESSANT MEDICATIONS

Change in body weight is a frequent symptom of major depression, most likely a result of alterations in appetite. Patients typically lose weight (1–3), although some do gain weight during a depressive episode (3–5). As a pharmacologic treatment, the tricyclic antidepressants remain, even after almost 40 years, the first choice of medication for the treatment of severe major depression throughout the world (6). Although very effective agents for restoration of normal mood, there are numerous side effects associated with this drug treatment, particularly unwanted and excessive weight gain. Previously, weight gain during antidepressant treatment had been interpreted as a positive sign of improvement, so prevalent and predictable was the effect. Such weight gain is of concern to both patient and clinician, as this is the reason often cited for medication non-compliance. It is important to point out that over the past 15 years, several newer medications of a different drug class, the selective serotonin reuptake inhibitors (SSRIs), have become available. These drugs are effective as antidepressants, usually (but not always, see below) without the side effect of weight gain, but with other problematic side effects (6,7).

International Textbook of Obesity. Edited by Per Björntorp.

Table 19.1 Drugs causing obesity

Antipsychotics	All subgroups
Antidepressants	Tricyclic antidepressants
	Lithium
	MAO inhibitors
Anticonvulsants	Valproate, carbamazepine
Antimigraine and antihistaminergic drugs	Cyproheptadine, flunarizine, pizotifen
Antidiabetic agents	Sulfonylurea agents, all insulin preparations, glitazones
Glucocorticoids	Pharmacological doses
Beta-blockers	Non-specific, e.g. propranolol
Sex hormones	Estrogen (high dose), megestrol acetate, tamoxifen
Other	Some antineoplastic agents

Table 19.2 Putative mechanisms involved in drug-induced obesity

- Decreased serotoninergic and dopaminergic activity
- Impaired mitochondrial beta-oxidation of fatty acids and other changes in substrate oxidation
- Reduced sympathetic nervous system activity
- Decreased energy expenditure
- Sedation
- Anticholinergic side effects causing dry mouth and increased intake of caloric beverages
- Altered activity of hypothalamic leptin and neuropeptide Y

Tricyclic Antidepressants

Two frequently prescribed tricyclic drugs, amitriptyline (8–11) and imipramine (11–13), have most often been associated with increasing body weight during treatment. Moreover, within the tricyclic drug class, amitriptyline appears to promote weight gain to a much greater degree than the others. Importantly, in a series of studies, no relationship between clinical response and weight gain was observed (9,11,13). In fact, weight change during drug treatment was not negatively correlated with that occurring at disease onset; that is, weight gain was not simply a reflection of weight lost during the depressive episode. These results suggest that drug-induced changes in weight probably result from a pharmacologic action of the drug independent of its effect on mood. The mechanism(s) by which tricyclic antidepressants promote weight gain are not well understood and can reflect changes in energy balance produced by increases in caloric intake, reductions in energy expenditure, or both. As described in the following sections, a reduction in energy expenditure is a key factor associated with the weight promoting effects of the tricyclic drugs, while changes in food intake probably contribute to a much smaller degree.

Tricyclics, Ingestive Behavior, and Weight Gain

Much of the available information on antidepressants and ingestive behavior has been based on abundant anecdotal accounts. Unlike metabolic rate, where reasonable quantitative analyses are achieved, evaluating feeding behavior in drug-treated patients is much more difficult. Prior to the studies by Fernstrom (11,13,14), several reports described the presence of food cravings, particularly for 'sweets' or carbohydrates, associated with weight gain in some patients treated with tricyclic antidepressants. The inference of these reports is that weight gain resulted from excessive food consumption, based on increased desire. Only an occasional published report, however, has actually attempted to examine this issue with any precision. Paykel et al. (8), who coined the term 'carbohydrate craving', reported a craving for 'carbohydrates' among patients treated with amitriptyline. However, the desired 'carbohydrate' foods reported contained substantial amounts of fat (sometimes more than the carbohydrate) and were uniformly sweet tasting, like chocolate and pastry. Berken et al. (12) observed an increase in 'sweets' consumption in some patients treated with antidepressants, although no further description of the desired foods was provided. Such changes in food preference were reported to be large, and obvious to both patient and clinician.

These early studies lacked an accurate nutritional basis for defining food groups and evaluating food preferences. For example, numerous definitions have been proposed for 'carbohydrate' foods (Table 19.3). This confusion in terminology indicates only that people eat *foods* not macronutrients, with many factors involved in preference. Certainly, once a food is eaten, the individual macronutrients are handled biochemically in the same manner, regardless of its presentation in the original food. However, the interesting and relevant study is to define which components of foods (e.g. macronutrient composition, sweetness, palatability) are driving the consumption behavior.

To address these questions a series of studies were conducted to determine how appetite changes during antidepressant treatment. A sound database for evaluating food preference changes during treatment was generated using a validated survey, the Pittsburgh Appetite Test (PAT) (14). The aims were to identify, systematically, the extent to which changes in food preference occur during tricyclic antidepressant treatment and how these might impact on subsequent weight gain. The PAT was not designed to quantitate food intake, but rather to focus on the issue of reported food cravings, and what foods these might be. Such information can help in identifying particular components generating food selection. This instrument can detect shifts in appetite and food preference, providing a reasonable index of eating attitudes and preferences. The food categories are based on macronutrient content and taste (i.e. a sugar-rich high fat food (chocolate) is different from a starch-rich high fat food (potato chips)) and were easily recognizable to the patients. Patients completed the PAT two to three times during the medication-free period, and then monthly during treatment with imipramine.

The results from the PAT at the end of 4 months of treatment (the period of time associated with the greatest incidence of weight gain) do not show marked changes in preference for calorically dense (high fat) foods with or without a sweet taste, nor for any of the foods in the other categories. Although no significant changes were noted in preference for sweets, a small percentage of patients (15%) did experience a notable change in preference toward carbohydrate-fat rich sweet tasting foods (13). It is important to point out that the craved food items contained *both* carbohydrate (mostly sucrose) and fat, while no preference was expressed for sweet foods containing sucrose and little fat (fruit, gum drops), nor for sweet foods without sucrose or fat (i.e. fruit, which contained fructose). It thus seems

unlikely that sweetness alone is the determinant of choice. Both sweetness and fat content apparently motivate preference in these patients, a result compatible with those obtained by Drewnowski and Greenwood in normal subjects (15). It is noteworthy that shifts in food preference toward carbohydrate-fat rich sweet foods are also found in another group: the actively ill depressed patient. A marked increase in cravings for these foods was present in more than a third of depressed patients (14).

Clinical outcome was not correlated with preference for sweet/fat food items: when comparing those with cravings to those without, no changes in clinical improvement were noted. Moreover, although substantial weight gain (> 5 lb (2 kg)) was noted in 43% of patients, neither weight gain nor the presence of obesity predicted who would seek such palatable, calorically dense foods (13).

Presently, it is unclear the extent to which increases in food intake, prompted by food cravings promote antidepressant-induced weight gain. Generally, a craving for sweet, calorically dense foods does not appear a significant problem for most treated patients, although this association can be seen in an occasional patient treated with a tricyclic medication, and could promote weight gain in the susceptible individual.

Tricyclics, Energy Expenditure, and Weight Gain

Alterations in energy expenditure can directly contribute to body weight change. Reductions in one or more compartments of energy expenditure (resting metabolic rate, diet-induced thermogenesis, exercise) can produce increases in body weight. Depressed patients treated with tricyclic medications might well produce weight gain via this mechanism, since these drugs might be predicted to alter sympathetic nervous system function and thus metabolic rate. Thus, the positive energy balance resulting in weight gain might be accounted for by a decrease in caloric utilization, making an individual more energy efficient and promoting weight gain. Resting metabolic rate (RMR) represents the greatest energy compartment, with at least 70% of daily energy use dedicated to maintenance of body systems (16); RMR probably accounts for an even greater proportion of calories in hospitalized patients due to their greater inactivity. Thus, should a

Table 19.3   Definitions of 'carbohydrate' foods

Carbohydrate/fat rich; sweet taste
Carbohydrate/fat rich; savory taste
Carbohydrate rich/low fat; sweet taste
Carbohydrate rich/low fat; savory taste
'Sweets'

reduction in energy expenditure occur during antidepressant treatment, RMR measurements are likely to reveal it. RMR is a technique which is reliable, and readily quantitated under controlled conditions. In one of the few clinical studies, a consistent reduction was found in the resting metabolic rate of patients treated with tricyclic antidepressants (17).

Because metabolic rate has a relatively wide range of 'normal' values, it is important to use each subject as his or her own control. Comparing triplicate measurements obtained during a 2-week medication-free period with those obtained during the second and fourth weeks of drug treatment, the drug-free, control measurements are quite reproducible, and RMR values are within the normal range for each patient's height and weight. After treatment with a tricyclic drug for 2–4 weeks, sizable reductions in RMR were observed (18). Consistent with the observed reductions in RMR is the notable decrease in diet-induced thermogenesis (DIT) (the naturally occurring increase in RMR after food ingestion) in some treated patients. Such reductions in RMR are remarkably large, and exceed by far changes in RMR produced by other stimuli. Exercise, for example, produces a 5–10% change in RMR, an effect considered to be robust. These results suggest that the magnitude of the change in RMR after drug treatment is physiologically important, and could have important ramifications in overall metabolic activity. Such changes, translated into calories, predict a reduction in daily caloric need of about 300–400 kcal/day. Thus, an individual might be expected to gain a pound every 10–14 days, independent of a change in food intake The reductions in DIT after a single meal, although modest (accounting for about 10–25 kcal), would likely be repeated every time food is ingested (four to seven times/day), supporting an additional contribution to the decline in energy expenditure. These results support the idea that reductions in caloric expenditure during drug treatment probably contribute to problematic weight gain. In fact, an increase in body weight would normally be ex-

pected to raise, not lower, RMR (16), suggesting further that the effect on metabolic rate is drug-related.

Although the underlying mechanism(s) eliciting changes in metabolic rate are presently unknown, it is apparent that alterations in caloric expenditure do contribute to weight change in patients treated with tricyclic medications. Because both RMR and diet-induced thermogenesis seem to be altered, it is reasonable to suggest that reductions in sympathetic nervous system (SNS) tone contribute to these effects.

Serotonin Specific Reuptake Inhibitors (SSRIs)

The SSRIs have proven to be effective treatment for depression, without the problematic side effect of excessive weight gain. The apparent lack of appetitive effects and perhaps an enhancement of resting metabolic rate contribute to the lack of weight gain observed. However, there are atypical responders to particular SSRIs, which do occasionally produce significant weight gain (19,20). This seems unrelated to changes in sympathetic tone, as reported for the tricyclic drugs. Thus, because the SSRI drugs are not usually associated with weight gain, this class of serotonergic drugs may be a more attractive treatment alternative, particularly in patients where drug-induced weight gain has been problematic.

SSRIs, Ingestive Behavior, and Weight Gain

For paroxetine, 2% of treated patients experienced weight gain over 6 weeks, while weight gain is highly variable by the end of one year (20). Thus, although the incidence is low, it is possible for susceptible individuals to experience some weight gain during treatment with paroxetine. Fisher *et al.* (21) reported an increase in weight during treatment with either sertraline or fluoxetine, while weight promoting properties of citalopram (22) have also been reported.

Multiple hypotheses exist to explain the incidence of SSRI-induced increases in body weight. Blockage of 5HT2C receptors can increase appetite (23) as demonstrated by the upregulation of these receptors in rat brain (24). Alternatively, dopamine (D2) receptors antagonized, indirectly by 5HT connections, can also increase appetite (as demonstrated for antipsychotics, see below). Histamine may also explain these effects, with H1 receptor antagonism also associated with an increase in appetite (22).

MONOAMINE OXIDASE (MAO) INHIBITORS

Weight gain has been described in a relation to older MAO inhibitors, whereas this side effect seems to be less prominent with the selective, reversible drugs such as meclobemide. These compounds may therefore represent an alternative treatment modality.

LITHIUM

Weight gain with lithium treatment is quite common, with estimates ranging between one-third and two-thirds of treated patients (25). Weight gain appears to be dose-related, and this side effect remains a leading reason for medication non-compliance (26). Interestingly, weight gain is more likely to occur in patients already overweight, and seems more problematic in female patients (25,27). The weight gain may be as much as 10 kg during a 2- to 10-year period.

The mechanism(s) responsible for lithium-induced weight gain are diverse and relatively inconsistent (25). These include increased appetite, increased fluid intake, altered energy metabolism and endocrine changes, including medication-induced hypothyroidism (28).

ANTIPSYCHOTIC MEDICATIONS

Weight gain as a side effect of antipsychotic treatment has been well documented for over 40 years (29,30) but its importance in the clinical management of chronic schizophrenia has been downplayed (31). Like antidepressants, it is also a common reason for medication non-compliance (31–33). Although numerous mechanisms have been proposed to explain such medication-induced weight gain, the mechanism(s) involved are even less clear than those for antidepressants; some data sup-

port a role for changes in appetite and food intake, as well as energy expenditure. Mefferd et al. (29) have suggested that increased appetite can account for weight gain, although this is poorly understood. It is possible that increases in thirst (resulting from the anticholinergic action of many drugs) result in increased caloric intake through increased fluid consumption (34), or from inactivity resulting from medication-related sedation (34), although these are presently only hypotheses.

Conventional Antipsychotics

Phenothiazines have been shown to be weight promoting during the chronic treatment of schizephrenia. Chlorpromazine (35), chlordiazepoxide (36) and thioridazine (36) increased weight significantly, compared to placebo. Ganguli (37) reported weight gain with haloperidol, thiothixane and fluphenazine. It has been suggested that weight gain is not proportional to dose, since depot injections of varying dosages did not correlate positively with weight gain (37–39). The weight gain can vary between 1–5 kg over several years to exorbitant weight increases in a few months of more than 28 kg, as illustrated in the cases shown in Figure 191.

Novel Antipsychotics

Clozapine is clearly associated with weight gain during treatment, and is among the greatest weight promoters of the antipsychotics (40,41), while molindone appears to be the only novel compound without weight promoting effects (41). Both clozapine and olanzapine appear to increase body weight through a leptin-mediated mechanism, since serum leptin levels increased during treatment with these compounds (42,43). A recent review ranked weight gain among the novel antipsychotics as follows: clozapine and olanzapine, risperidone and sertindole (44). The authors suggest a strong correlation with the histamine binding properties of these compounds (44) as a possible mechanism of action. Finally, weight gain and obesity may also arise in children after prenatal exposure to antipsychotic drugs such as haloperidol, which in the case reported by Breum (45) was prescribed as an

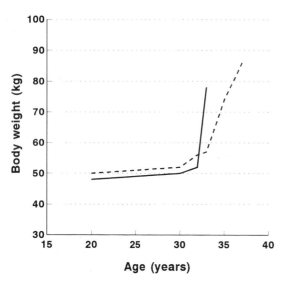

Figure 19.1 Two cases of drug-induced obesity in previously normal-weight women. Patient 1 (solid line) was treated with levomepromazine for only 7 months and increased her body weight by 28.7 kg. Patient 2 (dashed line) was treated for 4 years with chlorprothixene and was finally referred to a department of endocrinology due to 'unexplained' weight gain and a suspected endocrine 'disturbance'

antiemetic drug to an otherwise healthy pregnant female.

Weight Gain and Clinical Improvement

It has been suggested, as with antidepressants, that weight gain during neuroleptic treatment is a positive sign of improvement (3), and is necessary for a positive outcome, an obeservation confirmed by Leadbetter *et al.* (40). However, more recent data suggest that, in fact, weight gain is not necessary to achieve effective pharmacologic activity and improvement in symptoms (40,41).

ANTIEPILEPTIC DRUGS

Weight gain is one of the most prevalent side effects of several antiepileptic drugs, but has been particularly related with the use of valproate (valproic acid), a short-chain fatty acid widely used as an antiepileptic drug, and sometimes for the treatment of mania (46–49). In retrospective studies, treatment with valproate has been found to increase body weight by 4.0 to 7.5 kg in more than 60% of the patients (47,48). It has not been possible to detect any differences between weight-gainers and weight-stable patients with regard to family history, sex, age, reported appetite, duration, dosage or serum levels of valproate (48,50). The weight gain varies between different individuals and study populations, but might often amount to 20 kg and not infrequently resulting in discontinuation of the treatment (49). The pathogenetic mechanism is still largely unknown. Changes in thyroid hormones have earlier been proposed as an explanation (51), but a subsequent clinical study by Breum has not supported this theory (52). Valproate interferes with the gamma-amino butyric acid neurotransmitter system, which might affect the appetite regulation, but this remains unstudied. In one of the few physiological studies performed in patients before and during valproate treatment, it was not possible to demonstrate any significant differences in either energy intake obtained by food records or energy expenditure during a glucose load and under basal conditions (52). It has been suggested that a reduced beta-oxidation of fatty acids, as found in the above study, could be of etiological importance since valproic acid is known to enhance the excretion of carnitine, which is an essential cofactor for the transport of fatty acids across the mitochondrial membrane (53,54). The impact of valproate on serum leptin and insulin levels has also been measured, but it seems to reflect the obese state more than any specific effect of valproate treatment (55).

Animal studies are of limited interest due to difficulties in interpreting the results since drug treatment decreases food intake and enhances energy expenditure in many animals (56–58).

Weight gain is also a commonly described side effect to carbamazepine treatment of both epilepsy and mania. However, both the size of the problem as well as the number of studies are limited compared to valproate. In a study from the Veterans Affairs Epilepsy Cooperative Study Group it was shown that long-term treatment with carbamazepine was associated less frequently with weight gain more than 5.5 kg than with valproate (20% vs. 8%) (59). In susceptible individuals, the weight gain can be very pronounced and has been associated with a sharp increase in food intake and weight gain up to 15 kg over a few months (60). It is often necessary to stop the treatment before normal body weight can be achieved.

As with valproate, the mechanisms contributing to the weight gain are unknown, but since carbamazepine shares some chemical properties with tricyclic antidepressants it might affect body weight regulation through the same serotoninergic and noradrenergic pathways increasing the appetite, as suggested in some cases (60).

During the last decade, several new antiepileptic drugs have been introduced into clinical practice. One of those drugs, vigabatrin, is normally better tolerated than the older compounds, but has recently been shown to be more frequently associated with weight gain than carbamazepine (61). In contrast to this finding, weight gain has not been yet been described with lamotrigine and this drug may therefore represent an alternative treatment modality at least in some types of epilepsy.

ANTIANXIETY DRUGS

Benzodiazepine and its derivatives have in short-term experiments been shown to promote hyperphagia and weight gain in rodents due to an effect on dopamine D2 receptors (62) or gamma-amino butyric acid neurons (63), whereas long-term animal experiments have not been able to confirm these findings (64). Very few clinical human studies have been published reporting changes in body weight during treatment with anxiolytics. In a small study with myelopathy patients, a reduction or discontinuation of the diazepam medication in high doses resulted in a weight loss of 5 to 16 kg during a 10-month period. In a subgroup of the patients, who were reintroduced to the pharmacological treatment, body weight increased by 3 to 12 kg (65). However, in other larger human studies comparing various anxiolytics with other psychotropic drugs in subjects without severe physical handicaps, weight gain has not been reported as a side effect (66,67). Weight loss has also been described (68). Thus, in summary, benzodiazepines are unlikely to cause any significant weight gain in clinical practice.

ANTIMIGRAINE AND ANTIHISTAMINERGIC DRUGS

Weight gain is a common and early side effect of drugs such as sanomigran (69) and cyproheptadine (70) probably due to their combined antihistaminergic and serotonergic effect. The weight changes are, however, rather modest and the clinical importance of the problem is limited. Because to its ability to increase appetite attempts have been made to use cyproheptadine as a pharmacological support in the treatment of both anorexia nervosa (71) and cancer cachexia (72), but so far without encouraging results. Newer, non-sedating antihistaminergic agents such as loratadine and astemizole also produce weight gain, but to a lesser degree than the older compounds (73). The calcium antagonist flunarizine, used in migraine prophylaxis, has in several studies (74,75) been shown to increased appetite and induce a dose-dependent weight gain of up to 4 kg during the first months of the treatment period (74,76). The mechanism is not known, but an appetite stimulating effect involving brain dopamine and other central neurotransmitters has been suggested.

BETA-BLOCKERS

Treatment with non-specific beta-blockers, such as propranolol, has been associated with a modest, but sustained weight gain (77,78). In a large retrospective study of 3837 patients randomized to either propranolol or placebo treatment after a myocardial infarction, a weight gain of 2.3 kg was found after the first year in the beta-blocker treated patients compared to 1.2 kg in the placebo group. The difference between the groups remained during the following 2 years (77). The mechanism behind the weight gain is thought to be mediated through an effect on beta-receptors resulting in a reduction of the energy expenditure, including facultative thermogenesis, by approximately 200 kJ/day. In the recent UKPDS 39 substudy (79), atenolol and captopril were found to be equally effective in lowering blood pressure and reducing the risk of diabetic complications. However, the patients treated with atenolol showed a larger weight gain than those treated with captopril during a 9-year study period (3.4 kg vs. 1.6 kg). During the first 4 years of the study, the glycated haemoglobin was slightly higher in the atenolol group and more patients required additional glucose lowering treatment at the end of the study. It has been suggested (80,81) that beta-blockers might worsen the already impaired insulin sensitivity found in obese subjects, but the recent data from the UKPDS and other studies showed a reduced risk of cardiac events in beta-blocker treated patients (79).

INSULIN AND ORAL HYPOGLYCEMIC AGENTS

Intensive blood glucose control has, in large intervention trials, been shown to increase body weight in both type 1 and type 2 diabetic patients (82,83). In the Diabetes Control and Complications Trial (DCCT), intensive treatment with either multiple daily injections of insulin or continuous subcutaneous insulin infusion resulted in a 60% increased risk of a body weight more than 120% of the ideal body weight. On average, the intensively treated patients had a weight gain of 5 kg compared to the patients treated with conventional insulin regimens (82). Most of the weight changes appeared during the first year of treatment (82,84). In another DCCT substudy it was concluded that the changes in lipid levels and blood pressure that occur with excessive weight gain with intensive therapy were similar to those seen in the insulin resistance syndrome and may increase the risk of coronary artery disease in this subset of subjects with time (85). Not surprisingly, more female than male patients have been found to be worried about weight gain as a side effect and this may prove a significant impediment to the clinical implementation of intensive insulin treatments. It has been estimated that 70% of the weight gain can be accounted for by reduced glucosuria and that 30% is due to a reduction in energy expenditure by the reversal of the catabolic changes in carbohydrate, protein and lipid metabolism (86). Increased body weight has also been found in young type 1 patients on intensive therapy and might, especially in adolescent girls, influence adherence to good metabolic control regimens. (87,88).

In type 2 diabetes, the UKPDS study showed that weight gain was significantly higher in the intensive group (mean 5.4 kg) than in the conventional group (2.5 kg), and patients assigned to insulin had a greater gain in weight (6.5 kg) than those assigned to chlorpropamide (5.1 kg) or glibenclamide (3.2 kg) (83).

In contrast to these findings, a UKPDS substudy

with metformin in obese type 2 patients showed that the weight gain in metformin treated patients was similar to the conventional control group and less than the weight increases found in patients assigned to intensive treatment with insulin or sulphonylureas (89). In addition, patients who received metformin also had a more favorable outcome with respect to diabetes complications and mortality (89). If diabetes control cannot be achieved by metformin treatment alone, it should be combined with bedtime insulin since this treatment modality has been shown in a recent 12-month study to prevent weight gain and provide acceptable metabolic regulation (90). Also the newer glitazones have been associated with a modest, but significant, weight gain, although long-term data are still lacking.

ESTROGENS AND OTHER HORMONE DERIVATIVES

In earlier reports weight increases have been described in relation to older high dose hormonal contraceptives and weight gain is still one of the most prevalent complaints of women using oral hormonal contraceptives. However, the typical present day combination therapy contains only small doses of estrogen and progesterone and these compounds have not been associated with excessive weight gain apart from cyclic periods of moderate water retention in some individuals (91,92).

In postmenopausal women, several studies (93,94) have also demonstrated that hormone replacement therapy if anything may lead to a small weight reduction. This effect is not fully understood, but increased lipid oxidation seems to be of importance, whereas circulating leptin is not affected (95,96).

In contrast to these findings high to moderate doses of megestrol acetate have been shown to increase appetite and body weight in women with advanced cancer disease (97,98). Tamoxifen, a partial oestrogen receptor antagonist used in postmenopausal women with breast cancer, also promotes weight gain (99–101), but to a lesser extent when used as monotherapy (102).

These compounds, especially megestrol acetate, have therefore been suggested as adjuvant treatment in patients with cancer-induced cachexia (98). Other non-hormone antineoplastic agents such as cyclophosphamide and fluorouracil have also been associated with weight gain exceeding the pre-illness body weight in patients with early stage cancer disease (103). The mechanisms have not been elucidated and very few data are available.

GLUCOCORTICOSTEROIDS

Weight gain is a common adverse effect of long-term pharmacological treatment with glucocorticoids in patients not suffering from adrenal insufficiency (104–106). In a 12-month study of 109 patients with polymyalgia rheumatica/giant cell arteritis, a steroid-related dose-dependent weight increase of between 2 and 13 kg occurred in more than 50% of all patients (104). In a large retrospective study with 774 patients examined before and after liver transplantation, mean body mass index (BMI) increased from $24.8 \, kg/m^2$ initially to $28.1 \, kg/m^2$ in the second year after the operation (105). Of the 320 patients who were not obese before transplantation more than 20% became obese later. Interestingly, both donor and recipient BMIs were found to be risk factors for weight gain together with a high cumulative prednisolone dose. Other studies have suggested that intermittent use of glucocorticoids may diminish the weight gain (107), but data are not overwhelming. Glucocorticoid treatment also affects body fat distribution by predominantly increasing the abdominal fat tissue mass (108) and together with the more immediate effects on insulin resistance this may increase the risk for cardiovascular diseases and later diabetes.

The mechanisms behind glucocorticoid-induced weight increase is not fully understood, but it is well known that glucocorticosteroid hormones are important in obesity, since adrenalectomy will reverse or prevent the development of most forms of obesity in animals. It has been suggested that glucocorticoids may primarily exert an effect on energy balance through a stimulating effect on food intake since animal studies have shown that centrally injected glucocorticoids inhibit the hypothalamic effect of leptin and increase the activity of neuropeptide Y (NPY) (109,110). Central glucocorticoid infusion has also been shown to produce a marked decrease in the expression of uncoupling protein UCP1 and UCP3. In contrast to these results it was not possible to show any decrease in free-living energy expenditure or significant changes in substrate oxidation using the doubly labelled water method in healthy female volunteers taking 1 mg of betamethasone twice a day for 21 days (111). Other short-term human studies also failed to demonstrate an effect on energy expenditure or plasma leptin levels whereas energy intake was increased (112,113).

SUMMARY AND CONCLUSIONS

Weight gain associated with tricyclic antidepressant and certain antipsychotic medications is problematic for many treated patients, and often a reason for non-compliance. Such weight gain is associated, at least in part, with reductions in resting metabolic rate and diet-induced thermogenesis. Changes in food preference towards calorically dense ('fattening') sweet-tasting foods do not appear to affect a majority of patients treated with tricyclic medications, but can occur. When such preference changes do occur, though, they are not associated with the development or maintenance of obesity. Another class of antidepressants, specific serotonin reuptake inhibitors (SSRIs), have been used in the past few years as effective antidepressants, but do not promote weight gain during treatment, although this is occasionally seen. The antipsychotic medications often promote weight gain, particularly the conventional medications, but also some of the novel antipsychotics seem to have weight promoting effects. Although the mechanism(s) for antipsychotic-induced medications is poorly understood, increased caloric intake, a change in leptin response, and reduction in physical activity have all been proposed. Medication-induced weight gain is a significant problem for many treated patients, and the weight promoting effects of different psychiatric drugs should be considered in drug selection. A selection of the least weight promoting medication may promote drug compliance for many treated individuals, as well as avoid the comorbidities associated with increasing weight and obesity.

With respect to other drugs, the weight increases are often more modest, but can be a very serious problem with compounds used for chronic medication or long periods as with antiepileptic drugs such as valproate. The weight increases due to insulin or sulfonylurea agents not only might worsen the metabolic control in diabetic patients, but are also a major factor in non-compliance. So far only very few studies have been performed elucidating specific treatment possibilities in these groups of patients. Unfortunately, none of the current available anorectic agents have so far been studied in these groups of patients. Dietary advice, including avoidance of high calorie beverages, and lifestyle and exercise programs are still the fundamentals for the treatment of medication-induced weight gain. However, the recent advance in obesity research and especially the increased understanding of brain function may provide new possibilities for further treatment.

REFERENCES

1. Robinson RG, McHugh PR, Folstein MF. Measurement of appetite distrubances in psychiatric disorders. *J Psychiatr Res* 1975; **12**: 59–68.
2. Paykel ES. Depression and appetite. *J Psychosom Res* 1977; **21**: 401–407.
3. Mezzich JE, Raab JS. Depressive symptomology across the Americas. *Arch Gen Psychiatry* 1980; **37**: 818–823.
4. Stunkard AJ, Fernstrom MH, Price A, Frank E, Kupfer DJ. Direction of weight change in recurrent depression: A possible marker for subtypes of depression. *Arch Gen Psychiatry* 1990; **47**: 857–860.
5. Weissenburger JA, Rush AJ, Giles DE, Stunkard AJ. Weight change in depression. *Psychiatry Res* 1986; **17**: 275–283.
6. Rudorfer MV, Manji HK, Potter WZ. Comparative tolerability profiles of the newer versus older antidepressants. *Drug Saf* 1994; **10**: 18–46.
7. Kasper S, Fuger J, Moller H-J. Comparative efficacy of antidepressants. *Drugs* 1992; **43** (Suppl. 2): 11–23.
8. Paykel ES, Meuller PS, DeLa Vergne PM. Amitriptyline, weight gain, and carbohydrate craving. *Br J Psychiatry* 1973; **123**: 501–507.
9. Kupfer DJ, Coble PA, Rubenstein D. Changes in weight during treatment for depression. *Psychosom Med* 1979; **41**: 535–543.
10. Harris B, Young J, Hughes B. Appetite and weight duirng short-term antidepressant treament. *Br J Psychiatry* 1986; **145**: 645–648.
11. Fernstrom MH, Kupfer DJ. Antidepressant-induced weight gain: A comparison study of four medications. *Psychiatry Res* 1988; **26**: 265–271.
12. Berken GH, Weinstein D, Stern WC. Weight gain: A side effect of tricyclic antidepressants. *J Affect Disord* 1984; **7**: 133–138.
13. Fernstrom MH, Kupfer DJ. Imipramine treatment and preference for sweets. *Appetite* 1988; **10**: 149–155.
14. Fernstrom MH, Krowinski RL, Kupfer DJ. Appetite and food preference in depression: Effects of imipramine treatment. *Biol Psychiatry* 1987; **22**: 529–539.
15. Drewnowski A, Greenwood MRC. Cream and sugar: Human preferences for high-fat foods. *Physiol Behav* 1982; **30**: 629–633.
16. Garrow JS. *Energy Balance and Obesity in Man*, 2nd edn. Oxford: Elsevier-North Holland Press, 1978.
17. Fernstrom MH, Spiker DG, Epstein LH, Kupfer DJ. Resting metabolic rate is reduced in patients treated with antidepressants. *Biol Psychiatry* 1985; **20**: 688–692.
18. Fernstrom MH. Drugs that cause weight gain. *Obes Res* 1995; **3**(Suppl 4): 435–439.
19. Fogelson DL. Weight gain during fluoxetine treatment. *J Clin Psychopharmacol* 1991; **11**: 220–221.
20. Sussman N, Ginsburg DL. Weight gain associated with SSRIs. *Primary Psychiatry* 1988; **5**: 28–37.
21. Fisher S, Kent TA, Bryant SG. Postmarketing surveillance by patient self-monitoring: preliminary data for sertraline versus fluoxetine. *J Clin Psychiatry* 1991; **56**: 288–296.
22. Bouver CB, Harvey BH. Phasic craving for carbohydrate observed with citalopram. *Int Clin Psychopharmacol* 1996; **11**: 273–276.
23. Palvimaki EP, Roth BL, Majasuo H, *et al.* Interactions of selective serotonin receptor inhibitors with the serotonin 5HT2C receptor. *Psychopharmacology* 1996; **126**: 234– 240.
24. Laakso A, Palvimaki EP, Kuoppamaki M, *et al.* Chronic citalopram and fluoxetine treatments upregulate 5-HT2C receptors in the rat choroid plexus. *Neuropsy-chopharmacology* 1996; **15**: 143–151.
25. Ackerman S and Nolan LJ. Bodyweight gain induced by psychotropic drugs: incidence, mechanisms, and management. *CNS Drugs* 1998; **9**: 135–151.
26. John RE, McFarland BH. Lithium use and discontinuation in a health maintenance organization. *Am J Psychiatry* 1996; **153**: 993–1000.
27. Pijl H, Meinders AE. Bodyweight change as an adverse effect of drug treatment: mechanism and management. *Drug Saf* 1996; **14**: 329–342.
28. Holt RA, Maunder EMW. Is lithium-induced weight gain prevented by providing healthy eating advice at the commencement of lithium therapy? *J Nutr Hum Diet* 1996; **9**: 127–133.
29. Mefferd RB, Labrosse EH, Gawienowski AM, Williams R. Influence of chlorpromazine on certain biochemical variables of chornic male schizophrenics. *J Nerv Ment Dis* 1958; **127**: 167–179.
30. Planansky K, Heilizer F. Weight changes in relation to the characteristics of patients on chlorpromazine. *J Clin Exp Psychopathol* 1959; **20**: 53–57.
31. Silverstone T, Smith G, Goodall E. Prevalence of obesity in patients receiving depot antipsychotics. *Br J Psychiatry* 1988; **153**: 214–217.
32. Bernstein JG. Induction of obesity by psychotropic drugs. *Ann N Y Acad Med* 1988; **499**: 203–215.
33. Brady KT. Weight gain associated with psychotropic drugs. *South Med J* 1989; **82**: 611–617.
34. Stanton JM. Weight gain associated with neuroleptic medication: a review. *Schizophr Bull* 1995; **21**: 463–472.
35. Klett CJ, Caffey EM. Weight changes during treatment with phenothizaine derivatives. *J Neuropsychiatry* 1960; **2**: 102–108.
36. Holden JMC, Holden UP. Weight changes with schizophrenic psychosis and psychotropic drug therapy. *Psycho-*

somatics 1970; **11**: 551–561.

37. Ganguli R. Weight gain associated with antipsychotic drugs. *J Clin Psychiatry* 1999; **60**: (S2)20–24.

38. Johnson DA, Breen M. Weight changes with depot neuroleptic maintenance therapy. *Acta Psychiatr Scand* 1979; **59**: 525–528.

39. Cookson JC, Kennedy NM, Gribbon D. Weight gain and prolactin levels in patients on long-term antipsychotic medication: a double-blind comparative trial of haloperidol decanoate and fluphenazine decanoate. *Int Clin Psychopharmacol* 1986; **S1**: 41–51.

40. Leadbetter R, Shutty M, Pavalonis D, *et al*. Clozapine-induced weight gain: prevalence and clinical relevance. *Am J Psychiatry* 1982; **149**: 68–72.

41. Sachs GS, Guille C. Weight gain associated with the use of psychotropic medications. *J Clin Psychiatry* 1999; **60**(S2): 16–19.

42. Kraus T, Haack M, Schuld A, *et al*. Body weight and leptin plasma levels during treatment with antipsychotic drugs. *Am J Psychiatry* 1999; **156**: 312–314.

43. Bromel T, Blum WF, Ziegler A, *et al*. Serum leptin levels increase rapidly after initiation of clozapine therapy. *Mol Psychiatry* 1998; **3**: 76–80.

44. Wirshing DA, Wirshing WC, Kysar L, *et al*. Novel antipsychotics: comparison of weight gain liabilities. *J Clin Psychiatry* 1999; **60**: 358–363.

45. Breum L, Astrup AV, Quaade F. Increased appetite after prenatal haloperidol exposure—a case report. *Int J Obes* 1993; **10**: 609.

46. Convanis A, Gupta K, Jeavons PM. Sodium valproate: Monotherapy and polytherapy. *Epilepsia* 1982; **23**: 693–720.

47. Corman CL, Leung NM, Guberman AH. Weight gain in epileptic patients during treatment with valproic acid: a retrospective study. *Can J Neurol Sci* 1997; **24**: 240–244.

48. Dinesen H, Gram L, Andersen T, Dam M. Weight gain during treatment with valproate. *Acta Neurol Scand* 1984; **70**: 65–69.

49. Egger J, Brett EM. Effects of sodium valproate in 100 children with special reference to weight. *BMJ* 1981; **283**: 557–581.

50. Novak GP, Maytal J, Alshansky A, Eviatar L, Sy-Kho R, Siddique Q. Risk of excessive weight gain in epileptic children treated with valproate. *J Child Neurol* 1999; **14**: 490–495.

51. Bentsen KD, Gram L, Veje A. Serum thyroid hormones and blood folic acid during monotherapy with carbamazepine or valproate. *Acta Neurol Scand* 1983: 67: 235–241.

52. Breum L, Astrup A, Gram L, Andersen T, Stokholm KH, Christensen NJ, Werdelin L, Madsen J. Metabolic changes during treatment with valproate in humans: Implication for untoward weight gain. *Metabolism* 1992; **41**: 666–670.

53. Laub MC, Paetzke-Brunner, Jaeger G: Serum carnitine dyring valproic acid therapy: *Epilepsia* 1986; **27**: 559–562.

54. Editorial. Carnitine deficiency. *Lancet* 1990; 631–633.

55. Verrotti A, Basciani F, Morresi S, de Martino M, Morgese G, Chiarelli F. Serum leptin changes in epileptic patients who gain weight after therapy with valproic acid. *Neurology* 1999; **53**: 230–232.

56. Horton R, Rothwell NJ, Stock MJ. Chronic inhibition of Gaba Transaminase results in activation of thermogenesis and brown fat in the rat. *Gen Pharmacol* 1988; **19**: 403–405.

57. Coscina DV, Nobrega JN. Anorectic potency of inhibiting GABA transamination in brain studies of hypothalamic, dietary and genetic obesities. *Int J Obes* 1984; **8**: 191–200.

58. Wolden-Hanson T, Gidal BE, Atkinson RL. Evaluation of a rat model of valproate-induced obesity. *Pharmacotherapy* 1998; **18**: 1075–1081.

59. Mattson RH, Cramer JA, Collins JF. A comparison of valproate with carbamazepine for the treatment of complex partial seizures and secondarily generalized tonic-clonic seizures in adults. *N Engl J Med* 1992; **327**: 765–771.

60. Lampl Y, Eshel Y, Rapaport A, Sarova-Pinhas I. Weight gain, increased appetite, and excessive food intake induced by carbamazepine. *Clin Neuropharmacol* 1991; **14**: 251–255.

61. Chadwick D. Safety and efficacy of vigabatrin and carbamazepine in newly diagnosed epilepsy: a multicentre randomised double-blind study. Vigabatrin European Monotherapy Study Group. *Lancet* 1999; **354**: 13–19.

62. Rahminiwati M, Nishimura M. Diazepam-induced hyperphagia in mice is sensitive to quinpirole. *J Vet Med Sci* 1999; **61**: 777–780.

63. Cooper SJ. GABA and endorphin mechanism in relation to the effects of benzodiazepines on feeding and drinking. *Prog Neuropsychopharmacol Biol Psychiatry* 1983; **7**: 495–505.

64. Jing X, Wala EP, Sloan JW. The effect of chronic benzodiazepines exposure on body weight in rats. *Pharmacol Res* 1998; **37**: 179–189.

65. Frisbie JH, Aguilera EJ. Diazepam and body weight in myelopathy patients. *J Spinal Cord Med* 1995; **18**: 200–202.

66. Jokinen K, Koskinen T, Selonen R. Flupenthixol versus diazepam in the treatment of psychosomatic disorders: a double-blind, multi-centre trial in general practice. *Pharmatherapeutica* 1984; **3**: 573–581.

67. Bjertnaes A, Block JM, Hafstad PE, Holte M, Ottemo I, Larsen T, Pinder RM, Steffensen K, Stulemeijer SM. A multicentre placebo-controlled trial comparing the efficacy of mianserin and chlordiazepoxide in general practice patients with primary anxiety. *Acta Psychiatr Scand* 1982; **66**: 199–207.

68. Ostwald I, Adam K. Benzodiazepines cause small loss of body weight. *BMJ* 1980; **281**: 1039–1040.

69. Louis P, Spierings EL. Comparison of flunarizine (Sibelium) and pizotifen (Sanomigran) in migraine treatment: a double-blind study. *Cephalalgia* 1982; **2**: 197–203.

70. Toth K, Szonyi A. The appetite stimulating and weight gain promoting effect of peritol (cyproheptadine) examined on a great number of outpatients. *Ther Hung* 1976; **1**: 24–32.

71. Walsh BT, Devlin MJ. The pharmacologic treatment of eating disorders. *Psychiatr Clin North Am* 1992; **15**: 149–160.

72. Chlebowski RT, Palomares MR, Lillington L, Grosvenor M. Recent implications of weight loss in lung cancer management. *Nutrition* 1996; **12**(S1): S43–47.

73. Chervinsky P, Georgitis J, Banov C, Boggs P, Vande Souwe R, Greenstein S. Once daily loratadine versus astemizole once daily. *Ann Allergy* 1994; **73**: 109–113.

74. Martinez-Lage JM. Flunarizine (Sibelium) in the prophylaxis of migraine. An open, long-term, multicenter trial. *Cephalalgia* 1988; **8(S8)**: 15–20.

75. Sorensen PS, Larsen BH, Rasmussen MJ, Kinge E, Iversen H, Alslev T, Nohr P, Pedersen KK, Schroder P, Lademann A, et al. Flunarizine versus metoprolol in migraine prophylaxis: a double-blind, randomized parallel group study of efficacy and tolerability. *Headache* 1991; **31**: 650–657.

76. Centonze V, Magrone D, Vino M, Caporaletti P, Attolini E, Campanale G, Albano O. Flunarizine in migraine prophylaxis: efficacy and tolerability of 5 mg and 10 mg dose levels. *Cephalalgia* 1990; **10**: 17–24.

77. Rossner S, Taylor CL, Byington RP, Furberg CD. Long term propranolol treatment and changes in body weight after myocardial infarction. *BMJ* 1990; **300**: 902–903.

78. Shimell CJ, Fritz VU, Levien SL. A comparative trial of flunarizine and propranolol in the prevention of migraine. *S Afr Med J* 1990; **77**: 75–77.

79. UK Prospective Diabetes Study Group. Efficacy of atenolol and captopril in reducing risk of macrovascular and microvascular complications in type 2 diabetes: UKPDS 39. UK Prospective Diabetes Study Group. *BMJ* 1998; **317**: 713–720.

80. Jacob S, Rett K, Henriksen EJ. Antihypertensive therapy and insulin sensitivity: do we have to redefine the role of beta-blocking agents? *Am J Hypertens* 1998; **10**: 1258–1265.

81. Lithell HO. Insulin resistance and diabetes in the context of treatment of hypertension. *Blood Press* 1998; **S3**: 28–31.

82. The Diabetes Control and Complications Trial Research Group. The effect of intensive treatment of diabetes on the development and progression of long-term complications in insulin-dependent diabetes mellitus. *N Engl J Med* 1993; **329**: 977–986.

83. UK Prospective Diabetes Study (UKPDS) Group. Intensive blood-glucose control with sulphonylureas or insulin compared with conventional treatment and risk of complications in patients with type 2 diabetes (UKPDS 33). *Lancet* 1998; **352**: 837–853.

84. DCCT Research Group. Weight gain associated with intensive therapy in the diabetes control and complications trial. *Diabetes Care* 1988; **11**: 567–573.

85. Purnell JQ, Hokanson JE, Marcovina SM, Steffes MW, Cleary PA, Brunzell JD. Effect of excessive weight gain with intensive therapy of type 1 diabetes on lipid levels and blood pressure: results from the DCCT. Diabetes Control and Complications Trial. *JAMA* 1998; **280**: 140–146.

86. Carlson MG, Campbell PJ: Intensive insulin therapy and weight gain in IDDM. *Diabetes* 1993; **42**: 1700–1707.

87. Mortensen HB, Robertson KJ, Aanstoot HJ, Danne T, Holl RW, Hougaard P, Atchison JA, Chiarelli F, Daneman D, Dinesen B, Dorchy H, Garandeau P, Greene S, Hoey H, Kaprio EA, Kocova M, Martul P, Matsuura S, Schoenle EJ, Sovik O, Swift PG, Tsou RM, Vanelli M, Aman J. Insulin management and metabolic control of type 1 diabetes mellitus in childhood and adolescence in 18 countries. *Diabet Med* 1998; **15**: 752–759.

88. Morris AD, Boyle DI, McMahon AD, Greene SA, MacDonald TM, Newton RW. Adherence to insulin treatment, glycaemic control, and ketoacidosis in insulin-dependent diabetes mellitus. The DARTS/MEMO Collaboration. Diabetes Audit and Research in Tayside Scotland. Medicines Monitoring Unit. *Lancet* 1997; **350**: 1505–1510.

89. UK Prospective Diabetes Study (UKPDS) Group. Effect of intensive blood glucose control with metformin on complications in overweight patients with type 2 diabetes (UKPDS 34). *Lancet* 1998; **352**: 854–865.

90. Yki-Jarvinen H, Ryysy L, Nikkila K, Tulokas T, Vanamo R, Heikkila M. Comparison of bedtime insulin regimens in patients with type 2 diabetes mellitus. A randomized, controlled trial. *Ann Intern Med* 1999; **130**: 389–396.

91. Risser WL, Gefter LR, Barratt MS, Risser JM. Weight change in adolescents who used hormonal contraception. *J Adolesc Health* 1999; **24**: 433–436.

92. Rosenberg M. Weight change with oral contraceptive use and during the menstrual cycle. Results of daily measurements. *Contraception* 1998; **58**: 345–349.

93. Chmouliovsky L, Habicht F, James RW, Lehmann T, Campana A, Golay A. Beneficial effect of hormone replacement therapy on weight loss in obese menopausal women. *Maturitas* 1999; **32**: 147–153.

94. Weber-Diehl F, Unger R, Lachnit U. Triphasic combination of ethinyl estradiol and gestodene. Long-term clinical trial. *Contraception* 1992; **46**: 19–27.

95. Kristensen K, Pedersen SB, Vestergaard P, Mosekilde B, Richelsen L. Hormone replacement therapy affects body composition and leptin differently in obese and non-obese postmenopausal women. *J Endocrinol* 1999; **163**: 55–62.

96. Gambacciani M, Ciaponi M, Cappagli B, Piaggesi L, De Simone L, Orlandi R, Genazzani AR. Body weight, body fat distribution, and hormonal replacement therapy in early postmenopausal women. *J Clin Endocrinol Metab* 1997; **82**: 414–417.

97. Bruera E, Macmillan K, Kuehn N, Hanson J, MacDonald RN. A controlled trial of megestrol acetate on appetite, caloric intake, nutritional status, and other symptoms in patients with advanced cancer. *Cancer* 1990; **66**: 1279–1282.

98. Alexieva-Figusch J, van Gilse HA, Hop WC, Phoa CH, Blonk-van der Wijst J, Treurniet RE. Progestin therapy in advanced breast cancer: megestrol acetate—an evaluation of 160 treated cases. *Cancer* 1980; **46**: 2369–2372.

99. Hoskin PJ, Ashley S, Yarnold JR. Weight gain after primary surgery for breast cancer—effect of tamoxifen. *Breast Cancer Res Treat* 1992; **22**: 129–132.

100. Goodwin PJ, Panzarella T, Boyd NF. Weight gain in women with localized breast cancer—a descriptive study. *Breast Cancer Res Treat* 1988; **11**: 59–66.

101. Goodwin PJ, Ennis M, Pritchard KI, McCready D, Koo J, Sidlofsky S, Trudeau M, Hood N, Redwood S. Adjuvant treatment and onset of menopause predict weight gain after breast cancer diagnosis. *J Clin Oncol* 1999; **17**: 120–129.

102. Kumar NB, Allen K, Cantor A, Cox CE, Greenberg H, Shah S, Lyman GH. Weight gain associated with adjuvant tamoxifen therapy in stage I and II breast cancer: fact or artifact?. *Breast Cancer Res Treat* 1997; **44**: 135–143.

103. Demark-Wahnefried W, Winer EP, Rimer BK. Why women gain weight with adjuvant chemotherapy for breast cancer. *J Clin Oncol* 1993; **11**: 1418–1429.

104. Kyle V, Hazleman BL. Treatment of polymyalgia rheumatica and giant cell arteritis. II. Relation between steroid dose and steroid associated side effects. *Ann Rheum Dis* 1989; **48**: 662–666.

105. Everhart JE, Lombardero M, Lake JR, Wiesner RH, Zetterman RK, Hoofnagle JH. Weight change and obesity after liver transplantation: incidence and risk factors. *Liver*

Transpl Surg 1998; **4**: 285–296.

106. Prummel MF, Mourits MP, Blank L, Berghout A, Koornneef L, Wiersinga WM. Randomized double-blind trial of prednisone versus radiotherapy in Graves' ophthalmopathy. *Lancet* 1993; **342**: 949–954.

107. Curtis JJ, Galla JH, Woodford SY, Saykaly RJ, Luke RG. Comparison of daily and alternate-day prednisone during chronic maintenance therapy: a controlled crossover study. *Am J Kidney Dis* 1981; **1**: 166–171.

108. Horber FF, Zurcher RM, Herren H, Crivelli MA, Robotti G, Frey FJ. Altered body fat distribution in patients with glucocorticoid treatment and in patients on long-term dialysis. *Am J Clin Nutr* 1986; **43**: 758–769.

109. Zakrzewska KE, Cusin I, Stricker-Krongrad A, Boss O, Ricquier D, Jeanrenaud B, Rohner-Jeanrenaud F. Induction of obesity and hyperleptinemia by central glucocorticoid infusion in the rat. *Diabetes* 1999; **48**: 365–370.

110. Zakrzewska KE, Sainsbury A, Cusin I, Rouru J, Jeanrenaud B, Rohner-Jeanrenaud F. Selective dependence of intracerebroventricular neuropeptide Y-elicited effects on central glucocorticoids. *Endocrinology* 1999; **140**: 3183–3187.

111. Chong PK, Jung RT, Scrimgeour CM, Rennie MJ. The effect of pharmacological dosages of glucocorticoids on free living total energy expenditure in man. *Clin Endo-crinol (Oxf)* 1994; **40**: 577–581.

112. Tataranni PA, Larson DE, Snitker S, Young JB, Flatt JP, Ravussin E. Effects of glucocorticoids on energy metabolism and food intake in humans. *Am J Physiol* 1996; **271**: E317–325.

113. Tataranni PA, Pratley R, Maffei M, Ravussin E. Acute and prolonged administration of glucocorticoids (methylprednisolone) does not affect plasma leptin concentration in humans. *Int J Obes Relat Metab Disord* 1997; **21**: 327–330.

20

Pregnancy

Helen E. Harris

PHLS Communicable Disease Surveillance Centre, London, UK

FEMALE OBESITY

The prevalence of female obesity has increased steadily over the last 40 years in both the UK and the USA (1,2). Even during the last decade, the prevalence of female obesity (BMI > 30) in Britain rose from 8% in 1980 to 12% in 1987 (3). This increase led the British government to identify 'the reduction of obesity' as one of its main targets for health improvement (4), yet in spite of this initiative female obesity continues to rise and currently stands at 20% (5). Paradoxically, the increasing prevalence of obesity has occurred in the face of remarkable social pressure to be thin, and data from weight surveys consistently show more women than men to be affected (Figure 20.1). If pregnancy is a determinant of obesity, then this might explain the higher prevalence of obesity in women. The accelerated rate of weight gain observed among young women might also be a reflection of the current trend towards encouraging women to gain more weight during pregnancy (6).

PREGNANCY AS A CAUSE OF OBESITY: THE EVIDENCE

Women in developing countries often become progressively malnourished with successive pregnancies and this has been shown to lead to maternal depletion rather than maternal obesity (8,9). However, in developed countries most investigators report a net increase in body weight with pregnancy that may persist and even increase with successive pregnancies (10,11).

Anecdotal Evidence and Evidence from Case Series Studies

Pregnancy has long been thought to be aetiologically related to obesity (12) and as early as 1939, Greene (13) observed that some of his obese female patients: 'gained 15 to 25 pounds with each pregnancy, maintained the added weight, and thus became obese after three to six pregnancies.' By 1949, Sheldon (14) suggested that it was: 'a matter of common observation that women may at times develop a severe obesity after having a baby', and he coined the term 'maternal obesity' to describe this phenomenon. There is certainly a wealth of anecdotal evidence that pregnancy can lead to obesity, and evidence from case series studies suggests that obese women often cite pregnancy as a triggering life event for the development of their obesity (15–17). The results of such studies should, however, be interpreted with caution as women may retrospectively report pregnancy as a socially acceptable cause for an obesity that resulted from excessive energy intake. The validity of these studies can also depend on the accuracy with which obese women report their body weight (18). Although self-reported body weight is highly correlated with measured weight (19), there is considerable inter-individual variation in the accuracy with which it is reported. For example, Stevens-Simon *et al.* (19),

International Textbook of Obesity. Edited by Per Björntorp.

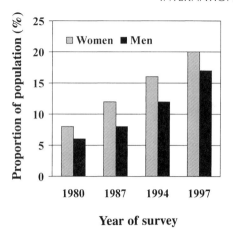

Figure 20.1 Prevalence of clinical obesity in the UK (from Jebb (7)). Reproduced by permission of Flour Advisory Bureau

found that women underestimated their body weight by an average of 1.3 kg. This figure, however, ranged from a mean over-report of 1.4 kg for women who were initially underweight (less than 90% of ideal weight-for-height) to a mean under-report of 5.0 kg for women who were initially over-weight (more than 120% of ideal weight-for-height). Therefore, women's desire to report a body weight that conforms to their own ideal or to perceived norms represents an important methodological limitation for studies that rely on self-reported in-formation. Nevertheless, case series studies provide the first level of evidence that pregnancy may trig-ger obesity, even if only in a small percentage of women.

Cross-sectional Studies that Examine the Effect of Pregnancy on Body Weight

More compelling evidence comes from cross-sec-tional surveys that examine the effect of childbear-ing on body weight (Table 20.1). Some of the very first systematic studies were based on demographic and industrial surveys of women's body weight (20–24). These surveys found that women with children had higher body weights than those with-out, and that maternal body weight increased with increasing parity (parity approximates to 'number of live births'). Since this time, there have been numerous other studies demonstrating the same association (25–28). Parity is, however, associated with a number of sociodemographic characteristics, such as higher maternal age, lower social class and

marriage, all of which are independently associated with an increased risk of weight gain (23,29). It is therefore possible that some, or all, of the observed effect of parity on body weight results from failure to control for the confounding effects of factors that are inherently associated with pregnancy but inde-pendently associated with weight gain.

A number of population-based cross-sectional studies (25,28), have employed stratification or multivariate statistical techniques to adjust for the confounding effects of age and other factors. In so doing, they reduce the possibility that any remain-ing differences in body weight between women of differing parity are simply the result of confounding. Williamson et al. (28) undertook one such analysis using data that had been collected during the first US National Health and Nutrition Examination Survey. This analysis showed that for women with children, body weight increases with each addi-tional live birth, even after accounting for a large number of known confounding factors (Figure 20.2). Women with three or more live births had higher mean body weight than women with fewer live births, with the greatest increases in mean body weight being associated with five or more live births. Such cross-sectional studies provide strong evidence that pregnancy is independently asso-ciated with persistent weight gain. However, it is probably not possible to control for all of the fac-tors that might be responsible for differences in energy balance between women. There might also be inherent, immeasurable, and therefore uncon-trollable, differences between women who choose to have children and those who have none.

Many cross-sectional studies are essentially op-portunistic analyses of large, readily available, epi-demiological data sets. They therefore often fail to control for many of the psychosocial and behav-ioural confounders associated with pregnancy, sim-ply because these data are not routinely collected on a national basis. As such, cross-sectional studies can rarely differentiate between the effects of child *bearing* and child *rearing* on body weight.

Longitudinal Studies that Examine the Effect of Pregnancy on Body Weight

Perhaps the best evidence comes from longitudinal studies that effectively use each woman as her own

Table 20.1   Cross-sectional studies that examined the relationship between parity and maternal body weight

Country	Date of data collection	Control for potential confounders	Sample size (n)	Reference
England	1945–55	1, 2	5081	Lowe and Gibson (23)
Scotland	—	1, 3	—	Thomson and Billewicz (30)
Sweden	1962–63	1b, 2, 4	378	Cederlöf and Kaij (31)
Netherlands	1980	1, 2, 3, 5, 6, 7, 8	2092	Baecke et al. (32)
United States	1968–69	1, 3, 7, 9	755	Lee-Feldstein et al. (33)
Sweden	1968–69	1, 2, 3, 5, 6, 10, 11, 12	1373	Noppa and Bengtsson (34)
Finland	1966–72	1, 2, 3, 6, 7, 13, 14	17688	Heliövaara and Aromaa (25)
Gambia	1978–79	15	139	Prentice et al. (35)
Wales	1965–79	1, 2, 3, 6, 14, 30	35556	Newcombe (26)
England and Scotland	1972	1, 2, 3, 6, 16	7013	Rona and Morris (29)
United States	1977–78	1, 2, 3, 5, 6, 9, 12, 14	1133	Forster et al. (36)
United States	1981	1, 3, 9, 14, 19, 20, 21, 31	514	Caan et al. (37)
Bangladesh	1975–78	1	2446	Chowdhury (38)
United States	1971–80	1, 3, 9	7414	Kumanyika (39)
United States	1984–87	1, 3, 26	1186	Kritz-Silverstein (40)
Sweden	Mid 1980's	1	2295	Öhlin and Rössner (41)
United States	—	1, 3, 29	87	Rodin et al. (42)
United States	1985	1, 2, 3, 5, 14	41184	Brown et al. (27)
United States	1976	3	113606	Manson et al. (43)
United States	1971–84	1, 2, 3, 5, 6, 14, 24, 25, 26, 29	2547	Williamson et al. (28)
United States	1991–92	1, 17	211	Hunt et al. (44)

Potential confounders: 1, maternal age; 2, marital status; 3, maternal height; 4, heterozygosity (monozygotic twins); 5, education; 6, occupation, social class and employment status; 7, urbanization; 8, religion and church attendance; 9, ethnicity; 10, size and housing; 11, husband's age; 12, income; 13, capacity for work; 14, smoking status; 15, fertility; 16, husband's BMI; 17, obesity during adolescence and adult life; 18, age at menopause and/or menopausal problems; 19, birthweight of previous child; 20, body weight during first pregnancy; 21, household size; 22, age at menarchy; 23, contraceptive and/or HRT use; 24, alcohol use; 25, physical activity; 26, medical history and health status; 27, family history of breast and/or endometrial cancer; 28, menstrual cycle rhythmicity; 29, dieting and weight cycling; 30, lactation; 31, Interbirth interval.
From Harris and Ellison (12). Reproduced by permission of the Nutrition Society.

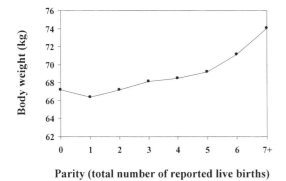

Parity (total number of reported live births)

Figure 20.2   The relationship between parity and body weight among women examined by Williamson et al. (28). Adjusted for the confounding effects of age, education, smoking status, drinking status, physical activity, health status, marital status, and dieting

control by comparing body weight after pregnancy with that recorded before conception. In this way, any differences in weight can be directly attributed to events that occurred during the intervening per-

iod. Provided an accurate measure of pre-pregnant weight is available, and that women are given sufficient time to lose the weight that they gain during pregnancy, longitudinal studies should be able to assess whether persistent changes in maternal body weight occur (12). They should also be able to establish whether pregnancy is responsible for any of the weight changes that are observed.

Intrinsic to this design is the need to quantify, and correct for, any weight gain that might have occurred during the study if the women had not become pregnant. Basal metabolic rate normally decreases by approximately 1% per year, and for an individual who maintains an identical lifestyle with regard to eating habits and exercise, this implies a weight increase of around 0.47 kg per year (45). One way to correct for this ageing-related weight gain in pregnant women is simultaneously to monitor the weight development of a (control) group of women who do not experience pregnancy (46–48). The weight gain of these women can then be used to

correct for ageing-related weight gain in the pregnant (case) women. In practice it is actually very
difficult to recruit an appropriate group of control
women since any differences in the amount of
weight gained by pregnant and non-pregnant
women might simply be the result of confounding.
For example, non-pregnant women *without*
children have been shown to gain more weight over
time than non-pregnant women *with* children (28).
To avoid these problems other researchers have
corrected for ageing-related gains by employing
multivariate statistical techniques to account for
the weight gain that is independently associated
with the study interval (49,50). In a pioneering study
by McKeown and Record (51), this problem was
overcome by using each woman's rate of weight
gain during the second year after delivery to correct
for the ageing-related weight gain during the period
of study.

There are a variety of longitudinal studies that
have examined the development of body weight
following pregnancy, and the results of those studies
whose primary aim was to assess the impact of
pregnancy on body weight are summarized in Table
20.2. A more exhaustive survey of studies published
up to 1995 is given by Harris and Ellison (12). A
critical review of these longitudinal studies (12) revealed three studies to be particularly robust
(28,46,48). The first of these studies formed part of
an extensive 4-year follow-up study monitoring the
development of obesity in young Dutch adults (46).
This study compared the changes in body mass
index (BMI) of a group of women who became
pregnant (cases) with the changes in BMI of a group
of women who did not fall pregnant (controls). All
pre-pregnant body weights were measured before
conception, and these measurements were taken at
least 9 months after any preceding pregnancy. The
follow-up measurements of body weight were
taken, on average, 12 months after delivery so that
all of the women in the study had sufficient time for
their body weight to return to its pre-pregnant level
before follow-up measurements of body weight
were taken. Rookus *et al.* (46) showed that the 40
cases gained, on average, $0.61 \pm 0.15 \, \text{kg/m}^2$ during
the study period, whereas the 400 non-pregnant
controls gained only $0.27 \pm 0.05 \, \text{kg/m}^2$, the crude
difference ($0.34 \pm 0.16 \, \text{kg/m}^2$) being statistically significant. However, after accounting for differences
in age, level of education, parity, giving up work,
smoking status and change in smoking status be-

tween the cases and the controls, the differential
change in BMI between the two groups was no
longer statistically significant ($0.15 \pm 0.21 \, \text{kg/m}^2$).

The second study by Smith *et al.* (48) examined
the relationship between pregnancy and persistent
changes in weight among young US women in a
prospective investigation that used data from the
CARDIA (Coronary Artery Risk Development in
Young Adults) study. In this study, measurements
of body weight were taken at a baseline examination in 1985–1986, at a second examination in
1987–1988, and again in 1990–1991. Women were
included in the study if they remained childless
throughout the three examinations (nulliparous
controls) or if they had a single pregnancy between
examinations 1 and 3 (primiparous or multiparous
cases, depending on their baseline parity). The
measurement of body weight taken at baseline served as the pre-pregnant weight, and all multiparous
cases were at least 12 months postpartum at baseline to exclude the effects of any previous pregnancies. Similarly, cases were excluded if they were not
at least 12 months postpartum at the time of examination 3, so that any expected return to pre-pregnancy weight should have occurred prior to the
follow-up examination. Their results showed that
black mothers having their first child gained 3.3 kg
more weight than black nulliparous control women
($P = 0.02$). Likewise, white mothers having their
first baby gained 2.3 kg more weight than white
nulliparous control women ($P = 0.03$). In contrast,
all those mothers who delivered a second or higher
order child during the period of study did not gain
significantly more weight as a result of their (later)
pregnancies than did the nulliparous controls.
Overall, mothers who experienced pregnancy
gained 0.92 kg more weight than the controls
(2.76 kg more for primiparous mothers, and 0.52 kg
less for multiparous mothers), which reduced to
0.80 kg after adjusting for a variety of confounders
(2.35 kg more for primiparous mothers, and 0.42 kg
less for multiparous mothers).

The third study by Williamson *et al.* (28) compared the weight development of mothers with both
parous and nulliparous controls. In this study Williamson *et al.* (28) presented results from the analysis
of a nationally representative cohort of US white
women aged 25–45 years, who were followed for
approximately 10 years from 1971–1975 to 1981–
1984. All pre-pregnant weights were measured before conception during the baseline examin-

Table 20.2 Longitudinal studies whose primary aim was to investigate the effect of pregnancy on maternal body weight

Country	Date of data collection	Type of pre-pregnant weight measurement	Postpartum follow-up	Control for ageing (kg/year)	Long-term weight gain $x \pm SEM\ (kg)^a$	No.	Reference
England	1949–50	Measured ≤ 28 weeks gestation	24 months	0.27	0.8 ± 0.0	289	McKeown and Record (51)
Scotland	1949–64	Measured 20 weeks gestation	18–108 months	~ 0.40	1.8 ± 0.1	3583	Billewicz and Thomson (52)
England	1965–75	Measured 20 weeks gestation	6 weeks	—	−0.2 ± 0.0	50	Beazley and Swinhoe (10)
United States	—	Self-report	6 weeks	—	2.7 ± 0.1	182	Olsen and Mundt (53)
Netherlands	1980–85	Measured before conception	12 months	0.40	1.6 ± 0.4	40	Rookus et al. (46)
United States	1959–65	Self-report	< 6 years	0.45	1.5 ± 0.1	7116	Greene et al. (49)
Sweden	Mid-1980s	Self-report	12 months	0.10	1.5 ± 0.1	1423	Öhlin and Rössner (54,55)
United States	—	Self-report	6–9 months	0.50	3.8 ± 0.9	37	Parham et al. (47)
United States	1989–90	Measured ~ 12 weeks gestation	~ 6 months	—	1.4 ± 0.2	489	Schauberger et al. (56)
United States	1988	Self-report	10–18 months	—	1.3	1592	Keppel and Taffel (57)
United States	1985–91	Measured before conception	12–60 months	0.76	5.3 ± 1.2	202	Smith et al. (48)
United States	1971–84	Measured before conception	24–156 months	0.38	1.7 ± 0.6	215	Williamson et al. (28)
United States	—	Self-report	7–12 months	—	5.0 ± 0.1	345	Boardley et al. (58)
United States	1985–88	Self-report	6 months	—	4.8 ± 0.5	274	Scholl et al. (59)
Canada	1979–89	Measured before conception	6 weeks	—	5.3 ± 0.3	371	Muscati et al. (60)
United States	—	Self-report	18 months	—	2.3 ± 0.8	75	Walker (61)
England	1980–93	Measured ≤ 13 weeks gestation	> 12 months	0.94	2.6 ± 0.3	243	Harris et al. (50)
United States	—	Self-report	18 months	—	3.0 ± 0.5	71	Janney et al. (62)
Iceland	—	Self-report	18–24 months	—	1.3 ± 0.4	175	Thorsdottir and Birgisdottir (63)
Hong Kong	—	Self-report	3–4 months	—	3.6 ± 0.2	272	To and Cheung (64)

^{a}Long-term maternal weight gain = (mean maternal body weight at follow-up) − (mean pre-pregnant body weight), and was uncorrected for ageing. Where necessary, standard errors of long-term maternal weight gain were calculated using the mean coefficients of variation for measurements of body weight recorded before and after pregnancy.
Data from Harris and Ellison (12)

ation at least 12 months after any preceding pregnancy. All women were at least 12 months postpartum by the time of follow-up interview. When compared to all women who did not give birth during the period of the study (both parous and nulliparous), and after controlling for a variety of confounding factors, the mean excess weight gain attributable to childbearing was 1.4 kg, 1.0 kg, and 1.8 kg, for women having one, two, and three live births, respectively. However, when nulliparous women were removed from the control group, these estimates increased to 1.7 kg, 1.7 kg, and 2.2 kg, respectively. The effect on weight gain of having two or three live births during the study period was similar to that of having only one live birth since none of the estimates were significantly different from each other. Among all parous women, the weight gain attributable to one additional live birth was 1.7 kg. Therefore, having one live birth during the study period increased the risk of becoming moderately overweight (BMI $\geq$ 27.3) by 60% and of becoming severely overweight (BMI $\geq$ 30.0) by 110%.

PATTERN AND VARIABILITY OF PREGNANCY-RELATED WEIGHT GAINS

Overall, robust longitudinal studies suggest that women experience *average* long-term weight gains of up to 3 kg in association with pregnancy. However, the pattern of weight change after pregnancy is not well documented and varies considerably between women.

Figure 20.3 shows the weight development of 1423 Swedish women from before pregnancy until 12 months postpartum (54). This graph shows the classical pattern of weight gain during pregnancy. After delivery, body weight falls until it begins to plateau-off at around 5–6 months postpartum. However, this overall picture disguises the marked differences in patterns of weight change that are observed between different women. A number of studies have found that pregnancy-related weight gains do not simply result from failing to lose weight retained following delivery, but that they also result from gaining additional weight after the baby is born (47,54,62,63,65). In a recent study (65), more than 60% of mothers reported returning to their pre-pregnant weight following pregnancy, al-

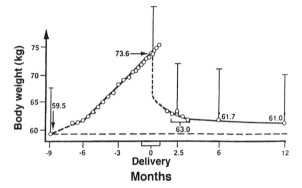

Figure 20.3 Body weight development of 1423 women in the Stockholm pregnancy and weight development study from pregnancy until 12 months postpartum. Data for mean values $\pm$ SD at conception, delivery, and 2.5, 6 and 12 months postpartum are shown; $\bigcirc$ = mean data from women weighed that particular week. From Öhlin and Rössner, (54)

though more than half of these women said that they had gained additional weight during the postpartum period, a phenomenon reported by 57% of the entire sample. While a component of this weight increase undoubtedly reflects the weight gain associated with ageing, it is likely that some of the additional weight gain results from changes in lifestyle that accompany pregnancy and motherhood which predispose some women to gain weight (65,66).

For the majority of women, pregnancy does not trigger obesity and most women can expect to regain their pre-pregnant weight within a year or so after the birth of their child (50,63,65). However, *average* weight gains mask the fact that around 10–15% of women remain at least 5 kg heavier after pregnancy than they were before conception (49,50,54,65). In a contemporary study of 243 first time mothers (50), no significant increase in mean maternal body weight was observed following pregnancy, yet the 10% of women with the highest pregnancy-related weight gains were nearly 9 kg (8.95 kg) heavier at least 1 year after delivery (Figure 20.4). Long-term weight changes following pregnancy have been shown to range from a weight loss of 13.6 kg to a weight gain of 29.5 kg (45,65,67), and this variability is a remarkably consistent feature of pregnancy-related weight changes. Such variability suggests that only certain women are at risk of maternal obesity.

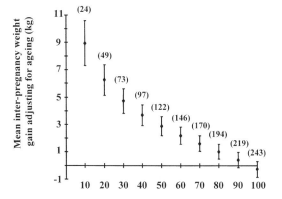

Figure 20.4 The distribution (decentiles) of inter-pregnancy weight change, after accounting for the effect of ageing at an estimated rate of 0.078 kg/month, among a group of 243 first time mothers (50). Error bars show 95% confidence intervals and sample size is shown in parentheses

RISK FACTORS FOR MATERNAL OBESITY

Since most women return (or get close) to their pre-pregnant weight after pregnancy (50), the compelling question is not *whether* women return to their pre-pregnant weight, but rather *which* women fail to return to their pre-pregnant weight and *why?* Several studies have revealed a variety of important risk factors that explain why some women experience persistent weight gains following pregnancy, while others remain unaffected. Broadly speaking, these risk factors can be split into four main groups:

- Risk factors associated with the period of pregnancy itself
- Risk factors associated with both the pregnancy *and* postpartum periods
- Risk factors associated with the postpartum period
- Pre-existing risk factors

Among those risk factors associated with the pregnancy itself, high weight gain *during* pregnancy (gestational weight gain) is probably the most important risk factor (49,50,54). Cessation of smoking during pregnancy has also been shown to trigger subsequent weight gain (49,54,65). Other studies suggest that lifestyle changes *following* pregnancy are more important than biological changes *during*

pregnancy in affecting body weight (41,65,66). This theory is compelling given the limited explanatory power of anthropometric and sociodemographic variables to explain the variable impact of pregnancy on maternal body weight. Further evidence for this view comes from the positive association between the number of children at home and overweight among fathers (29). Weight gain is not an isolated experience for mothers, but is intertwined with the emotional and social strands of their lives. There are therefore many psychosocial factors, like changes of body image and attitudes to weight gain, stress, social support and depression, which together can influence maternal energy balance (65,67). Factors more directly related to energy balance, such as the duration and intensity of breast-feeding, as well as changes in energy intake and activity, also play a part (41,56,65).

The last group of risk factors includes those maternal characteristics that predispose weight gain, even in the absence of pregnancy. Here, the principal risk factor is an already high pre-pregnant body weight (19,56,58). High body weight arises if the individual has a heritable predisposition to gain weight or if they maintain a lifestyle that predisposes weight gain (68). There are also a variety of sociodemographic factors like maternal age, parity, ethnicity, marital status, education and income, which have all been shown to be independently associated with weight gain (29,54,67,69,70). The principal risk factors for pregnancy-related weight gain are discussed in detail below.

Risk Factors Associated with the Period of Pregnancy

Weight Gain During Pregnancy

Excessive gestational weight gain is by far the most important risk factor associated with the period of pregnancy (50,61,71,72). This is of particular concern today as weight gain recommendations for pregnancy have recently increased (6). Following a review of the scientific literature published in the 1970s and 1980s, the US Institute of Medicine proposed new guidelines for maternal weight gain based on pre-pregnant body mass index (see Table 20.3). There is however, concern that these increased weight gain recommendations will do little to improve the birthweight of infants (their primary

Table 20.3 The US Institute of Medicine's (1990) recommended total weight gain ranges for pregnant women,[a] by pre-pregnancy body mass index (BMI)[b]

Weight-for-height category	Recommended total gain	
	kg	lb
Low (BMI < 19.8)	12.5–18.0	28.0–40.0
Normal (BMI 19.8–26.0)	11.5–16.0	25.0–35.0
High[c] (BMI > 26.0–29.0)	7.0–11.5	15.0–25.0

[a]Young adolescents and black women should strive for gains at the upper end of the recommended range. Short women (< 57 cm, or 62 in) should strive for gains at the lower end of the range.
[b]BMI is calculated using metric units.
[c]The recommended target weight gain for obese women (BMI > 29.0) is at least 6.0 kg (15 lb).
Reproduced by permission of the National Academy of Sciences (National Academy Press).

objective), and do more to contribute to obesity in the mother (59,60,73). Further evidence to support this view is now emerging: To and Cheung (64) showed that gestational gains greater than two standard deviations above the mean were not associated with any significant increase in birthweight, but that they were associated with higher postpartum weight retention. However, the results of studies which measure body weight too soon after delivery (53,57,60,64) should be interpreted with caution as they do not give women with high gestational gains enough time for their body weight to equilibrate after delivery (12). In this way, they can erroneously conclude that high weight gains during pregnancy predispose women to long-term weight gain. However, there are numerous studies which do give women sufficient time for body weight to stabilize following pregnancy (49,50,54,57,61–63), and all of these suggest that women with high gestational gains are at increased risk of long-term weight gain.

Greene et al. (49) investigated the effect of weight gain during pregnancy on maternal body weight in a group of 7116 US women. All women in this study had experienced more than one pregnancy so that their change in body weight from one pregnancy to the next could be examined. Inter-pregnancy weight gain was defined as pre-pregnant weight in the second study pregnancy minus pre-pregnant weight in the first study pregnancy. This measure of long-term weight gain was then compared to the gestational weight gains that the women experienced in their first study pregnancy. Figure 20.5 shows the mean gestational weight gain for 11 maternal weight gain groups plotted against the mean inter-pregnancy weight change. It is clear from this figure that women with high gestational weight gains are at greater risk of persistent weight gain when compared to women with relatively lower gestational weight gains. The authors concluded that gestational weight gains in excess of 9.1 kg were positively related to the amount of weight retained postpartum, and that: 'the more weight a woman gains, the more she retains'.

Similar results have been obtained in more recent studies. For example, Thorsdottir and Birgisdottir (63), in their study of women of normal BMI before pregnancy, showed that women with high gestational weight gains (18–24 kg) were, on average, 2.6 kg heavier (more than a year) after pregnancy than they were before, whereas women with comparatively moderate gestational gains (9–15 kg) weighed less after pregnancy than they did before. The almost universal observation that high gestational gain is positively associated with persistent weight gain is particularly disheartening since most women today experience gestational gains well in excess of 9.1 kg (47,50,54), and are indeed recommended to do so (6) (Table 20.3). It therefore appears that pregnancy is associated with a persistent increase in body weight simply because it is a period of positive energy balance during which some women gain excessive weight.

Smoking Cessation

Another group of women who are at increased risk of persistent weight gains following pregnancy are those who quit smoking (54). Statistics show that 38% of women in the UK are classified as smokers at conception and that 26% of these women will quit smoking during pregnancy (74). Öhlin and Rössner (54) showed that women who gave up smoking early in pregnancy gained significantly more weight during pregnancy than other groups. Women who did not start smoking again during the follow-up year experienced significantly greater long-term weight gains (3.4 kg) than did continuous smokers (0.9 kg) and non-smokers (1.5 kg; $P <$ 0.01), while women who resumed smoking within 6 months of delivery had long-term weight gains similar to those of non-smokers (1.4 kg). Smoking is known to increase basal metabolic rate by around 10% (75), and for this reason women who smoke

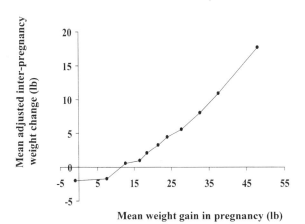

Figure 20.5 Mean weight change by mean weight gain in pregnancy for 11 prenatal weight gain groups, after adjusting for the effects of inter-pregnancy interval, smoking, gestation at registration, socioeconomic status, breast-feeding at hospital, complications of pregnancy, gravidity, maternal age, per cent ideal body weight, marital status, and race. From Greene *et al.* (49). Reprinted with permission from the American College of Obstetricians and Gynecologists (*Obstetrics and Gynecology* 1988; **71**: 701–707)

throughout pregnancy tend to have lower long-term weight gains than those who do not (49,54,56). For similar reasons, women who quit smoking during pregnancy are at greater risk of subsequent weight gain. While cigarette smoking is protective against weight retention postpartum, the observed benefit of smoking does not offset the toxic effects of cigarettes on the health of both the mother and her child (71).

Risk Factors Common to Both the Pregnancy and Postpartum Periods

Changes in Activity

Until recently (55,56,61,65), the potential effects of changes in activity on maternal body weight had received relatively little attention. Schauberger *et al.* (56) found that mothers who resumed work within 2 weeks of delivery retained significantly less weight by 6 months postpartum than did mothers who went back to work later. However, this relationship did not seem to be the result of differences in activity between working mothers and those who stayed at home, as there was no evidence of an association between activity and long-term weight gain. Öhlin and Rössner (55) also found no difference in long-

term weight gain between mothers with altered leisure activities following pregnancy, and neither they nor Harris *et al.* (65) found any association between returning to work and long-term maternal weight gain. Harris *et al.* (65) did, however, find long-term weight gains to be significantly greater (3.1 kg greater) among women who reported undertaking less exercise after pregnancy than they did before pregnancy. In this descriptive study, lack of opportunity, energy, time and money were commonly cited reasons for declines in activity postpartum.

One explanation for these equivocal findings is that the intensity of activity, and/or the nature of employment, determines the absolute importance of changes in activity and/or employment status for long-term weight gain. Alternatively, changes in energy intake might be more important than changes in activity patterns in the development of obesity among women with predominantly sedentary lifestyles, such as those in Western Europe. As with all reported behaviours, care must be taken when evaluating the possible influence of changes in activity on body weight after pregnancy. Reports of activity levels may be embellished pictures of reality, and when information on pre-pregnancy activity patterns are gathered retrospectively they may be subject to recall bias. In particular, retrospective recall of certain behaviours may often be biased if mothers misreport these behaviours as post-hoc justification for any weight gains they may have experienced. Likewise, the complex interrelationships between many behavioural characteristics (68) indicates the need for caution when evaluating the results of descriptive studies, since any relationships observed may simply be the result of confounding. For example, the relationship between reduced activity and long-term weight gain that was found by Harris *et al.* (65) in their descriptive study was not statistically significant after adjustment for the confounding effects of other factors including changes in: energy intake, access to food and body image, as well as parental obesity, social support, parity, maternal age, marital status, smoking status, gestational weight gain and pre-pregnant weight (68).

Changes in Energy Intake and Patterns of Eating

It has been shown that changes in dietary intake are a common characteristic of pregnancy and the postpartum period (50,55,76,77). A large proportion of new mothers stay at home for a time after birth, and whilst at home they often have greater access to food throughout more of the day than they had before they were pregnant (65,66). Among mothers participating in the Stockholm Pregnancy and Weight Development Study, those who displayed less well-structured eating patterns retained more weight by 1 year postpartum (55). Women who increased in body weight also reported that their energy intake had risen during pregnancy and the postpartum period because they ate larger portions and snacked more frequently. These women also skipped breakfast and lunch more regularly than women who put on less weight (55).

In a descriptive study by Harris *et al.* (65), more than 70% of mothers felt they ate differently from the way they did before they were pregnant. Mothers who felt they ate more after their children were born displayed significantly greater long-term weight gains (2.78 kg) than those who felt they had not increased the amount they ate (-1.15 kg). Although this association just failed to reach significance after accounting for the effects of confounding factors ($P = 0.08$; (68), this finding may be important since more than a fifth of the mothers in the group reported increasing their energy intake after the birth of their child. In this study, more than 13% of the mothers who reported increasing their energy intake were newly classified as overweight or obese (BMI > 26.0) after pregnancy (68). Mothers often report having to grab their meals when they can, and devoting more time to feeding their children than they do to preparing food for themselves (65). It is therefore possible that these changes in maternal eating habits and patterns of eating predispose some women to gain weight after pregnancy. It is important that women are aware of this possibility, so they can take steps to prevent these new behaviours from tracking into the future.

Dieting and Attitudes to Weight Gain

Studies show that between 13 and 52% of European women undertake some form of dieting during the first year after birth (54,65). There is, however, little evidence to suggest that these women are any more successful in returning to their pre-pregnant weight than are those who do not diet during the postpartum period (65). For some women, a previous history of dieting has been shown to be positively related to pregnancy-related weight gain (54) but this is not the case for all women (65). It is likely that the impact of dieting on body weight is just as difficult to predict after pregnancy as it is at any time in a woman's life, although some believe the immediate post-pregnancy period to be a better-than-average time to achieve a successful persistent weight loss (16,78,79). Some women do, however, appear to experience marked changes in their attitudes to weight gain both during and after pregnancy. For woman who normally restrain their eating to preserve their figures, the inevitable change of shape during pregnancy may serve as justification for 'letting themselves go'. Others believe they should 'eat for two' or fear that by depriving themselves they are depriving their child. In a recent UK study more than 40% of mothers felt it was inevitable that they retained some of the weight that they gained during pregnancy (65). In this study changes in attitude to weight gain were also assessed using the 'drive for thinness' sub-scale of the Eating Disorder Inventory (80). This scale contains seven questions that assess 'concern with dieting, preoccupation with weight, and entrenchment in an extreme pursuit of thinness'. Harris *et al.* (65) showed that mothers displayed significantly greater scores in their drive for thinness after pregnancy than they did before ($P < 0.001$). Interestingly, those mothers with an increased drive for thinness had not gained significantly more weight than those mothers who displayed no increase in drive for thinness after pregnancy. Such changes in attitudes to weight gain, which are independent of actual changes in body weight, are suggestive of an increased vulnerability to eating psychopathology during the postpartum period (81). For these women, pregnancy may represent an important 'risk period' for the development of obesity.

Change of Body Image

In Western society, the notion of beauty in women equates with being thin (82), and it is therefore not surprising that women are commonly concerned about their weight and shape both during and after pregnancy. Younger or primiparous women can be somewhat unrealistic in forecasting their expected postnatal weight, and the greater the difference between anticipated and actual postnatal weight, the greater the postnatal weight dissatisfaction (83). This may be important as others have found that, after accounting for the effects of potential confounders and known risk factors for maternal obesity, women who were more dissatisfied with their bodies after pregnancy were significantly more likely to have higher long-term weight gains than those who displayed no increase in dissatisfaction with their bodies after pregnancy ($P = 0.01$; (68)). This association suggests that either (i) increased body image dissatisfaction predisposes mothers to gain more weight in association with pregnancy or (ii) mothers who gain more weight following pregnancy are more dissatisfied with their bodies. Bivariate correlation analyses have shown mothers who were more dissatisfied with their bodies postpartum to be more likely to report an increase in energy intake following pregnancy. While it is impossible to determine the causal direction of these relationships, previous analyses have demonstrated significantly higher levels of depression among women with increased body dissatisfaction following pregnancy (68). The changes in body image that occur following pregnancy might therefore lead to depression and reduced self-esteem, which in themselves are known risk factors for increased energy intake (84), particularly among women (85,86).

Risk Factors Associated with the Postpartum Period

Breast-feeding

Breast-feeding has traditionally been thought to facilitate weight loss. In clinical practice, women are often instructed to try to breast-feed as much as possible to revert to normal weight after delivery (72). This seems logical since a full lactation requires about 500 kcal a day, which for many women in this age group may constitute around 20 to 25% of their daily energy requirement (72). In theory, the metabolic costs of lactation can be met in four main ways: women can either (1) increase their energy intake, (2) mobilize their energy stores, (3) increase their metabolic efficiency, (4) reduce their energy expenditure, or employ a combination of these four adaptations. From a nutritional point of view, it seems reasonable to assume that the adipose tissue that is stored during pregnancy provides energy for the child during the lactation period. However, it is evident from the literature that postpartum weight changes in breast-feeding women are highly variable both within and across populations (87).

Several studies have supported a positive influence of breast-feeding on weight loss (62,88,89), while others have shown a negative influence (26,46,90) or little influence at all (50,56,58,60,63,69,90–92). Overall, breast-feeding appears to have its greatest effect in the early months (54,62,87,89,91,93), yet by 12 months postpartum (after which time most women have stopped breast-feeding) the difference in weight loss between those who had been breast-feeding and those who had not is minimal (54,92,93). Only in the small numbers of women who breast-feed for lengthy periods (around 12 months), does breast-feeding appear to be related to increased weight loss (54,93).

In the Stockholm Pregnancy and Weight Development Study, Öhlin and Rössner (54) found breast-feeding to have only a minor influence on postpartum weight development: In this study a scoring system was constructed to reflect both the duration and intensity of breast-feeding. Their system gave every month of full lactation a score of 4 points, and every month with mixed feeding a score of 2 points. This score was then multiplied by the number of months during which women indicated that they breast-fed. This system made it possible to sum up periods of complete lactation with ensuing periods of partial lactation, and in this way a range from 10 to 48 points was obtained to give a rough estimate of the total energy expenditure for milk production. Although they found a significant relationship between lactation score and weight retention, the relationship was very weak ($r = -0.09$, $P < 0.01$). However, they were able to demonstrate that women with high lactation scores lost more weight during the first 6 months following delivery, but by the end of the year the difference between the groups was limited (Figure 20.6).

Insensitive definitions which fail to reflect the duration and intensity of breast-feeding are inevitably responsible for some of the conflicting results on the influence of breast-feeding on body weight. Likewise the paucity of data on energy intakes makes interpretation and inter-study comparisons difficult. Nevertheless, in most reports, rates of weight loss do not differ between breast-feeding and non-breast-feeding women, and only subtle short-term differences in body composition are observed following pregnancy (87). In those studies that demonstrate a statistically significant effect of breast-feeding on body weight, the contribution to the

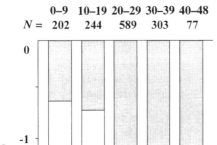

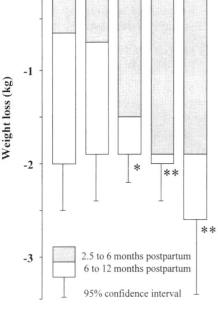

Figure 20.6 Weight loss (kg) from 2.5 months postpartum in groups with different lactation scores. * Differed from 0–9, 10–19 ($P < 0.05$). ** Differed from 0–9, 10–19 ($P < 0.01$). From Öhlin and Rössner (54). Reproduced by permission of MacMillan Press Ltd

overall variability in postpartum weight change is minor (87). In developed countries, it seems that changes in eating behaviour and lifestyle affect women in such a way that they use their adipose tissue storage only when food is not readily available. For example, several studies (94,95) indicate that well-nourished women with foods freely available do not necessarily mobilize body fat during lactation, but rather tend to cover the energy costs of lactation by an increased energy intake and possibly by decreased physical activity (96). In this way changes in eating behaviour patterns after delivery seem to counteract the inherent weight controlling potential of breast-feeding. This behaviour may go some way to explain why women from developed countries tend towards obesity following pregnancy, while women in developing countries tend towards maternal depletion. In developed countries, it is likely that the effects of breast-feeding on

body weight are sufficiently limited to warrant minimal emphasis on breast-feeding as a means of minimizing postpartum weight retention.

Psychosocial Factors: Depression, Self-esteem, Stress and Social Support

There are a number of other psychosocial factors, such as depression, self-esteem, stress and social support, that might also influence maternal energy balance after pregnancy. These risk factors have received relatively little attention and are notoriously difficult to measure. As such, absence of an association between any of these variables and weight gain does not always mean that no association exists. These factors rarely operate in isolation and usually form part of a complex milieu of social and emotional factors that make up a woman's life. Even when psychosocial variables, like these, are found to be related to a biological outcome, like body weight, questions necessarily arise about the processes that underlie the relationships. If data on psychosocial symptoms and postpartum weight are collected simultaneously, the direction of influence of any relationship is usually unclear. For example, women may experience depressive symptoms as a result of their weight *or* depressive symptoms may modify biological or behavioural processes that affect body weight. Therefore, the direction of these causal relationships is usually difficult to predict and most studies are only able to describe tentative associations between psychosocial variables and body weight. For these and other reasons, studies investigating the influence of psychosocial factors on body weight are scarce.

Some researchers have investigated the effects of stress on changes in body weight following pregnancy (65,67). However, these studies have found no association between life event stress or the stresses of parenting and long-term weight gain following pregnancy (65,67). However, both Walker (67) and Harris *et al.* (65) found high levels of stress and low levels of social support to be related to higher depressive symptoms, which in themselves have been shown to be related to long-term weight gain following pregnancy (67,83). Others have suggested that weight loss following delivery might depend upon the amount of social support each mother receives (97) and that women with little social support, who might feel isolated and lonely as a result, respond to their lack of support by compensatory 'comfort' eating. There is tentative evidence to support this view (67,68), although the mechanisms that underlie this association are far from clear. Other researchers have explored the effects of changes in self-esteem following pregnancy. Given the importance of body weight to perceived attractiveness, and the importance of attractiveness to a woman's self-image (82), it follows that a woman's satisfaction with her weight is likely to be a central aspect of her self-esteem. In a study by Walker (67), mothers were asked at 1 year postpartum whether their current body weight affected how they felt about themselves, and just less than half of the entire sample (47%) reported that their self-esteem had decreased. Reduced self-esteem and the normally inescapable demands imposed by motherhood can set the stage for depressive symptoms during the period after childbirth (67). In fact in Walker's study (67), those mothers with gains at 1 year postpartum of at least 5 kg reported high depressive symptoms more often than women with lesser gains (53% vs. 28%).

It is likely that psychosocial factors play an important role in the development of maternal body weight following pregnancy. However, well-designed prospective studies are needed if the effects of these factors are to be elucidated.

Pre-existing Risk Factors

Pre-pregnant Weight

Along with gestational weight gain, pre-pregnancy weight is the other variable that consistently shows a significant positive association with pregnancy-related weight gain (19,49,50,56,58). This suggests that women who enter pregnancy with an already high body weight are at greater risk of long-term weight gain than are women of lower body weight. Furthermore, the weight development of women who begin pregnancy overweight is known to be more variable (52,54,57,66). For example, Keppel and Taffel (57) showed that among normal weight women (BMI 19.8–26.0 kg/m^2) whose gestational gains were within the Institute of Medicine's recommended range (see Table 20.3), 20% retained 4 kg or more, while 29% lost weight by 10–18 months postpartum. In contrast, of the overweight women (BMI 26.1–29.0 kg/m^2) who gained as recommended, 38% retained 4 kg or more, while 33% lost weight.

This variability of pregnancy-related weight gains is a remarkably consistent feature of postpartum weight change in overweight women.

To some extent, the higher weight gains of heavier mothers may be the result of fundamental differences in physiology and/or lifestyle that place these women at increased risk of gaining more weight, irrespective of pregnancy. Differences in nutritional status (BMI) are the consequence of differences in physiological characteristics and/or lifestyles that cause some women to gain more weight than others. There are, however, two important points to consider. Firstly, overweight women are known to under-report their body weight to a greater extent than women of lower weight (18,19). Because weight retention is usually calculated as: body weight measured after pregnancy minus pre-pregnant weight, overweight women may appear to be retaining more weight than lighter women with the same weight retention, when calculations are based on self-reported pre-pregnant weight (50,58). This does not, however, explain the greater weight gains observed among overweight women in studies that rely on pre-pregnant body weights that are measured in early pregnancy (50,56). Secondly, the increased risk of weight retention observed among overweight women might simply be an artefact of longitudinal study design: for example, we might observe this relationship simply because heavier women gain more weight over a fixed period of time than lighter women, regardless of pregnancy. This would give the impression that overweight women are at greater risk of pregnancy-related weight gains, when in fact they are simply at greater risk of weight gain generally (98). With this in mind, there is little empirical evidence to suggest that overweight women are at any increased risk of *maternal* obesity when compared to women of lower body weight (98).

Heredity

Few studies have considered the effects of heredity on postpartum weight, and this represents an important oversight since heredity is considered to be one of the three most important factors determining body weight (99). More than 50 years ago clinicians noticed that mothers of the maternal obese had more often suffered from obesity after pregnancy than had mothers of women whose obesity was not pregnancy-related (14,100). These early observations suggested that a history of maternal obesity in a woman's mother might be a risk factor for pregnancy-related weight gain.

Harris *et al.* (68) assessed the relative importance of heritable characteristics and lifestyle in the development of body weight following pregnancy in a group of mothers from south-east London. In this study, 74 mothers of low antenatal risk who had been weighed during the first trimester of pregnancy were followed up 2.5 years after delivery. 'Heritable' predisposition to gain weight was assessed using the Silhouette Technique (101). This technique asks subjects to score the degree of obesity in their parents using a series of nine silhouette drawings showing bodies of increasing obesity, ranging from very thin to very obese (numbered in order from 1 to 9). This technique has been validated by correlation with BMI, as offspring's selected silhouettes of their mothers have been shown to correlate well with measured maternal BMI ($r = 0.74$: Sørenson and Stunkard (101)). After adjusting for the effects of potential confounders and known risk factors for maternal obesity, women who selected larger silhouettes to represent their biological mothers were significantly more likely to have higher long-term weight gains than those who selected thinner maternal silhouettes ($r^2 = 0.083$, $P = 0.004$; see Figure 20.7). Interestingly, long-term weight gain was not associated with the size of the biological father ($P = 0.50$). This shows that a 'heritable' predisposition to gain weight is independently associated with long-term weight gain following pregnancy, and suggests that some component of heredity might determine why some women gain more weight than others in association with pregnancy. A number of previous studies have shown that the familial resemblance of obesity has a genetic component which may be inherited (101–104), with twin and adoption studies indicating that genes play a major role (102). However, it is also possible that offspring 'inherit' lifestyles that predispose them to gain weight by adopting similar eating habits and exercise patterns to those of their parents. The absence of an association between long-term maternal weight gain and the size of the biological father (68) suggests that inherited maternal attitudes to body weight and weight gain, as well as postpartum lifestyle, might be more important than any genetic characteristic inherited from either parent. Nevertheless, it is likely that both processes have a role.

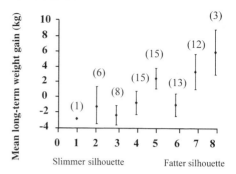

Figure 20.7 Mean long-term weight gains of 74 women according to the number of silhouette selected to represent their biological mother. Error bars show standard error about the mean and sample size is shown in parentheses. From Harris *et al.* (68). Reproduced with permission of the BMJ Publishing Group

Maternal Age

The results of studies on the modification of pregnancy-related weight gain by age are limited and conflicting. Some show no significant association between maternal age and weight gain following pregnancy (49,50,70), while others show a significant negative influence (54,62,63). Another recent study showed that among white women, younger compared to older women were found to be more likely to experience substantial pregnancy-related weight gains (defined as gains > 11.4 kg during the 10-year study period), while among black women, the opposite was true (105).

It seems logical to assume that older women might be at greater risk of pregnancy-related weight gain, as a direct consequence of the reduced metabolic efficiency that accompanies advancing age. Older mothers may also be less concerned about slimness than younger women (63). Janney *et al.* (62) showed that age rather than parity influenced the rate of postpartum weight retention after a first or second pregnancy. In this study, older women were shown to be significantly less likely to return to their pre-pregnant weight than younger women. They also had slower rates of weight loss than their younger counterparts. The significant interaction between maternal age and time since delivery is illustrated in Figure 20.8 (62). This model suggests that for women who experience pregnancy between the ages of 20 and 35 years, regaining pre-pregnant weight would be anticipated, but for women who

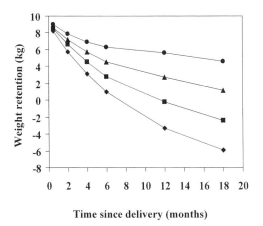

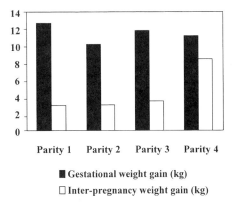

Figure 20.8 Predicted weight retention curves for women of various ages (hypothetical married women who fully breast-fed for 6 months and gained 15.9 kg during pregnancy). ●, 40 years; ▲, 35 years; ■, 30 years; ◆, 25 years. From Janney *et al.* (62). Reproduced by permission of the American Society for Nutritional Sciences

Figure 20.9 Independent relationships between weight gain and parity (data from Harris *et al.* (70). Adjusted for the effects of smoking status, alcohol consumption, socioeconomic status, breast-feeding at hospital, maternal age, nulliparous BMI, marital status, birth weight, plus (for analyses of inter-pregnancy weight gain only) gestational weight gain, and inter-pregnancy interval

experience pregnancy between the ages of 35 and 40 years, an average weight retention of up to 5 kg is predicted by 18 months postpartum. Öhlin and Rössner (54) also reported age to be more strongly related to long-term weight gain ($P < 0.05$) than was parity, and among primiparous women, those in the oldest age group (≥ 36 years) retained significantly more weight (2.9 kg) than did younger women (1.4 kg). Given the current trend toward delayed childbearing (106), the risk of weight retention among mothers over the age of 35 certainly warrants further examination.

Parity

The interaction between parity and body weight is complex and highly confounded with maternal age because older women tend to have more children than younger women (25). After accounting for differences in maternal age, an effect of parity on body weight is only consistently observed at high parities (28,52,70).

Harris *et al.* (70) investigated the independent relationship between parity and maternal weight gain in a group of 523 multiparous women from south-east London. In this repeat-pregnancy study, the change in maternal body weight from the beginning of one pregnancy to the beginning of the next was examined, and parity was found to be indepen-

dently associated with both gestational weight gain and inter-pregnancy weight gain (Figure 20.9). These relationships suggest that first-time mothers are at risk of long-term weight gain because they gain the most weight *during* pregnancy, and high gestational weight gain is in itself a risk factor for long-term weight gain (49,50,57). However, women of higher parity (4 +) seemed to be at risk of long-term weight gain because they gained more weight in association with pregnancy, irrespective of the amount of weight they gained *during* pregnancy. Therefore, for women of parity 3 or less, the association between maternal body weight and parity appeared to be the result of cumulative weight gains during successive pregnancies. For women of higher parity, the association between maternal body weight and parity was partly the cumulative effect of excess gestational weight gains from successive pregnancies, and partly the result of gaining more weight in association with later pregnancies.

It could be that the increase in weight gain observed with increasing parity is the result of women of higher parity having their pregnancies at older ages 'when weight gain is the norm' (66). However, more sophisticated analyses have shown the effects of parity on body weight to be independent of maternal age (28,70). Alternatively, mothers of high parity might gain more weight in association with pregnancy as a result of differential effects of motherhood at different parities. For example,

Dodge and Silva (107) showed that the pressures of child rearing increased with family size. In their study, the numbers of symptoms reported by mothers concerning physical ill health (including changes in body weight) were found to be positively correlated with the number of children living at home. Similarly, the numbers of symptoms concerning psychological ill health (including anxiety and depression) were significantly correlated with the number of children at home, especially in mothers with children of pre-school age. Since many women respond to stress by increasing their energy intake (85,86), this might explain why mothers with larger families tend to gain more weight than do mothers with fewer children. It is also conceivable that different demographic groups, who are at greater risk of weight gain, are selected into this high parity group and that the observed association is simply the result of uncontrolled confounding. The variable success of investigators to control for the effects of socioeconomic status might therefore explain why other researchers have found no effect of parity on weight development after pregnancy (49,54,60).

Ethnicity

To date, the relationship between ethnicity and maternal body weight has largely been restricted to a few national studies of white and black US women (48,57,69). These studies consistently show pregnancy-related weight gains to be greater in African-Americans than in white women (105), and at any level of weight gain, black women are seen to retain more weight postpartum than white women (48,57,58,61,69).

Data from the 1988 National Maternal and Infant Health Survey show that among women of normal BMI, black mothers are more than twice as likely than white mothers to retain at least 9 kg postpartum (69). This difference was shown to persist after adjustment for differences in maternal age, parity, gestational weight gain, infant birth weight, height, BMI, marital status and social class. The reasons for this differential impact of pregnancy on body weight among women from different ethnic backgrounds are not clear. A possible explanation has been suggested by researchers who examined national data on energy intakes before, during and after pregnancy (108). In this study, the reported energy intakes of non-lactating white women ap-

peared to decrease after pregnancy, whereas for black women, mean increases of more than 300 kcal over pre-pregnant intakes were reported by 3 months postpartum. This finding is consistent with others which suggest that black women are not necessarily at increased risk of gaining weight, but rather that they are less likely to lose it (58,109). Other studies have shown that factors related to postpartum weight retention differ by ethnic group: For example, married white mothers appear to have a lower risk of excess weight retention than unmarried white mothers, but among black mothers, marital status was unrelated to weight retention (69). In a similar way, high parity predicted retained weight for black but not white mothers (69). These and other observations suggest that ethnicity is probably just a proxy for social, economic, environmental, cultural and other factors that influence a woman's body weight following pregnancy.

Marital Status, Education, Income and Socioeconomic Status

Greater weight retention has been observed among unmarried women when compared to married women (49,62,68,69). Janney et al. (62) showed that unlike married women, unmarried women had a pattern of weight gain rather than weight loss, and Harris et al. (70), in their study of 523 multiparous English women, also showed marital status to be significantly related to long-term weight gain. After adjusting for the influence of confounding factors, Harris et al. (70) found that unmarried mothers retained significantly more weight (4.0 kg) than married mothers (3.15 kg) by at least 1 year postpartum. In this context it is likely that marital status serves as a proxy for socioeconomic status and/or social support. However, others have found no effect of marital status on long-term weight gain following pregnancy (54).

Marital status is just one of many component measures of socioeconomic status, and the relationships between the various measures of socioeconomic status and pregnancy-related weight gain are complex and inconsistent. Most studies show women with lower incomes or less education to be at increased risk of retaining weight postpartum (61,67,69,90). However, others that have measured socioeconomic status by occupation or social class have found no significant associations (49,50,54,70). As with many health outcomes, it is likely that the poorest members of society will be at greatest risk of maternal obesity.

PREVENTION AND TREATMENT OF MATERNAL OBESITY

It is often said that 'prevention is better than cure', but in the context of pregnancy, this cannot be taken as read. Because excessive gestational weight gain is probably the most important risk factor for maternal obesity, restricting the amount of weight that women gain should theoretically help to reduce the burden of obesity-related disease in women. However, restricting weight gain during pregnancy presents health care workers with a dilemma: weight restriction may help to diminish the risk of maternal obesity, but may also affect the development of the growing child. In any event, advocating weight restriction during pregnancy may be a moot point, because there is little empirical evidence to suggest that weight gain is easy to modify during pregnancy (110). Mothers routinely report difficulties in complying with dietary instructions during pregnancy (111,112) because they usually experience a 'surge of appetite' during pregnancy (113) which is difficult to overcome (Dieckmann 1952 in Hytten (113)).

Even if it were possible or beneficial to modify the amount of weight women gain during pregnancy to reduce the prevalence of maternal obesity, the association between fetal development *in utero* and health later on in life (114–117) should make clinicians extremely cautious when recommending weight restriction during pregnancy, even for those mothers whose gains appear excessive. Restricting weight gain during pregnancy may have undesirable consequences not only for the fetus, but for the generations that follow as the effects of inadequate biological development *in utero* can establish the biological parameters within which individuals will function later in life (115,117). For these reasons, it would seem more appropriate to address the problem of pregnancy-related weight gains soon after the birth, at a time when fetal growth cannot be compromised. At this time it would also be appropriate to forewarn mothers of the changes in lifestyle that accompany motherhood which can encourage further weight gain.

During the postpartum period women are offered little advice (66). Many are only likely to see a physician for a 6-week check-up, and at this time women may be receptive to advice about their own health as they recognize their responsibility for a new life (66). In this setting, it could be made clear that permanent weight gain need not be a consequence of pregnancy, and that lifestyle changes rather than biological changes may be a more important cause of pregnancy-related weight gains (66).

Helping mothers to establish appropriate exercise routines should be an important component of postpartum care. In recent years, exercise has been shown to be beneficial to health, and postpartum women are no exception (106). Unfortunately there are many barriers to regular exercise for a mother with a new baby, and perhaps other young children at home. The cost of child care and formal exercise often makes these pursuits prohibitive, and for many there are difficulties in accessing leisure facilities (65). Likewise, lack of time, particularly for working mothers, often makes participation in exercise difficult following pregnancy (65). Even walking can jeopardize personal safety and cause fear among mothers who live in areas of high crime (106). Consequently, health care providers should discuss exercise needs individually and set realistic goals that are tailed to the individual's needs (106).

Women should be given realistic advice about postpartum weight change as well as assistance in beginning or maintaining lifestyles that will promote health and an appropriate body weight. For some new mothers, dealing with the demands of an infant, running a household, and in many cases holding a job as well, make dieting and other weight loss strategies seem overwhelming (61). Health care providers should therefore have a supportive attitude to ensure that concerns about weight management are balanced with concerns about maternal self-esteem. The following five recommendations should go some way to reduce the burden of disease associated with maternal obesity:

- Women should be encouraged to eat to appetite during pregnancy by consuming a varied and balanced diet, but be advised that it is not necessary to 'eat for two' in order to provide the appropriate nutrients for their growing child.
- Mothers should be given assistance in beginning or maintaining lifestyles that will promote health and an appropriate body weight at the time of

their 6-week postpartum check-up.
- Mothers should be forewarned of the changes in eating habits that often accompany pregnancy and motherhood which predispose weight gain so they can take steps to prevent these new behaviours from tracking into the future.
- Mothers should be encouraged to maintain or establish appropriate exercise routines with realistic goals that are tailored to the individual's needs.
- Mothers should be given realistic advice about postpartum weight change so that they do not have unrealistic expectations about weight loss following delivery.

REFERENCES

1. National Center for Health Statistics. *Health, United States, 1995*. Hyattsville, MD: Public Health Service, 1996: 183.
2. Office for National Statistics. *The Health of Adult Britain 1841–1994*, vol. 1. London: The Stationery Office, 1997: 112–113.
3. British Nutrition Foundation. *The Nature and Risks of Obesity: Briefing Paper—27*. London: The British Nutrition Foundation, 1992.
4. Department of Health. *The Health of the Nation: a Strategy for Health in England*. London: HMSO, 1992.
5. Prescott-Clarke P, Primatesta P. *Health Survey for England 1997*. HMSO, 1999.
6. US Institute of Medicine. *Nutrition During Pregnancy*. Washington DC: National Academy Press, 1990.
7. Jebb S. *The Weight of the Nation: Obesity in the UK*. Commissioned by the Bread for Life Campaign. The Flour Advisory Bureau, 1999.
8. Merchant K, Martorell R, Haas JD. Consequences for maternal nutrition of reproductive stress across consecutive pregnancies. *Am J Clin Nutr* 1990; **52**: 616–620.
9. Khan KS, Chien PFC, Khan NB. Nutritional stress of reproduction. A cohort study over two consecutive pregnancies. *Acta Obstet Gynecol Scand* 1998; **77**: 395–401.
10. Beazley JM, Swinhoe JR. Body weight in parous women: is there any alteration between successive pregnancies? *Acta Obstet Gynecol Scand* 1979; **58**: 45–47.
11. Samra JS, Tang LCH, Obhrai MS. Changes in body weight between consecutive pregnancies. *Lancet* 1988; **ii** (8625): 1420–1421.
12. Harris HE, Ellison GTH. Do the changes in energy balance that occur during pregnancy predispose parous women to obesity? *Nutr Res Rev* 1997; **10**: 57–81.
13. Greene JA. Clinical study of the etiology of obesity. *Ann Intern Med* 1939; **12**: 1797–1803.
14. Sheldon JH. Maternal obesity. *Lancet* 1949; **ii**: 869–873.
15. Mullins A. Overweight in pregnancy. *Lancet* 1960; **i**: 146–147.
16. Bradley PJ. Does pregnancy cause obesity? *Med J Aust* 1989; **151**: 543–544.
17. Rössner S. Pregnancy, weight cycling and weight gain in obesity. *Int J Obes* 1992; **16**: 145–147.
18. Harris HE, Ellison GTH. Practical approaches for estimating pre-pregnant body weight. *J Nurse Midwif* 1998; **43**: 97–101.
19. Stevens-Simon C, Roghmann KJ, McAnarney ER. Relationship of self-reported prepregnant weight and weight gain during pregnancy to maternal body habitus and age. *J Am Diet Assoc* 1992; **92**: 85–86.
20. Cathcart EP, Bedale EM, Blair C, Macleod K, Weatherhead M. The physique of women in industry. *Rep Industr Fatig Res Bd* 1927; (Lond) 44.
21. US Department of Agriculture. *Women's Measurements for Garment and Pattern Construction*. USDA Misc Publ, 1941: 454.
22. Kemsley WFF. Weight and height of a population in 1943. *Ann Eugen* 1950; **15**: 161–183.
23. Lowe CR, Gibson JR. Changes in body weight associated with age and marital status. *BMJ* 1955; **2**: 1006–1008.
24. Karn MN. Considerations arising from weight and some other variables recorded in the survey of women's measurements. *Ann Hum Genet* 1957; **22**: 385–390.
25. Heliövaara M, Aromaa A. Parity and obesity. *J Epidemiol Comm Health* 1981; **35**: 197–199.
26. Newcombe RG. Development of obesity in parous women. *J Epidemiol Comm Health* 1982; **36**: 306–309.
27. Brown JE, Kaye SA, Folsom AR. Parity-related weight change in women. *Int J Obes* 1992; **16**: 627–631.
28. Williamson DF, Madans J, Pamuk E, Flegal KM, Kendrick JS, Serdula MK. A prospective study of childbearing and 10-year weight gain in US white women 25 to 45 years of age. *Int J Obes* 1994; **18**: 561–569.
29. Rona RJ, Morris RW. National Study of Health and Growth: social and family factors and overweight in English and Scottish parents. *Ann Hum Biol* 1982; **9**: 147–156.
30. Thomson AM, Billewicz WZ. Maternal weight for height. *Proc Nutr Soc* 1965; **24**: 14–20.
31. Cederlöf R, Kaij L. The effect of childbearing on body weight: a twin control study. *Acta Psychiatr Scand Suppl* 1970; **219**: 47–49.
32. Baecke JAH, Burema J, Frijters JER, Hautvast JGAJ, Van der Wiel-Wetzels WAM. Obesity in young Dutch adults: I, socio-demographic variables and body mass index. *Int J Obes* 1983; **7**: 1–12.
33. Lee-Feldstein A, Harburg E, Hauenstein L. Parity and blood pressure among four race-stress groups of females in Detroit. *Am J Epidemiol* 1980; **111**: 356–366.
34. Noppa H, Bengtsson C. Obesity in relation to socioeconomic status. A population study of women in Göteborg, Sweden. *J Epidemiol Comm Health* 1980; **34**: 139–142.
35. Prentice AM, Whitehead RG, Roberts SB, Paul AA. Long-term energy balance in child-bearing Gambian women. *Am J Clin Nutr* 1981; **34**: 2790–2799.
36. Forster JL, Bloom E, Sorensen G, Jeffery RW, Prineas RJ. Reproductive history and body mass index in black and white women. *Prev Med* 1986; **15**: 685–691.

37. Caan B, Horgen DM, Margen S, King JC, Jewell NP. Benefits associated with WIC supplemental feeding during the interpregnancy interval. *Am J Clin Nutr* 1987; **45**: 29–41.

38. Chowdhury AKMA. Changes in maternal nutritional status in a chronically malnourished population in rural Bangladesh. *Ecol Fd Nutr* 1987; **19**: 201–211.

39. Kumanyika S. Obesity in black women. *Epidemiol Rev* 1987; **9**: 31–50.

40. Kritz-Silverstein D, Barrett-Connor E, Wingard DL. The effect of parity on the later development of non-insulin dependent diabetes mellitus or impaired glucose tolerance. *N Engl J Med* 1989; **321**: 1214–1219.

41. Öhlin A, Rössner S. Factors related to body weight changes during and after pregnancy: The Stockholm Pregnancy and Weight Development Study. *Obes Res* 1996; **4**: 271–276.

42. Rodin J, Radke-Sharpe N, Rebuffé-Scrive M, Greenwood MRC. Weight cycling and fat distribution. *Int J Obes* 1990; **14**: 303–310.

43. Manson JE, Rimm EB, Colditz GA, Stampfer MJ, Willett WC, Arky RA, Rosner B, Hennekens CH, Speizer FE. Parity and incidence of non-insulin-dependent diabetes mellitus. *Am J Med* 1992; **93**: 11–18.

44. Hunt SC, Daines MM, Adams TD, Heath EM, Williams RR. Pregnancy weight retention in morbid obesity. *Obes Res* 1995; **3**: 121–130.

45. Rössner S. Weight gain in pregnancy. *Hum Reprod* 1997; **12** (Suppl 1): 110–115.

46. Rookus MA, Rokebrand P, Burema J, Deurenberg P. The effect of pregnancy on the body mass index 9 months postpartum in 49 women. *Int J Obes* 1987; **11**: 609–618.

47. Parham ES, Astrom MF, King SH. The association of pregnancy weight gain with the mother's postpartum weight. *JAMA* 1990; **90**: 550–554.

48. Smith DE, Lewis CE, Caveny JL, Perkins LL, Burke GL, Bild DE. Longitudinal changes in adiposity associated with pregnancy. *JAMA* 1994; **271**: 1747–1751.

49. Greene GW, Smiciklas-Wright H, Scholl TO, Karp RJ. Postpartum weight change: How much of the weight gained in pregnancy will be lost after delivery? *Obstet Gynecol* 1988; **71**: 701–707.

50. Harris HE, Ellison GTH, Holliday M, Lucassen E. The impact of pregnancy on the long term weight gain of primiparous women in England. *Int J Obes* 1997; **21**: 747–755.

51. McKeown T, Record RG. The influence of reproduction on body weight in women. *J Endocrinol* 1957; **15**: 393–409.

52. Billewicz WZ, Thomson AM. Body weight in parous women. *Br J Prev Soc Med* 1970; **24**: 97–104.

53. Olsen LC, Mundt MH. Postpartum weight loss in a nurse-midwifery practice. *J Nurs Midwif* 1986; **31**: 177–181.

54. Öhlin A, Rössner S. Maternal body weight development after pregnancy. *Int J Obes* 1990; **14**: 159–173.

55. Öhlin A, Rössner S. Trends in eating patterns, physical activity and socio-demographic factors in relation to post-partum body weight development. *Br J Nutr* 1994; **71**: 457–470.

56. Schauberger CW, Rooney BL, Brimer LM. Factors that influence weight loss in the puerperium. *Obstet Gynecol* 1992; **79**: 424–429.

57. Keppel KG, Taffel SM. Pregnancy-related weight gain and retention: Implications of the 1990 Institute of Medicine Guidelines. *Am J Public Health* 1993; **83**: 1100–1103.

58. Boardley DJ, Sargent RG, Coker AL, Hussey JR, Sharpe PA. The relationship between diet, activity, and other factors, and postpartum weight change by race. *Obstet Gynecol* 1995; **86**: 834–838.

59. Scholl TO, Hediger ML, Schall JI, Ances IG, Smith WK. Gestational weight gain, pregnancy outcome and postpartum weight retention. *Obstet Gynecol* 1995; **86**: 423–427.

60. Muscati SK, Gray-Donald K, Koski KG. Timing of weight gain during pregnancy: promoting fetal growth and minimising maternal weight retention. *Int J Obes* 1996; **20**: 526–532.

61. Walker LO. Predictors of weight gain at 6 and 18 months after childbirth: A pilot study. *J Obstet Gynecol Neonatal Nurs* 1996; **25**: 39–48.

62. Janney CA, Zhang D, Sowers M. Lactation and weight retention. *Am J Clin Nutr* 1997; **66**: 1116–1124.

63. Thorsdottir I, Birgisdottir BE. Different weight gain in women of normal weight before pregnancy: postpartum weight and birth weight. *Obstet Gynecol* 1998; **92**: 377–383.

64. To WWK, Cheung W. The relationship between weight gain in pregnancy, birth weight and postpartum weight retention. *Aust NZ J Obstet Gynaecol* 1998; **38**: 176–179.

65. Harris HE, Ellison GTH, Clement S. Do the psychosocial and behavioural changes that accompany motherhood influence the impact of pregnancy on long-term weight gain? *J Psychosom Obstet Gynaecol* 1999; **20**: 65–79.

66. Lederman SA. The effect of pregnancy weight gain on later obesity. *Obstet Gynecol* 1993; **82**: 148–155.

67. Walker LO. Weight and weight-related distress after childbirth: relationships to stress, social support, and depressive symptoms. *Journal of Holistic Nursing* 1997; **15**: 389–405.

68. Harris HE, Ellison GTH, Clement S. The relative importance of heritable characteristics and lifestyle in the development of maternal obesity. *J Epidemiol Comm Health* 1999; **53**: 66–74.

69. Parker J, Abrams B. Differences in postpartum weight retention between black and white mothers. *Obstet Gynecol* 1993; **81**: 768–774.

70. Harris HE, Ellison GTH, Holliday M. Is there an independent association between parity and maternal weight gain? *Ann Hum Biol* 1997; **24**: 507–519.

71. Crowell, DT. Weight change in the postpartum period. A review of the literature. *J Nurse Midwif* 1995; **40**: 418–423.

72. Rössner S, Öhlin A. Pregnancy as a risk factor for obesity: Lessons from the Stockholm pregnancy and weight development study. *Obes Res* 1995; **3**: 267s–275s.

73. Lawrence M, McKillop FM, Durnin JVGA. Women who gain more fat during pregnancy may not have bigger babies: implications for recommended weight gain during pregnancy. *Br J Obstet Gynaecol* 1991; **98**: 254–259.

74. OPCS. *Survey of Infant Feeding Practice*. London: HMSO, 1992.

75. Rössner S. Cessation of cigarette smoking and body weight increase. *Acta Med Scand* 1986; **219**: 1–2.

76. Olsen F, Frische G, Poulsen AO, Kirchheiner H. Changing smoking, drinking, and eating behaviour among pregnant women in Denmark. Evaluation of a health campaign in a local region. *Scand J Soc Med* 1989; **17**: 277–280.

77. Clissold TL, Hopkins WG, Seddon RJ. Lifestyle behaviours during pregnancy. *NZ Med J* 1991; **104**: 111–113.

78. Craddock D. Association for the study of obesity. *Int J Obes* 1980; **4**: 186.

79. Bradley PJ. Conditions recalled to have been associated with weight gain in adulthood. *Appetite* 1985; **6**: 235–241.

80. Garner DM, Olmsted MP, Polivy J. Development and validation of a multidimensional eating disorder inventory for anorexia nervosa and bulimia. *Int J Eat Disord* 1983; **2**: 15–34.

81. Stein A, Fairburn CG. Eating habits and attitudes in the postpartum period. *Psychosom Med* 1996; **58**: 321–325.

82. Rodin J, Silberstein L, Striegel-Moore R. Women and weight: A normative discontent. In: Sonderegger TB (ed.) *Psychology and Gender*. Lincoln: University of Nebraska Press, 1985.

83. Jenkin W, Tiggemann M. Psychological effects of weight retained after pregnancy. *Women and Health* 1997; **25**: 89–98.

84. DiPietro L, Anda RF, Williamson DF, Stunkard AJ. Depressive symptoms and weight change in a national cohort of adults. *Int J Obes* 1992; **16**: 745–753.

85. Pine CJ. Anxiety and eating behaviour in obese and nonobese American Indians and White Americans. *J Pers Soc Psychol* 1985; **49**: 774–780.

86. Grunberg NE, Straub RO. The role of gender and taste class in the effects of stress on eating. *Health Psychol* 1992; **11**: 97–100.

87. Butte NF, Hopkinson JM. Body composition changes during lactation are highly variable among women. *J Nutr* 1998; **128**: 381S–385S.

88. Dewey KG, Heinig MJ, Nommsen LA. Maternal weight-loss patterns during prolonged lactation. *Am J Clin Nutr* 1993; **58**: 162–166.

89. Kramer FM, Stunkard AJ, Marshall KA, McKinney S, Liebschutz J. Breast-feeding reduces maternal lower-body fat. *J Am Diet Assoc* 1993; **93**: 429–433.

90. Potter S, Hannum S, McFarlin B, Essex-Sorlie D, Campbell E, Trupin S. Does infant feeding method influence postpartum weight loss? *J Am Diet Assoc* 1991; **91**: 411–446.

91. Brewer MM, Bates MR, Vannoy LP. Postpartum changes in maternal weight and body fat depots in lactating versus nonlactating women. *Am J Clin Nutr* 1989; **49**: 259–265.

92. Dugdale AE, Eaton-Evans J. The effect of lactation and other factors on post-partum changes in body-weight and triceps skinfold thickness. *Br J Nutr* 1989; **61**: 149–153.

93. Johnston EM. Weight changes during pregnancy and the postpartum period. *Prog Fd Nutr Sc* 1991; **15**: 117–157.

94. van Raaij JMA, Vermaat-Miedemaa SH, Schonk CM, Peek MEM, Hautvast JGAJ. Energy requirements of pregnancy in the Netherlands. *Lancet* 1987; **ii**: 953–955.

95. Sohlström A, Forsum E. Changes in adipose tissue volume and distribution during reproduction in Swedish women as assessed by magnetic resonance imaging. *Am J Clin Nutr* 1995; **61**: 287–295.

96. Sadurskis A, Kabir N, Wager J, Forsum E. Energy metabolism, body composition and milk production in healthy Swedish women during lactation. *Am J Clin Nutr* 1988; **48**: 44–49.

97. Gillen RS. Does pregnancy cause obesity? *Med J Aust* 1990; **152**: 112.

98. Harris HE, Ellison GTH, Richter LM, DeWet T, Levin J. Are overweight women at increased risk of obesity following pregnancy? *Br J Nutr* 1998; **79**: 489–494.

99. Miller WC, Lindeman AK, Wallace J, Niederpruem M. Diet composition, energy intake, and exercise in relation to body fat in men and women. *Am J Clin Nutr* 1990; **56**: 426–30.

100. Richardson JS. The treatment of maternal obesity. *Lancet* 1952; **i**: 525–528.

101. Sørensen TIA, Stunkard AJ. Does obesity run in families because of genes? An adoption study using silhouettes as a measure of obesity. *Acta Psychiatr Scand* 1993; **370**: 67–72 (Suppl).

102. Stunkard AJ, Sørensen TIA, Hanis C, Teasdale TW, Chakrabarty R, Schull WJ, *et al.* An adoption study of human obesity. *N Engl J Med* 1986; **314**: 193–198.

103. Sørensen TIA, Price RA, Stunkard AJ, Schulsinger F. Genetics of obesity in adult adoptees and their biological siblings. *BMJ* 1989; **298**: 87–90.

104. Sørensen TIA, Holst C, Stunkard AJ, Skovgaard LT. Correlations of body mass index of adult adoptees and their biological and adoptive relatives. *Int J Obes* 1992; **16**: 227–236.

105. Wolfe WS, Sobal J, Olson CM, Frongillo EA, Williamson DF. Parity-associated weight gain and its modification by sociodemographic and behavioural factors: a prospective analysis in US women. *Int J Obes* 1997; **21**: 802–810.

106. Parker J. Postpartum weight change. *Clin Obstet Gynecol* 1994; **37**: 528–537.

107. Dodge J, Silva PA. A study of mothers' health. *NZ Med J* 1980; **91**: 353–355.

108. Murphy SP, Abrams BF. Changes in energy intakes during pregnancy and lactation in a national sample of US women. *Am J Public Health* 1993; **83**: 1161–3.

109. Kahn HS, Williamson DF, Stevens JA. Race and weight change in US women: The roles of socioeconmic factors in young adult women. *Am J Public Health* 1991; **34**: 139–142.

110. Ellison GTH, Harris HE. The efficacy and cost-effectiveness of prenatal nutrition counselling for appropriate weight gain and improving birth weight: Two caveats. *J Am Diet Assoc* 1996; **96**: 448–449.

111. Light HK, Fenster C. Maternal concerns during pregnancy. *Am J Obstet Gynecol* 1974; **118**: 46–50.

112. Orr RD, Simmons JJ. Nutritional care in pregnancy: The patient's view. II. Perceptions, satisfaction, and response to dietary advice and treatment. *J Am Diet Assoc* 1979; **75**: 131–136.

113. Hytten FE. Is it important or even useful to measure weight gain in pregnancy? *Midwifery* 1990; **6**: 28–32.

114. Barker DJP, Bull AR, Osmond C, Simmonds SJ. Fetal and placental size and risk of hypertension in adult life. *BMJ* 1990; **301**: 259–262.

115. Barker DJP, Godfrey KM, Osmond C, Bull A. The relation of fetal length, ponderal index and head circumference to blood pressure and the risk of hypertension later in life. *Paediatr Perin Epidemiol* 1992; **6**: 35–44.

116. Law CM, Barker DJP, Osmond C, Fall CHD, Simmonds SJ. Early growth and abdominal fatness in adult life. In:

Barker DJP (ed.) *Fetal and Infant Origins of Adult Disease*. London: British Medical Journal Publications, 1992: 291–296.

117. Wadsworth MEJ, Kuh DJL. Childhood influences on adult health: A review of recent work from the British 1946 national birth cohort study, the MRC National survey of Health and Development. *Paediatr Perin Epidemiol* 1997; **11**: 2–20.

21

Social and Cultural Influences on Obesity

Jeffery Sobal

Cornell University, Ithaca, New York, USA

INTRODUCTION

Obesity may be defined as the condition of having high levels of stored body fat. Relative body weight is commonly used to describe obesity, and people who are obese are commonly described as being overweight. Obesity and overweight are complex biopsychosocial phenomena that are shaped by many factors, including a variety of social and cultural influences.

This chapter will examine patterns of fatness and thinness using social science perspectives to frame, review, and discuss social and cultural influences on obesity. Framing the influences on obesity first involves examining the larger social contexts of culture and history, and then considering the more specific social characteristics of individuals. Societal mechanisms involved in energy intake and energy expenditure will be discussed in light of their collective contribution to rising levels of body weight. Finally, conclusions about the social aspects of weight will be presented.

SOCIAL CONTEXTS

Two major social contexts provide overarching perspectives for framing obesity: culture and history. The culture within which a person lives is likely to be the most powerful influence on their eating patterns, activity levels, and body weight. Within each culture, conditions change (sometimes dramatically) over time, and historical period is also a strong influence on levels of fatness and thinness of individuals and populations.

Culture

Culture is the learned system of categories, rules, and plans that people use to guide their behaviors (1,2). A person's culture permeates every aspect of their life, including how they think about fatness and thinness, eating behaviors, activity patterns, and all other facets of living in the world.

Cultural values and norms about body weight vary considerably. Anthropologists estimate that there have been fewer than 8000 cultures that have existed in the world (3), although we only have information about a minority of all cultures that have existed. Information about body weight levels and weight beliefs is not available for the vast majority of cultures. Archaeological evidence about body weight is rare because body fat tissue is not well preserved over long periods of time.

Ancient representations of human figures such as drawings and sculptures provide some information about weight beliefs or ideals, but not necessarily actual weight patterns or fatness norms. The 25 000-year-old Venus of Willendorf is a tiny female statuette with a huge stomach and large, pendulous breasts that is often suggested to be a maternal or

International Textbook of Obesity. Edited by Per Björntorp.

fertility icon, and is an artifact widely discussed as evidence about past cultural preferences for plump body shapes for women (4). However, this figure is not necessarily representative of all icons of the same era because that period is unique and the place it originated from is dissimilar from other ancient cultures (5).

Holocultural analyses examine large samples of cultures (1), but few such investigations have examined perceptions about body weight. Brown and Konner (6) found that information about weight ideals was not available for most cultures, although among the 38 cultures that had data about female shape ideals, 81% (31) preferred plumpness or moderate fat rather than thinness or extreme obesity. Anderson *et al.* (7) also examined cross-cultural data and also found that 81% (50 of 62 cultures for which data was available) preferred fatter individuals. Ritenbaugh (8) suggests that the condition of obesity and the rejection of fatness may be a culture-bound phenomenon (9), meaning that it is particular to contemporary postindustrial societies and not culturally recognized by other societies. Overall, cross-cultural analyses suggest that most cultures in the world have valued moderate fatness and avoided extreme thinness.

People who live in economically developed societies are more likely to be obese than their counterparts in developing societies (10). Modernization is the complex set of social changes that occur as societies shift from being 'traditional' to 'modern' (11). Modernization involves shifts in modes of economic production for whole societies, which has substantial impacts on energy expenditure of human populations. Primary production extracts raw materials from the environment in agriculture, hunting and fishing, gathering, timbering, etc., and traditionally drew energy largely from muscles of humans and animals. Secondary production transforms raw materials into manufactured products, and on a mass scale typically draws energy from fossil, hydrological, or other fuels. Tertiary production provides services to consumers, and is not as dependent on physical energy sources as primary and secondary production. As whole societies shift from being based on primary to secondary to tertiary production as they modernize, the energy expenditure of most people in the population decreases dramatically. Examples from across the globe reveal that people are becoming fatter in modernizing societies (12,13).

Comparisons between various contemporary developed societies reveal substantial differences in body weight (14–16) that may be associated with modernization but also reflect cultural differences. For example, cultural differences between the USA and France in values about food and body weight have strongly shaped the prevalence of obesity in those two cultures (17). Cultural predispositions to obesity exist, with life in contemporary postindustrial cultures more likely to lead members of those cultures to become obese (5).

Migration between cultures places people into new food systems and new social and built environments, and has important health consequences (18). Zelensky (19) proposed that a migration transition is occurring, where people are travelling and moving more frequently and over longer distances. While migration flows occur between most areas of the world, the major migration streams tend to move from less developed to more developed societies. People in these dominant migration streams tend to gain weight after migration (20). The loss of the buffering effects of the traditional culture of many migrants puts them at further risk of illness if they gain weight in a new society (21). Specific mechanisms for relationships between migration and weight vary, with the relative contribution of energy intake and energy expenditure being specific to the circumstances of particular individuals and groups coming from distinctive origins to unique destinations. Also, the relative contributions of selection versus causation (22) are not clearly understood for migration, with a need for further investigation of the extent that migrants have a differential predisposition for weight change or whether the new environments of immigrants changes their weights.

Acculturation occurs as people become socialized into another culture (23,24). Acculturation is a multidimensional phenomenon, and can operate differently for various domains such as social relationships, behaviors, values, and other topics (25). Studies in the USA suggest that acculturation is associated with increases in body weight (26,27). The relationship between relative body weight and acculturation often varies among particular ethnic subgroups, with US Hispanic migrant groups having acculturation more strongly associated with weight for Mexican Americans and less for Cuban Americans and Puerto Ricans (20).

Overall, culture and the dynamics of culture

changes are a crucial influence on the way people live, operating as a strong determinant of energy intake and expenditure. Culture also shapes values, attitudes, and beliefs about fatness and thinness, providing a basis for how people interpret their own body weights and the weights of others. The dynamics of larger cultural changes and individual acculturation and migration reveal the overwhelming importance of culture in body weight and obesity.

History

Historical changes occur as societies move through time, and clear temporal shifts have occurred in body weight and values about obesity in many societies. However, valid and representative population data about actual body weight are rare for time periods prior to the mid-1900s, so conclusions about historical changes in actual weight prior to that time are problematic. Some historical records of weights of select populations do exist, such as military recruits (28), but these are not necessarily generalizable to the broader population. Insurance company data began to provide broader population level historical information in the twentieth century (29,30), but still offered limited generalizability because of the select population that is covered by insurance policies (31). Only with the advent of national nutrition surveys in developed societies beginning in about the 1960s did solid prevalence data about weight become historically available, such as the US National Health and Nutrition Examination Surveys (NHANES) (32). Despite data limitations, several interpretations of historical patterns in weight can be developed.

Obesity appears to be increasing for most societies of the world during the second half of the twentieth century (33–36). The increase has not necessarily been an evenly progressing secular trend over time, with the historical periods in the late 1940s and in the 1970s revealing cohort and history shifts towards higher prevalence of obesity (37). Some observers label this a global obesity epidemic (38–41).

Information is available about historical changes in social values concerning body weight. In Europe and America prior to 1900, plumpness was valued as insurance against consumptive illness (17). The major transition point when public attitudes moved from valuing or accepting fatness to desiring or seeking thinness appears to be around the beginning of the twentieth century (15). Many types of diets and other weight loss strategies began to be widely available and used after 1900 (42–44). During the second half of the twentieth century, social ideals have increasingly emphasized the value of slimness for women, as evidenced in the increasingly thinner body shapes of idealized women's roles such as beauty pageant winners (45,46) and fashion models (47).

The rejection of fatness has escalated since the beginning of the twentieth century, but is grounded in a prior history of stigmatization of obese individuals both in Europe and in Asia (48). A moral model for thinking about obesity was pervasive in developed societies for most of the twentieth century, treating fatness as badness rather than sickness (49). However, since the 1950s there has been a medicalization of obesity that cast it as an illness rather than a consequence of moral failures of individuals (49).

Overall, historical patterns exist for body weight and attitudes about body weight, and those patterns have been continually changing. Globalization of Western culture is a strong influence on food, eating, and weight (11), and this is leading to a high prevalence of obesity across the world. This suggests that it is essential to frame obesity within historical as well as cultural contexts to fully understand the causes and consequences of fatness and thinness.

SOCIAL CHARACTERISTICS

Many social characteristics of individuals are associated with body weight in postindustrial societies. The social epidemiology of body weight can be usefully examined in relationship to 12 fundamental social characteristics of individuals: sex/gender, age/life stage, race/ethnicity, employment, occupation, income, education, household size, marital status, parenthood, residential density, and region. While there is well-established information about the social epidemiology of body weight for some of these characteristics, for others weight patterns are less clear. The specific mechanisms for most have yet to be well understood.

The relationship of each of these 12 characteristics with body weight will be discussed in the following sections. Most of the discussion will focus on patterns in developed societies at the beginning of the twenty-first century, where more research has been conducted, although some cultural and historical contrasts will be made.

Sex/Gender

Sex refers to the ascribed biological status of being female or male (as differentiated by anatomy and physiology), while gender refers to the achieved social status of being a woman or man (as constructed by psychosociocultural factors). Clear sexual dimorphism exists in body weight, with females generally having more stored body fat than males and being more likely than males to be obese (5,34). Many sex differences are physiological and linked to reproductive functioning (50), with more overall subcutaneous fat present in females and the distribution of body fat deposits being greater in lower body for females and upper body for males.

Beyond biological sex differences in body fat, substantial social and psychological gender differences exist with respect to weight in many societies, with fatness and thinness being more likely to be female and feminist issues (51). Women are judged by and more concerned about their physical appearance than men, with body weight and body shape a major criterion for judging female attractiveness (52–54). Among the public, weight concerns are based more on appearance than health motivations, particularly among women (55). Stigmatization of body weight is more prevalent and severe for women than men (56), leading to pressures in postindustrial societies that make body weight a 'normative discontent' for most women (57).

Overall, sex and gender are overriding characteristics when considering obesity. The prevalence and meaning of weight are so different for men and women that much obesity research is done only on one sex or the other, and most data about weight is presented separately for males and females. Clearly, body weight and obesity are gendered issues.

Age/Life Stage

Age refers to the chronological time since an individual's birth, and life stage refers to the social roles and expectations that exist for people of a given age. In contemporary postindustrial societies, body weight and obesity tend to increase as a person ages, and then decline in the last decades of a person's life (5,35). This leads to an inverted 'U' or 'J' shaped pattern in body weight as a person ages. The prevalence of obesity tends to be lowest among the youngest and oldest segments of the adult population (58). The highest weight gain occurs in both genders between age 25 and 34 (59). Elderly people typically experience weight loss in their later years. Weight changes with age vary among individuals, and for most people weight gains appear to be small and continuous over time (60).

Explaining patterns in the relationship of weight and age is complex, involving many considerations. Aging involves biological as well as psychosocial components, both of which are important influences on body weight. It is difficult to disentangle the relative contribution of biology versus social influences on patterns of weight by age. Metabolic arguments support the tendency to gain weight up to adulthood and lose it as a person becomes elderly.

Mechanisms involved in shaping body weight vary by age. Activity levels of younger people tend to be higher, and decline as people age (61). Eating patterns also vary throughout the life course (62), influencing the caloric intake of individuals and consequently their body weight.

Life stage differences exist in social norms about body shape ideals, with young people emphasizing slimness more than older people (52,63). As people proceed through their life course, they exhibit a personal weight trajectory that is subject to social expectations about age-appropriate standards for body weight (62). Concern about weight varies across life stages for women, with greater concern among younger than older women (64). However, it appears that concerns about body weight are more tied with women's self-esteem among middle-aged women (age 30 to 49), suggesting that weight concern may be less problematic among most younger and older women.

Overall, age and life stage are consistently associated with body weight and obesity, with younger and older people being thinner and less likely to be obese. The mechanisms for these relationships have yet to be clearly delineated, involving a combination of physiological changes, activity levels, and caloric intake.

Race/Ethnicity

Race refers to physiological subgroups that exhibit biological variations in human populations, while ethnicity refers to the different cultures and subcultures in human societies, particularly complex societies that are multiethnic. When differences in racial/ethnic groups occur, attribution of these differences to biological versus social factors is extremely problematic. This is especially true for body weight, where racial/ethnic differences exist in obesity in many societies. Adding to the complexity of this issue are the differential patterns in socioeconomic status and other variables among racial/ethnic groups (65).

Many investigations in the USA have reported ethnic patterns in body weight and obesity, with minority groups typically being more likely to be obese than the majority and some variation between minority groups (35,66). A meta-analysis of American ethnic differences in body weight (67) found complex patterns in weight variations between ethnic groups. Overall, Polynesians had the highest mean relative body weights, followed by blacks, Caucasians, Thais and others. However, percent body fat did not precisely correspond with weight levels.

The mechanisms for ethnic variations in body weight are problematic, with no consensus about the relative contribution of genetics, activity levels, or caloric intake differences (68,69). Ethnic variations in caloric intake and physical activity have been reported (70), but these are confounded by other factors such as socioeconomic status or residential location.

Beliefs, perceptions, and attitudes about weight differ among ethnic groups in many societies. In the USA, many minority ethnic groups tend to be more accepting of higher body weights than those in the white majority ethnic group (58). Specific differences in ethnic groups in the way that they deal with weight need to be examined and considered as an important factor in the etiology and epidemiology of fatness and thinness.

Overall, ethnicity is a characteristic that is important to consider in relationship to obesity, but presents complex questions about how and why is associated with weight. The ethnic compositions of populations are continually changing, and ethnic groups are migrating and acculturating, making ethnicity a problematic aspect of the social patterns of obesity.

Employment

Employment involves work paid for by wages or salary in the labor force, and may be full-time or part-time. A person's work role is a major social identity for most adults, with almost all men and the majority of women participating in the labor force in most contemporary postindustrial societies. One of the most significant changes in industrialized societies in the second half of the twentieth century is the entry of the majority of adult women into the labor force.

Many aspects of employment are relevant to body weight and obesity (71). Employment provides financial resources through income, and also access and opportunities for using health care services. Many jobs include health benefits and risks, some related to body weight such as involvement in healthy levels of physical activity or the stress of working varying schedules in 'shift work' (72). An important aspect of employment is that working usually imposes an organized structure on people's lives and provides a social world that is different from the family and household social network.

Despite the potential relevance of work to patterns of body weight, relatively little explicit attention has focused on patterns of work and weight. However, employment information is reported in studies of other aspects of weight. Some studies in postindustrial societies find that women who are not employed are more likely to be obese than their counterparts who participate in the labor force (73). Unemployed men have been reported to be underweight (74). Fuller analysis of employment and employment transitions such as entering the workforce, changing jobs, and retiring need to be conducted to understand their role in body weight and obesity.

Overall, even though the majority of adults in developed societies are employed outside the home, there is a dearth of information about how employment influences obesity. Mechanisms for activity level and caloric intake from employment are not well worked out, so employment and obesity deserves additional research attention in the future.

Occupation

Occupation is the type of work that a person performs in a society. The occupations are diverse, and can be classified on many dimensions relevant to body weight. While occupation has not been a focus in most of the weight literature, differences in weight levels and the prevalence of obesity do occur. Women in low prestige jobs tend to be more obese, but the relationship between occupation and weight is less consistent for men (75).

Energy intake is not necessarily determined by occupation, although jobs that are related to food preparation (such as cooks, clerks in businesses that sell food, etc.) may provide eating opportunities that facilitate overeating. Some occupations also have obligations for employees to eat to perform their jobs, such as salespeople who are expected to take clients to meals, etc. Another aspect of some occupations related to energy intake is whether they are structured to permit, enhance, or prevent eating on the job. Some jobs are flexible about eating at work, while others rigidly provide set times where eating can occur. Many worksites offer foodservice to their employees, which provides a source of calories that may either facilitate or prevent obesity, depending on how the foodservice is used.

Energy expenditure varies considerably by occupation. Some jobs involving high levels of energy expenditure over extended durations of time, while others involve minimal physical activity for long periods. On this basis, some workers expend many calories over the course of their workday and may be underweight, while others spend long sedentary hours at work that can contribute to obesity. Occupations also vary in the flexibility they offer to workers to engage in recreational exercise. Some jobs encourage workers to exercise before, during, and after their workday, and even provide worksite recreational facilities and organized exercise programs. By contrast, other jobs offer no opportunities or facilitation of exercise for their employees.

Another occupational consideration is selection of people into particular jobs because of their weight. Occupational prestige tends to be inversely associated with relative body weight, especially for women, with higher status occupations having thinner workers (10). There is considerable documentation of weight discrimination during the hiring process against the entry of obese individuals into many jobs, particularly those with higher prestige

and public visibility (76–78). Additionally, upward occupational mobility is limited or restricted for obese individuals due to weight discrimination in the promotion process (79–81). This suggests that body weight influences occupation, in addition to occupation influencing body weight, and that the disentanglement of those two causal processes is difficult.

Overall, the high proportion of both men and women who participate in the labor force in postindustrial societies and the long hours that are spent at the worksite suggest that occupation has the potential to become an important factor in the prevalence and treatment of obesity. Occupations provide lifestyles that play a role in eating, exercise, and weight management. Weight and work are topics that need to be examined more completely in the future.

Income

Income is the wages and other benefits provided through employment, as well as from other sources such as investments, inheritance, and government assistance programs. Income provides resources that can influence energy intake and expenditure, which in turn shape body weight.

One of the most consistent patterns in the obesity literature is the direct association between income and body weight in men and women in developing nations, and the inverse association between income and weight among women (and perhaps men) in developed societies (10). There is some debate about whether the direction of causality operates as income influencing weight, weight influencing income, or both (71). Income provides opportunities to exercise control over many aspects of life, including diet and activity levels, and can be used to seek the thin ideal that exists in most postindustrial societies. Low income levels produce stress, which may lead some people to store more body fat as insurance against difficult times in the future, and others to seek solace from their troubles through the comfort of eating.

Energy intake appears to have an inverted 'U' shaped relationship with income, with the lowest and highest income groups ingesting fewer kilocalories of food than middle income individuals (70). Income facilitates control over energy intake by providing resources that permit a person to select foods. Resources are an important consideration in making food choices (82,83). Having adequate income allows someone to focus on other aspects foods than cost, such as health and caloric value. People who experience hunger or food insecurity may overeat when food is available, which leads lower income groups in some societies to be more likely to be obese (84). In postindustrial societies, people with higher incomes have the resources to purchase more expensive low-fat or dieting products to attempt to control their weight, as well as to enroll in sometimes costly weight control classes and programs.

Energy expenditure is generally inversely associated with income at work because most higher paying professions require less caloric activity on the job than the manual, physical labor of many low paying jobs. However, those with higher incomes are more likely to have the resources to afford living in low crime neighborhoods where they can safely participate in outdoor recreational activities. Higher income individuals also can afford to pay for recreational exercise equipment, classes, coaching, travel, etc.

Overall, income is a powerful predictor of body weight levels and obesity. In postindustrial societies, higher income women in particular are thinner and less likely to be obese. Income provides many resources that permit people to avoid or overcome obesity, and needs to be considered in examining patterns of obesity and interventions to prevent or reduce obesity.

Education

Education is usually seen as the amount of formal schooling that a person has experienced. Education provides knowledge about eating, nutrition, activity, health, and weight that is used in assessing food and activity choices and in managing body weight. Education also socializes people into the dominant norms of society about fatness and thinness, providing them with motivations as well as skills to conform to cultural weight expectations.

In developing societies men and women with the most education tend to be heavier than their peers, although often not fat by the standards of developed societies (10). In postindustrial societies and groups, people with the highest levels of education are least likely to be obese (66). The relationship between education and body weight appears to be bidirectional in postindustrial societies (71). People with lower education have less knowledge about nutrition, activity, and weight, and are more likely to become obese. Additionally, obese people are more likely to be discriminated against in acquiring greater education because they are excluded from admission to various educational opportunities (56).

Energy intake is not clearly associated with education in postindustrial societies (70). People with the lowest levels of education are more likely to eat higher fat foods and less likely to consume fruits and vegetables, but also may experience lower food intake.

Energy expenditure is inversely associated with education (61). People who have the least education tend to have jobs that involve more manual labor and those with the most education have more mental and interactional labor included in their daily work. Energy use in recreational activities is more frequent among those with higher education, who are more likely to participate in sports and exercise programs specifically to manage body weight.

Overall, education is one of the strongest predictors of body weight and obesity in populations, with more highly educated people being thinner. The knowledge, thinking skills, and normative socialization acquired through education appear to be important in preventing gaining of body weight during adulthood, and dealing with weight gains that do occur. Public investments in education for the population may be one of the most effective ways to limit the development and lower the prevalence of obesity.

Household Size

Household size is the number of people that a person resides with in their household or home. Household size is related to eating patterns, activity levels, and body weight, particularly among some portions of the population such as the elderly. In particular, living alone is a risk factor for problematic eating, activity levels, and body weight.

Little research attention has been given to household size, weight, and obesity among the general population. Among the elderly, however, living alone can be a risk for undernutrition and insufficient body weight even though the collective findings of studies of eating alone and weight are mixed (85).

Energy intake does not necessarily vary by household size (70). However, energy intake is influenced by the presence of others. Commensality is important in encouraging adequate food intake (86), and people who eat alone frequently do not eat enough to maintain body weight levels (87). A body of work on social facilitation concludes that there is a direct relationship between the number of people who are present at meals and the amount that people consume (88). This suggests that household size may influence energy intake, with the more people who live in a dwelling unit the more calories they each consume.

Energy expenditure may be influenced by household size in various ways. Interacting with other individuals involves additional activity beyond being alone. Such interaction may lead to expending more energy among people in larger households. Especially if there are children in a household, people spend more time moving around than when others are not present.

Overall, the number of people with whom a person lives has the potential to influence their caloric intake, activity level, and values about body weight. A particular concern exists for people living alone. However, these relationships between household size and weight have not been a focus of past research and deserve more attention in the future.

Marital Status

Marital status is related to body weight and obesity in many different ways (89). Obese people are stigmatized, which produces problems in dating and attracting marital partners (90,91) and in maintaining partners in marriage (92). Entering and terminating marriage are significant life events when people renegotiate eating and activity patterns which often lead to weight changes (93,94). Obese people enter marriage later (95) and marry heavier partners (96), which is evidence that success in the marriage market is a problem for large individuals, particularly women. Married men, but not necessarily women, weigh more than unmarried individuals (55,73).

People tend to gain weight after entering marriage (93,94,97,98), and married couples tend synchronically to gain and lose weight together (99). People who terminate their marriages tend to lose weight (97,98,100). Overall, entering into marriage is more difficult for obese people, being married is associated with higher body weight, and terminating marriage is associated with weight loss.

Energy intake differs between married and unmarried individuals. Spouses eat the majority of their meals and snacks together both at home and away from home, so that people consume most of their calories with their marital partner. Marriage structures people's eating patterns, providing regular meals and commensal partners. Partners involved in a marriage perceive an obligation to eat with their spouse, sometimes consuming calories that they would not have eaten if they did were not married (101). Men in postindustrial societies cite getting married as one of the most significant reasons that they gained weight and are overweight (102).

Energy expenditure is also influenced by marital status (61,94). The social obligation to spend time together as spousal partners presents an opportunity cost for many forms of individualistic exercise activities (although many partners participate together in sports and recreation). Unmarried people sometimes engage in recreational physical activity to remain thin to attract a desirable partner and also as a form of social activity to interact with other people.

Overall, marriage structures people's lives, provides social obligations for eating and activities, and includes normative perceptions about body weight and shape. This suggests that marital status is a predictor of body weight levels, and that interventions to change or maintain body weights should consider marriage and perhaps be structured around marital partners (103).

Parenthood

Parenthood is having children, involving pregnancy and childbirth among women and the raising of children for both men and women. Being a parent is an important role in many people's lives, and there has been considerable interest in the relationship between having children and body weight.

Adult women in postindustrial societies cite having a child as one of the major reasons that they gained weight and are overweight (102). Many studies have examined postpartum weight retention (controlling for age and other factors), and the consensus of research in postindustrial societies is that a direct association exists between parity and weight but that the effect is small, about an average gain per birth of about one kilogram (2.2 pounds) (104). However, these averages vary widely, with some women gaining and retaining considerable weight after childbirth while others lose weight (105). The association between parity and body weight is modified by many sociodemographic and behavioral factors, with women who are minority, rural, lower socioeconomic status, unemployed, unmarried, and getting little physical activity at greater potential risk of parity-associated weight retention (106,107).

Many questions about parenthood and body weight remain unresolved. While epidemiological studies show that some weight gain is associated with each additional child, the source of this gain is not clear. Williamson *et al.* (105) made the conceptual distinction between the contribution of *childbearing* and *childrearing* to weight gain after pregnancy. Childbearing contributes to weight gain largely through physiological processes involved in pregnancy and childbirth, while childrearing contributes to weight gain largely by changes in the social aspects of households when raising children such as changes in the family food system and parental physical activity patterns (108). Current studies have not been able to distinguish between the relative contributions of childbirth versus parenting to postpartum weight retention, and it is up to future researchers to disentangle those mechanisms. Overall, while women with more children are more likely to have higher body weights and be obese, the patterns and dynamics of this relationship have yet to be fully understood.

Energy intake of pregnant women typically increases as they gain weight during pregnancy (104). These higher calorie consumption patterns may establish longstanding food choice trajectories that persist after the pregnancy for some women but not others (62). During childrearing, many parents consume additional calories as they have special children's foods available in addition to adult foods, as well as when they consume foods uneaten by their children to avoid wasting the foods. All of these factors suggest that childbearing and childrearing provide risks of increased caloric consumption by mothers (and possibly fathers) that may contribute to weight gain and maintenance of higher body weights by people in the parental role.

Energy expenditure can differ for parents compared to people who do not have children, with childrearing demands and opportunity costs playing a role in parental physical activities. Considerable energy expenditure is often required in the process of caring for children, and childrearing may lead to greater energy expenditure among people who previously were not very physically active during their leisure time. By contrast, for people involved in regular recreational activities the time demands for rearing children can present an opportunity cost that may diminish their voluntary exercise levels and lead to decreasing energy expenditure. The energy demands and time obligations of childrearing can influence both mothers and fathers, and may vary for particular individuals.

Overall, being a parent is a significant role, and includes a myriad of components that can influence parental body weights. Many women attribute weight gains to parental involvement, but it is currently not clear whether this is from bearing or rearing children or how much of any weight patterns associated with parenthood are due to caloric intake or energy expenditure.

Residential Density

Residential density refers to whether a person lives in a rural, suburban, or urban area. Rural and urban may be conceptualized as opposite points on a continuum of residential density, or rural, suburban, and urban areas may be seen as categorically different types of communities. While there have been some studies that provide some data on rural–urban differences in weight and obesity, little specific analysis has examined variations in body weight by residential density, although some investigations provide rural–urban data as descriptive information during the course of studying other issues.

Analysis of rural–urban weight differences in the USA using national data found that rural women are slightly more likely to be obese than their metropolitan counterparts (109). There was an overall gradient in rural–urban weight without controlling for other variables that revealed that urban men and women had higher relative body weights. However, it is crucial to control for other attributes that also vary between rural and urban areas, such as income, education, age, etc., to attempt to distinguish between inherent rural–urban differences versus compositional differences. When other variables were controlled, the rural–urban differences persisted but were weak for women, and were not present for men.

Energy intake varies somewhat between rural and urban areas, with rural residents having slightly higher caloric intakes (70). Higher population density provides a more diverse foodscape, with more opportunities to eat from a variety of food sources. Rural food options tend to be more limited, and lower calorie foods may not be as available as in suburban or urban areas.

Energy expenditure was traditionally very high in rural areas, due to the large percentage of the population involved in farmwork and the need to walk long distances to engage in social activities. With the rise of the automobile, rural and suburban residents tend to drive at least as much, if not more, than their metropolitan counterparts.

The context a person lives in provides social norms and attitudes about weight. The body shape comparisons between people in cities encourages people to strive for thinness (110). Appearance may be more important for the high number of fleeting interactions in urban areas, with more multifaceted relationships occurring between people in places with lower population density.

Overall, it appears that a relationship exists between obesity and rural–urban residence, with a slight tendency for rural people to have higher body weights even when controlling for other variables. This may be partly due to activity levels, and partly to caloric intake. The attitudes and values in urban areas may underlie these differences, with an emphasis on thinness in cities leading people there to more actively control their weight.

Region

Region is the particular place where people live. Geographers specialize in studying regionality, and use several levels of scale to conceptualize differences in regions of the world, a continent, a nation, or a city. Only scattered data exist on regional variations in obesity and body weight. An important consideration in examining spatial patterns such as regional differences is the need to differentiate between inherent regional qualities that determine differences in weight, such as eating patterns or activity levels, and compositional differences in the inhabitants of a region, such as when young or lower income people predominate in a particular place. Determinative versus compositional effects can be examined by controlling for key variables in multivariate analyses, and this currently has not been well sorted out for regional patterns of obesity.

In the USA, government studies of obesity during the 1990s reported that it was most concentrated in the south and southeast, but as the entire US population became fatter obesity spread in most regions of the country (66). In Brazil, the more economically developed southern region of the country had greater prevalence of obesity (111). Neighborhoods in a Scottish city exhibited different levels of weight, suggesting that obesity prevention efforts would benefit from focusing on place of residence (112).

Energy intake variations by geographical region have been reported in some studies (65). Geographical location is associated with dietary patterns. Cuisines and taste ratings (113) are widely recognized as having regional differences, but it is less clear whether caloric intake varies between geographical regions.

Energy expenditure may vary among the populations of geographical regions, but it is difficult to clearly establish reasons for such variations. Some may be climactic, some due to regional differences in the composition of the population, and some to specific regional attitudes and norms about physical activity.

Overall, region is strongly influenced by the economic status associated with different places, which in turn appears to influence diet, activity, and body weight. However, more research on this topic is needed to identify systematic patterns.

SOCIETAL MECHANISMS

Many social mechanisms have been proposed to explain variations in weight between individuals, groups, societies, and time periods. These mechanisms reflect modifications in energy intake and energy output. Two major societal mechanisms that influence body weight involve large-scale shifts that are occurring in most societies: (1) food system transformations are modifying energy intake, and (2) built environment efficiencies are reducing levels of physical activity.

Food System Transformations

The food system is the complex of activities that provides crops, foodstuffs, and foods to the population as a source of caloric energy and nutrients (114). Significant food system transformations have occurred over time (11) and have had important influences on energy intake and body weight. Technology has greatly increased the volume, diversified the content, and increased the variety of the food supply in many areas of the world. Overall, the food system has moved from offering relatively few calories per person to being a calorically abundant system. An increasing proportion of the calories in the food system are from fat (115). For example, in the USA today there are approximately 3800 kilocalories available per capita, almost twice the requirement for adults. The food system can be divided into six major stages that will be discussed here in relationship to their contribution to increasing caloric intake of the populations of postindustrial societies: production, processing, distribution, acquisition, preparation, and consumption.

Food production in ancient societies involved only hunting and gathering. Those societies experienced fluctuations and uncertainties in maintaining an adequate and constant food supply (116). Famines were common and always a threat to society, leading to an ever-present risk of inadequate caloric intake. Over 10 000 years ago the agricultural revolution led to a more stable food supply that produced surplus foods to insure a constant energy stream in the face of environmental vicissitudes, and create a supply of surplus foods that freed an increasing proportion of society from involvement in food production. The industrial revolution in agriculture beginning in the 1800s further increased food surplus production, permitting the majority of society to forsake food production to pursue other tasks. Currently, industrial and postindustrial societies produce up to twice the number of calories

per capita that can be consumed by members of those societies (115). Thus food production has led to an extremely abundant availability of calories in postindustrial food systems.

Food processing changes crops into foodstuffs and foods. Food processing procedures increase the palatability and durability of foods, preventing the waste of crops and enhancing the desirability of foods for consumption and reducing spoilage. Food processing often involves manufacturing procedures that increase the caloric levels and caloric density of foods over their unprocessed forms, adding to the energy content of the food supply (11). For example, many food manufacturing processes add sugar and fat to raw foodstuffs to produce higher calorie prepared and preserved food products. Thus food processing has tended to increase the caloric density of the food system, typically by adding sugars and fats.

Food distribution has undergone major changes over time that are making food almost universally available and accessible, deterring people from running out of food and facilitating higher levels of energy consumption. The proliferation of institutions offering food such as grocery stores, restaurants, vending machines, take away or carry out foods, food delivery, mobile food vendors, catering, etc., has made it rare to be in a place where food is not available. The ease of obtaining food at all hours of the day or night in almost all places has removed barriers to eating for almost everyone (although because of social inequalities a small portion of society experiences food insufficiency and food insecurity (84)). The increasing durability of food products has also overcome barriers of time and space in making calories more available to virtually all people at all times in postindustrial societies (11). The portion sizes of food in foodservice operations are also increasing, distributing more calories in individual servings than in the past (38). Thus food distribution makes calories beyond basic energy needs available to almost all people at all times in most places in developed societies.

Food acquisition is the procurement of foods from various distribution outlets in raw, processed, and prepared forms. Increasingly, food purchases have been processed foods that have fats and sugars added and are ready to eat, encouraging immediate consumption of energy dense foods. Consumers also are more likely to eat foods prepared by others in commercial establishments, with half of the US food expenditures spent eating away from home (117), making consumers less aware of the ingredients and caloric content of the foods they eat. Thus easy acquisition of tasty foods without awareness of their ingredients facilitates the increased likelihood of obtaining higher levels of calories when foods are acquired from the food system by individuals.

Food preparation manipulates foodstuffs into foods using a variety of methods. Foodstuffs are increasingly likely to have some preparation steps already performed commercially prior to personal cooking, decreasing the human energy expenditure involved in cooking and making ingredients and caloric content less obvious to food preparers. Cooking methods vary in the number of calories they add to foods, with many techniques involving heating foodstuffs in fats or oils which adds to the caloric content and density of the foods that are prepared. Thus food preparation methods often add calories (particularly as fat) to the food system, increasing caloric intakes of individuals who eat these foods.

Food consumption involves selection, serving, and ingesting foods. Many social food events occur in contemporary societies, providing obligations to ingest calories in foods. Consumption patterns are often divided into meals and snacks between meals, with an increase in the prevalence of snacking across the day (118). Research findings about eating frequency and body weight are mixed. Several studies suggest a gendered relationship where women who eat more frequently have higher body weights, but men who eat more often have lower body weights (119). Thus the more universal availability and accessibility of prepared foods has created a system that facilitates consumption of food energy, which may be linked to eating frequency.

Overall from production to consumption, contemporary food systems increasingly deliver a higher amount of caloric energy that is more easily and cheaply available to more people than ever before. Current trends suggest that ingestible calorie supplies beyond basic metabolic needs are moving towards being universally available across time, place, and people, with a decreasing minority of the population experiencing hunger. Globalization of production, processing, and distribution increase caloric availability, and advances in communication and transportation facilitate caloric acquisition, preparation, and consumption. On a societal scale, these changes have produced an increasingly fattening food system that contributes to a rising prevalence of obesity.

Built Environment Efficiencies

Humans have modified their physical environments in many ways, including the development and use of many forms of technology to modify clothing, housing, transportation, worksites, communications, and other areas. Natural environments have many features that require people to expend energy by temperature regulation, sheltering from exposure to the elements (sun, precipitation, wind), moving between places, etc. With economic modernization, built environments have expanded to house an increasingly larger scope of human activities. An ever-rising amount of each person's life is spent in built spaces that are shielded from requirements to expend energy to cope with natural forces. Within built environments, technological developments have continually made life tasks more efficient. The sum of all these changes has led to lower energy expenditures by humans because of built environment efficiencies, and these contribute to increased body weights and more obesity.

Clothing has become more energy efficient and more widely available, which has decreased energy expenditure needed to maintain body temperature for the majority of the population (120). The industrial revolution developed mass production of cloth, permitting the population to keep warm efficiently through days and nights in a manner never before possible. Clothing is often taken for granted in contemporary postindustrial societies, even though it saves the expenditure of calories compared with the cruder and less task-specific clothing of hundreds or thousands of years ago.

Two important aspects of the human built environment that have greatly decreased energy are housing and furniture. Housing structures have evolved new materials and forms that increasingly separate built from natural environments. Efficient heating and cooling systems combined with improved insulation of structures separate humans from the world outside of their dwellings and vehicles. Precisely and automatically controlled temperatures decrease the need for people to generate body heat to keep themselves warm in cold weather. Air conditioning permits obese people with high levels of insulating body fat to remain comfortable in cool weather. Lighting permits people to spend more time inside. Clocks coordinate people's activities (121), minimizing the time spent standing and waiting for others.

Widely available, ergonomically designed and inexpensive furniture (with backs rather than just seats) permits people to conserve energy by sitting rather than standing for an increasing proportion of their waking hours. Padded furniture is more comfortable, making it more attractive to sit for longer periods and causing less energy to be used in fidgeting and shifting positions to vary body position to remain comfortable.

Workplace environments have undergone and are continuing to undergo huge transformations in energy expenditure requirements. People increasingly travel to work in vehicles rather than walking. Occupational activity levels decreased substantially with the industrial revolution, which increasingly substituted mechanically produced energy for human generated energy. Much technological development is geared toward more efficient (and therefore more productive and profitable) workplace activities, substituting mechanical devices for human muscles and minimizing the time and effort of human input required (122). All of these workplace efficiencies have moved worktime for an increasing proportion of the population from being a period of high energy expenditure to being a sedentary part of the day where few calories are expended above those needed to sit (or sometimes stand).

Recreational activity levels of populations have changed significantly over time. An increasing amount of leisure became available as childhood and adolescence became shielded from adult work responsibilities, work weeks shortened, and vacations lengthened. However, the overall energy expenditure of people during their leisure time has tended to be low. Sedentary activities increasingly became available to fill available leisure, including reading, radio, television, and other mass forms of passive consumption that involved little caloric expenditure. Sports and games moved from being active participation to passive spectator activities (although there has been a resurgence in widespread public exercise and sport participation in recent decades among a minority of the population).

Two built environment changes that are cited as particularly significant contributions to population levels of obesity are automobiles and television. The automobile and related motor powered vehicles such as buses, trucks, motorcycles, etc., were broadly introduced and popularized in the early twentieth century, and revolutionized human activity levels. Human muscle powered transport for more than short distances declined rapidly with the introduction of automobiles. The built environment became designed around automobiles, and task-oriented walking more than short distances became an increasingly unusual activity for most people. Personal energy expenditure for transportation is rapidly being minimized for most people in postindustrial societies.

Television was developed and widely diffused in the middle of the twentieth century, attaining almost universal penetration into the households of people in developed societies (and more recently in developing societies). Television rapidly took up an increasing number of waking hours of the majority of the population, with the US average of over 3 hours of daily viewing constituting the third most frequent use of time (after sleep and work or school) (123). Technological developments in television made it an increasingly attractive activity (with more channels, clearer and colored pictures, and linkage with videotape players) that required progressively less activity (with remote control units used for changing channels and sound levels).

Obesity researchers frequently cite television as a major contributor to higher body weight levels (124). The amount of television viewing is directly associated with body weight in studies of children and adults. Television influences body weight through both decreased energy expenditure and increasing energy intake (125). Energy output reductions occur because the sedentary activity of watching television displaces more active pursuits (126). Energy input increases occur because advertisements on television encourage consumption of high calorie and high fat foods (127).

Children are a special audience deemed to be particularly vulnerable to the influence of television (128). Children are high users of television (2–4 hours/day in the USA), and exhibit high attention levels to television. Television programming that targets children includes a majority of advertisements for food, particularly sweets, cereals, snacks, and soft drinks (129). Children's food purchase requests are related to time spent viewing television (127).

In prior historical time periods, most people engaged in physical labor in their jobs, and used what leisure time they had to rest and recover from workday tasks. Currently, energy expenditure beyond resting metabolic rates must increasingly occur by means of voluntary exercise, where people are purposively active during their 'leisure' time for reasons of health promotion and expending energy to lose weight. However, Western cultures have no concept for 'activity hunger' (130), and the idea of voluntarily engaging in leisure time physical activity to control body weight has lagged behind cultural values about increased energy intake. These cultural and historical discrepancies have contributed to the rising prevalence of obesity.

Built environment efficiencies exert a cumulative and pervasive effect in decreasing human energy expenditure. On a societal scale, these changes have produced increasingly fattening human environments that contribute to a rising prevalence of obesity in individuals and populations.

CONCLUSION

Obesity is a complex, dynamic, and multidimensional biosocial phenomenon, a synergistic product of the interaction between physiology and the social world. Levels of obesity must be seen within their cultural and historical contexts, with each particular society and time period establishing broad conditions within which body weight levels occur for the population. In specific times and places, the social demographics of individuals are important influences on body weight patterns (131). It is also important to recognize that food systems and human environments have become increasingly 'obesi-genic' in their continual increase in caloric availability and activity efficiency (38).

Consideration of the contributions of food system changes to the prevalence of obesity suggests that it is important to consider occurrences 'upstream' in the calorie supply in searching for society-level mechanisms and intervention opportunities for body weight modification of populations. On a societal scale, producing less food and processing foods in ways that are lower in caloric density may decrease obesity in society. The prevalence and types of food supply channels providing food energy to consumers may also be major determinants of the prevalence of obesity among the public,

although distribution of food to all of the population to prevent hunger and food insecurity is also a problem.

Consideration of the contributions of built environment changes to the prevalence of obesity suggest that a focus on the role of energy expenditure on body weight is warranted, particularly in everyday activities. Analysis of national data in several developed nations suggests that small energy reductions can have dramatic influences on the prevalence of obesity, and such changes in energy expenditure can account for the recent rises in obesity of the broader population (132,133). The body weight consequences of a continually developing quest for more efficient activities in all domains of life must be examined. As less energy is required to live, more energy must be voluntarily expended to achieve metabolic balance with caloric intake. The adoption of widespread daily recreational activity equal to the energy savings from efficiencies in the built environment has not been readily accepted by the population, and this presents a major dilemma for future patterns in body weight and interventions to change them.

The major paradigms used in conceptualizing obesity have been biological and psychological, which provide crucial insights but are not exhaustive of ways to think about body weight. Social analysis considers issues beyond behavior and past physiology, applying social science thinking to offer additional insights about the prevalence and patterns of fatness and thinness. Understanding the contributions of culture, history, and sociology to patterns of body weight can help reframe thinking about the influences on obesity in ways that can generate new insights for research and practice.

REFERENCES

1 Sobal J. Cultural comparison research designs in food, eating, and nutrition. *Food Quality and Preference* 1998; 9(6): 385–392.
2. Spradley JP (ed.) *Culture and Cognition: Rules, Maps, and Plans.* Prospect Heights, IL: Waveland Press, 1987.
3. Otterbein KF. Sampling and samples in cross-cultural studies. *Behav Sci Res* 1976; 11(2): 107–121.
4. Bray GA. Obesity: Historical development of scientific and cultural ideas. In: Björntorp P, Brodoff BN (eds) *Obesity.* Philadelphia: JB Lippincott, 1992: 281–293.
5. Brown PJ. Culture and the evolution of obesity. *Hum Nature* 1991; 2(1): 31–57.

6. Brown PJ, Konner M. An anthropological perspective on obesity. *Ann N Y Acad Sci* 1987; **499**: 29–46.

7. Anderson JL, Crawford CB, Nadeau J, Lindberg T. Was the Dutchess of Windsor right? A cross-cultural review of the socioecology of ideals of female body shape. *Ethol Sociobiol* 1992; **13**: 197–227.

8 Ritenbaugh C. Obesity as a culture-bound syndrome. *Culture, Medicine, and Psychiatry* 1982; **6**: 347–361.

9. Simons RC, Hughes CC. (eds). *The Culture-bound Syndromes: Folk Illnesses of Psychiatric and Anthropological Interest*. Boston: Kluwer Academic, 1985.

10. Sobal J, Stunkard AJ. Socioeconomic status and obesity: A review of the literature. *Psychol Bull* 1989; **105**(2): 260–275.

11. Sobal, J. Food system globalization, eating transformations, and nutrition transitions. In: Grew R (ed.) *Food in Global History*. Boulder, CO: Westview Press, 1999.

12. Hodge AM, Dowse GK, Koki G, Mavo B, Aplers MP, Zimmet PZ. Modernity and obesity in coastal and highland Papua New Guinea. *Int J Obes* 1995; **19**: 154–161.

13. Paeratakul S, Popkin BM, Keyou G, Adair LS, Stevens J. Changes in diet and physical activity affect the body mass index of Chinese adults. *Int J Obes* 1998; **22**: 424–431.

14. Epstein FH, Higgins M. Epidemiology of obesity. In: Björntorp P, Brodoff BN (eds) *Obesity*. Philadelphia, PA: JB Lippencott, 1992: 330–342.

15. Stearns PN. *Fat History: Bodies and Beauty in the Modern West*. New York: New York University Press, 1997.

16. Laurier D, Guiguet M, Chau NP, Wells JA, Valleron A. Prevalence of obesity: A comparative survey in France, the United Kingdom, and the United States. *Int J Obes* 1992; **16**: 563–572.

17. Stearns PN. Children and weight control: Priorities in the United States and France. In: Sobal J, Maurer D. (eds) *Weighty Issues: Fatness and Thinness as Social Problems*. Hawthorne, NY: Aldine de Gruyter, 1999: 11–30.

18. Kasl SV, Berkman L. Health consequences of the experience of migration. *Ann Rev Public Health* 1983; **4**: 69–90.

19. Zelensky W. The hypothesis of the mobility transition. *Geographical Review* 1971; **61**: 219–249.

20. Khan LK, Sobal J, Martorell R. Acculturation, socioeconomic status, and overweight in US Hispanics. *Int J Obes* 1997; **21**: 91–96.

21. Janes CR, Pawson IG. Migration and biocultural adaptation: Samoans in California. *Soc Sci Med* 1986; **22**: 821–834.

22. Goldman N. Social factors and health: The causation-selection issue revisited. *Proc Nat Acad Sci* 1994; **91**: 1251–1255.

23. Keefe SE, Padilla AM. *Chicano Identity*. Albuquerque, NM: University of New Mexico Press, 1987.

24. Padilla AM (ed.). *Acculturation: Theory, Models, and Some New Findings*. Boulder, CO: Westview Press, 1980.

25. Lee S, Sobal J, Frongillo EA. Acculturation and health in Korean Americans. *Soc Sci Med* 2000; **51**: 159–173.

26. Pawson IG, Martorell R, Mendoza FE. Prevalence of overweight and obesity in US Hispanic populations. *Am J Clin Nutr* 1991; **53**: 1522S–1528S.

27. Popkin BM, Udry JR. Adolescent obesity increases significantly in second and third generation U.S. immigrants: The National Longitudinal Study of Adolescent Health. *J Nutr* 1998; **128**(4): 701–706.

28. Cuff T. The Body Mass Index values of mid nineteenth-century West Point cadets. *Historical Methods* 1993; **26**:

171–181.

29. Trends in average weights and heights of men: An insurance experience. *Statistical Bulletin of the Metropolitan Life Insurance Company* 1966; **47**: 11–13.

30. Trends in Average weights and heights of men: An insurance experience. *Statistical Bulletin of the Metropolitan Life Insurance Company* 1970; **51**: 6–7.

31. Bennett W, Gurin J. *The Dieter's Dilemma*. New York: Basic Books, 1982.

32. Abraham S. *Obese and Overweight Adults in the United States*. Vital and Health Statistics. Series 11, No. 230. DHHS Pub. No. 83-1680. Public Health Service. Washington DC: US Government Printing Office, 1983.

33. Seidell JC. Obesity in Europe: Scaling an epidemic. *Int J Obes* 1995; **19**(Suppl 3): S1–S4.

34. Kuczmarski RJ, Flegal KM, Cambell SM, Johnson CL. Increasing prevalence of overweight among US adults: The National Health and Nutrition Examination Surveys, 1960–1991. *JAMA* 1994; **272**: 205–211.

35. Flegal KM, Carrol MD, Kuczmarski RJ, Johnson CL. Overweight and obesity trends in the United States: prevalence and trends, 1960–1994. *Int J Obes* 1998; **22**: 39–47.

36. Harlan WR, Landis JR, Flegal KM, David CS, Miller ME. Secular trends in body mass in the United States: 1960–1980. *Am J Epidemiol* 1988; **128**: 1065–1074.

37. Thomsen BL, Ekstrom CT, Sorensen TIA. Development of the obesity epidemic in Denmark: Cohort, time and age effects among boys born 1930–1975. *Int J Obes* 1999; **23**: 693–701.

38. Hill JO, Peters JC. Environmental contributions to the obesity epidemic. *Science* 1998; **280**: 1371–1390.

39. Jeffery RA, French SA. Epidemic obesity in the United States: are fast food and television viewing contributing? *Am J Public Health* 1998; **88**: 277–280.

40. Rippe JM. The obesity epidemic: A mandate for a multidisciplinary approach. *J Am Diet Assoc* 1998; **98**(10, Supplement 2): S5–54.

41. World Health Organization. Obesity—Preventing and Managing a Global Epidemic. Geneva: World Health Organization, 1998.

42. Levenstein H. *Paradox of Plenty: A Social History of Eating in Modern America*. New York: Oxford University Press, 1993.

43. Schwartz H. *Never Satisfied: A Cultural History of Diets, Fantasies, and Fat*. New York: Free Press, 1986.

44. Seid RP. *Never Too Thin: Why Women Are at War with Their Bodies*. New York: Prentice Hall, 1989.

45. Garner DM, Garfinkle PE, Schwartz D. Cultural expectations of thinness in women. *Psychol Rep* 1980; **47**: 483–491.

46. Wiseman C, Gray JJ, Mosimann JE, Ahrens AH. Cultural expectations of thinness in women: An update. *Int J Eating Disord* 1992; **11**: 85–89.

47. Morris A, Cooper T, Cooper PJ. The changing shape of female fashion models. *Int J Eating Disord* 1989; **8**: 593–596.

48. Stunkard AJ, LaFleur WR, Wadden TA. Stigmatization of obesity in medieval times: Asia and Africa. *Int J Obes* 1998; **22**: 1141–1144.

49. Sobal J. The medicalization and demedicalization of obesity. In: Maurer D and Sobal J (eds) *Eating Agendas: Food and Nutrition as Social Problems*, Hawthorne, NY: Aldine de Gruyter, 1995: 67–90.

50. Caro TM, Sellen DW. The reproductive advantages of fat in women. *Ethol Sociobiol* 1990; **11**: 51–66.

51. Bordo S. *Unbearable Weight: Feminism, Western Culture, and the Body*. Berkeley: University of California Press, 1993.

52. Pliner P, Chaiken S, Flett G. Gender differences in concern with body weight and physical appearance over the life span. *Pers Soc Psychol Bull* 1990; **16**(2): 263–273.

53. Sobal J, Maurer D. (eds) *Weighty Issues: Fatness and Thinness as Social Problems*. Hawthorne, NY: Aldine de Gruyter, 1999.

54. Sobal J, Maurer D (eds). *Interpreting Weight: Social Management of Fatness and Thinness*. Hawthorne, NY: Aldine de Gruyter, 1999.

55. Hayes D, Ross CE. Concern with appearance, health beliefs, and eating habits. *J Health Soc Behav* 1987; **28**: 120–130.

56. Sobal J. Sociological analysis of the stigmatisation of obesity. In: Germov J, Williams L (eds) *A Sociology of Food and Nutrition: Introducing the Social Appetite*. Melbourne: Oxford University Press, 1999: 187–204.

57. Rodin J, Silberstein L, Striegel-Moore R. Women and weight: A normative discontent. In: Nebraska Symposium on Motivation. Lincoln: University of Nebraska Press, 1984: 267–303.

58. Rand CSW, Kuldau JM. The epidemiology of obesity and self-defined weight problem in the general population: Gender, race, age, and social class. *Int J Eating Disord* 1990; **9**(3): 329–343.

59. Williamson DF, Khan HS, Remington PL, Anda RF. The 10-year incidence of overweight and major weight gain in US adults. *Arch Intern Med* 1990; **150**: 665–672.

60. Heitmann BL, Garby L. Patterns of long-term weight changes in overweight developing Danish men and women aged between 30 and 60 years. *Int J Obes* 1999; **23**: 1074–1078.

61. Martinez-Gonzales MA, Martinez JA, Hu FB, Gibney MJ, Kearney J. Physical inactivity, sedentary lifestyle and obesity in the European Union. *Int J Obes* 1999; **23**: 1192–1201.

62. Devine CM, Bove C, Olson CM. Continuity and change in women's weight orientations through pregnancy and the postpartum period: The influence of life course trajectories and transitional events. *Soc Sci Med* 1999; **50**: 567–582.

63. Lamb CS, Jackson LA, Cassiday PB, Priest DJ. Body figure preferences of men and women: A comparison of two generations. *Sex Roles* 1993; **28**: 345–358.

64. Tiggemann M, Stevens C. Weight concerns across the lifespan: Relationship to self-esteem and feminist identity. *Int J Eating Disord* 1999; **26**: 103–106.

65. Winkleby MA, Kraemer HC, Ahn DK, Varady AN. Ethnic and socioeconomic differences in cardiovascular disease risk factors: Findings for women from the Third National Health and Nutrition Examination Survey, 1988–1994. *JAMA* 1998; **280**: 356–362.

66. Mokdad AH, Serdula MK, Dietz WH, Bowman BA, Marks JS, Koplan JP. The spread of the obesity epidemic in the United States, 1991–1998. *JAMA* 1999; **282**(16): 1519–1522.

67. Deurenberg P, Yap M, Staveren WA. Body mass index and percent body fat: A meta analysis among different ethnic groups. *Int J Obes* 1998; **22**: 1164–1171.

68. Kumanyika SK. Obesity in minority populations: An epidemiologic assessment. *Obes Res* 1994; **2**: 166–182.

69. Kumanyika SK. Understanding ethnic differences in energy balance: Can we get there from here? *Am J Clin Nutr* 1999; **70**: 1–2.

70. Windham CT, Wyse BW, Hansen RG, Hurst RL. Nutrient density of diets in the USDA Nationwide Food Consumption Survey, 1977–1978: I. Impact of socioeconomic status on dietary density. *J Am Diet Assoc* 1983; **82**(1): 28–82.

71. Sobal J. Obesity and socioeconomic status: A framework for examining relationships between physical and social variables. *Med Anthropol* 1991; **13**(3): 231–247.

72. Amelsvoort LGPM, Schouten EG, Kok FJ. Duration of shiftwork related to body mass index and waist to hip ratio. *Int J Obes* 1999; **23**: 973–978.

73. Sobal J, Rauschenbach B, Frongillo E. Marital status, fatness, and obesity. *Soc Sci Med* 1992; **35**(7): 915–923.

74. Montgomery SM, Cook DG, Bartley MJ, Wadsworth MEJ. Unemployment, cigarette smoking, alcohol consumption, and body weight in young British men. *Eur J Public Health* 1998; **8**(1): 21–27.

75. Pagan JA, Davila A. Obesity, occupational attainment, and earnings. *Soc Sci Quart* 1997; **78**: 756–770.

76. Larkin JC, Pines HA. No fat persons need apply: Experimental studies of the overweight stereotype and hiring preference. *Sociology of Work and Occupations* 1979; **13**: 379–385.

77. Matusewitch E. Employment discrimination against the overweight. *Personnel J* 1983; **62**: 446–450.

78. Roe D, Eickwort KR. Relationships between obesity and associated health factors with unemployment among low income women. *J Am Med Women's Assoc* 1976; **31**: 193–204.

79. Averett S, Korenman S. The economic reality of the Beauty Myth. *J Hum Resources* 1996; **31**(2): 304–330.

80. Loh ES. The economic effects of physical appearance. *Soc Sci Quart* 1993; **74**(2): 420–438.

81. Register CA, Williams DR. Wage effects of obesity among young workers. *Soc Sci Quart* 1990; **71**: 130–141.

82. Falk LW, Bisogni CA, Sobal J. Food choice processes of older adults. *J Nutr Educ* 1996; **28**: 257–265.

83. Furst T, Connors M, Bisogni CA, Sobal J, Winter Falk L. Food choice: A conceptual model of the process. *Appetite* 1996; **26**(3): 247–265.

84. Olson CM. Nutrition and health outcomes associated with food insecurity and hunger. *J Nutr* 1999; **129**: 521S–524S.

85. Mahajan KH, Schafer E. Influence of selected psychosocial factors on dietary intake in the elderly. *J Nutr Elderly* 1993; **12**(4): 21–31.

86. Sobal J. Sociability and meals: Facilitation, commensality, and interaction. In: Meiselman H (ed.) *The Meal*. Gaithersburg, MD: Aspen Publishers, 2000: 119–133.

87. McIntosh WA, Shifflett PA, Picou JS. Social support, stressful events, strain, dietary intake and the elderly. *Med Care* 1989; **27**: 140–153.

88. de Castro JM, Brewer EM. The amount eaten in meals by humans is a power function of the number of people present. *Physiol Behav* 1992; **51**: 121–125.

89. Sobal J. Marriage, obesity and dieting. *Marriage and Family Review* 1984; **7**: 115–139.

90. Kallen D, Doughty A. The relationship of weight, the self

perception of weight, and self esteem with courtship behavior. *Marriage and Family Review* 1984; **7**: 93–114.

91. Sobal J, Nicolopoulos V, Lee J. Attitudes about weight and dating among secondary school students. *Int J Obes* 1995; **19**: 376–381.

92. Margolin L, White L. The continuing role of physical attractiveness in marriage. *J Marriage and the Family* 1987; **49**: 21–27.

93. Craig PL, Truswell AS. Dynamics of food habits of newly married couples: Food related activities and attitudes toward food. *J Nutr Hum Diet* 1988; **1**: 409–419.

94. Craig PL, Truswell AS. Dynamics of food habits of newly married couples: Weight and exercise patterns. *Aust J Nutr Diet* 1990; **47**: 42–46.

95. Gortmaker SL, Must A, Perrin JM, Sobol AM, Dietz WH. Social and economic consequences of overweight in adolescence and young adulthood. *N Engl J Med* 1993; **329**: 1008–1012.

96. Sackett DL, Anderson GD, Milner R, Feinleib M, Kannel WB. Concordance for coronary risk factors among spouses. *Circulation* 1975; **52**: 589–595.

97. Kahn HS, Williamson DF. The contributions of income, education, and changing marital status to weight change among US men. *Int J Obes* 1990; **14**: 1057–1068.

98. Kahn HS, Williamson DF, Stevens JA. Race and weight changes in U.S. Women: The roles of socioeconomic status and marital status. *Am J Public Health* 1991; **81**: 319–323

99. Garn S, LaVelle M, Pilkington JJ. Obesity and living together. *Marriage and Family Review* 1984; **7**: 33–47.

100. Rauschenbach B, Sobal J, Frongillo E. The influence of change in marital status on weight change over one year. *Obes Res* 1995; **3**(4): 319–327.

101. Kemner D, Anderson AS, Marshall DW. Living together and eating together: Changes in food choice and eating habits during the transition from single to married/cohabiting. *Sociol Rev* 1998; **46**: 48–72.

102. Bradley PJ. Conditions recalled to have been associated with weight gain in adulthood. *Appetite* 1985; **6**: 235–241.

103. Burke V, Giangiulio N, Gillam HF, Beilin LJ, Houghton S, Milligan RAK. Health promotion in couples adapting to a shared lifestyle. *Health Educ Res* 1999; **14**(2): 269–288.

104. IOM—Institute of Medicine. *Nutrition During Pregnancy: Weight Gain, Nutrient Supplements*. Washington DC: National Academy Press, 1990.

105. Williamson DF, Madans J, Pamuk E, Flegal KM, Kendrick JS, Serdula MK. A prospective study of childbearing and 10-year weight gain in US white women 25 to 45 years of age. *Int J Obes* 1994; **18**: 561–569.

106. Wolfe WS, Sobal J, Olson CA, Frongillo EA. Parity-associated body weight: Modification by sociodemographic and behavioral factors. *Obes Res* 1997; **5**(2): 131–141.

107. Wolfe WS, Sobal J, Olson CA, Frongillo EA, Williamson D. Parity-associated weight gain and its modification by sociodemographic and behavioral factors: A prospective analysis of US Women. *Int J Obes* 1997; **21**: 802–810.

108. Devault K. *Feeding the Family: The Social Organization of Caring as Gendered Work*. Chicago: University of Chicago Press, 1991.

109. Sobal J, Troiano RP, Frongillo EA. Rural–urban differences in obesity. *Rural Sociology* 1996; **61**(2): 289–305.

110. Allon N. *Urban Lifestyles*. Dubuque, IA: Wm. C. Brown, 1979.

111. Sichieri R, Coitinho DC, Leao MM, Recine E, Everhart JE. High temporal, geographic, and income variation in body mass index among adults in Brazil. *Am J Public Health* 1994; **84**(5): 793–798.

112. Ellaway A, Anderson A, McIntyre S. Does area of residence affect body size and shape? *Int J Obes* 1997; **21**: 304–308.

113. Gerding AL. Taste ratings of obese people, and taste preferences based on geographical location. *Bull Psychonomic Soc* 1992; **30**(6): 509–510.

114. Sobal J, Khan LK, Bisogni CA. A conceptual model of the food and nutrition system. *Soc Sci Med* 1998; **47**(7): 853–863.

115. Drenowski A, Popkin BM. The nutrition transition: New trends in the global diet. *Nutr Rev* 1997; **55**: 31–43.

116. Rothberg RI, Rabb TK. *Hunger and History: The Impact of Changing Food Production and Consumption Patterns on Society*. New York: Cambridge University Press, 1983.

117. Dumagan JC, Hackett JW. Almost half of the food budget is spent eating out. *Food Rev* 1995; January–April: 37–39.

118. Senauer B, Asp E, Kinsey J. *Food Trends and the Changing Consumer*. St Paul, MN: Eagan Press, 1991.

119. Drummond SE, Crombie NE, Cursiter MC, Kirk TR. Evidence that eating frequency is inversely related to body weight status in male, but not female, non-obese adults reporting valid dietary intakes. *Int J Obes* 1998; **22**: 105–112.

120. Watkins SM. *Clothing: The Portable Environment*. Ames: Iowa State University Press, 1995.

121. Mumford L. *Technics and Civilization*. New York: Harcourt, Brace, and World, 1963.

122. Kanigel R. *The One Best Way: Fredrick Winslow Taylor and the Enigma of Efficiency*. New York: Penguin Putnam, 1999.

123. Huston AC, Donnerstein E, Fairchild H, Feshbach N, Katz P, Murray J, Rubinstein E, Wilcox B, Zuckerman D. *Big World, Small Screen: The Role of Television in American Society*. Lincoln, NE: University of Nebraska Press, 1992.

124. Dietz WH, Strasburger VC. Children, adolescents, and television. *Curr Probl Pediatr* 1991; **21**: 8–31.

125. Taras HL, Sallis JF, Patterson TL, Nader PR, Nelson JA. Television's influence on children's diet and physical activity. *J Devel Behav Pediatr* 1989; **10**: 176–180.

126 Buchowski MS, Sun M. Energy expenditure, television viewing, and obesity. *Int J Obes* 1996; **20**: 236–244.

127. Goldberg M. A quasi-experiment assessing the effectiveness of TV advertising directed to children. *J Marketing Res* 1990; **27**: 445–454.

128. Andersen RE, Crespo CJ, Bartlett SJ, Cheskin LJ, Pratt M. Relationship of physical activity and television watching with body weight and level of fatness among children: Results from the third National Health and Nutrition Examination Survey. *JAMA* 1998; **279**(12): 938–942.

129. Kotz D, Story M. Food advertisements during children's saturday morning television programming: Are they consistent with dietary recommendations? *J Am Diet Assoc* 1994; **94**(11): 1296–1300.

130. Ritenbaugh C. *Nutrition, Obesity, and Body Image*: A Cross-Cultural Update. Washington DC: Progress report on Healthy People 2000. March, 1997.

131. Sobal J, Devine CM. Social aspects of obesity: influences,

consequences, assessments, and interventions. In: Dalton S. (ed). *Overweight and Weight Management*. Gaithers-burg, MD: Aspen Publishers, 1997: 312–331.

132. Prentice AM, Jebb SA. Obesity in Britain: Gluttony or sloth? *B M J* 1995; **11**(7002): 437–439.

133. Seidell JC. Time trends in obesity: An epidemiological per-spective. *Horm Metab Res* 1997; **29**: 155–158.

22

Cessation of Smoking and Body Weight

Kenneth D. Ward, Robert C. Klesges and Mark W. Vander Weg

University of Memphis Center for Community Health, Memphis, Tennessee, USA

The health consequences of cigarette smoking are well established (1). Smoking has been linked to many serious health problems including cancer, coronary heart disease, stroke, and chronic obstructive pulmonary disease (2). As a result, smoking has been determined to be the single most preventable cause of death in Western society (3). Each year, an estimated 419 000 people in the United States die from smoking-related diseases (4), making it responsible for approximately one in every five deaths (2). Although overall smoking rates have declined over the past 30 years in the United States, nearly 26% of the population continue to smoke (5), including 3.1 million adolescents (6).

One of the many factors which may encourage smoking, despite health risks, is the influence of smoking on body weight. There is considerable evidence that the weight-controlling properties associated with cigarette smoking influence decisions to smoke. For example, the relationship between smoking and weight control has been linked to the initiation of smoking (7,8). In a study examining the relationship between weight concerns and cigarette smoking, French *et al.* (9) found that concerns about weight were associated with a greater likelihood of smoking initiation among female adolescents over a 1-year period. The relationship between smoking and body weight is also related to smoking maintenance in adults. Smoking for weight control is frequently reported, particularly by women (7,10,11). Additionally, individuals who are concerned about gaining weight are often more reluctant to quit smoking (12,13). Finally, concerns about gaining weight have been associated with failure to quit smoking (14,15) and relapse (7,16) although these effects appear to be equivocal (17–19).

WEIGHT DIFFERENCES BETWEEN SMOKERS AND NON-SMOKERS

It is well established that middle-aged and older smokers weigh less than comparably aged non-smokers. In a review of 29 cross-sectional studies evaluating weight and smoking status, smokers weighed an average of 3.4 kg less than non-smokers (1,20,21). Weight differences between smokers and non-smokers tended to be greater for moderate smokers (compared to light or heavy smokers), older smokers, and women (20). Although most studies have been conducted in American populations, similar weight differences between smokers and non-smokers (as well as a more pronounced weight-control effect for women compared to men) were reported from the World Health Organization MONICA project, which assessed weight and smoking status in 69 000 individuals from 42 populations (22).

This weight-attenuating effect of smoking, observed in adults after decades of smoking, is small or non-existent in adolescent and young adult smokers. In a biracial sample of 6751 seventh grade students (average age of 13 years), daily smokers had a significantly *higher* body mass index (BMI) than non-smokers (21.61 vs. 20.56 kg/m², respectively) (23). Among 1926 members of this sample who were followed prospectively for 4 years, those who began smoking had greater increases in body weight for 2 years after initiation of smoking compared to non-smokers, especially white females after one year of smoking, and black males after 2 years of smoking. For those youths who smoked three or more years, body weight was virtually identical compared to those who never smoked (24). In a cross-sectional study of more than 31 000 young adult military recruits, smoking had no relationship to body weight in females, and a very small effect of body weight reduction in males, averaging less than 1 kg (25). Finally, Klesges *et al.* (26), in a 7-year prospective study of more than 4000 black and white young adults (18–30 years of age at baseline), reported that smoking produced a small attenuation of weight gain among Blacks (2.6 kg over 7 years, or 0.4 kg per year, adjusted for gender, baseline weight, age, education, physical fitness, alcohol intake, and fat intake). In contrast, smoking had no weight-attenuating effect among white men or women in this study, the latter being the group most likely to report smoking to control body weight (10). In summary, smokers weigh 3–4 kg less than non-smokers, on average, after many years of smoking. However, smoking has minimal impact on body weight in young smokers.

WEIGHT CHANGE AFTER SMOKING CESSATION

Smoking cessation reliably produces weight gain in both women and men, although the magnitude of this gain, and the mechanisms involved are less clear (20,27). In the 1970s, a commonly reported but empirically unsupported estimate was that one-third of quitters gain weight, one-third remain the same, and one-third lose weight (28). Based on a review of 43 longitudinal studies, conducted primarily during the 1970s and 1980s, the average weight gain was estimated at 2.8 kg (0.8 to 8.2 kg) during the first year after cessation, with women tending to gain more than men (21). Another review around this time estimated post-cessation weight gain using only methodologically rigorous studies (1). Fifteen longitudinal investigations which included a control group of continuing smokers, a minimum follow-up length of 1 month, and a sample size of at least 10 quitters were examined. The average sample size of the reviewed studies was 1348 subjects with an average follow-up length of 2 years. The weight gain among quitters was considerably greater than that of continuing smokers (mean of 2.1 vs. 0.4 kg, respectively). Seventy-nine percent of quitters in this review experienced a weight gain (range of 58–87% among studies) compared to 56% of continuing smokers. Overall, the risk of weight gain after cessation was 45% greater for quitters compared to continuing smokers (RR = 1.45, CI = 1.31, 1.75). The prevalence of major weight gain (> 4.5 kg) was relatively low (20.3% vs. 0.8% for quitters and continuing smokers, respectively), but quitters were 90% more likely to experience major weight gain.

A large study of smoking cessation and weight gain in a national cohort (27) avoided several limitations common to previous studies, including short follow-up periods and reliance on self-reports of body weight. Subjects were more than 9000 participants in the First National Health and Nutrition Examination Survey (NHANES I) who were interviewed during the years 1971–1975 and re-interviewed during 1982–1984. Consistent with previous reports, women tended to gain more weight than men. The average weight gain attributable to smoking cessation (i.e difference in weight gain between quitters and continuing smokers), adjusted for age, race, education, alcohol, illnesses related to weight change, baseline weight, and physical activity was 2.8 kg for men and 3.8 kg for women. Major weight gain (> 13 kg) occurred in 9.8% of men and 13.4% of women. The relative risk of major weight gain for quitters, compared to continuing smokers, was 8.1 (CI = 4.4, 14.9) in men and 5.8 (3.7, 9.1) in women. Risk of major weight gain in women was greater for those who were initially underweight, younger (25–54 years vs. 55–74 years), physically inactive, and parous.

These NHANES I data also indicated that post-cessation weight gain was greater in Blacks than in Whites, with black women and black men being 3.3 times and 2.9 times more likely, respectively, to experience major weight gain compared to other ethnic groups (27). Similar ethnic differences were observed recently in a 7-year prospective study of smoking and weight change among 5115 black and white young adults (26). Weight gain attributable to smoking cessation over a 7-year period in a large biracial cohort was 6.6 kg for Blacks compared to 4.2 kg for Whites. While 36.3% of white quitters experienced major weight gain ($\geq$ 10 kg) over the 7-year follow-up, more than half of Blacks (52.3%) had major weight gain.

A prospective analysis of weight gain and smoking status among 121 700 nurses followed for 8 years (1976–1984) (29) found a mean attributable weight gain of 1.4 kg among quitters who had smoked < 25 cigarettes/day and 2.8 kg for those who had smoked > 25 cigarettes/day. Weight gain of 5 kg or more occurred in 14.2% of continuous smokers compared to 21.7% of women who had quit for less than 2 years. Consistent with the results of Williamson et al. (27), weight gain after cessation was positively associated with greater amount smoked, younger age, and initial lower weight.

Post-cessation weight gain does not appear to continue indefinitely, but causes weight to 'catch up' to that of non-smokers. Among both men and women in the NHANES I follow-up study reported by Williamson et al. (27) quitters weighed significantly less than never-smokers at baseline, but did not differ significantly after approximately 10 years of follow-up. Similarly, risk of major weight gain decreases over time. Williamson et al. (27) reported that for women, the odds of gaining > 13 kg for sustained quitters, compared to continuing smokers, was 6.9, 8.8, and 4.2 for those quit 1 to 3 years, 4 to 6 years, and 7 to 12 years, respectively. For men, risk of major weight gain was 3.1, 11.8, and 7.9 for those quit 1 to 3 years, 4 to 6 years, and 7 to 12 years, respectively. In the Nurses' Health Study, the incidence of 5 kg or more of weight gain was higher among women who had quit for $\leq$ 2 years compared to continuous smokers (21.7% vs. 14.2%), but incidence dropped to 16.0% and 17.1% among women quit for 2–4 years and 4–6 years, respectively. Among a cross-sectional study of more than 7000 Japanese workers (30), the risk of being overweight (BMI > 25) was compared among former smokers and never-smokers. No differences in risk of being overweight were found between never-smokers and former light smokers (1–24 cigarettes/day) regardless of number of years quit. However, among former heavy smokers ($\geq$ 25 cigarettes/day), those who had quit 2–4 years previ-

ously were nearly twice as likely to be overweight as never-smokers (OR = 1.88, 95% CI = 1.05–3.35) but no significant differences in risk of overweight between former and never-smokers were observed for those quit 5–7 years (OR = 1.32, CI = 0.74–2.34) or 8–10 years (OR = 0.66, CI = 0.33–1.31). Thus, smoking cessation, on average, causes weight to increase to levels typically experienced by non-smokers, and the risk of major weight gain also decreases as a function of time quit.

As noted above, available evidence from several prospective studies indicates that the magnitude of weight gain attributable to smoking cessation was on the order of 2 to 4 kg. There is reason to believe that these studies may have underestimated actual weight gain. One issue is that these estimates were based on studies conducted during the 1970s and 1980s. Individuals who have quit smoking in the past few years may be more nicotine dependent and have higher tobacco intake, two factors which increase the risk of post-cessation weight gain (27,29). Another issue is that few studies have been designed specifically to assess the effects of smoking cessation on weight gain prospectively and have relied on self-reports of smoking status and weight (1). In addition, studies have typically used point-prevalence estimates of smoking status rather than sustained abstinence. Two recent studies indicated that the magnitude of post-cessation weight gain may be higher than these previous estimates. Nides et al. (31) evaluated post-cessation weight gain in a sample of 691 sustained quitters from the Lung Health Study. Sustained quitting yielded weight gains 50–100% higher than the average weight gain reported in earlier studies (5.3 kg for women and 5.5 kg for men at the 1-year follow-up).

A recent study (32) compared the magnitude of weight gain using both point prevalence and sustained quitting definitions of abstinence. Subjects were 196 women and men followed prospectively for 1 year. Smoking status was validated biochemically and actual weights were obtained at each follow-up assessment. Those who met the criteria for point-prevalent abstinence (abstinent at the 1-year follow-up but no abstinence at one or more of the previous follow-ups) gained an average of 3.0 kg, which was very similar to previous estimates. However, subjects with sustained abstinence gained almost double this amount—5.9 kg. Thus, recent estimates of post-cessation weight gain, using more sophisticated methodologies, have indicated that

weight gain may be higher than previously estimated. It is common practice to advise smokers
that the typical 2 to 3 kg post-cessation weight gain,
while cosmetically unappealing, does not affect
health status (29). However, if the *average* weight
gain following smoking cessation is actually 6 kg, a
substantially higher proportion of quitters than
previously thought may experience major weight
gain.

MECHANISMS OF POST-CESSATION WEIGHT GAIN

The exact mechanisms underlying post-cessation
weight gain still are not well understood. According
to the principles of energy balance, smoking cessation must lead to either an increase in energy intake,
and/or a decrease in energy expenditure (viz., metabolic rate, physical activity) to promote weight gain
(33).

Physical Activity

The available data indicate that physical activity
does not play a role in the relationship between
smoking and body weight (20,33,34). Cross-sectional studies comparing activity levels in smokers
and non-smokers have failed to find discrepancies
that would account for the difference in body
weight between the two groups (20,35). In fact, studies finding a relationship between smoking status
and physical activity have typically found smokers
to be *less* active than non-smokers (36–38). Additionally, physical activity does not appear to decrease following smoking cessation (33,39–41).
Those studies finding changes following smoking
cessation have reported *increases* in physical activity (42–44). Thus, physical activity does not appear
to figure independently in either the difference in
body weight between smokers and non-smokers, or
in post-cessation weight gain.

Dietary Intake

Energy intake appears to play an important, although complicated, role in the relationship between smoking and body weight (34). Despite the
fact that they tend to have lower body weights,
smokers consume as much, or *more* energy than
non-smokers (37,45,46).

Additionally, smoking cessation is associated
with increased energy intake, at least acutely. Several studies of short-term cessation (1 day to 7
weeks) have documented increases in total energy
(41,47–49) although negative findings also have
been reported (39,43,50). Despite considerable
variability in methodology, studies typically show
an immediate increase in energy intake of 250 to 300
kilocalories per day following smoking cessation
(51,52).

Long-term changes in intake following smoking
cessation, however, have been less consistent (52).
Unfortunately, few studies have examined changes
in energy intake beyond a few months post-cessation. One study, however, assessed changes in dietary intake among women who quit smoking for a
period of 1 year. Caan *et al.* (53) found increases of
163 and 125 kcal/day at 1 and 6 months post-cessation, respectively. Levels of energy intake had returned to baseline, however, by the 1-year follow-
up. These results suggest that increases in energy
intake following smoking cessation probably do
not extend much beyond 6 months, which may help
to account for the fact that most of the weight that is
gained after quitting smoking occurs within this
time period (32,53–55).

In addition to short-term increases in total energy intake, smoking cessation has been associated
with changes in specific components of dietary intake. Selective increases in dietary fat (56), carbohydrates (57), sucrose (56,58), and alcohol (41) have
been observed following smoking cessation. Overall, increases in dietary intake after smoking cessation appear to be due to between-meal snacking,
rather than from a general increase in food consumption during meals. Gilbert and Pope (59)
found that energy intake from meals was similar
during 24-hour periods of *ad libitum* smoking and
abstinence, but that intake from between-meal
snacks increased 50% in men and 94% in women
during abstinence.

Given that women generally have greater concerns about post-cessation weight gain, as well as
greater actual weight gain, gender differences in the
mechanisms of post-cessation weight gain are of
major interest. There is evidence that changes in
energy intake associated with smoking cessation
may differ by gender, but the exact relationship is

unclear. While several studies have reported differences in energy intake as a function of gender, they have disagreed on the nature of the relationship. Klesges et al. (39), for example, found increased intake of polyunsaturated and monounsaturated fat in women during a week of abstinence, but no changes in dietary intake for men. Conversely, Hatsukami et al. (60) observed a greater increase in total energy intake in men than women following 4 days of cessation. Hall et al. (56) found that both women and men increased their intake of total energy, fat, and sucrose immediately after quitting. Men decreased their average total energy intake by nearly 1000 kcal from the first week after cessation to 4 months (3014 to 2119 kcal) and maintained this lower level at 6 months (2035 kcal). In contrast, total energy intake by women remained stable (1841, 2077, and 1867 kcal at 1 week, 4 months, and 6 months, respectively). Increased energy intake predicted weight gain at 6 months for women, but not for men. Thus, information on the influence of gender on changes in energy intake following smoking cessation is incomplete, but suggests significant and sustained post-cessation energy intake increases in women, which are associated with weight gain.

Metabolic Rate

Studies examining the relationship between smoking and metabolic rate have been inconclusive. There is considerable indirect evidence that metabolic factors influence the weight-controlling properties of smoking. The fact that smokers are no more active than non-smokers and consume as much or more energy, yet weigh less, suggests that metabolism may play a role in the relationship between smoking and body weight (34).

Several studies have documented acute metabolic increases due to smoking or nicotine administration (61–64). At least one study did not find any acute effect of smoking on metabolic rate (65) and in general, there appears to be tremendous individual variation in the metabolic response to smoking and smoking cessation (1,62). There is evidence that the acute effects of smoking may be more pronounced during light physical activity than during rest (63,66), at least among men, and for normal weight smokers than the obese (61). Thus, it is possible that

the acute metabolic effects of smoking may factor into the difference in body weight between smokers and non-smokers, although it remains unclear whether these effects are strong and persistent enough to have a substantial impact on body weight.

Studies that have directly examined the chronic metabolic effects of smoking have produced inconsistent results. Cross-sectional studies comparing resting energy expenditure (REE) in smokers and non-smokers have typically found little or no differences between the groups (38,67). The few studies that did find differences failed to control for the thermic effects of nicotine by allowing smokers to smoke before the assessments, which could have resulted in an overestimation of the chronic effects of smoking on metabolic rate (68).

Only a few prospective studies have examined metabolic changes during long-term smoking cessation, and conflicting results have been found. Moffatt and Owens (40) compared changes in metabolic rate among 36 women who quit for 60 days ($n = 12$), quit but relapsed 30 to 60 days post-cessation ($n = 6$), continued smoking ($n = 8$), or were non-smokers ($n = 10$). Resting metabolic rate (RMR) was assessed as oxygen uptake at baseline, 30 and 60 days post-cessation. At baseline, RMR was higher in smokers than non-smokers. No changes in RMR were observed for non-smokers or continuing smokers. Smoking cessation resulted in a 16% decrease in RMR at day 30. Both relapsers and abstinent subjects showed trends for RMR to rebound toward baseline at day 60. Despite the trend for RMR to return toward baseline, weight continued to increase throughout the 60-day follow-up. The authors estimated that 39% of the weight gain among quitters was attributable to change in RMR. Dallosso and James (50) reported a 4% decrease in resting metabolic rate following smoking cessation, although the change was only significant when expressed per kilogram of body weight.

In contrast, Stamford et al. (49) did not find changes in oxygen consumption in 13 subjects who quit smoking for 48 days. Additionally, a recent study (69) assessed 24-hour energy expenditure in a respiratory chamber and basal metabolic rate among eight smokers (four men and four women) during regular smoking and after 4 to 8 weeks of abstinence. No significant differences were observed between smoking and non-smoking assessments for either measure of energy expenditure, suggesting that smoking cessation does not produce any chronic alteration in metabolic rate. Other studies also have failed to find chronic changes in resting energy expenditure (REE) after quitting smoking (70–72). Thus, the relationship between smoking and REE remains unclear. One possible explanation is that changes in REE following smoking cessation are influenced by moderators, such as ethnicity or gender. Most studies investigating this relationship have consisted of small, homogeneous samples, making it impossible to investigate these variables. Thus, there is a need to examine changes in REE following smoking cessation in large, diverse samples.

Simultaneously examining the influence of all three energy balance variables would be helpful in understanding the relative contribution of each component. However, to date, only five prospective studies have examined the influence of smoking cessation on all three components of energy balance. Four of these studies utilized relatively short follow-up periods (14 to 60 days). Vander Weg et al. (73) examined changes in energy balance in 95 male and female smokers during 2 weeks of abstinence from smoking. Energy intake increased significantly following cessation (344 kcal/day). There were no changes, however, in REE or physical activity. Stamford et al. (49) examined changes in body weight and energy balance in 13 women following 48 days of abstinence from smoking. There were no changes in either physical activity or REE. Energy intake, however, did increase by an average of 227 kilocalories/day. Perkins et al. (41) investigated changes in energy balance in seven female smokers over a 3-week period consisting of a week of smoking, a week of abstinence, and a return to smoking. Energy intake increased significantly during the week of abstinence, primarily due to an increase in alcohol consumption. REE also changed over the 3-week period. A non-significant decrease in REE was observed during abstinence, followed by a significant increase upon return to smoking. There were no changes in physical activity. Finally, Moffatt and Owens (40) examined changes in energy balance in 18 women who quit smoking for 30 to 60 days. Consistent with the other studies, physical activity did not change as a function of smoking status, while energy intake increased significantly following cessation. However, unlike the three previous studies, smoking cessation was associated

with a significant decrease in REE.

Klesges et al. (55) assessed the relationships of all three major components of energy balance and weight gain during 12 months of abstinence—the longest follow-up period to be examined to date. The sample included 42 subjects (22 women, 20 men) with biochemically verified sustained abstinence over the 12-month following period. Weight gain among women was predicted by lower baseline REE, higher baseline total energy intake, and increased carbohydrate intake over the year. However, changes in energy balance components (dietary intake, physical activity, and REE) did not predict weight gain among women. Furthermore, no energy balance variables predicted weight gain for men. Future research should attempt to examine more fully potential gender differences in energy balance changes that predict weight gain during extended smoking cessation.

In summary, increases in energy intake appear to be the most consistent energy balance change following smoking cessation. There is no evidence that changes in physical activity generally contribute to post-cessation weight gain. While removal of the acute increases in metabolic rate caused by smoking may also contribute somewhat to post-cessation weight gain, long-term changes in metabolic rate after smoking cessation do not occur reliably.

PREVENTION OF POST-CESSATION WEIGHT GAIN

Numerous behavioral and pharmacologic interventions have been developed during the past 10 years in an attempt to reduce or prevent post-cessation weight gain (see reviews by Perkins et al. (74); Perkins (75)). These efforts may seem misguided given that weight gain after quitting smoking is rather modest (typically not higher than 6 kg, on average) and less health-damaging than continued smoking. Furthermore, the *actual* amount of weight gain has been shown to be unrelated to outcome in some studies (76,77) or to predict continued abstinence in others (54). However, as discussed above, many smokers, particularly women, report using smoking as a weight-control strategy, and fear of gaining weight as a reason for not attempting to quit. As such, adjunct treatments that effectively address these concerns clearly are needed to optimize smoking cessation interventions. Below, both be-havioral and pharmacologic strategies will be de-scribed.

Diet and Exercise Interventions

Because of the evidence that most of the cessation-induced weight gain is due to increased eating, it has been widely accepted that efforts to prevent this weight gain through dieting will improve absti-nence. However, there is little direct support for this assumption and some evidence supporting the op-posite notion, that attempting to prevent moderate weight gain after quitting may be detrimental. Hall et al. (78) supplemented an intensive behavioral smoking cessation program (seven $1\frac{1}{2}$ hour sessions over 2 weeks) with either (1) a behavioral weight control program (five sessions over 4 weeks consist-ing of daily weight and calorie monitoring, encour-agement to engage in aerobic exercise $\geq$ 3 times per week, and behavioral self-management prin-ciples, (2) a non-specific weight control program (group therapy providing support and information on diet and exercise), or (3) standard treatment control (a printed information packet on nutrition and exercise). Unexpectedly, subjects in both weight control conditions had lower abstinence rates at end of treatgment and 1 year follow-up than those in the standard treatment. Also, weight gain was not attenuated in either of the weight control conditions relative to standard treatment, at either 6 weeks or 1 year post-treatment.

Pirie et al. (79) randomized 417 female smokers in a 2 × 2 design to receive nicotine gum vs. no gum crossed with weight control counseling vs. no weight control counseling. All four groups received behavioral smoking cessation counseling. Weight control counseling involved counseling to modestly reduce caloric intake and increase activity. At 12 months, abstinence rates were highest among sub-jects receiving nicotine gum only, and lowest in those who received nicotine gum plus the weight control programs.

Results from both of these large, well-conducted investigations suggest that adding a weight control component to an already intensive smoking cessa-tion intervention provides too complicated an ap-proach that overwhelms participants. Attempts to focus one's attention simultaneously on weight con-

trol and smoking abstinence may actually lead to failure to accomplish either. Another possible rea-son for the failure of these interventions to prevent weight gain is that reducing energy intake may lead to the loss of another powerful reinforcer (in addi-tion to nicotine), which in turn encourages smoking. Consistent with this hypothesis is that food depri-vation increases the self-administration of several drugs in animals, including nicotine (74). It may also be that eating helps to attenuate nicotine with-drawal symptoms (74). This is consistent with the results of two studies that have found that both food (80) and glucose tablets (81) reduced cravings for cigarettes during abstinence from smoking.

If the failure of these interventions to prevent weight gain is due to cognitive overload from simul-taneously trying to change two behaviors, then de-laying the weight control intervention until after smoking cessation had been achieved would be ex-pected to prevent weight gain more effectively. This hypothesis is supported in preliminary data from 291 women enrolled in a 16-week behavioral smok-ing cessation/weight gain prevention trial (82). Sub-jects were randomized to receive the weight control intervention early in the program (first 8 weeks), late in the program (last 8 weeks), or to no weight control component. Although cessation outcomes did not differ among the three groups, at both 6 and 9 months post-cessation, subjects who received the weight control intervention late gained less weight than either control subjects or those who received the intervention early. These data suggest that a behavioral intervention can reduce post-cessation weight gain, without undermining smoking cessa-tion, by delaying the weight management compo-nent.

Although promoting adherence to regular physi-cal activity is challenging, there is evidence that incorporating physical activity into smoking cessa-tion interventions can reduce post-cessation weight gain. In a prospective observational study of 9306 nurses who were regular smokers at baseline, change in weight over 2 years was evaluated as a function of changes in smoking status and physical activity levels. Among women smoking 1–24 ciga-rettes/day at baseline, those who quit without changing their exercise level gained an average of 2.3 kg more than women who continued to smoke. In contrast, women who quit gained an excess of only 1.8 kg if they increased exercise by 8–16 MET-hours/week (equivalent to 1–2 hours of vigorous activity/week), and only 1.3 kg if they increased exercise by more than 16 MET-hours/week (83).

A recently published clinical trial randomized 281 sedentary women to receive either a 12-week behavioral smoking cessation program with either vigorous aerobic exercise (three 1-hour supervised sessions of aerobic activity per week for 12 weeks) or an equal time contact control condition (health education lectures and discussions) (84). At the end of treatment, subjects in the exercise condition gained less weight than control subjects (3.05 vs. 5.40 kg, respectively). However, the groups did not differ in the magnitude of weight gain at 12 months follow-up. Unfortunately, only 10% of subjects in the exercise condition continued with regular exercise throughout the 1-year follow-up period. Thus, while exercise appears to be helpful strategy to prevent post-cessation weight gain, longer treatment periods probably are needed to sustain its effect. It is likely, however, that such an intensive approach is not appealing to many smokers. In this study, a high proportion (68%) of eligible smokers chose not to participate, and substantial loss to follow-up occurred.

Perkins et al. (74) have argued that weight gain early after cessation, even if somewhat attenuated by a weight control intervention, may be enough to discourage continued efforts to remain abstinent. While there is clear evidence that integrating a weight control component into smoking cessation interventions can *attenuate* weight gain, these programs have not entirely *prevented* weight gain. However, one study indicates that behavioral change is capable of entirely preventing weight gain, albeit in highly controlled circumstances (military boot camp) (85). Participants were 332 Air Force recruits (227 men, 105 women) undergoing 6 weeks of basic military training. A total ban on smoking was strictly enforced throughout training, and recruits underwent a rigorous program of strenuous daily physical activity (aerobics, calisthenics, drilling, marching, etc.) and *ad libitum* access to food at meals but no access to snack foods or between-meal eating. At the end of training, all recruits tended to lose weight, although non-smokers lost marginally more than did smokers (0.89 vs. 0.03 kg, respectively, $P = 0.07$). Thus, under an 'ideal' treatment environment involving increased physical activity and prohibition of snacking, post-cessation weight gain can be eliminated.

Given that post-cessation weight gain tends to be modest and does not predict success at quitting, Perkins (74) has suggested treating weight *concerns* rather than weight gain per se, as a potentially useful intervention. Perkins and colleagues are testing this hypothesis in an ongoing clinical trial, where a cognitive–behavioral intervention is used to challenge attitudes and perceptions regarding weight and body image. The goals of the intervention are to tolerate a modest increase in snacking and not to overreact emotionally to a modest weight increase.

Pharmacologic Interventions

Several pharmacologic strategies to prevent post-cessation weight gain have been evaluated, including nicotine replacement, and both serotonin-enhancing and catecholamingeric drugs. Several clinical trials have found that nicotine gum attenuates post-cessation weight gain, at least during treatment (77,86–88). Furthermore, these effects appear to be dose-dependent (86,88). For example, Doherty et al. (86) examined weight gain through 90 days post-cessation among 79 abstinent cigarette smokers who were randomized to either placebo or 2 mg or 4 mg of nicotine gum. Nicotine gum was shown to suppress weight gain in a dose-dependent fashion. At 90 days post-cessation, placebo gum users gained 3.7 kg, compared to 2.1 kg and 1.7 kg for subjects receiving 2 mg and 4 mg of nicotine gum, respectively. A similar dose-dependent effect on weight gain was observed when the percentage of baseline cotinine levels replaced during treatment was correlated with weight gain.

Unfortunately, the weight-control benefits of nicotine gum appear to persist for only as long as the gum is used. Among patients treated with 2 mg nicotine gum in a hospital-based smoking cessation clinic, those who quit successfully for one year gained less weight if they continued to use the gum throughout the year (mean weight gain of 3.1 kg) compared to successful quitters who discontinued use of the gum (5.2 kg) (87).

In contrast to nicotine gum, the weight-attenuating effects of transdermal nicotine ('the patch') have been less consistent. In a quantitative review of four clinical trials, both placebo and transdermal nicotine groups gained weight during the periods of study, with no differences between conditions (89).

Several other studies, however, have reported reduced weight gain among patients treated with transdermal nicotine relative to placebo. For example, Abelin et al. (90) randomized patients to transdermal nicotine or placebo. After 3 months, those in the placebo group gained 4.4 kg, compared to only 0.1 kg in those receiving active treatment. Jorenby et al. (91) also examined post-cessation weight changes among patients randomized to 21 mg transdermal nicotine or placebo. Those treated with transdermal nicotine gained significantly less weight after 4 weeks (1.85 kg) than those receiving placebo (2.88 kg). Finally, Allen et al. (92) compared post-cessation weight changes among participants receiving three doses of transdermal nicotine (7, 14 and 21 mg) or placebo. Weight changes after 6 weeks were 2.5 kg (placebo), 2.03 kg (7 mg), 1.98 kg (14 mg), and 1.85 kg (21 mg), with those receiving 21 mg of transdermal nicotine gaining significantly less weight than those assigned to placebo. Thus, while some studies have reported transdermal nicotine to be associated with reduced post-cessation weight gain compared to placebo, others have found no weight attenuating effects.

Perkins (75) proposed three possible explanations for the weight-gain-attenuating benefits of nicotine gum compared to the patch. First, the differing route of administration of gum allows gum to produce more variable change in blood nicotine levels and allows for self-titration of dose. Second, the sensory and/or behavioral effects of nicotine gum may be incompatible with or otherwise discourage eating. Third, self-selection of subjects may occur in studies utilizing nicotine gum vs. patch. Nicotine gum places greater behavioral demands on subjects (in terms of frequency of chewing, following behavioral instructions) which may be related to motivational level or ability/willingness to perform other behaviors necessary to prevent weight gain.

Another possibility is that the typical doses of nicotine obtained from the patch may be insufficient to reduce weight gain. Transdermal nicotine has been found to reduce post-cessation increases in total energy, carbohydrate, and fat intake in a dose-dependent fashion (93). Additionally, in a clinical trial comparing three dosages of transdermal nicotine (11, 22, 44 mg/day) among 70 subjects, weight change over 8 weeks of patch use was negatively correlated with percentage of cotinine replacement ($r = -0.38$, $P = 0.012$) (94). Unfortunately, no studies have directly compared the weight-gain-attenuating effects of nicotine gum vs. patch at equivalent doses. One clinical trial, however, compared a combination of nicotine gum and nicotine patch (combined condition) vs. nicotine gum and placebo patch (gum only), used for 18 weeks (95). At 12 months post-treatment, weight gain was attenuated in subjects in the combined condition compared to those in the gum only condition (2.7 kg vs. 4.0 kg, respectively). Although the percentage of cotinine replaced was not measured in the study, the greater weight attenuation in the combined condition suggests a weight control benefit to the patch, possibly due to greater total dosage of nicotine replacement. Collectively, these findings suggest that the amount of nicotine that is replaced, rather than the method of administration, may have the greater impact on post-cessation weight gain.

Two newer nicotine replacement products, a nasal spray and an inhaler, have recently become commercially available in the United States. Similar to results with gum and patch, nicotine nasal spray has been shown to attenuate weight gain, but only during the period of usage. Sutherland et al. (96) randomly assigned 227 smokers to 4 weeks of group supportive treatment plus either active nicotine spray or placebo nicotine spray. Recommended duration of nasal spray usage was 3 months, but subjects were allowed to continue use beyond this time. At 12 months post-cessation, those in the placebo spray condition gained an average of 5.8 kg. Weight gain among those subjects in the active spray condition who discontinued use of spray at the end of the treatment period was similar to placebo subjects (5.5 kg). In contrast, subjects who were still using the active spray at the 12-month follow-up gained only 3.0 kg.

Two placebo-controlled clinical trials of the nicotine inhaler have examined short- and long-term effects on weight gain. Tonnesen et al. (97) found no difference in weight gain between conditions at either 6 weeks or one year post-cessation. Another study, however, found non-significant trends for the inhaler, compared to placebo inhaler, to attenuate weight gain at 2 weeks post-cessation (0.6 kg vs. 1.2 kg, respectively, $P = 0.07$) and 12 months post-cessation (4.5 kg vs. 5.6 kg, respectively, $P = 0.09$) (98).

Other studies have examined non-nicotine pharmacologic strategies to prevent weight gain. Phenylpropanolamine (PPA), a catecholaminergic drug, has been found to prevent weight gain completely during 2 weeks of smoking abstinence (99). Over 4 weeks of cessation, PPA was shown to reduce weight gain by more than 50% (100). Thus, while PPA shows promise as an adjuctant pharmacologic treatment to prevent post-cessation weight gain, no published studies have yet evaluated its long-term efficacy.

A few studies have evaluated the effects of dexflenfluramine and fluoxetine, both serotonin-enhancing drugs, on post-cessation weight gain. In a study of 31 overweight female smokers, Spring et al. (57) demonstrated that dexfenfluramine prevented weight gain (and actually led to a small weight loss, averaging 0.8 kg) during 4 weeks of smoking abstinence compared to placebo. In another small, short-term clinical trial, fluoxetine was shown to prevent weight gain entirely (mean weight change $= -0.6$ kg) compared to placebo (3.3 kg increase) among smokers who significantly reduced their nicotine intake (101). Spring et al. (102) compared the efficacy of dexfenfluramine and fluoxetine in preventing post-cessation weight gain. Subjects were 144 normal weight women, randomized to dexfenfluramine (30 mg), fluoxetine (40 mg), or placebo for 14 weeks. At 1 month post-cessation the placebo group gained more weight than either of the drug groups. By 3 months post-cessation the dexfenfluramine group had gained significantly less weight (1.0 kg) compared to either the placebo (3.5 kg) or fluoxetine (2.7 kg) groups. By 6 months post-cessation, however, weight gain was similar among the three groups. Both of these studies suggested that the weight-gain-attenuating effects of serotonin-enhancing drugs was related to suppression of the usual increases in energy intake observed after smoking cessation, particularly carbohydrates.

A recent study (103) compared the effects of two dosages of fluoxetine (30 mg vs. 60 mg) to placebo on post-cessation weight gain. During treatment, weight gain among placebo subjects was greater (2.61 kg) than that of subjects receiving either 30 mg of fluoxetine (1.33 kg) or 60 mg (1.25 kg). However, after discontinuing the drug, subjects who received 60 mg of fluoxetine had greater weight gain (6.5 kg) than subjects receiving either 30 mg of fluoxetine (3.6 kg) or placebo (4.7 kg). Thus, similar to the effects of nicotine replacement, serotoninergic drugs minimize post-cessation weight gain, but only for the duration of drug treatment. Unfortunately,

however, the observed dose-dependent weight rebound after discontinuation of fluoxetine indicates the drug may have limited utility for the long-term prevention of post-cessation weight gain.

Two recent studies examined the effect of bupropion on post-cessation weight gain. Hurt et al. (104) compared weight gain among patients treated for 7 weeks with three doses of bupropion (100,150, and 300 mg) or placebo. Weight change was found to be negatively associated with dose following 6 weeks of cessation. Weight gain among those receiving placebo averaged 2.9 kg, compared with 2.3 kg among those receiving either 100 or 150 mg of bupriopion, and 1.5 kg for those in the 300 mg group. No group differences in weight gain, however, were observed at the 6-month follow-up. Jorenby et al. (105) examined post-cessation weight changes among participants in a 2 (300 mg bupropion vs. placebo) × 2 (transdermal nicotine patch vs. placebo) randomized clinical trial. Those in the combined treatment group (i.e. bupriopion plus transdermal nicotine) gained significantly less weight at 6 weeks (1.1 kg) than those in either the bupropion only (1.7 kg) or double placebo (2.1 kg) groups, and a similar but non-significant trend was observed for the patch-only group (1.6 kg). No differences in weight gain among treatment groups existed at 6 months follow-up, however. Thus, while bupropion may help to reduce post-cessation weight gain in the short term, the weight-attenuating effects do not appear to last beyond the duration of treatment.

CONCLUSIONS

It is clear that smokers weigh less than non-smokers (averaging 3 to 4 kg) after many years of smoking. However, among adolescents and young adults, weight differences between smokers and non-smokers are small or non-existent, and smoking initiation is *not* associated with weight loss. In contrast, smoking cessation reliably produces weight gain. In several large prospective studies, weight gain attributable to smoking cessation has averaged 2 to 4 kg, and has been greater in women, Blacks (compared to Whites), younger smokers, those who weigh less prior to quitting, and those who smoke more (27,34). On average, quitting smoking increases one's weight to a level that would be expected for a non-smoker. Although some individuals experience major weight gain (10 kg or so) after quitting smoking, this occurs in a relatively small proportion of quitters—generally fewer than 20%. Post-cessation weight gain seems to be largely related to increases in energy intake, particularly high fat and carbohydrate between-meal snacking (74). Loss of the acute metabolic-enhancing effects of nicotine may also partly contribute to weight gain, but the bulk of evidence argues against a chronic effect of smoking cessation on metabolism (33).

It may seem ironic that there currently is so much interest in developing smoking cessation interventions that effectively reduce or eliminate post-cessation weight gain, given that weight gain generally is modest, and is certainly less health-damaging than continued smoking. However, many smokers, particularly women, have serious concerns about post-cessation weight gain which contribute to decisions not to attempt quitting, or to relapse once cessation has been attempted (74). As such, cessation interventions that are effective at preventing weight gain may encourage smokers to quit, and may provide additional motivation to remain quit. Behavioral strategies involving restriction of energy intake and increased physical activity generally have failed to prevent weight gain, and have also impeded cessation efforts, possibly because individuals become overwhelmed at changing two behaviors simultaneously. Staggering the interventions, such that weight control efforts are not attempted until smoking cessation is firmly established, shows promise of attenuating weight gain (82). Additionally, several pharmacologic interventions, including nicotine replacement and serotoninergic and catecholaminergic agents, have been shown to reduce post-cessation weight gain, although this effect is limited to the duration of drug treatment. More work is needed to improve the efficacy of both behavioral and pharmacologic approaches to reduce post-cessation weight gain, and combining behavioral and pharmacologic strategies may be a promising approach to eradicating this tenacious problem.

REFERENCES

1. US Department of Health and Human Services. *The Health Benefits of Smoking Cessation: a Report of the Surgeon General.* Rockville (MD): US Department of Health and Human Services, Public Health Service, Center for Disease Control, Center for Health Promotion and Education, Office on Smoking and Health, 1990. DHHS publication no. (CDC) 90-8416.

2. Centers for Disease Control and Prevention. Cigarette smoking-attributable mortality and years of potential life lost—United States, 1990. *Morbid Mortal Weekly Rep* 1993; **33:** 645–649.

3. Centers for Disease Control and Prevention. Perspectives in disease prevention and health promotion smoking-attributable mortality and years of potential life lost—United States, 1984. *Morbid Mortal Weekly Rep* 1997; **42**(33): 444–451.

4. American Cancer Society. *Cancer Facts & Figures—1995.* Atlanta, GA: Author.

5. National Center for Health Statistics. *Health, United States, 1996–1997.* Hyattsville (MD): Public Health Service, 1997.

6. US Department of Health and Human Services. Preventing tobacco use among young people: a report of the Surgeon General. Atlanta, Georgia: US Department of Health and Human Services, Public Health Service, Centers for Disease Control and Prevention, National Center for Chronic Disease Prevention and health Promotion, Office on Smoking and Health, 1994.

7. Klesges RC, Klesges LM. Cigarette smoking as a dieting strategy in a university population. *Int J Eating Disorder* 1988; **7**(3): 413–419.

8. Tucker LA. Cigarette smoking intentions and obesity among high school males. *Psychol Rep* 1983; **52:** 530.

9. French SA, Perry CL, Leon GR, Fulkerson JA. Weight Concerns, dieting behavior, and smoking initiation in adolescents: A prospective epidemiologic study. *Am J Public Health* 1994; **84:** 1818–1820.

10. Camp DE, Klesges RC, Relyea G. The relationship between body weight concerns and adolescent smoking. *Health Psychol* 1993; **12:** 24–32.

11. Gerend MA, Boyle RG, Peterson CB, Hatsukami DK. Eating behavior and weight control among women using smokeless tobacco, cigarettes, and normal controls. *Addict Behav* 1998; **23**(2): 171–178.

12. Klesges RC, Somes G, Pascale RW, Klesges LM, Murphy M, Brown K, Williams E. Knowledge and beliefs regarding the consequences of cigarette smoking and their relationship to smoking status in a biethnic sample. *Health Psychol* 1988; **7**(15): 387–401.

13. Weekley CK, Klesges RC, Reylea G. Smoking as a weight-control strategy and its relationship to smoking status. *Addict Behav* 1992; **17:** 259–271.

14. Klesges RC, Brown K, Pascale RW, Murphy M, Williams E, Cigrang JA. Factors associated with participation, attrition, and outcome in a smoking cessation program at the workplace. *Health Psychol* 1988; **7**(6): 575–589.

15. Meyers AW, Klesges RC, Winders SE, Ward KD, Peterson BA, Eck LH. Are weight concerns predictive of smoking cessation? A prospective analysis. *J Consult Clin Psychol* 1997; **65**(3): 448–452.

16. Richmond RL, Kehoe L, Webster IW. Weight change after smoking cessation in general practice. *Med J Aust* 1993; **158:** 821–822.

17. French SA, Jeffery RW, Klesges LM, Forster JL. Weight concerns and changes in smoking behavior over two years

in a working population. *Am J Public Health* 1995; **85**(5): 720–722.

18. French SA, Jeffrey RW, Pirie PL, McBride CM. Do weight concerns hinder smoking cessation efforts? *Addict Behav* 1992; **17**(3): 219–226.

19. Jeffery RW, Boles SM, Strycker LA, Glasgow RE. Smoking-specific weight gain concerns and smoking cessation in a working population. *Health Psychol* 1997; **16**(5): 487–489.

20. Klesges RC, Mayers AW, Klesges LM, LaVasque ME. Smoking, body weight, and their effects on smoking behavior: A comprehensive review of the literature. *Psychol Bull* 1989; **106**(2): 204–230.

21. US Department of Health and Human Services. *The Health Consequences of Smoking: Nicotine Addiction: a Report of the Surgeon General*. Rockville(MD): US Department of Health and Human Services, Public Health Service, Center for Disease Control, Center for Health Promotion and Education, Office on Smoking and Health, 1988. DHHS publication no. (CDC) 88-8406.

22. Molarius A, Seidell JC, Kuulasmaa K, Dobson AJ, Sans S. Smoking and relative body weight: an international perspective from the WHO MONICA Project. *J Epidemiol Community Health* 1997; **51**: 252–260.

23. Klesges RC, Robinson LA, Zbikowski SM. Is smoking associated with lower body mass in adolescents?: a large-scale biracial investigation. *Addict Behav* 1998; **23**(1): 109–113.

24. Cooper TV, Klesges RC, Robinson L, Zbikowski SM. A prospective evaluation of the relationship between smoking and body mass index in an adolescent, biracial cohort. (Manuscript under review)

25. Klesges RC, Zbikowski SM, Lando HA, Haddock CK, Talcott GW, Robinson LA. The relationship between smoking and body weight in a population of young military personnel. *Health Psychol* 1998; **17**(5): 454–458.

26. Klesges RC, Ward KD, Ray JW, Cutter G, Hilner J, Jacobs DR, Wagenknecht L. The prospective relationships between smoking and weight in a young biracial cohort: The Coronary Artery Risk Development in Young Adults study. *J Consult Clin Psychol* 1998; **66**(6): 987–993.

27. Williamson DF, Madans J, Anda RF, Kleinman JC, Giovino GA, Byers T. Smoking cessation and severity of weight gain in a national cohort. *N Engl J Med* 1991; **324**(11): 739–745.

28. US Department of Health, Education, and Welfare. *The Smoking Digest: Progress Report on a Nation Kicking the Habit*. US Department of Health, Education, and Welfare, Public Health Service, National Institute of Health, Office of Cancer Communications, National Cancer Institute, 1977.

29. Colditz GA, Segal MR, Myers AH, Stampfer MJ, Willett W, Speizer FE. Weight change in relation to smoking cessation among women. *J Smoking Relat Dis* 1992; **3**(2): 145–153.

30. Mizoue T, Ueda R, Tokui N, Hino Y, Yoshimura T. Body mass decrease after initial gain following smoking cessation. *Int J Epidemiol* 1998; **27**: 984–988.

31. Nides M, Rand C, Dolce J, Murray R, O'Hara P, Voelker H, Connett J. Weight gain as a function of smoking cessation and 2-mg nicotine gum use among middle-aged smokers with mild lung impairment in the first 2 years of the Lung Health Study. *Health Psychol* 1994; **13**(4): 354–361.

32. Klesges RC, Winders SE, Meyers AW, Eck LH, Ward KD, Hultquist CM, Ray JW, Shadish RW. How much weight gain occurs following smoking cessation? A comparison of weight gain using both continuous and point prevalence abstinence. *J Consult Clin Psychol* 1997; **65**(2): 286–291.

33. Perkins KA. Weight gain following smoking cessation. *J Consult Clin Psychol* 1993; **61**(5): 768–777.

34. Klesges RC, Meyers AW, Winders SE, French SN. Determining the reasons for weight gain following smoking cessation: current findings, methodological issues, and future directions for research. *Ann Behav Med* 1989; **11**(4): 134–143.

35. Klesges RC, Stein RC, Hultquist CM, Eck LH. Relationship between smoking status, body composition, energy intake, and physical activity among adult males. *J Subst Abuse* 1992; **4**: 47–56.

36. Blair SN, Jacobs DR, Powell KE. Relationships between exercise or physical activity and other health behaviors. *Public Health Rep* 1985; **100**(2): 172–180.

37. Klesges RC, Eck LH, Isbell TR, Fulliton W, Hanson CL. Smoking status: effects on the dietary intake, physical activity, and body fat of adult men. *Am J Clin Nutr* 1990; **51**: 784–789.

38. Marks BL, Perkins KA, Metz KF, Epstein LH, Robertson RJ, Goss FL, Sexton JE. Effects of smoking status on content of caloric intake and energy expenditure. *Int J Eating Disord* 1991; **10**(4): 441–449.

39. Klesges RC, Eck LH, Clark EM, Meyers AW, Hanson CL. The effects of smoking cessation and gender on dietary intake, physical activity, and weight gain. *Int J Eating Disord* 1990; **9**(4): 435–445.

40. Moffatt RJ, Owens SG. Cessation from cigarette smoking: changes in body weight, body composition, resting metabolism, and energy consumption. *Metabolism* 1991; **40**(5): 465–470.

41. Perkins KA, Epstein LH, Pastor S. Changes in energy balance following smoking cessation and resumption of smoking in women. *J Consult Clin Psychol* 1990; **58**(1): 121–125.

42. Perkins KA, Rohay J, Meilahn EN, Wing RR, Matthews KA, Kuller LH. Diet, alcohol, and physical activity as a function of smoking status in middle-aged women. *Health Psychol* 1993; **12**(5): 410–415.

43. Rodin JR. Weight change following smoking cessation: the role of food intake and exercise. *Addict Behav* 1987; **12**(4): 303–317.

44. Streater JA, Sargent RG, Wards DS. A study of factors associated with weight change in women who attempt smoking cessation. *Addict Behav* 1989; **14**(5): 523–530.

45. Albanes D, Jones DY, Micozzi MS, Mattson ME. Associations between smoking and body weight in the US population: analysis of NHANES II. *Am J Public Health* 1987; **77**(4): 439–444.

46. Fehily AM, Phillips KM, Yarnell JWG. Diet, smoking, social class, and body mass index in the caerphilly Heart Disease Study. *Am J Clin Nutr* 1984; **40**: 827–833.

47. Hatsukami DK, Hughes JR, Pickens RW, Svikis D. Tobacco withdrawal symptoms: an experimental analysis. *Psychopharmacology* 1984; **84**: 231–236.

48. Leischow SJ, Stitzer ML. Effects of smoking cessation on caloric intake and weight gain in an impatient unit. *Psychopharmacology* 1991; **104**(4): 522–526.

49. Stamford BA, Matters S, Fell RD, Papenek P. Effects of smoking cessation on weight gain, metabolic rate, caloric consumption, and blood lipids. *Am J Clin Nutr* 1986; **43**(4): 486–494.

50. Dallosso HM, James WPT. The role of smoking in the regulation of energy balance. *Int J Obes* 1984; **8**: 365–375.

51. Leischow SJ, Stitzer ML. Smoking cessation and weight gain. *Br J Addiction* 1991; **86**: 577–581.

52. Perkins KA. Effects of tobacco smoking on caloric intake. *Br J Addiction* 1992; **87**: 193–205.

53. Caan B, Coates A, Schaeger C, Finkler L, Sternfeld B, Corbett K. Women gain weight one year after smoking cessation while dietary intake temporarily increases. *J Am Diet Assoc* 1996; **96**(11): 1150–1155.

54. Hall SM, Ginsberg D, Jones RT. Smoking cessation and weight gain. *J Consult Clin Psychol* 1986; **54**(3): 342–346.

55. Klesges RC, Winders SE, Meyers A, Eck LH, Hultquist C, Ward K, Peterson BA, Johnson K. Mechanisms of weight gain following smoking cessation: a large prospective investigation. *Ann Behav Med* 1997; **19**(Supplement): S066.

56. Hall SM, McGee R, Tunstall C, Duffy J, Benowitz N. Changes in food intake and activity after quitting smoking. *J Consult Clin Psychol* 1989; **57**(1): 81–86.

57. Spring B, Wurtman J, Gleason R, Wurtman R, Kessler K. Weight gain and withdrawal symptoms after smoking cessation: a preventive intervention using d-fenfluramine. *Health Psychol* 1991; **10**(3): 216–223.

58. Perkins KA, Epstein LH, Sexton JE, Pastor S. Effects of smoking cessation on consumption of alcohol and sweet, high-fat foods. *J Subst Abuse* 1990; **2**: 287–297.

59. Gilbert RM, Pope MA. Early effects of quitting smoking. *Psychopharmacology* 1982; **78**: 121–127.

60. Hatsukami D, LaBounty L, Hughes J, Laine D. Effects of tobacco abstinence on food intake among cigarette smokers. *Health Psychol* 1993; **12**(6): 499–502.

61. Audrain JE, Klesges RC, Klesges LM. Relationship between obesity and the metabolic effects of smoking in women. *Health Psychol* 1995; **14**(2): 116–123.

62. Klesges RC, DePue K, Audrain J, Klesges LM, Meyers AW. Metabolic effects of nicotine gum and cigarette smoking: potential implications for postcessation weight gain? *J Consult Clin Psychol* 1991; **59**(5): 749–752.

63. Perkins KA, Epstein LH, Marks BL, Stiller RL, Jacob RG. The effect of nicotine on energy expenditure during light physical activity. *N Engl J Med* 1989; **320**: 898–903.

64. Perkins KA, Epstein LH, Stiller RL, Marks BL, Jacob RG. Acute effects of nicotine on metabolic rate in cigarette smokers. *Am J Clin Nutr* 1989; **50**: 545–550.

65. Warwick PM, Chapple RS, Thomson ES. The effect of smoking two cigarettes on resting metabolic rate with and without food. *Int J Obes* 1987; **11**(3): 229–237.

66. Hultquist CM, Meyers AW, Whelan JP, Klesges RC, Peacher-Ryan H, DeBon MW. The effect of smoking and light activity on metabolism in men. *Health Psychol* 1995; **14**(2): 124–131.

67. Jensen EX, Fusch CH, Jaeger P, Pehein E, Horber FF. Impact of chronic cigarette smoking on body composition and fuel metabolism. *J Clin Endocrinol Metab* 1995; **80**: 2181–2185.

68. Perkins KA. Metabolic effects of cigarette smoking. *J Appl Physiol* 1992; **72**: 401–409.

69. Warwick PM, Edmundson HM, Thomson ES. No evidence for a chronic effect of smoking on energy expenditure. *Int J Obes* 1995; **19**: 198–201.

70. Burse RL, Bynum GD, Pandolf KB, Goldman RF, Sims EAH, Danforth ER. Increased appetite and unchanged metabolism upon cessation of smoking with diet held constant (Abstract). *Physiologist* 1975; **18**: 157.

71. Cursiter M, Jennett S. The effect of smoking cessation on energy expenditure and body weight (Abstract). *Proc Nutr Soc* 1992; **51**: 48A.

72. Robinson S, York DA. The effect of cigarette smoking on the thermic response to feeding. *Int J Obes* 1986; **10**(5): 407–417.

73. Vander Weg MW, Klesges RC, Clemens LH, Meyers AW, Pascale RW. The relationships between ethnicity, gender, and short-term changes in energy balance following smoking cessation. *Int J Behav Med* (in press).

74. Perkins KA, Levine MD, Marcus MD, Shiffman S. Addressing women's concerns about weight gain due to smoking cessation. *J Subst Abuse Treat* 1997; **14**(2): 173–182.

75. Perkins KA. Issues in the prevention of weight gain after smoking cessation. *Ann Behav Med* 1994; **16**(1): 46–52.

76. Killen JD, Fortmann SP, Newman B. Weight change among participants in a large-sample minimal-contact smoking relapse prevention trial. *Addic Behav* 1990; **15**: 323–332.

77. Gross J, Stitzer ML, Maldonado J. Nicotine replacement: effects on postcessation weight gain. *J Consult Clin Psychol* 1989; **57**(1): 87–92.

78. Hall SM, Tunstall CD, Vila KL, Duffy J. Weight gain prevention and smoking cessation: cautionary findings. *Am J Public Health* 1992; **82**(6): 799–803.

79. Pirie P, McBride CM, Hellerstedt W, Jeffery RW, Hatsukami D, Allen S, Lando H. Smoking cessation in women concerned about weight. *Am J Public Health* 1992; **82**(9): 1238–1243.

80. Ogden J. Effects of smoking cessation, restrained eating, and motivational states on food intake in the laboratory. *Health Psychol* 1994; **13**(2): 114–121.

81. West R, Hajek P, Burrows S. Effect of glucose tablets on craving for cigarettes. *Psychopharmacology* 1990; **101**: 555–559.

82. Spring B, Pingitore R, Johnsen L, Pergadia M, Richmond M, Gunnarsdottir D, Corsica J, Mills M, Crayton J. Promoting smoking cessation and reducing weight gain. *Ann Behav Med* 1999; **21**(Suppl): S091.

83. Kawachi I, Troisi RJ, Rotnitzky AG, Coakley EH, Colditz GA. Can physical activity minimize weight gain in women after smoking cessation? *Am J Public Health* 1996; **86**: 999–1004.

84. Marcus BH, Albrecht AE, King TK, Parisi AF, Pinto BM, Roberts M, Niaura RS, Abrams DB. The efficacy of exercise as an aid for smoking cessation in women: a randomized controlled trial. *Arch Intern Med* 1999; **159**: 1229–1234.

85. Talcott GW, Fiedler ER, Pascale RW, Klesges RC, Peterson AL, Johnson RS. Is weight gain after smoking cessation inevitable? *J Consult Clin Psychol* 1995; **63**(2): 313–316.

86. Doherty K, Militello FS, Kinnunen T, Garvey AJ. Nicotine

gum dose and weight gain after smoking cessation. *J Consult Clin Psychol* 1996; **64**(4): 799–807.

87. Hajek P, Jackson P, Belcher M. Long-term use of nicotine chewing gum: occurrence, determinants, and effect on weight gain. *JAMA* 1988; **260**(11): 1593–1596.

88. Leischow SJ, Sachs DPL, Bostrom AG, Hansen MD. Effects of differing nicotine-replacement doses on weight gain after smoking cessation. *Arch Fam Med* 1992; **1**: 233–237.

89. Li Wan Po A. Transdermal nicotine in smoking cessation: a meta-analysis. *Eur J Clin Pharmacol* 1993; **45**: 519–528.

90. Abelin T, Buehler A, Muller P, Vesanen K, Imhof PR. Controlled trial of transdermal nicotine patch in tobacco withdrawal. *Lancet* 1989; **1**: 7–10.

91. Jorenby DE, Hatsukami DK, Smith SS, Fiore MC, Allen S, Jensen J, Baker TB. Characterization of tobacco withdrawal symptoms: transdermal nicotine reduces hunger and weight gain. *Psychopharmacology* 1996; **128**: 130–138.

92. Allen SS, Hatsukami D, Gorsline J, the Transdermal Nicotine Study Group. Cholesterol changes in smoking cessation using the transdermal nicotine system. *Prev Med* 1994; **23**: 190–196.

93. Hughes JR, Hatsukami DK. Effects of three doses of transdermal nicotine on post-cessation eating, hunger and weight. *J Subst Abuse* 1997; **9**: 151–159.

94. Dale LC, Schroeder DR, Wolter TD, Croghan IT, Hurt RD, Offord KP. Weight change after smoking cessation using variable doses of transdermal nicotine replacement. *J Gen Intern Med* 1998; **13**: 9–15.

95. Puska P, Korhonen HJ, Vartiainen E, Urjanheimo E-L, Gustavsson G, Westin A. Combined use of nicotine patch and gum compared with gum alone in smoking cessation: a clinical trial in North Karelia. *Tobacco Control* 1995; **4**: 231–235.

96. Sutherland G, Stapleton JA, Russell MAH, Jarvis MJ, Hajek P, Belcher M, Feyerabend C. Randomised controlled trial of nasal nicotine spray in smoking cessation. *Lancet* 1992; **340**: 324–329.

97. Tonnesen P, Norregaard J, Mikkelsen K, Jorgensen S, Nilsson F. A double-blind trial of a nicotine inhaler for smoking cessation. *JAMA* 1993; **269**(10): 1268–1271.

98. Hjalmarson A, Nilsson F, Sjostrom L, Wiklund O. The nicotine inhaler in smoking cessation. *Arch Intern Med* 1997; **157**: 1721–1728.

99. Klesges RC, Klesges LM, Meyers AW, Klem ML, Isbell T. The effects of phenylpropanolamine on dietary intake, physical activity, and body weight after smoking cessation. *Clin Pharmacol Ther* 1990; **47**: 747–754.

100. Klesges RC, Klesges LM, DeBon M, Shelton ML, Isbell TR, Klem ML. Effects of phenylpropanolamine on withdrawal symptoms. *Psychopharmacology* 1995; **119**: 85–91.

101. Pomerleau OF, Pomerleau CS, Morrell EM, Lowenbergh JM. Effects of fluoxetine on weight gain and food intake in smokers who reduce nicotine intake. *Psychoneuroendocrinology* 1991; **16**(5): 433–440.

102. Spring B, Wurtman J, Wurtman R, el-Khoury A, Goldberg H, McDermott J, Pingitore R. Efficacies of dexfenfluramine and fluoxetine in preventing weight gain after smoking cessation. *Am J Clin Nutr* 1995; **62**(6): 1181–1187.

103. Borrelli B, Spring B, Niaura R, Kristeller J, Ockene JK, Keuthen NJ. Weight suppression and weight rebound in ex-smokers treated with fluoxetine. *J Consult Clin Psychol* 1999; **67**(1): 124–131.

104. Hurt RD, Sachs DPL, Glover ED, Offord KP, Johnston JA, Lowell LC, Khayrallah MA, Schroeder, DR, Glover PN, Sullivan CR, Croghan UT, Sullivan PM. A comparison of sustained release bupropion and placebo for smoking cessation. *N Engl J Med* 1997; **337**(17): 1195–1202.

105. Jorenby DE, Leischow SJ, Nides MA, Rennard SI, Johnston JA, Hughes AR, Smith SS, Muramoto ML, Daughton DM, Doan K, Fiore MC, Baker TB. A controlled trial of sustained-release bupropion, a nicotine patch, or both for smoking cessation. *N Engl J Med* 1999; **340**(9): 685–691.

Part V

Complications

23

Visceral Obesity and the Metabolic Syndrome

Roland Rosmond

Sahlgrenska University Hospital, Göteborg, Sweden

INTRODUCTION—EPIDEMIOLOGY

The association between obesity and type 2 (non-insulin-dependent) diabetes mellitus has been recognized for several decades. It has now been shown that obesity is also associated with cardiovascular disease (CVD) and stroke. Population-based follow-up studies have revealed this concealed link, bringing the importance of obesity as an independent risk factor for cardiovascular morbidity and mortality to the forefront. However, at first, it was assumed that only severe obesity was as powerful a risk indicator of CVD and stroke as other, established risk factors such as hypercholesterolaemia and high blood pressure.

Retrospectively, it is now possible to identify why these studies failed to highlight the impact of excess body fat on cardiovascular morbidity. First, in analysing epidemiological data, it is common to adjust for the effect of some variables believed to distort the results, and in the case of obesity, adjustments were made for comorbidities such as dyslipidaemia, hypertension, insulin resistance and impaired glucose tolerance. However, these adjustments are biologically and clinically implausible, since obesity without such comorbidities is a rare condition. Furthermore, severe non-orthogonality is introduced in the statistical analyses since these comorbidities are highly correlated. Another problem with these early studies was that obesity, defined as increased body fat mass, was treated as one homogeneous entity. Human obesity has repeatedly been subjected to subdivisions with the clinical intuition that this is not one single disease, but rather a symptom of several underlying conditions, to some extent similar to diseases such as anaemia–polyglobulinaemia, where red blood cells vary in amount and quality for a number of underlying reasons.

Human obesity is characterized by a wide variation in the distribution of excess body fat, and the distribution of fat affects the risks associated with obesity as well as the kinds of comorbidities that result. In the 1920s the idea emerged, under Kretschmer's influence (1), that the pychnic type of body build was associated with abdominal obesity, gout, apoplexia and impaired glucose tolerance. Vague extended these observations further and labelled obesity types android (male-type) and gynoid (female-type), and noted that, although gender-specific in general, women might have android obesity and vice versa (2). Nevertheless, the android type of obesity carries a greater risk for disease in both men and women.

In addition to the pioneering attempts by Kretschmer and Vague to categorize obesity, recent developments have confirmed the higher prevalence of dyslipidaemia, insulin resistance and hypertension in abdominal, central obesity in comparison with the more peripherally distributed, gluteofemoral obesity (3,4), The techniques for the assessment of adipose tissue in these studies were

International Textbook of Obesity. Edited by Per Björntorp.

simpler than those employed by Vague (2), and included the ratio of waist and hip circumferences (WHR). Central obesity is thus more strongly associated with comorbidities in various systems than is peripheral obesity. This is particularly evident when intra-abdominal, visceral fat depots are enlarged (5,6).

The results of prospective epidemiological studies presented a major breakthrough in the significance of this type of categorization of obesity. These studies showed that WHR contributes independently to the risk of type 2 diabetes, CVD and stroke in both men and women, and is as powerful a predictor as other established risk factors for these diseases. Moreover, these studies showed that general obesity, measured as body mass index (BMI, weight (kg)/height^2 [m^2]), was not necessarily a part of this health hazard (7,8).

Subsequent studies have indicated other health consequences of central obesity such as cancer of the endometrium (9), breast (10) and ovaries (9) in women, and the prostate in men (11). The respiratory function when measured in obese subjects reveals many abnormalities, and one of the most extreme is the Pickwickian hypoventilation syndrome. Obstructive sleep apnoea is also common in obesity, and about 50% of subjects with this disorder are moderately to severely abdominally obese (12). Cholelithiasis and obesity has been documented in several studies (11), and hepatic steatosis occurs in about 68–94% of obese individuals (13).

PATHOGENETIC ASPECTS

These statistical observations imply a major, fundamental, systematic pathogenetic background to abdominal, visceral fat accumulation and its associated multiple comorbidities. From a clinical point of view, there is a perceptible resemblance between this condition and that of Cushing's syndrome. In fact, subjects with abdominal, visceral obesity share many of the metabolic, hormonal, circulatory and behavioural findings observed in Cushing's syndrome. It may therefore be suspected that the regulation of cortisol secretion is involved in the syndrome of visceral obesity (5,14).

Studies driven by this hypothesis suggested that urinary cortisol output was elevated with elevated WHR (15). Although statistically significant, the original findings were strongly influenced by a few extreme observations. It is also clear that the cortisol output is frequently normal or even low in subjects with elevated WHR (Figure 1 in reference 15). Results of other studies indicated that when the hypothalamic-pituitary-adrenal (HPA) axis, regulating cortisol secretion, was stimulated at the levels of the adrenals with adrenocorticotrophic hormone (ACTH), the pituitary with corticotrophin-releasing hormone (CRH) and the hypothalamic centres by laboratory stress, the total urinary output of cortisol appeared to be elevated in subjects with high WHR (15,16). However, the challenges at the different levels of the HPA axis were performed with maximal doses of ACTH and CRH. The use of such doses provides information about the responsiveness rather than sensitivity of the regulatory system. Maximal stimulation rarely, if ever, occurs under ordinary, everyday life conditions, and these results therefore had minor significance for the issue addressed.

METHODOLOGICAL DEVELOPMENTS

The idea that frequent or persistent challenges of the HPA axis may constitute a base for pathophysiological consequences in the periphery of the body stems from the central role played by the HPA axis in homeostatic processes. Although biologically plausible, this complex hypothesis has been difficult to study in humans (17), presumably as a result of several inherent problems.

The pattern of ACTH and cortisol variations shows an early morning peak, declining levels during the daytime and minimal secretory activity in the evening. This secretory pattern is brought about by the nervous system. There is, however, no sharp distinction between the endocrine and nervous systems, and in the hypothalamus and the pituitary there is a close connection between these two systems that integrates the two into one control unit. The CRH-secreting neurons, located within the paraventricular nuclei (PVN) (18), receive afferent regulatory signals from different parts of the brain. Stimulatory inputs arise from the suprachiasmatic nucleus (the regulator of circadian rhythms), the amygdala and the raphe nuclei (19,20), while inhibitory inputs on CRH secretion arise in the hippocampus and in the locus coeruleus. The CRH neurons are excitatory, influenced by cholinergic and serotoninergic central pathways (21). Inhibitory effects are exerted by γ-aminobutyric acid (GABA) (20). Catecholamines can exert both inhibitory and excitatory effects (22). Furthermore, stimulation of hypothalamic opioid peptide (POMC-producing) neurons will inhibit the release of CRH from the PVN (23).

In summary, the central nervous system provides inputs in terms of registrations by the senses, modified by experience and coping ability, and the integrated resulting signals transferred to the hypothalamus. These afferent signals are balanced by endocrine feedback regulation, mediated via glucocorticoid receptors (GR) in the hippocampus and the amygdala (24–26). Feedback information allows the HPA axis to adjust appropriately the cortisol secretion from the adrenals.

When measurements are performed aimed at elucidating the natural, spontaneous, everyday activity of the HPA axis, several prerequisites have to be considered. The regulation of the HPA axis is greatly affected by environmental disturbances. For instance, the artificial milieu of a laboratory or a hospital may distort normal activity, and even minor venepuncture per se can significantly increase cortisol concentration in serum. Urinary cortisol measurements offer a tool to circumvent this source of bias. However, urinary measurements do not reveal the secretory pattern of cortisol, which is, as will be seen in the following, vital information. Moreover, the technique is usually restricted for practical reasons to inpatients.

The assessment of cortisol in saliva provides several advantages over blood cortisol measurements, as the collection procedure is non-invasive and stress free, making it ideal for use in psychoneuroendocrinological research. Since salivary cortisol sampling is laboratory independent, it can be applied under a variety of field settings. It is well documented that salivary cortisol provides the clinician with a reliable tool for examination of pathological conditions characterized by abnormal cortisol secretion (27–30). Cortisol is lipid-soluble which enables the molecule to diffuse rapidly to the acinar cells of the salivary glands via the bloodstream, and then pass easily through these cells into saliva. Neither maximal stimulation of saliva flow (28) nor minimal secretion of saliva following medication with anticholinergic side effects influences the concentration of cortisol in saliva (27). Moreover, corti-

sol in saliva represents the unbound ('free') hormone fraction, and reflects accurately the free fraction of cortisol in plasma, despite the conversion of cortisol to cortisone in saliva by 11β-hydroxysteroid dehydrogenase (31).

To obtain a biochemical evaluation of the HPA axis activity and regulation that is as complete as possible several details are essential. A normal diurnal variation is a pattern in which cortisol levels are high and varying in the morning and from 1600 hours to midnight less than 75% of the morning values. This must be recorded together with the total cortisol levels. Since the HPA axis is subject to periodic or cyclic changes (19), the measurement of cortisol levels at various times of the day to determine the presence or absence of a circadian rhythm is crucial. Furthermore, the response to external stimuli is informative, and the physiological input by food intake can be measured, if the stimulus is standardized. Various centrally occurring challenges of the HPA axis, in terms of stress, are of fundamental importance, and as stressors are perceived differently, individual coping ability has to be taken into account. This is accomplished by reports by the proband of perceived stress.

In addition to these measurements of basal and stimulated HPA axis activity, the response to exogenous glucocorticoids is required to detect abnormal feedback regulation of ACTH and cortisol secretion (32). Conventionally dexamethasone is given in a dose of 1 mg, which is usually followed by a complete inhibition of ACTH and cortisol secretion, except in subjects with Cushing's syndrome. Preliminary examinations showed that utilizing a low dose (0.5 mg × 1) of dexamethasone (33) reveals mild abnormalities in the ability of the central glucorticoid receptor (GR) to control the HPA axis by feedback inhibition that cannot be discovered with the conventional dose of 1 mg (15).

In summary, these different characteristics of the HPA axis activity and regulation were measured by a series of saliva sampling during the day, in which cortisol levels were measured. A sample was obtained in the morning (0800–0900 hours), then at 1145 hours, and 30, 45 and 60 minutes after a standardized lunch at 1200 hours, 1700 hours, and finally just before bedtime. Within these periods, relatively small changes in unstimulated cortisol values occur and therefore a satisfactory estimation of the circadian rhythm can be acquired (34). The circadian rhythm of cortisol secretion was estimated as the variability of cortisol secretion. By addition of all measured values, a measurement of total cortisol secretion was obtained. The response to lunch was calculated as the peak of cortisol after lunch. Stress-related cortisol secretion was calculated as the response of cortisol to simultaneously reported perceived stress. Finally, the low dose ($0.5\,mg \times 1$) dexamethasone suppression test was performed similarly at home.

METHODOLOGICAL COMPARISONS

The concentration of cortisol in saliva, although approximately 30–50% lower (34), correlates closely with the concentration of free cortisol in serum ($r \approx 0.90$). Consequently, salivary cortisol measurements are an excellent index of the total, free cortisol concentration in serum as well as in urine in both normal and pathological conditions (27–30).

Cortisol has effects at nearly all levels in the human body, including an important role in lipid and glucose metabolism. Cortisol also inhibits most inflammatory processes (35), increases the left ventricular work index (36), and increases glomerular filtration rate, renal blood flow and potassium and acid excretion (37,38).

Centralization of body fat is most likely an effect of cortisol, as clearly seen in Cushing's syndrome, exhibited as severe truncal obesity. After successful therapy, the somatic features of Cushing's syndrome disappear (39). This provides evidence that cortisol may have a most potent stimulatory effect on central, visceral fat accumulation. Further evidence suggests that cortisol, in the presence of insulin, activates the main gateway for lipid accumulation in adipocytes, the lipoprotein lipase (LPL) enzyme, by actions on the processes of transcription and post-translation (40,41). Moreover, under these conditions the activity of the lipid mobilization system is low (41). These metabolic processes are mediated throughout the GR in adipose tissue. High activity in the lipid accumulating pathway together with low activity of lipid mobilization, exerted by cortisol, will be most pronounced is visceral fat depots due to the high density of GR (42). In light of this clinical and interventional evidence, strengthened by experimental studies, it is thus obvious that cortisol plays a major role as an aetiological factor in visceral fat accumulation.

With this background, it becomes relevant to determine to what extent salivary cortisol levels correlate to centrally localized body fat. Furthermore, it has been assumed that measurements of body fat centralization reflect a persistent, inappropriate cortisol secretion and related endocrine phenomena (43). In support of this assumption, anthropometric measurements were also correlated to the salivary cortisol assessments.

The presence of a normal circadian rhythm (variability) and feedback regulation (dexamethasone) of the HPA axis, along with an adequate response to stimuli (lunch), shows significant correlations with waist circumference (W) and abdominal sagittal diameter (D) (Table 23.1). The same results are also seen with an abnormal HPA axis, characterized by low variability and poor feedback regulation. Total cortisol secretion, however, showed no statistically significant relationship to the measurements of central obesity (W and D). In fact, total cortisol secretion even showed a negative association with WHR.

In conclusion, these findings suggest that the relationship between cortisol and central obesity can be entirely unveiled provided that the HPA axis is subjected to external stimulus or challenges, and that the total cortisol secretion per se is inappropriate for such purposes.

The BMI, an estimation of the total body fat mass regardless of regional distribution, showed several significant relationships to the functional status of the HPA axis. This indicates an association between general obesity, measured as BMI, and the HPA axis. This is further supported by means of structural equation modelling (path analysis) where a direct link between the HPA axis function and BMI was found (44). Given this information, together with previous studies (45) suggesting leptin resistance in obesity, we performed analyses of leptin with similar results—namely, an increase in leptin concentration is associated with elevated BMI (46). In addition, recent studies imply that cortisol may give rise to such a leptin resistance (47–49). There is thus a prospect that leptin concentrations are influenced by the HPA axis, and that increased total cortisol secretion with a normal axis, and evoked cortisol secretion by various stimulis with an abnormal axis (Table 23.1), may actually induce obesity. This would explain the well-known clinical observation that hypercortisolism, as in Cushing's syndrome or as an effect of corticosteroid

Table 23.1 Correlations between the function of the hypothalamic-pituitary-adrenal (HPA) axis and anthropometric measurements in middle-aged men

	BMI	WHR	W	D
Normal HPA axis				
Total cortisol level (nmol/L)	$-0.13\,(P = 0.035)$	$-0.08\,(P = 0.196)$	$-0.09\,(P = 0.153)$	$-0.11\,(P = 0.068)$
Cortisol after lunch (nmol/L)	$0.16\,(P = 0.005)$	$0.03\,(P > 0.200)$	$0.22\,(P < 0.001)$	$0.18\,(P = 0.001)$
Stress-related cortisol	$0.01\,(P > 0.200)$	$0.01\,(P > 0.200)$	$-0.01\,(P > 0.200)$	$0.17\,(P = 0.002)$
Abnormal HPA axis				
Total cortisol level (nmol/L)	$0.01\,(P > 0.200)$	$-0.10\,(P = 0.001)$	$-0.05\,(P = 0.087)$	$0.04\,(P = 0.190)$
Cortisol after lunch (nmol/L)	$0.14\,(P < 0.001)$	$0.07\,(P = 0.003)$	$0.10\,(P < 0.001)$	$0.15\,(P < 0.001)$
Stress-related cortisol	$0.35\,(P < 0.001)$	$0.41\,(P < 0.001)$	$0.37\,(P < 0.001)$	$0.44\,(P < 0.001)$

BMI, body mass index (kg/m^2); WHR, waist-to-hip circumference ratio; W, waist circumference (cm); D, abdominal sagittal diameter (cm). Modified from references 67–69.

therapy, is followed by obesity, whereas deficient secretion of cortisol, as in Addison's disease, is followed by anorexia. Moreover, in experimental models, obesity is frequently associated with an elevated adrenal secretion of cortisol, and upon adrenalectomy weight loss is successfully achieved (50).

In previous studies (7,8), the WHR was presumed to reflect an abnormal cortisol secretion, and as seen in Table 23.1, this assumption appears to be valid when the HPA axis is provoked by physiological challenge (lunch) or perceived stress. However, other endocrine perturbations are also involved in the syndrome of visceral obesity, as will be discussed later.

These results may be summarized as follows. Measurements of regional fat distribution by WHR, W or D, when elevated, are sufficient and useful indicators of adaptations of HPA axis activity, particularly when the axis is provoked by external stimuli. The accompanying neuroendocrine changes, however, do not necessarily comprise an elevated total cortisol secretion. Furthermore, the results support the anthropometric measurements (WHR, W, and D) as useful tools for large-scale population and epidemiological studies when HPA axis activity measurements in a clinical setting are not feasible.

In conclusion, the WHR may thus be substituted theoretically by HPA axis abnormalities when interpreting studies where the WHR displays a powerful independent risk factor for mortality and morbidity. In addition, factors related to the WHR such as low socioeconomic status (51,52), alcohol and smoking (53,54), and psychiatric ill health (55–57), may accordingly be substituted by HPA axis perturbations, known to arise after frequently repeated or chronic stress (25).

SUBGROUPING OF VISCERAL OBESITY WITH THE METABOLIC SYNDROME

Visceral obesity is associated with other endocrine abnormalities than that of cortisol. Indeed, visceral obese individuals with the metabolic syndrome may have all the hormonal abnormalities of the elderly, suggesting that this condition may be a sign of premature ageing (58). The most common deficiencies are those of growth hormone (GH) and sex steroids (59). Whereas men have low testosterone levels (60), women have irregular menstrual cycles (61). Functionally, the growth axis and the reproductive axis are influenced at many levels by the HPA axis. Prolonged activation of the HPA axis thus leads to suppression of GH secretion as well as inhibition of sex steroids (23,62).

These endocrine abnormalities have a profound effect on peripheral tissues. While cortisol promotes accumulation of visceral fat and insulin resistance in muscle tissue, the GH and sex steroids, often in concert, do the opposite (42). Low GH and sex steroid secretions will thereby multiply the pathogenetic effects of cortisol. In fact, there is evidence that low concentrations of GH and sex steroids without HPA axis perturbations may cause such effects. As a result, visceral obesity with the metabolic syndrome may originate on the basis of the following endocrine subgroups: one characterized by HPA axis perturbation, the other characterized by low secretion of GH and sex steroid, and finally, a combination of both these events.

This issue was addressed in a recently performed cohort study of middle-aged men (44). Subgroups were constructed based on the current clinical definition of low testosterone and insulin-like growth factor I (IGF-I), a mediator of the major actions of GH (63), and the dexamethasone suppression test as a measurement of the feedback regulation system. In the total cohort of men ($N = 284$), assessments of visceral obesity correlated strongly and consistently with all metabolic parameters except total and low density lipoprotein cholesterol. Furthermore, visceral obesity was found to be associated with elevated blood pressure and heart rate. Identical findings appeared within the subgroup characterized by HPA axis perturbation, defined as a blunted response to dexamethasone. This was also the case in the subgroup characterized by low secretion of testosterone and IGF-I. These results support the concept of endocrine subgrouping of visceral obesity with the metabolic syndrome.

In addition to these analyses, structural equation modelling (path analysis) was performed to examine potential causal models between the endocrine (testosterone and IGF-I), the anthropometric (WHR and D), and selected metabolic measurements (insulin and triglycerides). The results obtained are summarized in Figure 23.1. A blunted response to dexamethasone, that is, a HPA axis characterized by poor feedback regulation, was directly associated with low concentrations of testosterone and IGF-I as well as elevated levels of insulin. Low testosterone and IGF-I in turn was linked to increased WHR and D, and these anthropometric measurements were associated with hyperinsulinaemia, which was related to elevated levels of triglycerides. This chain of events suggests that HPA axis perturbations contribute to the outgrowth of central obesity and insulin resistance. The latter is also further influenced by central obesity measured as WHR or D. Figure 23.1 illustrates the impact of low testosterone and IGF-I on centralization of body fat stores. Thus, input into this chain of events, resulting in metabolic aberrations, may occur at different levels: the HPA axis, isolated testosterone and IGF-I deficiency, or by visceral obesity itself. This interpretation is in excellent agreement with the endocrine subgrouping of the metabolic syndrome as discussed above.

In summary, these findings suggest the possibility

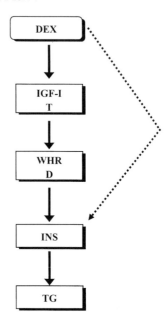

Figure 23.1 Summary of path analyses. DEX, blunted dexamethasone (0.5 mg × 1) suppression of cortisol secretion (nmol/L); IGF-I, insulin-like growth factor I (μg/L); T, testosterone (nmol/L); WHR, waist-to-hip circumference ratio; D, abdominal sagittal diameter (cm); INS, insulin (mU/L); TG, triglycerides (mol/L). Modified from reference 44

that visceral obesity with the metabolic syndrome may originate from other sources than primary perturbations of the HPA axis. For instance, primary deficiency of GH or testosterone might result in the metabolic syndrome; after adequate hormonal replacement therapy, the anthropometric, metabolic and circulatory abnormalities of the metabolic syndrome are successfully restored (64–66). This suggests a causal relationship between such endocrine deficiencies and visceral obesity with the metabolic syndrome.

SUBGROUPING OF THE HPA AXIS PERTURBATIONS

Throughout recently performed studies (67–70), we have been able to single out subgroups of the functional status of the HPA axis within a general population of non-cushingoid middle-aged men. The first group was characterized by a high morning cortisol peak, a normal circadian rhythm (variability) and feedback regulation (dexamethasone) along

Table 23.2 Stages of the hypothalamic-pituitary-adrenal axis status and feedback regulation with peripheral consequences

Stages	Endocrine Status	Feedback regulation	Peripheral consequences
I. Steady-state	Normal	Normal	None
II. Acute stress	High cortisol	Normal	↑ Accumulation of visceral fat ↑ Glucose, fatty acids and triglycerides
III. Repeated stress	High → Low cortisol Normal → Low GH and sex steroids	Normal → Blunted	Visceral obesity Metabolic syndrome Elevated BP
IV. Chronic stress	Low cortisol Low GH and sex steroids	Blunted	Visceral obesity Metabolic syndrome Elevated BP and HR

GH, growth hormone; BP, blood pressure; HR, heart rate.

with a brisk cortisol response to lunch. Such men are in general lean, measured as BMI and WHR, with higher values of IGF-I than average, and low total and low density lipoprotein (LDL) cholesterol as well as blood pressure.

The other group identified was characterized by the absence of a morning cortisol peak and circadian rhythm, a blunted suppression of cortisol by overnight low dose dexamethasone and a poor lunch-induced cortisol response. Such men suffer from obesity with a predominance of centrally located body fat, low testosterone and IGF-I concentrations, high glucose, insulin, triglycerides, total and LDL cholesterol, blood pressures and heart rate, while high density lipoprotein cholesterol is low. These relationships are all highly statistically significant (P values < 0.001), and consistent with the current opinion about the health consequences of an abnormally functioning HPA axis (17). Such men thus have visceral obesity with metabolic syndrome, including hypercholesterolaemia and hypertension. This is in contrast to men with a normal HPA axis function, and further emphasizes the importance of the HPA axis for human health (17,67–70).

In an attempt to highlight the importance of the HPA axis in human health, we performed multidimensional scaling analyses of the anthropometric, metabolic and circulatory risk factors for CVD, type 2 diabetes and stroke (70). Under the influence of an abnormal HPA axis, as described above, all these risk factors congregate into one distinct, strongly intercorrelated cluster (70). This indicates an overriding direct control of the conventional risk factors by such HPA axis perturbations.

STAGES OF THE HPA AXIS FUNCTIONAL STATUS

The above subgroups of the functional status of the HPA axis represent extremes in terms of the resiliency of the HPA axis. Although strongly genetically determined (71), environmental and social factors also affect the circadian rhythm of the HPA axis (72). The question arises whether there are time- and stress-related changes in patterns of HPA axis activity and regulation, and if it is possible to tentatively define stages of such HPA axis affliction. A *first stage* then would be a normal function of the HPA axis, defined as a normal circadian rhythm with high morning and low afternoon–evening cortisol levels, and normal feedback control of GRs. Total cortisol output is regulated within the normal range and this is associated with optimal health. A *second stage* is seen upon acute stress where central regulation of HPA axis rhythm is maintained as well as the feedback control. The growth and reproductive axes are not affected. Cortisol secretion will, however, be elevated with peripheral consequences if prolonged. A *third stage* appears when frequently repeated stress challenges the central regulation of HPA axis function. The GRs will be downregulated (26,73), resulting in a poor feedback control of ACTH and cortisol secretion. The elevated cortisol secretion will then eventually become low. This prolonged activation of the HPA axis will also suppress the GH and sex steroid secretions (23). The peripheral consequences will now be a full-blown metabolic syndrome. A *fourth and final stage* is that of chronic stress, with a 'burn-out' of central regulatory systems (25,26,74), resulting in a net decrease of cortisol output and inhibition of other endocrine axes resulting in a metabolic syndrome. These stages are summarized in Table 23.2.

GENETIC ASPECTS

As discussed above, the glucocorticoid feedback effects exerted on the pituitary and the hippocampus become blunted during stages III and IV. The feedback is initiated by binding of steroid to regulatory gene elements (75), and the feedback suppression is mediated by glucocorticoid receptors (GR) in the hippocampus (25,26). Studies *in vivo*, and *in vitro*, in cells from chronically stressed rats, have shown that the sensitivity of the HPA axis to inhibition by cortisol is impaired (76,77). When the HPA axis is subjected to prolonged elevation of cortisol levels as in chronic stress, the GRs gradually loses their function, ending up in a presumably irreversible neurodegenerative condition (74). Such hippocampal damage has been observed in individuals with Cushing's syndrome (78), a condition also characterized by hypercortisolism.

A dose–response study of inhibition by dexamethasone administration has shown that feedback regulation in subjects with visceral obesity is diminished (33), in parallel with a blunted function of GR in adipose tissue (Ottosson *et al.*, unpublished data). The latter study indicates the possibilities of both a decreased responsiveness and sensitivity of the GRs. Consequently, the GR gene (GRL), located in chromosome 5 and consisting of 10 exons with a minimum size of 80 kilobases (kb) (79), has been partially sequenced. However, no abnormalities in the DNA-binding (exon 2) or steroid binding (exon 9) domains of the GRL have been revealed (unpublished data). Nevertheless, the recent discovery that a *Bcl*I GRL polymorphism is associated with elevated cortisol concentrations in response to metabolic stress has raised the possibility that mutations may decrease the sensitivity to cortisol feedback (46). With the restriction enzyme *Bcl*I two alleles with fragment lengths of 4.5 and 2.3 kb are discoverable. The 4.5 kb allele is known to be associated with visceral obesity and insulin resistance (80,81). Furthermore, individuals carrying the 4.5 kb allele have higher leptin values (46). While the *Bcl*I restriction enzyme cleaves the GRL in the first intron the functional role of the polymorphism, if

any, is uncertain. However, a polymorphism in an intron may interfere with splicing of primary mRNA or serves as an index for functionally important polymorphisms in neighbouring gene domains, including the promotor region. With the restriction enzyme *Tth*III1, a variant of the 5'-flanking region of the GRL is discoverable as two alleles with fragment lengths of 3.4 and 3.8 kb (82). Individuals carrying the 3.8 kb allele have higher total and evening cortisol levels with trends for elevated levels over the day (82). This polymorphism is localized in the 5'-flanking region of the GRL gene locus, probably in the promotor region of the gene, and may therefore be involved in the regulation of GR density.

HYPERTENSION

Hypertension is closely related to the metabolic syndrome (43,83), and since hypertension is statistically associated with insulin (84), several authors have postulated that hyperinsulinaemia is related to blood pressure independently of body fat mass (85–87). However, hyperinsulinaemia is not found in all obese subjects and not all hypertensive subjects are obese (88). Recent studies have revealed that visceral obesity and HPA axis perturbations are independently related to blood pressure, and that insulin and insulin resistance may account for only a part of this association (89). This suggests that hypertension with accompanying, observed increases in heart rate may have a central origin. Although the pathophysiology of essential hypertension is still unclear, it is generally accepted that activation of the central sympathetic nervous system can increase blood pressure (90,91). We have suggested that the simultaneous activation of the sympathetic nervous system and the HPA axis might be mediated via a common arousal of hypothalamic centres (69). Such a hypothalamic arousal syndrome may provide an excitatory influence on both the sympathetic nervous system, resulting in hypertension, and the HPA axis, resulting in visceral obesity with the metabolic syndrome. This would explain the statistical relationship between hypertension and insulin resistance as well as the kinds of metabolic abnormalities that result.

ENVIRONMENTAL FACTORS INFLUENCING THE HPA AXIS

This overview has explored the pathophysiological consequences of an evoked, excessive perturbation of one of the principal axes of neuroendocrine response in the human body. In the following section, the environmental factors that influence the HPA axis will be reviewed.

A common, powerful group of activators are those included under the concept of stress. The origin of the concept of stress in biology and medicine is unknown. Investigations of stress rise from the recognition by Claude Bernard in 1878 that all living processes exist in a 'milieu interieur', formed by organic liquid that surrounds all of the tissue elements. Cannon elucidated the mechanisms of maintaining physiological factors within certain limits and coined the term 'homeostasis' and defined it as 'the coordinated physiological process which maintains most of the steady states in the organisms' (92). He describes a 'critical stress' level that produces a 'breaking strain' that results in failure to maintain homeostasis, and he adopts the terms 'stress' and 'strain' as they are used in physics. Selye extended Cannon's concept of homeostasis to include the responses mediated by the HPA axis and proposed a new concept of stress, 'general adaptation syndrome, or GAS'; a single stereotypic response elicited by any demand upon the body (93). For scientific purpose, he defined stress 'as the state which manifests itself by the GAS'.

As the homeostasis is constantly threatened by internal or external adverse factors, stressors, stress is usually defined as a state of threatened homeostasis (17). There are physical stressors such as cold, trauma, fever and infection; psychological stressors such as social subordination, anxiety and depression (94).

Traits of anxiety and depression have a predictive association with visceral obesity in both men and women (55,56). Furthermore, alcohol consumption and smoking are common among subjects with elevated WHR (51,52). In addition, we have recently identified a number of psychosocial and socioeconomic handicaps in this condition (51,52). The most prominent factors are divorce, solitude, poor economy and low education, unemployment, and problems at work when employed. Interestingly, socioeconomic inequality and low educational have

recently been shown to be associated with elevated stress-related cortisol secretion as well as visceral obesity (95). Moreover, we have identified a subgroup of elevated WHR and D, where a blunted dexamethasone response is found, associated with traits of anxiety and depression as well as personality disorders (57,96).

It has been suggested that persistent psychosocial and socioeconomic handicaps constitute a base for stress, resulting in frequent challenges of the HPA axis (43). Although biologically plausible, this hypothesis has been difficult to study in humans. In primates other than humans, a diminished feedback regulation of the cortisol secretion, suppression of the reproductive axis, and depressive behaviour follow exposure to standardized, moderate psychosocial stress (97,98). Moreover, such social stress is associated with visceral obesity, insulin resistance, dyslipidaemia, hypertension and coronary artery atherosclerosis (97,98). Thus, these results bear a striking resemblance to that of humans subjected to psychosocial stress, followed by visceral obesity with metabolic syndrome. These studies then provide a solid experimental groundwork for the hypothesis that psychosocial stress and socioeconomic subordination is indeed inducing the metabolic syndrome.

CONCLUSIONS

The concept of a neuroendocrine background to visceral obesity and the metabolic syndrome has been confirmed and strengthened considerably as well as modified by the recently obtained results presented in this overview. Above all, the multiple features of this syndrome have been possible to describe in terms of stages of the HPA axis perturbations and other associated endocrine abnormalities. A truly striking end result is the powerful interaction of the HPA axis with human health and disease (99). Visceral obesity has a remarkable predictive power for prevalent diseases such as type 2 diabetes, CVD, stroke, gallbladder disease, sleep apnoea, hypertension, dyslipidaemia and insulin resistance (relative risk ≥ 3).

Psychosocial and socioeconomic impairments are most likely important triggers for the perturbations of the HPA axis observed, and may have a particularly strong impact on individuals with a predisposing genetical vulnerability.

REFERENCES

1. Kretschmer E. *Physique and Character*. New York: Harcourt, 1936. (Originally published in German, 1921.)

2. Vague J. La differenciation sexuelle, facteur déterminant des formes d'obésité. *Presse Méd* 1947; **55**: 339–341.

3. Krotkiewski M, Björntorp P, Sjöström L, Smith U. Impact of obesity on metabolism in men and women. Importance of regional adipose tissue distribution. *J Clin Invest* 1983; **72**: 1150–1162.

4. Kissebah AH, Vydelingum N, Murray R, Evans DJ, Hartz AJ, Kalkhoff RK, *et al*. Relation of body fat distribution to metabolic complications of obesity. *J Clin Endocrinol Metab* 1982; **54**: 254–260.

5. Björntorp P. The associations between obesity, adipose tissue distribution and disease. *Acta Med Scand Suppl* 1987; **723**: 121–134.

6. Kissebah AH, Krakower GR. Regional adiposity and morbidity. *Physiol Rev* 1994; **74**: 761–811.

7. Larsson B, Svärdsudd K, Welin L, Wilhelmsen L, Björntorp P, Tibblin G. Abdominal adipose tissue distribution, obesity, and risk of cardiovascular disease and death: 13 year follow up of participants in the study of men born 1913. *Br Med J* 1984; **288**: 1401–1404.

8. Lapidus L, Bengtsson C, Larsson B, Pennert K, Rybo E, Sjöström L. Distribution of adipose tissue and risk of cardiovascular disease and death: a 12 year follow up of participants in the population study of women in Gothenburg, Sweden. *Br Med J* 1984; **289**: 1257–1261.

9. Lapidus L, Helgesson O, Merck C, Björntorp P. Adipose tissue distribution and female carcinomas. A 12-year follow-up of participants in the population study of women in Gothenburg, Sweden. *Int J Obes* 1988; **12**: 361–368.

10. Schapira DV, Clark RA, Wolff PA, Jarrett AR, Kumar NB, Aziz NM. Visceral obesity and breast cancer risk. *Cancer* 1994; **74**: 632–639.

11. Pi-Sunyer FX. Comorbidities of overweight and obesity: current evidence and research issues. *Med Sci Sports Exerc* 1999; **31** (11 Suppl): S602–608.

12. Grunstein R, Wilcox I, Yang TS, Gould Y, Hedner J. Snoring and sleep apnoea in men: association with central obesity and hypertension. *Int J Obes Relat Metab Disord* 1993; **17**: 533–540.

13. Bray GA. Complications of obesity. *Ann Intern Med* 1985; **103**: 1052–1062.

14. Björntorp P. Abdominal obesity and the development of noninsulin-dependent diabetes mellitus. *Diabetes Metab Rev* 1988; **4**: 615–622.

15. Mårin P, Darin N, Amemiya T, Andersson B, Jern S, Björntorp P. Cortisol secretion in relation to body fat distribution in obese premenopausal women. *Metabolism* 1992; **41**: 882–886.

16. Pasquali R, Cantobelli S, Casimirri F, Capelli M, Bortoluzzi L, Flamia R, *et al*. The hypothalamic-pituitary-adrenal axis in obese women with different patterns of body fat distribution. *J Clin Endocrinol Metab* 1993; **77**: 341–346.

17. Chrousos GP, Gold PW. A healthy body in a healthy mind—and vice versa—the damaging power of 'uncontrollable' stress. *J Clin Endocrinol Metab* 1998; **83**: 1842–1845.

18. Kiss A, Skultetyova I, Jezova D. Corticotropin-releasing hormone synthesizing neurons in the hypothalamic paraventricular nucleus of rats neonatally treated with monosodium glutamate can respond to different stress paradigms. *Neurol Res* 1999; **21**: 775–780.

19. Chrousos GP. Ultradian, circadian, and stress-related hypothalamic-pituitary-adrenal axis activity—a dynamic digital-to-analog modulation. *Endocrinology* 1998; **139**: 437–440.

20. Bernardis LL, Bellinger LL. The dorsomedial hypothalamic nucleus revisited: 1998 update. *Proc Soc Exp Biol Med* 1998; **218**: 284–306.

21. Fuller RW. The involvement of serotonin in regulation of pituitary-adrenocortical function. *Front Neuroendocrinol* 1992; **13**: 250–270.

22. Al-Damluji S. Adrenergic control of the secretion of anterior pituitary hormones. Baillière's *Clin Endocrinol Metab* 1993; **7**: 355–392.

23. Chrousos GP. Stressors, stress, and neuroendocrine integration of the adaptive response. The 1997 Hans Selye Memorial Lecture. *Ann N Y Acad Sci* 1998; **851**: 311–335.

24. Jacobson L, Sapolsky R. The role of the hippocampus in feedback regulation of the hypothalamic- pituitary-adrenocortical axis. *Endocr Rev* 1991; **12**: 118–134.

25. McEwen BS. Protective and damaging effects of stress mediators. *N Engl J Med* 1998; **338**: 171–179.

26. McEwen BS. Stress and the aging hippocampus. *Front Neuroendocrinol* 1999; **20**: 49–70.

27. Cook N, Harris B, Walker R, Hailwood R, Jones E, Johns S, *et al*. Clinical utility of the dexamethasone suppression test assessed by plasma and salivary cortisol determinations. *Psychiatry Res* 1986; **18**: 143–150.

28. Kahn JP, Rubinow DR, Davis C, Kling M, Post RM. Salivary cortisol: a practical method for evaluation of adrenal function. *Biol Psychiatry* 1988; **33**: 335–349.

29. Aardal-Eriksson E, Karlberg BE, Holm AC. Salivary cortisol—an alternative to serum cortisol determinations in dynamic function tests. *Clin Chem Lab Med* 1998; **36**: 215–222.

30. Castro M, Elias PC, Quidute AR, Halah FP, Moreira AC. Out-patient screening for Cushing's syndrome: the sensitivity of the combination of circadian rhythm and overnight dexamethasone suppression salivary cortisol tests. *J Clin Endocrinol Metab* 1999; **84**: 878–882.

31. Kirschbaum C, Hellhammer DH. Salivary cortisol in psychoneuroendocrine research: recent developments and applications. *Psychoneuroendocrinology* 1994; **19**: 313–333.

32. Liddle GW. Tests of pituitary-adrenal suppressibility in the diagnosis of Cushing's syndrome. *J Clin Endocrinol Metab* 1960; **20**: 1539–1560.

33. Ljung T, Andersson B, Bengtsson Å, Björntorp P, Mårin P. Inhibition of cortisol secretion by dexamethasone in relation to body fat distribution: a dose-response study. *Obes Res* 1996; **4**: 277–282.

34. Kirschbaum C, Hellhammer DH. Salivary cortisol in psychobiological research: an overview. *Neuropsychobiology* 1989; **22**: 150–169.

35. Sternberg EM. Neural-immune interactions in health and disease. *J Clin Invest* 1997; **100**: 2641–2647.

36. Duprez D, De Buyzere M, Paelinck M, Rubens R, Dhooge W, Clement DL. Relationship between left ventricular mass index and 24-h urinary free cortisol and cortisone in essential

arterial hypertension. *J Hypertens* 1999; **17**: 1583–1588.

37. Kaji DM, Thakkar U, Kahn T. Glucocorticoid-induced alterations in the sodium potassium pump of the human erythrocyte. *J Clin Invest* 1981; **68**: 422–430.

38. Noda Y, Yamada K, Igic R, Erdos EG. Regulation of rat urinary and renal kallikrein and prekallikrein by corticosteroids. *Proc Natl Acad Sci U S A* 1983; **80**: 3059–3063.

39. Lönn L, Kvist H, Ernest I, Sjöström L. Changes in body composition and adipose tissue distribution after treatment of women with Cushing's Syndrome. *Metabolism* 1994; **43**: 1517–1522.

40. Fried SK, Russell CD, Grauso NL, Brolin RE. Lipoprotein lipase regulation by insulin and glucocorticoid in subcutaneous and omental adipose tissue of obese women and men. *J Clin Invest* 1993; **92**: 2191–2198.

41. Ottosson M, Vikman-Adolfsson K, Enerbäck S, Olivecrona G, Björntorp P. The effects of cortisol on the regulation of lipoprotein lipase activity in human adipose tissue. *J Clin Endocrinol Metab* 1994; **79**: 820–825.

42. Björntorp P, Rosmond R. Visceral obesity and diabetes. *Drugs* 1999; **58** (Suppl 1): 13–18.

43. Björntorp P. Visceral obesity: a 'civilization syndrome'. *Obes Res* 1993; **1**: 206–222.

44. Rosmond R, Björntorp P. The interactions between hypothalamic-pituitary-adrenal axis activity, testosterone, insulin-like growth factor I and abdominal obesity with metabolism and blood pressure in men. *Int J Obes Relat Metab Disord* 1998; **22**: 1184–1196.

45. Considine RV, Sinha MK, Heiman ML, Kriauciunas A, Stephens TW, Nyce MR, *et al.* Serum immunoreactive-leptin concentrations in normal-weight and obese humans. *N Engl J Med* 1996; **334**: 292–295.

46. Rosmond R, Chagnon YC, Holm G, Chagnon M, Pérusse L, Lindell K, *et al.* A glucocorticoid receptor gene marker is associated with abdominal obesity, leptin and dysregulation of the hypothalamic-pituitary-adrenal axis. *Obes Res* 2000; **8**: 211–218.

47. Zakrzewska KE, Cusin I, Sainsbury A, Rohner-Jeanrenaud F, Jeanrenaud B. Glucocorticoids as counterregulatory hormones of leptin: towards an understanding of leptin resistance. *Diabetes* 1997; **46**: 717–719.

48. Cizza G, Lotsikas AJ, Licinio J, Gold PW, Chrousos GP. Plasma leptin levels do not change in patients with Cushing's disease shortly after correction of hypercortisolism. *J Clin Endocrinol Metab* 1997; **82**: 2747–2750.

49. Newcomer JW, Selke G, Melson AK, Gross J, Vogler GP, Dagogo-Jack S. Dose-dependent cortisol-induced increases in plasma leptin concentration in healthy humans. *Arch Gen Psychiatry* 1998; **55**: 995–1000.

50. York DA. Peripheral and central mechanisms regulating food intake and macronutrient selection. *Obes Surg* 1999; **9**: 471–479.

51. Rosmond R, Lapidus L, Björntorp P. The influence of occupational and social factors on obesity and body fat distribution in middle-aged men. *Int J Obes Relat Metab Disord* 1996; **20**: 599–607.

52. Rosmond R, Björntorp P. Psychosocial and socio-economic factors in women and their relationship to obesity and regional body fat distribution. *Int J Obes Relat Metab Disord* 1999; **23**: 138–145.

53. Kvist H, Hallgren P, Jönsson L, Pettersson P, Sjöberg C, Sjöström L, Björntorp P. Distribution of adipose tissue and muscle mass in alcoholic men. *Metabolism* 1993; **42**: 569–573.

54. Samaras K, Campbell LV. The non-genetic determinants of central adiposity. *Int J Obes Relat Metab Disord* 1997; **21**: 839–845.

55. Rosmond R, Lapidus L, Mårin P, Björntorp P. Mental distress, obesity and body fat distribution in middle-aged men. *Obes Res* 1996; **4**: 245–252.

56. Rosmond R, Björntorp P. Psychiatric ill-health of women and its relationship to obesity and body fat distribution. *Obes Res* 1998; **6**: 338–345.

57. Rosmond R, Björntorp P. Endocrine and metabolic aberrations in men with abdominal obesity in relation to anxiodepressive infirmity. *Metabolism* 1998; **47**: 1187–1193.

58. Björntorp P, Rosmond R. Perturbations of the hypothalamic-pituitary-adrenal axis and the metabolic syndrome in ageing. *Growth Horm IGF Res* 1999; **9** (Suppl A): 121–123.

59. Björntorp P, Holm G, Rosmond R. The pathogenesis of the metabolic syndrome. In: Ailhaud G and Guy-Grand B (eds) *Progress in Obesity Research*, vol. 8. London: John Libbey, 1999: 555–565.

60. Seidell JC, Björntorp P, Sjöström L, Kvist H, Sannerstedt R. Visceral fat accumulation in men is positively associated with insulin, glucose, and C-peptide levels, but negatively with testosterone levels. *Metabolism* 1990; **39**: 897–901.

61. Björntorp P. The android woman—a risky condition. *J Intern Med* 1996; **239**: 105–110.

62. Ono N, Samson WK, McDonald JK, Lumpkin MD, Bedran de Castro JC, McCann SM. Effects of intravenous and intraventricular injection of antisera directed against corticotropin-releasing factor on the secretion of anterior pituitary hormones. *Proc Natl Acad Sci U S A* 1985; **82**: 7787–7790.

63. Lee PD, Durham SK, Martinez V, Vasconez O, Powell DR, Guevara-Aguirre J. Kinetics of insulin-like growth factor (IGF) and IGF-binding protein responses to a single dose of growth hormone. *J Clin Endocrinol Metab* 1997; **82**: 2266–2274.

64. Mårin P, Holmäng S, Gustafsson G, Jönsson L, Kvist H, Elander A, *et al.* Androgen treatment of abdominally obese men. *Obes Res* 1993; **1**: 245–251.

65. Johannsson G, Mårin P, Lönn L, Ottosson M, Stenlöf K, Björntorp P, *et al.* Growth hormone treatment of abdominally obese men reduces abdominal fat mass, improves glucose and lipoprotein metabolism, and reduces diastolic blood pressure. *J Clin Endocrinol Metab* 1997; **82**: 727–734.

66. Tibblin G, Adlerberth A, Lindstedt G, Björntorp P. The pituitary-gonadal axis and health in elderly men: a study of men born in 1913. *Diabetes* 1996; **45**: 1605–1609.

67. Rosmond R, Dallman MF, Björntorp P. Stress-related cortisol secretion in men: relationships with abdominal obesity and endocrine, metabolic and hemodynamic abnormalities. *J Clin Endocrinol Metab* 1998; **83**: 1853–1859.

68. Rosmond R, Holm G, Björntorp P. Food-induced cortisol secretion in relation to anthropometric, metabolic and hemodynamic variables in men. *Int J Obes Relat Metab Disord* 2000; **24**: 416–422.

69. Björntorp P, Holm G, Rosmond R. Hypothalamic arousal, insulin resistance and Type 2 diabetes mellitus. *Diabet Med* 1999; **16**: 373–383.

70. Rosmond R, Björntorp P. The hypothalamic-pituitary-ad-

renal axis activity as a predictor of cardiovascular disease, Type 2 diabetes and stroke. *J Intern Med* **248**: 239–244.

71. Linkowski P, Van Onderbergen A, Kerkhofs M, Bosson D, Mendlewicz J, Van Cauter E. Twin study of the 24-h cortisol profile: evidence for genetic control of the human circadian clock. *Am J Physiol* 1993; **264**: E173–181.

72. Dallman MF. Stress update. Adaptation of the hypo-thalamic-pituitary-adrenal axis to chronic stress. *Trends Endocrinol Metab* 1993; **4**: 62–69.

73. Sapolsky RM, Krey LC, McEwen BS. Stress down-regulates corticosterone receptors in a site-specific manner in the brain. Endocrinology 1984; **114**: 287–292.

74. Uno H, Eisele S, Sakai A, Shelton S, Baker E, DeJesus O, *et al.* Neurotoxicity of glucocorticoids in the primate brain. *Horm Behav* 1994; **28**: 336–348.

75. Dayanithi G, Antoni FA. Rapid as well as delayed inhibitory effects of glucocorticoid hormones on pituitary adrenocor-ticotropic hormone release are mediated by type II glucocor-ticoid receptors and require newly synthesized messenger ribonucleic acid as well as protein. *Endocrinology* 1989; **125**: 308–313.

76. Young EA, Akil H. Paradoxical effect of corticosteroids on pituitary ACTH/β-endorphin release in stressed animals. *Psychoneuroendocrinology* 1988; **13**: 317–323.

77. Dallman MF, Akana SF, Scribner KA, Bradbury MJ, Walker C-D, Strack AM, *et al.* Stress, feedback and facili-tation in the hypothalamo-pituitary-adrenal axis. *J Neuroendocrinol* 1992; **4**: 517–526.

78. Starkman MN, Gebarski SS, Berent S, Schteingart DE. Hip-pocampal formation volume, memory dysfunction, and cor-tisol levels in patients with Cushing's syndrome. *Biol Psychiatry* 1992; **32**: 756–765.

79. Encio IJ, Detera-Wadleigh SD. The genomic structure of the human glucocorticoid receptor. *J Biol Chem* 1991; **266**: 7182–7188.

80. Weaver JU, Hitman GA, Kopelman PG. An association between a BclI restriction fragment length polymorphism of the glucocorticoid receptor locus and hyperinsu-linaemia in obese women. *J Mol Endocrinol* 1992; **9**: 295–300.

81. Buemann B, Vohl M-C, Chagnon M, Chagnon YC, Gagnon J, Pérusse L, *et al.* Abdominal visceral fat is associated with a BclI restriction fragment length polymorphism at the glucocorticoid receptor gene locus. *Obes Res* 1997; **5**: 186–192.

82. Rosmond R, Chagnon YC, Chagnon M, Pérusse L, Bouchard C, Björntorp P. A polymorphism on the 5′-flank-ing region of the glucocorticoid receptor gene locus is asso-ciated with basal secretion of cortisol in men. *Metabolism*

2000; **49**: 1197–1199.

83. Reaven GM. Banting lecture 1988. Role of insulin resistance in human disease. *Diabetes* 1988; **37**: 1595–1607.

84. Reisin E, Messerli FG, Ventura HO, Frohlich ED. Renal haemodynamic studies in obesity hypertension. *J Hypertens* 1987; **5**: 397–400.

85. Modan M, Halkin H, Almog S, Lusky A, Eshkol A, Shefi M, *et al.* Hyperinsulinemia. A link between hypertension obesity and glucose intolerance. *J Clin Invest* 1985; **75**: 809–817.

86. Haffner SM, Miettinen H, Gaskill SP, Stern MP. Metabolic precursors of hypertension. The San Antonio Heart Study. *Arch Intern Med* 1996; **156**: 1994–2000.

87. Fagot-Campagna A, Balkau B, Simon D, Ducimetière P, Eschwège E. Is insulin an independent risk factor for hyper-tension? The Paris Prospective Study. *Int J Epidemiol* 1997; **26**: 542–550.

88. Schmidt MI, Watson RL, Duncan BB, Metcalf, P, Brancati FL, Sharrett AR, *et al.* Clustering of dyslipidemia, hy-peruricemia, diabetes, and hypertension and its association with fasting insulin and central and overall obesity in a general population. *Metabolism* 1996; **45**: 699–706.

89. Rosmond R, Björntorp P. Blood pressure in relation to obesity, insulin and the hypothalamic-pituitary-adrenal axis in Swedish men. *J Hypertens* 1998; **16**: 1721–1726.

90. Henry JP. Biological basis of the stress response. *Integr Physiol Behav Sci* 1992; **27**: 66–83.

91. Folkow B. Physiological organization of neurohormonal responses to psychosocial stimuli: implications for health and disease. *Ann Behav Med* 1993; **15**: 236–244.

92. Cannon WB. *The Wisdom of the Body.* New York: WW Norton, 1939.

93. Selye H. *The Stress of Life.* New York: McGraw Hill, 1956.

94. McEwen BS, Stellar E. Stress and the individual. Mechanism leading to disease. *Arch Intern Med* 1993; **153**: 2093–2101.

95. Rosmond R, Björntorp P. Occupational status, cortisol se-cretory pattern and visceral obesity in middle-aged men. *Obes Res* 2000; **8**: 445–450.

96. Rosmond R, Eriksson E, Björntorp P. Personality disorders in relation to anthropometric, endocrine and metabolic fac-tors. *J Endocrinol Invest* 1999; **22**: 279–288.

97. Jayo JM, Shively CA, Kaplan JR, Manuck SB. Effects of exercise and stress on body fat distribution in male cynomol-gus monkeys. *Int J Obes Relat Metab Disord* 1993; **17**: 597–604.

98. Shively CA, Laber-Laird K, Anton RF. Behavior and physi-ology of social stress and depression in female cynomolgus monkeys. *Biol Psychiatry* 1997; **41**: 871–882.

99. Björntorp P, Rosmond R. Hypothalamic origin of the meta-bolic syndrome X. *Ann N Y Acad Sci* 1999; **892**: 297–307.

24

Obesity and Type 2 Diabetes Mellitus

Allison M. Hodge, Maximilian P. de Courten and Paul Zimmet

International Diabetes Institute, Caulfield, Victoria, Australia

INTRODUCTION

Obesity has reached epidemic proportions globally, and all evidence suggests that the situation is likely to get worse (1). In developed regions such as Europe (2), the USA (3), and Australia (4,5) the prevalence is high and increasing but in some developing countries even more extreme situations exist (6,7). Coincident with the high rates of obesity, the prevalence of type 2 (non-insulin-dependent) diabetes is also escalating, and this increase is expected to continue, so that by the year 2010 it is predicted that a total of 216 million people worldwide will have type 2 diabetes (8).

Obesity and type 2 diabetes are lifestyle-related conditions and it seems likely that changes in diet and physical activity associated with increased affluence can influence diabetes risk both directly, and indirectly through obesity. The link between degree of obesity and diabetes that has been observed may be complicated by other factors such as duration of obesity, body fat distribution, physical activity, age, diet composition, ethnicity, genetic susceptibility to type 2 diabetes and obesity, weight loss associated with diabetes, and possibly fetal and early infant growth rate; many of which can be considered risk factors for obesity as well as contributing to type 2 diabetes risk independently of

obesity. Thus at any level of obesity, the degree to which other risk factors for type 2 diabetes contribute will determine the overall risk of developing, and the age of onset of, diabetes.

To estimate the effects of obesity on type 2 diabetes it is necessary that the influence of the above mentioned factors are understood, and that a standardized definition is used for obesity and diabetes.

What is Obesity?

Obesity may be simply defined as the degree of body fat storage associated with elevated health risks (1). Due to the difficulties of measuring body fat under field conditions the practical definition of obesity for adults is based on body mass index (BMI) (1). It should be noted that adult BMI cut-points are not considered appropriate for children. Body mass index, also known as Quetelet's index, is calculated as an individual's weight (kg)/height^2 (m^2).

Various cut-points and measures of obesity have been used in the past, but a World Health Organization (WHO) consultation on obesity proposed a system of classification based on BMI (1) (Table 24.1), which is similar to classifications used in a number of past studies.

International Textbook of Obesity. Edited by Per Björntorp.
© 2001 John Wiley & Sons, Ltd.

Table 24.1 BMI classification in adults

Classification	BMI kg/m²)	Risk of comorbities
Underweight	< 18.5	Low (but increased risk of other clinical problems)
Normal range	18.5–24.9	Average
Overweight	≥ 25.0	
Pre-obese	25.0–29.9	Increased
Obese class I	30.0–34.9	Moderate
Obese class II	25.0–39.9	Severe
Obese class III	≥ 40.0	Very severe

Measuring Body Fat Distribution

Compared with subcutaneous adipose tissue, abdominal adipose tissue is more strongly linked to metabolic changes, including insulin resistance and glucose intolerance. The contribution of abdominal and subcutaneous adipose tissue to central obesity cannot be sufficiently determined using only anthropometric methods. Nonetheless, variations in anthropometrically evaluated body fat distribution contribute to the risk of cardiovascular disease (9–12) and type 2 diabetes (13–24) independent of overall obesity.

A number of methods have been used to assess body fat distribution, including subscapular/triceps skinfold ratio, waist/hip circumference ratio, waist/thigh circumference ratio, and more recently waist circumference alone. The preference for circumference measurements over skinfolds reflects the difficulty of reliably measuring skinfolds, especially in obese individuals. Waist-to-hip ratio (WHR) has now been accepted as a means of assessing abdominal fat distribution clinically and in epidemiological surveys. Cut-points indicating high risk vary between studies but commonly used criteria, at least for Caucasians, are WHR ≥ 1.0 in men and ≥ 0.85 in women (1). It is unlikely that universal cut-points for waist circumference will be developed due to variations between ethnic groups in the risk associated with a particular measurement (1). In a study of Dutch men and women the following waist measurements were found to be associated with a substantially increased risk of metabolic complications: ≥ 102 cm in men or ≥ 88 cm in women (1). Waist circumference can be used as a screening tool for identifying individuals at risk of obesity-related illness (1). It is also preferred to WHR for tracking changes in an individual over time, as WHR is less strongly correlated to weight change, and may in fact increase with weight loss in certain subgroups (smokers, black vs. white men, and anyone with WHR below the median at baseline) (25).

It is important when using circumference measurements that standard anatomical locations are used. The WHO (26) recommends the following methods.

Abdominal Circumference

The subject stands with feet 25–30 cm apart, weight evenly distributed. Measurement is taken midway between the inferior margin of the last rib and the crest of the ilium in a horizontal plane. The measurer sits by the side of the subject and fits the tape snugly but not compressing soft tissues. Circumference is measured to nearest 0.1 cm.

Hip (Buttocks) Circumference

Wearing only non-restrictive briefs or underwear, or a light smock over underwear, the subject stands erect with arms at the sides and feet together. The measurer sits at the side of the subject so that the level of the maximum extension of the buttocks can be seen, and places the tape measure around the buttocks in a horizontal plane. The tape is held snugly but not compressing soft tissues. Circumference is measured to the nearest 0.1 cm.

RISK FACTORS FOR TYPE 2 DIABETES

Table 24.2 presents the known modifiable and non-modifiable risk factors or aetiological determinants associated with type 2 diabetes (27). The overall risk of type 2 diabetes must be assessed on the basis of all of these. Because of the additive effect of different risk factors and determinants, individuals with high levels of non-obesity risk may develop type 2 diabetes without becoming obese, while in other cases obesity alone may be sufficient to lead to diabetes. Generalized and central obesity are just two of the interrelated risk factors associated with type 2 diabetes, and of the modifiable lifestyle factors are probably the most important in terms of size and consistency of effect.

Table 24.2 Aetiological determinants and risk factors of type 2 diabetes

A. Genetic factors
Genetic markers, family history, thrifty gene hypothesis etc.

B. Demographic determinants
Sex, age, ethnicity

C. Behavioural and lifestyle-related risk factors
Obesity (including distribution of obesity, duration)
Physical inactivity
Diet
Stress
Urban lifestyle

D. Metabolic determinants and intermediate risk categories of type 2 diabetes
Impaired glucose tolerance, impaired fasting glucose
Insulin resistance
Other components of the metabolic syndrome
Pregnancy-related determinants (parity, gestational diabetes, diabetes in offspring of women with diabetes during pregnancy, intrauterine environment)

Obesity and Type 2 Diabetes

The association between obesity and type 2 diabetes has been observed in both cross-sectional (13–19, 28–33) and prospective studies (20–23, 31,34–38) across various populations. Obesity confers a minimum 3- to 10-fold risk of type 2 diabetes (39) and it is estimated that type 2 diabetes risk could be reduced by 50–75% by control of obesity (40). Weight loss associated with the onset of diabetes (36,41) means that the association of obesity with type 2 diabetes prevalence is generally weaker than its association with incidence. For example, in an Israeli study, the main determinant of the incidence of type 2 diabetes over a 10-year study period was the BMI at baseline, rather than the BMI at follow-up when glucose tolerance was measured (38). Incident impaired glucose tolerance was associated with both concurrent and prior BMI, as would be expected if weight loss only occurs after glucose tolerance has deteriorated to frank diabetes.

In a study of Pima Indians baseline BMI was also strongly related to the incidence of type 2 diabetes but there was little association between diabetes prevalence and concurrent obesity (42). In a small subgroup of subjects of that study with BMI data from 4 years before diagnosis to 2 years after, there was a clear pattern of weight gain preceding diag-nosis, followed by weight loss after diagnosis. Older participants developed diabetes at a lower BMI than younger individuals, suggesting that age-related deterioration in insulin sensitivity enables the development of diabetes at lower levels of adiposity than required for the development of diabetes in younger subjects.

In contrast to the results in Pima Indians, Tai *et al.* (31) found that BMI was similarly associated with the prevalence or 4-year cumulative incidence of diabetes, with odds ratios of 1.12 and 1.14 respectively for a 1 unit increase in BMI in slim (mean BMI 23 kg/m^2) Chinese.

If diagnosis is made early in the natural history of diabetes before weight loss occurs it could be expected that a stronger positive association between BMI and prevalent type 2 diabetes would be observed.

The Importance of Duration and Changes in Obesity for Risk of Type 2 Diabetes

Although the duration of obesity is considered important in determining the risk of obesity associated conditions, including type 2 diabetes, there is little information available to quantify this relationship. Even in most prospective studies that actual onset of obesity is not measured and can only be estimated by recall. Moreover, if weight is changing it is difficult to differentiate between the effects of the degree and duration of obesity.

In the above mentioned large study in Israel, Modan *et al.* (38) found that obesity lasting for less than 10 years was not associated with a major increase in diabetes incidence compared with that in subjects who had remained slim (BMI < 23 kg/m^2). The risk of type 2 diabetes was increased in subjects who had lost weight to reach a specific BMI class relative to those who had remained stable within that class, while those with a stable BMI had in turn a greater risk of type 2 diabetes than those who had increased their BMI class, indicating that weight gain per se was not associated with increased risk of type 2 diabetes (38). Similar results were observed in the multiethnic population of Mauritius. For any level of BMI at 5 years of follow-up, the highest prevalence of type 2 diabetes was associated with weight loss since baseline, and the lowest with weight gain, while those whose weight had remained stable had an intermediate risk. Comparing the weight gainers with weight maintainers in both studies suggests that the stable group were at greater risk due to their longer duration at the higher current BMI.

In one of the few reports to actually examine the levels of glucose tolerance associated with different duration of self-reported obesity (based on percentage of standard weight ranging from 14 to 137% overweight), Ogilvie (43) observed that it took 5 to 18 years of obesity for glucose intolerance to develop, and 12 to 38 years for diabetes to occur. In contrast to other studies, the degree of obesity was not associated with glucose tolerance. In a more recent study, Felber *et al.* (44,45) examined fasting plasma glucose levels and glucose storage capacity in relation to obesity duration cross-sectionally in 67 moderately obese subjects (mean ideal body weight $150 \pm 3\%$). Participants with a duration of obesity less than 17 years generally had low fasting glucose concentrations and high rates of glucose uptake, while beyond this time fasting glucose began to increase and glucose storage capacity to fall. The time when fasting glucose began to rise and glucose uptake declined was considered the onset of type 2 diabetes; thus the results were interpreted as showing that at least 17 years of moderate obesity was required before type 2 diabetes developed. It seems likely that the actual level of obesity and other risk factors would affect the duration of obesity that had to be experienced before glucose tolerance deteriorated to diabetes.

Evidence for a specific effect of weight gain on type 2 diabetes comes from two American studies, where self-reported weight gain throughout adulthood or immediately prior to the study period was associated with increased risk of diabetes independent of BMI in early adulthood (34,35); although weight gain was no longer significant if attained BMI was controlled for. However, if the effect of weight gain is modelled controlling for attained BMI, it is effectively modelling duration, as obese people who have not gained weight also have a longer duration of obesity (46). This emphasizes the difficulty in delineating the effects of current BMI, duration of BMI, and weight gain. Harris (47) also indicated that weight gain between 25 and 50 years of age was a risk factor for type 2 diabetes, and Di Pietro *et al.* (48) have shown a rapid weight gain between puberty and age 25 years in a cohort of Swedish adults who were overweight in childhood and went on to develop diabetes. Weight gain also preceded type 2 diabetes in Pima Indians (36,42).

However, as mentioned earlier weight change had little effect on risk of type 2 diabetes in the Israeli study, and most of the incident cases of type 2 diabetes had not changed weight over 10 years of follow-up, and BMI had been at $27\,\mathrm{kg/m^2}$ or greater for at least the period of the study (38).

The effect of weight gain on diabetes incidence was quantified in a follow-up study of the baseline NHANES (National Health and Nutrition Examination Survey) cohort in the USA (49). The 9-year diabetes incidence, as determined from death certificates, hospitalization and nursing home records, increased by 4.5% for every kilogram of weight gained. This was after controlling for a number of factors including baseline BMI, but not BMI at diagnosis. From this result it was estimated that the average weight gain of 3.6 kg recorded between NHANES II and NHANES III could theoretically give rise to a 16% increase in diabetes incidence between 1990 and 2000.

Mechanisms Linking Obesity and Glucose Intolerance

Numerous mechanisms have been proposed linking obesity and glucose intolerance. Most obese individuals with type 2 diabetes are also insulin resistant, while lean subjects with type 2 diabetes are likely to have a defect in insulin secretion. A continuum between obese glucose tolerant, obese glucose intolerant, obese diabetic with hyperinsulinaemia, and obese diabetes with hypoinsulinaemia has been proposed by Golay *et al.* (45) and is supported by the work of others (50,51). Deficiency in glucose storage as glycogen is evident in each of these groups of obese subjects. The first step in both glucose storage and oxidation is through glucose 6-phosphate. Glucose storage proceeds under the action of glycogen synthase and mobilization is controlled by glycogen phosphorylase. Glucose oxidation proceeds via glycolysis to the citric acid cycle. In obesity there are increased circulating levels of free fatty acids (FFAs) and elevated lipid oxidation. This results in metabolic products (acetyl-CoA and citrate) which inhibit glucose mobilization. Intracellular glycogen therefore accumulates, inhibiting glycogen synthase and glucose storage (45). This occurs independent of the positive effect of hyperglycaemia and hyperinsulinaemia on glucose storage.

As long as glucose tolerance is normal in obesity,

the negative effect of increased intracellular glycogen on glucose uptake is smaller than the positive effect of hyperinsulinaemia and hyperglycaemia. Glucose intolerance occurs when the stimulating effects of increased glucose and insulin can no longer overcome the resistance to glucose storage—hence resulting in continuous hyperglycaemia. A vicious cycle develops with higher fasting glycaemia inhibiting glucose storage and inhibition of glucose storage causing hyperglycaemia (45).

Initially hyperglycaemia is accompanied by an increased insulin response to a glucose load, but eventually β-cell response becomes insufficient, and although basal insulin levels may still be elevated in comparison to lean subjects, insulin response to a glucose load or meal is diminished and hyperglycaemia persists (45,50,51).

This simplified account provides a framework within which the association between obesity and type 2 diabetes can be understood. The lowering of fat stores with weight loss enables mobilization of glycogen and therefore increased uptake of glucose for storage. In the short term, an energy-deficient diet or exercise will also improve glucose uptake by facilitating glycogen mobilization without any change in body fat content. Weight gain, as well as current weight, has been considered a risk factor for type 2 diabetes. At any level and duration of BMI, extra body fat could tip the balance to impaired glucose uptake. Behavioural factors resulting in weight gain, such as dietary changes or reduced physical activity, may also promote the development of type 2 diabetes.

Fat Distribution and Type 2 Diabetes

Abdominal fat, especially the visceral rather than subcutaneous depots, is strongly associated with the metabolic complications of obesity (52). Kissebah has recently reviewed the current understanding of the relationship between abdominal adiposity and metabolic changes leading to insulin resistance and glucose intolerance, elevated blood pressure and dyslipidaemia (52). Microcirculatory changes in blood flow may contribute to insulin resistance, along with a primary neurohumoral dysregulation, enhanced by genetically or environmentally overactive 'arousal systems'. The increased lipolysis associated with visceral adipose tissue, and the resultant increase in FFA flux to the liver, may impair hepatic insulin extraction, while increased androgenic hormones in centrally obese women could also contribute to insulin resistance (52). There are several issues pertinent to the relationship between fat distribution and diabetes.

Independent Effects of Overall and Central Obesity

Anthropometric measures of body fat distribution (e.g. waist-to-hip ratio (WHR), subscapular-to-triceps skinfold ratio (STR), waist-to-thigh ratio) or computed tomography (CT) scan measures are associated with risk of diabetes, in both longitudinal (20–23) and cross-sectional (13–19,24,32,53) studies. The effects of fat distribution are generally independent of measures of overall fatness (13–23) and may be even more important.

Using a variety of markers of fat distribution, prevalence studies in Asian Indians (17,18), English Caucasians (18), Pima Indians (36), American Caucasians (24) and American Hispanics (24) have demonstrated that overall body fat is less closely associated with type 2 diabetes than is body fat distribution.

In addition, some studies indicated that the effect of fat distribution is greater in more obese individuals (16,21,53). Exceptions occurred in Mauritius, where there was no apparent effect of BMI on the prevalence of type 2 diabetes across tertiles of WHR (14), and in American men (16), where the effect of WHR was higher in the leaner individuals. In both these studies the general level of BMI was not extreme. In the Pima Indians, an extremely obese population, the effect of fat distribution was diminished with increased BMI or age (36). It may be that a threshold amount of body fat is required before the effects of fat distribution become apparent, and that after a certain level of obesity, the deposition of fat in peripheral depots diminishes the importance of central fat.

Longitudinal studies are less consistent. Among men of the Normative Aging Study who were followed over 18 years, fat distribution as measured by the ratio of abdominal circumference/hip breadth was a stronger predictor of both type 2 diabetes and impaired glucose tolerance than was BMI (23), but in prospective studies of Swedish men (20), and women (21), BMI and WHR were of similar importance.

The tendency for markers of fat distribution to be more strongly associated with prevalence of type 2 diabetes than is BMI in cross-sectional studies could be explained by decreases in BMI, but not WHR, associated with the onset of diabetes. Unpublished analyses from a prospective study in Mauritius show a fall in BMI but not WHR, over 5 years in people with diabetes.

Gender, Fat Distribution and Diabetes

Overall the literature suggests that both general adiposity and distribution of fat deposits are independently important risk factors for type 2 diabetes, in both men and women. However, some studies suggest that there are gender differences in the relative importance of overall fatness and fat distribution. In general, fat distribution appeared to be less important in men than women in comparison with overall fat measure (14–16,54), This observation led Haffner et al. (54) to propose a plateau effect of centrality, in this case measured STR, whereby above a certain level of STR, i.e. that achieved in most men, there was no further increase in rates of type 2 diabetes.

Fat deposition in men is generally abdominal; thus waist circumference or WHR will correlate more strongly with overall obesity, and the range of fat distribution may be limited, compared to women. These factors may explain statistically the lack of an independent association of prevalence of type 2 diabetes with fat distribution in men, rather than their higher degree of abdominal obesity as suggested above.

In summary, both overall obesity and fat distribution contribute to the risk of type 2 diabetes, but their relative importance may vary in relation to whether incidence or prevalence is considered, the gender of the individuals examined or their degree of obesity. However, strategies to reduce type 2 diabetes risk via diet and physical activity can reduce both overall and abdominal obesity and improvements in both should be sought. For management of obesity, waist circumference rather than WHR is probably a better measure of benefit, as weight loss and decrease in abdominal adipose tissue, can occur without changes in WHR.

Ethinicity and Body Fat Distribution

There is evidence to suggest that in some ethnic groups the risk associated with a central distribution of body fat is relatively low. Among non-Hispanics in Colorado the diabetes risks associated with BMI, triceps and subscapular skinfold thicknesses, family history and income were similar to those found in Hispanics. However, a 1 unit increase in either WHR or STR was associated with a greater increase in risk of type 2 diabetes among non-Hispanic whites than among Hispanics (28). Similarly, upper body obesity was more closely associated with higher levels of plasma insulin and glucose, and reduced insulin sensitivity, in obese Caucasian compared to African-American women (55). This metabolic study, along with the study of Marshall et al. (28), suggest that Caucasians may be more susceptible to the effects of fat distribution than some other ethnic groups.

Genetic Factors and Type 2 Diabetes

There is clearly a genetic component to type 2 diabetes as indicated by twin studies, familial clustering of cases, and at the population level, by apparent ethnic differences in diabetes susceptibility with several genes assumed to contribute.

Individual Level

At the individual level, family history of type 2 diabetes can be used as an index of genetic predisposition to diabetes. A number of studies, examining different populations, have suggested that lean individuals with type 2 diabetes have a greater load of susceptibility genes. Thus individuals with a strong family history of type 2 diabetes do not need to accumulate large fat depots to achieve the same level of risk as those with less genetic susceptibility but a higher degree of obesity.

In Japanese men with a family history of type 2 diabetes it appeared that elevated prior or current obesity was not as strongly associated with type 2 diabetes as in men with no family history (56). Lemieux et al. (57) showed that among 'normal' glucose tolerant men with relatively high levels of insulin or glucose or both following an oral glucose tolerance test (OGTT), that is those at high risk of progression to diabetes, those with no family history of diabetes had a mean BMI at age 20 which was $2.6\,kg/m^2$ higher than those with a family history of type 2 diabetes. Using a different approach, Kuzuya and Matsuda found that patients with type 2 diabetes who had a definite history of obesity had a significantly ($P < 0.01$) lower prevalence of family history of diabetes (32%) than those who had not been obese (50%) (58). Similarly, the siblings of lean diabetics tended to have a higher prevalence of type 2 diabetes than the siblings of obese diabetics in the study of Lee et al. (59), while Hanson et al. (60) observed that the odds ratio for type 2 diabetes in the offspring of obese diabetic parents was 0.6 compared with offspring of lean diabetic parents. Among elderly diabetic men in the Zutphen (Netherlands) study, there was no difference in the degree or duration of obesity in those with a family history of type 2 diabetes or those with no family history (61). This lack of interaction could be related to the older age of these men, 69–90 years. If, as reported by Kuzuya (58) and Lee (59), family history of diabetes is associated with earlier onset of diabetes, it is possible that men with a strong family history and young onset of type 2 diabetes will have already died, which could bias the results. Ohlson et al. (21) also did not find any statistically significant interaction between obesity and family history of diabetes in Swedish men.

Population Level

Comparisons between different ethnic groups indicate residual differences in the prevalence of type 2 diabetes even after adjusting for BMI and other risk factors (28,62). Such differences may be attributed to a variety of factors, including increased genetic susceptibility, increased levels of other risk factors that were not considered, or the inability of anthropometric methods to accurately assess overall fat mass and distribution. Asian Indians, for example, appear to have an elevated risk of type 2 diabetes compared with members of other ethnic groups, even when BMI is at a similar or lower level (63–65). This is explained to some extent by differences in body fat distribution (66) which mean that Indian BMIs are not equivalent, regarding risk for diabetes, to BMIs of other ethnic groups. Fijian Indians had lower BMI than Melanesians, but their triceps skinfold thicknesses were greater, suggesting a higher body fat content in Indians (65). Indians also had a greater mean WHR than Europeans for the same level of BMI (18). In a comparison of young European and Polynesian women in New

Zealand it was found that a BMI of $30 \, kg/m^2$ for a European was equivalent, in terms of body fat content, to a BMI of about $34 \, kg/m^2$ for a Polynesian (67); therefore the effect of similar BMI on risk of type 2 diabetes may differ between these ethnic groups. Swinburn et al. (68) previously reported that resistance measured by a bioelectrical impedance device was lower in Polynesians than Caucasians at any level of weight (adjusted for height and age), also implying a lower body fat content. On the other hand, a recent study of Chinese and Dutch adults found similar relationships between BMI and body fat in both populations (69), suggesting that differences between ethnic groups are not universal.

Diet, Obesity and Type 2 Diabetes

Diet is associated with risk of type 2 diabetes through its effect on obesity, and more specifically, dietary components such as fat, sugar and fibre have long been implicated in the development of type 2 diabetes (70). The importance of diet, independent of obesity, in at least some studies, indicates that among subjects with similar BMIs, the risk of type 2 diabetes could be modified by their usual diet.

In the San Luis Valley Diabetes Study, total fat intake was predictive of type 2 diabetes over 1–3 years of follow-up in 123 individuals with impaired glucose tolerance, independent of BMI (71). After adjusting for a number of dietary, anthropometric and metabolic risk factors the odds ratio for type 2 diabetes associated with a 40 g increment in total fat intake was around 7; however, saturated fat intake was not a predictor. In a cross-sectional analysis of baseline data from the same study the evidence was also in support of total fat being associated with type 2 diabetes (72).

Tsunehara et al. have published cross-sectional (73) and prospective (74) data on diet and type 2 diabetes in Japanese American men indicating an association with animal fat, which is consistent with the results of a study on Seventh Day Adventists showing relationships between meat consumption and diabetes (75), although these studies did not control for obesity. In the Finnish and Dutch cohorts of the Seven Countries Study, total fat, saturated fat, monounsaturated fat and cholesterol were higher 20 years before diagnosis in men with diabetes compared with men who were normal or had impaired glucose tolerance (76). After adjustment for past BMI and other factors, total fat was still significantly associated with 2-h post-load glucose level.

Beneficial effects of fish on glucose tolerance have also been noted and it is believed that ω-3 fatty acids may be protective (77), although in one study this was only if accompanied by moderate physical activity (78). Thus the evidence for fat quantity and type being involved in the development of type 2 diabetes is expanding and is supported by studies on the effects of lipid composition of cell membranes on insulin sensitivity (79).

Two reports published in 1997, based on the long-running Health Professionals Follow-Up Study (80) and Nurses Health Study (81), concluded that diets with a high glycaemic load and low content of cereal fibre increased the risk of type 2 diabetes independently of BMI, in men and women respectively; the authors recommended that grains be consumed in a minimally refined form to reduce the risk of diabetes. The risk of developing type 2 diabetes for men and women in the top tertile of glycaemic load and the lowest for cereal fibre intake was twice that of those with low glycaemic load and high cereal fibre intake.

Nevertheless, a number of other studies have been unable to show any associations between diet and type 2 diabetes (82–85). However, it is clearly important to get some idea of dietary composition in order to evaluate the type 2 diabetes risk in individuals. The magnitude of the effect of diet on risk of type 2 diabetes is estimated as being of similar order as that of BMI; thus it should not be ignored.

Physical Activity, Obesity and Type 2 Diabetes

Obesity and physical activity have been found to be independently associated with both prevalence (14,86) and incidence (87–91) of type 2 diabetes in men and women. Physical activity may lower the risk of type 2 diabetes via reduced total body fat (86,87,89–93) and less abdominally distributed fat (86,89,92,93), and/or through its action in improving insulin sensitivity (92,93). These mechanisms are closely linked, but the independent effects of activity and obesity suggest that physical activity can modify the risk of type 2 diabetes at any given level of obesity.

In prospective studies where the effect of physical activity on type 2 diabetes risk has been shown to be independent of obesity, the benefits of physical activity were similar for lean and obese subjects among men and women in Malta (91), and women in the Nurses Health Study (87). In two studies of Caucasian American men, the effect of physical activity was strongest for more obese men and nonexistent in the leanest men (88,90), in contrast to the findings of the Honolulu Heart Study, where only the leaner men were protected by physical activity (89). These conflicting results cannot be explained by very different BMI levels in the different populations, but levels of other risk factors may be important. Gender may also modify the interaction between obesity and physical activity.

The relative risk of type 2 diabetes in less active individuals depends also on the levels of activity being compared, as well as many other factors. In the studies discussed above the relative risks ranged from 1.1 for the Pennsylvania Alumni (88), to 2.6 in Malta (91), of similar magnitude to the risks associated with obesity.

Fetal and Early Infant Nutrition, Obesity and Type 2 Diabetes

Hales and colleagues have proposed that poor intrauterine nutrition, and perhaps poor nutrition in early infancy, reflected in low birthweights and decreased rates of postnatal growth, can increase the risk of type 2 diabetes and cardiovascular diseases in later life, through either reducing pancreatic β-cell capacity, or increasing insulin resistance (94,95). The effects of low birthweight on insulin resistance (96) or the insulin resistance syndrome (97) appear to be enhanced by adult obesity. Thus for adults with a ponderal index at birth of $\leq 20.6 \, kg/m^3$, the degree of insulin resistance ($t_{1/2}$ min) ranged from 18 to 31 at adult BMI increased, compared with a range of 14 to 19 for those with a ponderal index at birth of $> 25 \, kg/m^3$ (96). Data in support of the so-called 'thrifty phenotype' hypothesis have been reported in Europeans (96–101), Indians (102), Mexican Americans (97), Australian Aborigines

(103) and Native Americans (104), although at least two studies in Europeans have failed to show the expected associations (105,106).

A recent review of studies into associations between fetal and/or infant growth and adult chronic disease concludes that the reported associations may be biased rather than causal, with possible selection bias due to loss to follow-up and confounding by socioeconomic factors (107). New evidence for a genetic explanation of the link between fetal growth and adult diabetes comes from Dunger *et al.* (108), with the observation that variation in the expression of the insulin gene is associated with size at birth.

Whatever the mechanism for the association of low birthweight with adult disease, and McCance *et al.* have suggested that the observations can be explained by more conventional genetic hypotheses (104), the association is strong in a number of ethnically varied populations and hence its effects may contribute to differences in risk of type 2 diabetes seen in people with similar levels of adult obesity.

Leptin, Obesity and Type 2 Diabetes

While it is now accepted that human obesity is generally associated with elevated circulating leptin levels (109), and in many studies leptin is correlated with insulin levels (110–114) or insulin resistance (115,116), it is not clear whether leptin has a role in glucose intolerance in humans. In the leptin deficient *ob/ob* mouse treatment with leptin lowered glucose and insulin concentrations in the blood independently of weight loss (117,118). The leptin treated animals also increased physical activity and metabolic rate to 'normal' levels (117) and this may have enhanced insulin sensitivity and glucose uptake via increased glycogen mobilization as discussed above, or increased glucose uptake by some insulin-independent mechanism which would result in reduced insulin levels (118). Leptin may also influence insulin secretion in *ob/ob* mice via neuropeptide Y (NPY) (119) or by direct action on β-cells (120,121).

In humans, in contrast to rats and mice, insulin does not have an acute effect on leptin levels (111,113,122), although chronic hyperinsulinaemia appears to be associated with elevated leptin levels (111,123,124), perhaps due to adipocyte hyper-

trophy (111). On the other hand, there is some evidence for leptin influencing insulin sensitivity. In isolated human liver cells leptin antagonizes insulin signalling (125), and in the Israeli sand rat (*Psammomys obesus*), a polygenic animal model of type 2 diabetes, leptin has been reported to inhibit insulin binding to adipocyte insulin receptors (126).

A number of studies have reported on leptin levels in diabetic versus non-diabetic individuals; after adjusting for obesity there is no consistent picture with no difference being found in Polynesians in Western Samoa (110), Mexican Americans (127), Finnish men (123), American men and women (128) and German men and women (129) who mostly appear to have type 2 diabetes. Clément *et al.* (130) have found lower leptin levels in morbidly obese, poorly controlled diabetes compared with controlled diabetes or non-diabetics with similar levels of obesity. The low leptin levels in poorly controlled subjects may have been associated with lower insulin levels in this group.

Although the development of obesity in humans is unlikely to be linked to a defect in the OB gene as in the *ob/ob* mouse, in two related cases OB mutations in the homozygous form were reported to result in severe leptin deficiency and obesity (131). Recently, a rare mutation in exon 16 of OB-R was identified in humans. This alteration was found to result in morbid obesity and endocrine abnormalities in individuals homozygous for the mutation (132).

Leptin resistance, as observed in the *db/db* mouse and *fa/fa* rat which have a single mutation in the leptin receptor gene, has not been demonstrated yet in humans (133) and it may be that leptin resistance is due to a defect in body mass regulation downstream of leptin. It may also be that leptin is not important in preventing obesity in humans as it is in *ob/ob* mice, and merely reflects fat stores. In a small study of Pima Indians, low leptin levels predicted weight gain (134), but in a population-based study of Mauritians we were unable to find any association between high (leptin resistance) or low (leptin deficiency) leptin levels and weight gain over 5 years (135). Consistent with human evolutionary pressure, it has been suggested that leptin may have a more important role in protecting against the effects of undernutrition (136–138), especially in relation to reproduction (139–141), rather than preventing overnutrition. In this case it may have little relevance to type 2 diabetes, but more research is

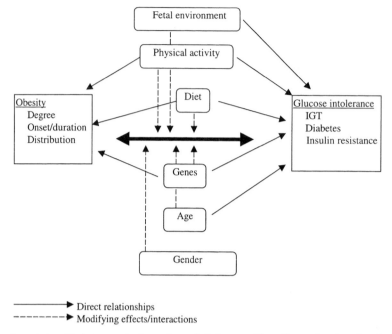

Figure 24.1   The complex relationship between obesity and type 2 diabetes mellitus, illustrating the roles of other risk factors. IGT, impaired glucose tolerance

needed to determine whether leptin has a role in the development of diabetes.

CONCLUSION

Obesity, and central obesity in particular, are known to be important risk factors for development of type 2 diabetes. As discussed in this review, the association between obesity and type 2 diabetes may be modified by diet, physical activity, duration of obesity and other factors (Figure 24.1).

Obesity and diabetes are interlinked through several mechanisms, and some of the relations are complicated by methodological issues surrounding assessment of obesity and study design. In a multifactonal setting comprising environmental (including behavioural) and genetic factors, where risk factors and outcome can both influence each other, data derived from epidemiological studies describing average effects can only provide a rough estimate of an individual's risk of developing type 2 diabetes.

On the other hand, reducing an individual's risk from obesity should reflect the complexity of the relationship between obesity and type 2 diabetes, and other risk factors for type 2 diabetes must also be considered. Thus all individuals at a similar level of obesity should not necessarily be treated in the same way.

REFERENCES

1. World Health Organization. *Obesity: Preventing and Managing the Global Epidemic*. Geneva: World Health Organization, 1998.
2. Björntorp P. Obesity. *Lancet* 1997; **350**: 423–426.
3. Kuczmarski R, Flegal K, Campbell S, Johnson C. Increasing prevalence of overweight among US adults: the National Health and Nutrition Examination Surveys. *JAMA* 1994; **272**: 205–211.
4. Risk Factor Prevalence Study Management Committee. *Risk Factor Prevalence Study: Survey No 2 1983*. Canberra: National Heart Foundation of Australia and Australian Institute of Health, 1984.
5. Risk Factor Prevalence Study Management Committee. *Risk Factor Prevalence Study: Survey No 3 1989*. Canberra: National Heart Foundation of Australia and Australian Institute of Health, 1990.
6. Hodge AM, Dowse GK, Zimmet PZ, Collins VR. Preva-

lence and secular trends in obesity in Pacific and Indian Ocean island populations. *Obes Res* 1995; **3**(Suppl. 2): 77s–87s.

7. Hodge AM, Dowse GK, Zimmet PZ. Obesity in Pacific populations. *Pacific Health Dialog* 1996; **3**(1): 77–86.

8. Amos A, McCarty D, Zimmet P. The rising global burden of diabetes and its complications: Estimates and projections to the year 2010. *Diebet Med* 1997; **14**(Suppl 5): S1–S85.

9. Lapidus L, Bengtsson C, Larsson B, Pennert K, Rybo E, Sjöström L. Distribution of adipose tissue and risk of cardiovascular disease and death: a 12 year follow up of participants in the population study of women in Gothenburg, Sweden. *BMJ* 1984; **289**: 1257–1261.

10. Larsson B, Svardsudd K, Welin L, Welhelmsen L, Björntorp P, Tibblin G. Abdominal adipose tissue distribution, obesity, and risk of cardiovascular disease and death: 13 year follow up of participants in the study of men born in 1913. *BMJ* 1984; **288**: 1401–1404.

11. Filipovský J, Ducimetière P, Darné B, Richard J. Abdominal body mass distribution and elevated blood pressure are associated with increased risk of death from cardiovascular diseases and cancer in middle-aged men. The results of a 15-to 20-year follow-up in the Paris prospective study. *Int J Obes* 1993; **17**: 197–203.

12. Prineas R, Folsom A, Kaye S. Central adiposity and increased risk of coronary artery disease mortality in older women. *Ann Epidemiol* 1993; **3**: 34–41.

13. Haffner S, Stern M, Hazuda H, Pugh J, Paterson J. Do upper-body and centralized adiposity measure different aspects of regional body-fat distribution? Relationship to non-insulin dependent diabetes mellitus, lipids, and lipoproteins. *Diabetes* 1987; **36**: 43–51.

14. Dowse G, Zimmet P, Gareeboo H, *et al.* Abdominal obesity and physical inactivity as risk factors for NIDDM and impaired glucose tolerance in Indian, Creole and Chinese Mauritians. *Diabetes Care* 1991; **14**: 271–282.

15. Chou P, Liao M-J, Shih-Tzer T. Associated risk factors of diabetes in Kin-Hu, Kinmen. *Diabetes Res Clin Pract* 1994; **26**: 229–235.

16. Schmidt M, Duncan B, Canani L, Karohl C, Chambless L. Associations of waist-hip ratio with diabetes mellitus. Strength and possible modifiers. *Diabetes Care* 1992; **15**: 912–914.

17. Shelgikar K, Hockaday T, Yajnik C. Central rather than generalized obesity is related to hyperglycaemia in Asian Indian subjects. *Diabet Med* 1991; **8**: 712–717.

18. McKeigue P, Pierpoint T, Ferrie J, Marmot M. Relationship of glucose intolerance and hyperinsulinaemia to body fat pattern in South Asians and Europeans. *Diabetologia* 1992; **35**: 785–791.

19. Collins V, Dowse G, Toelupe P, *et al.* Increasing prevalence of NIDDM in the Pacific island population of Western Samoa over a 13-year period. *Diabetes Care* 1994; **17**: 288–296.

20. Lundgren H, Bengtsson C, Blohme G, Lapidus L, Sjöström L. Adiposity and adipose tissue distribution in relation to incidence of diabetes in women: results from a prospective population study in Gothenburg, Sweden. *Int J Obes* 1989; **13**: 413–423.

21. Ohlson L-O, Larsson B, Svardsudd K, *et al.* The influence of body fat distribution on the incidence of diabetes mellitus. 13.5 years of follow-up of the participants in the study of men born in 1913. *Diabetes* 1985; **35**: 1055–1058.

22. Haffner SM, Stern MP, Mitchell BD, Hazuda HP, Patterson JK. Incidence of type II diabetes in Mexican Americans predicted by fasting insulin and glucose levels, obesity and body-fat distribution. *Diabetes* 1990; **39**: 283–288.

23. Cassano P, Rosner B, Vokonas P, Weiss S. Obesity and body fat distribution in relation to the incidence of non-insulin-dependent diabetes mellitus. *Am J Epidemiol* 1992; **136**: 1474–1486.

24. Sosenko J, Kato M, Soto R, Goldberg R. A comparison of adiposity measures for screening of non-insulin dependent diabetes mellitus. *Int J Obes* 1993; **17**: 441–444.

25. Caan B, Armstrong M, Selby J, *et al.* Changes in measurements of body fat distribution accompanying weight change. *Int J Obes* 1994; **18**: 397–404.

26. WHO Expert Committee. *Physical Status: the Use and Interpretation of Anthropometry.* Geneva: World Health Organization, 1995.

27. de Courten M, Bennett P, Tuomilehto J, Zimmet P. Epidemiology of NIDDM in non-Europids. In: Alberti KGMM, Zimmet P, DeFronzo RA (eds) *International Textbook of Diabetes Mellitus*, 2nd edn. Chichester: John Wiley, 1997.

28. Marshall J, Hamman R, Baxter J, *et al.* Ethnic differences in risk factors associated with the prevalence of non-insulin-dependent diabetes mellitus. *Am J Epidemiol* 1993; **137**: 706–718.

29. Skarfors E, Selinus K, Lithell H. Risk factors for developing non-insulin dependent diabetes: a 10 year follow-up of men in Uppsala. *BMJ* 1991; **303**: 755–760.

30. Shaten B, Smith G, Kuller L, Neaton J. Risk factors for the development of Type II diabetes among men enrolled in the Usual Care group of the Multiple Risk Factor Intervention Trial. *Diabetes Care* 1993; **16**: 1331–1339.

31. Tai T-Y, Chuang L-M, Wu H-P, Chen C-J. Association of body build with non-insulin-dependent diabetes mellitus and hypertension among Chinese adults: A 4-year follow-up study. *Int J Epidemiol* 1992; **21**(3): 511–517.

32. Van Noord P, Seidell J, Den Tonkelaar I, Baanders-Van Halewijn E, Ouwehand I. The relationship between fat distribution and some chronic diseases in 11825 women participating in the DOM-Project. *Int J Epidemiol* 1990; **19**: 564–570.

33. Hartz A, Rupley D, Rimm A. The association of girth measurements with disease in 32,856 women. *Am J Epidemiol* 1984; **119**: 71–80.

34. Colditz GA, Willett WC, Stampfer MJ, *et al.* Weight as a risk factor for clinical diabetes in women. *Am J Epidemiol* 1990; **132**(3): 501–513.

35. Chan J, Rimm E, Colditz G, Stampfer M, Willett W. Obesity, fat distribution, and weight gain as risk factors for clinical diabetes in men. *Diabetes Care* 1994; **17**: 961–966.

36. Knowler W, Pettitt D, Saad M, Charles M, Nelson R, Howard B. Obesity in the Pima Indians: its magnitude and relationship with diabetes. *Am J Clin Nutr* 1991; **53**: 1543S–1551S.

37. Charles M, Fontbonne A, Thibult N, Warnet J-M, Rosselin G, Eschwege E. Risk factors for NIDDM in white population. Paris Prospective Study. *Diabetes* 1991; **40**: 796–799.

38. Modan M, Karasik A, Halkin H, *et al.* Effect of past and concurrent body mass index on prevalence of glucose intolerance and type 2 (non-insulin dependent) diabetes and on insulin response. The Israeli study of glucose intolerance, obesity and hypertension. *Diabetologia* 1986; **29**: 82–89.

39. Zimmet P, Alberti K. Leptin: Is it important in diabetes? *Diabet Med* 1996; **13**: 501–503.

40. Manson J, Spelsberg A. Primary prevention of non-insulin-dependent diabetes mellitus. *Am J Prev Med* 1994; **10**: 172–184.

41. Sicree R, Zimmet P, King H, Coventry J. Weight change amongst Nauruans over 6.5 years extent, and association with glucose intolerance. *Diabetes Res Clin Pract* 1987; **3**: 327–336.

42. Knowler W, Pettitt D, Savage P, Bennett P. Diabetes incidence in Pima Indians: contributions of obesity and parental diabetes. *Am J Epidemiol* 1981; **113**: 144–156.

43. Ogilvie R. Sugar tolerance in obese subjects. A review of sixty-five cases. *Q J Med* 1935; Series 2, **4**: 345–358.

44. Felber J, Golay A, Jéquier E, *et al.* The metabolic consequences of long-term human obesity. *Int J Obes* 1988; **12**: 377–389.

45. Golay A, Munger R, Felber J-P. Obesity and NIDDM: the retrograde regulation concept. *Diabetes Rev* 1997; **5**: 69–82.

46. Colditz G, Willett W, Rotnitzky A, Manson J. Weight gain as a risk factor for clinical diabetes mellitus in women. *Ann Intern Med* 1995; **122**: 481–486.

47. Harris MI. Impaired glucose tolerance in the US population. *Diabetes Care* 1989; **12**: 464–474.

48. DiPietro L, Mossberg H-O, Stunkard A. A 40-year history of overweight children in Stockholm: life-time overweight, morbidity, and mortality. *Int J Obes* 1994; **18**: 585–590.

49. Ford E, Williamson D, Liu S. Weight change and diabetes incidence: Findings from a national cohort of US adults. *Am J Epidemiol* 1997; **146**: 214–222.

50. Hansen B, Bodkin H. Heterogeneity of insulin responses: phases leading to Type 2 (non-insulin-dependent) diabetes mellitus in the rhesus monkey. *Diabetologia* 1986; **29**: 713–719.

51. Dowse G, Zimmet P, Collins V. Insulin levels and the natural history of glucose intolerance in Nauruans. *Diabetes* 1996; **45**: 1367–1372.

52. Kissebah A. Central obesity: measurement and metabolic effects. *Diabetes Rev* 1997; **5**: 8–20.

53. Hartz A, Rupley D, Kalkhoff R, Rimm A. Relationship of obesity to diabetes: influence of obesity level and body fat distribution. *Prev Med* 1983; **12**: 351–357.

54. Haffner S, Stern M, Hazuda H, Rosenthal M, Knapp J, Malina R. Role of obesity and fat distribution in non-insulin-dependent diabetes mellitus in Mexican Americans and Non-Hispanic whites. *Diabetes Care* 1986; **9**: 153–561.

55. Dowling H, Pi-Sunyer F. Race-dependent health risks of upper body obesity. *Diabetes* 1993; **42**: 537–543.

56. Fujimoto W, Leonetti D, Newell-Morris L, Shuman W, Wahl P. Relationship of absence or presence of a family history of diabetes to body weight and body fat distribution in type 2 diabetes. *Int J Obes* 1991; **15**: 111–120.

57. Lemieux S, Després J-P, Nadeau A, Prud'homme D, Tremblay A, Bouchard C. Heterogeneous glycaemic and insulinaemic responses to oral glucose in non-diabetic men: Interactions between duration of obesity, body fat distribu-

tion and family history of diabetes mellitus. *Diabetologia* 1992; **35**: 653–659.

58. Kuzuya T, Matsuda A. Family history of diabetes among Japanese patients with type 1 (insulin-dependent) and type 2 (non-insulin-dependent) diabetes. *Diabetologia* 1982; **22**: 372–374.

59. Lee E, Anderson P, Jr, Bryan J, Bahr C, Coniglione T, Cleves M. Diabetes, parental diabetes, and obesity in Oklahoma Indians. *Diabetes Care* 1985; **8**: 107–113.

60. Hanson R, Pettit D, Bennett P, *et al.* Familial relationships between obesity and NIDDM. *Diabetes* 1995; **44**: 418–422.

61. Boer J, Feskens E, Kromhout D. Characteristics of non-insulin-dependent diabetes mellitus in elderly men: Effect modification by family history. *Int J Epidemiol* 1996; **25**: 394–302.

62. Stern M, Gaskill S, Hazuda H, Gardner L, Haffner S. Does obesity explain excess prevalence of diabetes among Mexican Americans? Results of the San Antonio Heart Study. *Diabetologia* 1983; **14**: 272–277.

63. Mather H, Keen H. The Southall diabetes survey: prevalence of known diabetes in Asians and Europeans. *BMJ* 1985; **291**: 1081–1084.

64. Simmons D, Williams DR, Powell MJ. Prevalence of diabetes in a predominantly Asian community: preliminary findings of the Coventry diabetes study. *BMJ* 1989; **298**: 18–21.

65. Zimmet P, Taylor R, Ram P, *et al.* The prevalence of diabetes and impaired glucose tolerance in the biracial (Melanesian and Indian) population of Fiji: a rural–urban comparison. *Am J Epidemiol* 1983; **118**: 673–688.

66. Hodge AM, Dowse GK, Collins VR, *et al.* Abdominal fat distribution and insulin levels only partially explain adverse cardiovascular risk profile in Asian Indians. *J Cardiovasc Risk* 1996; **3**: 263–270.

67. Rush E, Plank L, Laulu M, Robinson S. Prediction of percentage body fat from anthropometric measurements: comparison of New Zealand European and Polynesian young women. *Am J Clin Nutr* 1997; **66**: 2–7.

68. Swinburn B, Craig P, Daniel R, Dent D, Strauss B. Body composition differences between Polynesians and Caucasians assessed by bioelectrical impedance. *Int J Obes* 1996; **20**: 889–894.

69. Deurenberg P, Keyou G, Hautvast J, Jingzhong W. Body mass index as predictor for body fat: comparison between Chinese and Dutch adult subjects. *Asia Pacific J Clin Nutr* 1997; **6**: 102–105.

70. West K. *Epidemiology of Diabetes and its Vascular Lesions.* New York: Elsevier, 1978.

71. Marshall JA, Hoag S, Shetterly S, Hamman RF. Dietary fat predicts conversion from impaired glucose tolerance to NIDDM. *Diabetes Care* 1994; **17**(1): 50–56.

72. Marshall JA, Hamman RF, Baxter H. High-fat, low-carbohydrate diet and the etiology of non-insulin-dependent diabetes mellitus: The San Luis Valley Diabetes Study. *Am J Epidemiol* 1991; **134**: 590–603.

73. Tsunehara CH, Leonetti DL, Fujimoto WY. Diet of second-generation Japanese-American men with and without non-insulin-dependent diabetes. *Am J Clin Nutr* 1990; **52**: 731–738.

74. Tsunehara CH, Leonetti DL, Fujimoto WY. Animal fat and cholesterol intake is high in men with IGT progressing

to NIDDM. *Diabetes* 1991; **40**(Suppl 1): 427A.

27. Snowden DA, Phillips RL. Does a vegetarian diet reduce the risk of diabetes? *Am J Public Health* 1985; **75**: 507–512.

76. Feskens EJ, Virtanen SM, Räsänen L, *et al.* Dietary factors determining diabetes and impaired glucose tolerance: A 20-year follow-up of the Finnish and Dutch cohorts of the Seven Countries. Study. *Diabetes Care* 1995; **18**(8): 1104–1112.

77. Feskens EJ, Bowles CH, Kromhout D. Inverse association between fish intake and risk of glucose intolerance in normoglycemic elderly men and women. *Diabetes Care* 1991; **14**(11): 935–941.

78. Dunstan D, Mori T, Puddey I, *et al.* The independent and combined effects of aerobic exercise and dietary fish intake on serum lipis and glycemic control in NIDDM: a randomized controlled study. *Diabetes Care* 1997; **20**: 913–921.

79. Storlein L, Baur L, Kriketos A, *et al.* Dietary fats and insulin action. *Diabetologia* 1996; **39**: 621–631.

80. Salmerón J, Ascherio A, Rimm EB, *et al.* Dietary fiber, glycemic load, and risk of NIDDM in men. *Diabetes Care* 1997; **20**(4): 545–550.

81. Salmerón J, Manson JE, Stampfer MJ, Colditz GA, Wing AL, Willet WC. Dietary fiber, glycemic load, and risk of non-insulin-dependent diabetes mellitus in women. *JAMA* 1997; **277**(6): 472–477.

82. Hodge AM, Dowse GK, Zimmet PZ. Diet does not predict incidence or prevalence of non-insulin-dependent diabetes in Nauruans. *Asia Pac J Clin Nutr* 1993; **2**: 35–41.

83. Hodge A, Montgomery J, Dowse G, Mavo B, Watt T, Zimmet P. A case-control study of diet in newly diagnosed non-insulin-dependent diabetes mellitus in the Wanigela people of Papua New Guinea. *Diabetes Care* 1996; **19**: 457–462.

84. Kahn H, Herman J, Medalie J, Neufeld H, Riss E, Goldbourt U. Factors related to diabetes incidence: a multivariate analysis of two years observation on 10,000 men, The Israel Ischaemic Heart Disease Study. *J Chron Disord* 1971; **23**: 617–629.

85. Lundgren H, Bengtsson C, Blohmé G, *et al.* Dietary habits and incidence of noninsulin-dependent diabetes mellitus in a population study of women in Gothenberg, Sweden. *Am J Clin Nutr* 1989; **49**: 708–712.

86. Kriska A, LaPorte R, Pettitt D, *et al.* The association of physical activity with obesity, fat distribution and glucose intolerance in Pima Indians. *Diabetologia* 1993; **36**: 863–869.

87. Manson J, Rimm E, Stampfer M, *et al.* Physical activity and incidence of non-insulin-dependent diabetes mellitus in women. *Lancet* 1991; **338**: 774–778.

88. Helmrich SP, Ragland DR, Leung RW, Paffenbarger RS. Physical activity and reduced occurrence of non-insulin-dependent diabetes mellitus. *N Engl J Med* 1991; **325**: 147–152.

89. Burchfiel C, Sharp D, Curb J, *et al.* Physical activity and incidence of diabetes: The Honolulu Heart Program. *Am J Epidemiol* 1995; **141**: 360–368.

90. Manson J, Nathan D, Krolewski A, Stampfer M, Willett W, Hennekens C. A prospective study of exercise and incidence of diabetes among US male physicians. *JAMA* 1992; **268**: 63–67.

91. Schranz A, Tuomilehto J, Marti B, Jarrett R, Grabaukas V,

Vassallo A. Low physical activity and worsening of glucose tolerance: results from a 2-year follow-up of a population sample in Malta. *Diabetes Res Clin Practice* 1991; **11**: 127–136.

92. Houmard J, McCulley C, Roy L, Bruner R, McCammon M, Israel R. Effects of exercise training on absolute and relative measurements of regional adiposity. *Int J Obes* 1994; **18**: 243–248.

93. Bouchard C, Després J-P, Tremblay A. Exercise and obesity. *Obes Res* 1993; **1**: 133–147.

94. Hales CN, Barker DJP. Type 2 (non-insulin-dependent) diabetes mellitus: The thrifty phenotype hypothesis. *Diabetologia* 1992; **35**: 595–601.

95. Hales C, Desai M, Ozanne S. The thrifty phenotype hypothesis: How does it look after 5 years? *Diabet Med* 1997; **14**: 189–195.

96. Phillips D, Barker D, Hales C, Hirst S, Osmond C. Thinness at birth and insulin resistance in adult life. *Diabetologia* 1994; **37**: 150–154.

97. Valdez R, Athens M, Thompson G, Bradshaw B, Stern M. Birthweight and adult health outcomes in a beiethnic population in the USA. *Diabetologia* 1994; **37**: 624–631.

98. Hales CN, Barker DJP, Clark PMS, *et al.* Fetal and infant growth and impaired glucose tolerance at age 64. *BMJ* 1991; **303**: 1019–1022.

99. Fall C, Osmond C, Barker D, Clark P, Hales C. Fetal and infant growth and cardiovascular risk factors in women. *BMJ* 1995; **310**: 428–432.

100. Leon DA, Koupiliva I, Lithell HO, *et al.* Failure to realise growth potential in utero and adult obesity in relation to blood pressure in 50 year old Swedish men. *BMJ* 1996; **312**: 401–406.

101. Poulsen P, Vaag A, Kyvik K, Møller Jensen D, Beck-Nielsen H. Low birth weight is associated with NIDDM in discordant monozygotic and dizygotic twin pairs. *Diabetologia* 1997; **40**: 439–446.

102. Yajnik C, Fall C, Vaidya U, *et al.* Fetal growth and glucose and insulin metabolism in four-year-old Indian children. *Diabet Med* 1995; **12**: 330–336.

103. Hoy W, Kyle E, Rees M, *et al.* Birth weight, adult weight and insulin levels: associations in an Australian Aboriginal (AA) community. *The First World Conference on Prevention of Diabetes and its Complications.* Lyngby, Denmark, 1996: 80.

104. McCance D, Pettitt D, Hanson R, Jacobsson L, Knowler W, Bennett P. Birth weight and non-insulin dependent diabetes: thrifty genotype, thrifty phenotype, or surviving small baby genotype? *BMJ* 1994; **308**: 942–945.

105. Alvarsson M, Efendic S, Grill V. Insulin responses to glucose in healthy males are associated with adult height but not with birth weight. *J Intern Med* 1994; **236**: 275–279.

106. Cook JT, Levy JC, Page RC, Shaw AG, Hattersley AT, Turner RC. Association of low birth weight with β cell function in the adult first degree relatives of non-insulin dependent diabetic subjects. *BMJ* 1993; **306**: 302–306.

107. Joseph K, Kramer M. Review of the evidence on fetal and early childhood antecedents of adult chronic disease. *Epidemiol Rev* 1996; **18**: 158–174.

108. Dunger D, Ong K, Huxtable S, *et al.* Associations of the *INS* VNTR with size at birth. *Nat Genet* 1998; **19**: 98–100.

109. Matson CA, Wiater MF, Weigle DS. Leptin and the regula-

tion of body adiposity: A critical review. *Diabetes Rev* 1996; **4**(4): 488–508.

110. Zimmet P, Hodge A, Nicolson M, *et al.* Serum leptin concentration, obesity, and insulin resistance in Western Samoans: cross sectional study. *BMJ* 1996; **313**: 965–969.

111. Kolaczynski JW, Nyce MR, Considine RV, *et al.* Acute and chronic effects of insulin on leptin production in humans. Studies in vivo and in vitro. *Diabetes* 1996; **45**: 699–701.

112. Wabitsch M, Jensen PB, Blum WF, *et al.* Insulin and cortisol promote leptin production in cultured human fat cells. *Diabetes* 1996; **45**: 1435–1438.

113. Dagogo-Jack S, Fanelli C, Paramore D, Brothers J, Landt M. Plasma leptin and insulin relationships in obese and nonobese humans. *Diabetes* 1996; **45**: 695–698.

114. Zimmet P, Collins V, de Courten M, *et al.* Is there a relationship between leptin and insulin sensitivity independent of obesity? A population-based study in the Indian Ocean nation of Mauritius. *Int J Obes* 1998; **21**: 171–177.

115. Segal KR, Landt M, Klein S. Relationship between insulin sensitivity and plasma leptin concentration in lean and obese men. *Diabetes* 1996; **45**: 988–991.

116. Haffner S, Miettinen H, Mykkänen L, Karhapää P, Rainwater D, Laakso M. Leptin concentrations and insulin sensitivity in normoglycemic men. *Int J Obes* 1997; **21**: 393–399.

117. Pelleymounter M, Cullen M, Baker M, *et al.* Effects of the *obese* gene product on body weight regulation in *ob/ob* mice. *Science* 1995; **269**: 540–543.

118. Schwartz M, Baskin D, Bukowski T, *et al.* Specificity of leptin action on elevated blood glucose levels and hypothalamic neuropeptide Y gene expression in *ob/ob* mice. *Diabetes* 1996; **45**: 531–535.

119. Stephens T, Basinski M, Bristow P, *et al.* The role of neuropeptide Y in the antiobesity action of the obese gene product. *Nature* 1995; **377**: 530–532.

120. Emilsson V, Liu Y-L, Cawthorne M, Morton N, Davenport M. Expression of the functional leptin receptor mRNA in pancreatic islets and direct inhibitory action of leptin on insulin secretion. *Diabetes* 1997; **46**: 313–316.

121. Kieffer T, Heller R, Leech C, Holz G, Habener J. Leptin suppression of insulin secretion by activation of ATP-sensitive K^+ channels in pancreatic β-cells. *Diabetes* 1997; **46**: 1087–1093.

122. Gabriel M, Jinagouda S, Boyadjian R, Kades W, Ayad M, Saad M. Is leptin the link between obesity and insulin resistance? *Diabetes* 1996; **45**(Suppl 2): 51A.

123. Malmström R, Taskinen M-R, Karonen S-L, Yki-Järvinen H. Insulin increases plasma leptin concentrations in normal subjects and patients with NIDDM. *Diabetologia* 1996; **39**: 993–996.

124. Utriainen T, Malmström R, Mäkimattila S, Yki-Järvinen H. Supraphysiological hyperinsulinemia increases plasma leptin concentrations after 4 h in normal subjects. *Diabetes* 1996; **45**: 1364–1366.

125. Cohen B, Novick D, Rubinstein M. Modulation of insulin activities by leptin. *Science* 1996; **274**: 1185–1188.

126. Walder K, Filippis A, Clark S, Zimmet P, Collier G. Leptin inhibits insulin binding in isolated rat adipocytes. *Diabetologia* 1997; **40**(Suppl 1): A176.

127. Haffner S, Stern M, Miettinen H, Wei M, Gingerich R. Leptin concentrations in diabetic and nondiabetic Mexican-Americans. *Diabetes* 1996; **45**: 822–824.

128. Sinha M, Ohannesian J, Heiman M, *et al.* Nocturnal rise of leptin in lean, obese, and non-insulin-dependent diabetes mellitus subjects. *J Clin Invest* 1996; **97**: 1344–1347.

129. McGregor G, Desaga J, Ehlenz K, *et al.* Radioimmunological measurement of leptin in plasma of obese and diabetic human subjects. *Endocrinology* 1996; **137**: 1501–1504.

130. Clément K, Lahlou N, Ruiz J, *et al.* Association of poorly controlled diabetes with low serum leptin in morbid obesity. *Int J Obes* 1997; **21**: 556–561.

131. Montague C, Farooqi I, Whitehead J, *et al.* Congenital leptin deficiency is associated with severe early-onset obesity in humans. *Nature* 1997; **387**: 903–908.

132. Clément K, Vaisse C, Lahlou N, *et al.* A mutation in the human leptin receptor gene causes obesity and pituitary dysfunction. *Nature* 1998; **392**: 398–401.

133. Considine RV, Considine EL, Williams CJ, Hyde TM, Caro JF. The hypothalamic leptin receptor in humans. Identification of incidental sequence polymorphisms and absence of the *db/db* mouse and *fa/fa* rat mutations. *Diabetes* 1996; **45**: 992–994.

134. Ravussin E, Pratley RE, Maffei M, *et al.* Relatively low plasma leptin concentrations precede weight gain in Pima Indians. *Nat Med* 1997; **3**(1): 238–240.

135. Hodge A, de Courten M, Zimmet P. Leptin levels do not predict weight gain: A prospective study. *Diabetologia* 1997; **40**(Suppl 1): A262.

136. Ahima RS, Prabakaran D, Mantzoroz C, *et al.* Role of leptin in the neuroendocrine response to fasting. *Nature* 1996; **382**: 250–252 (Letter).

137. Schwartz M, Seeley R. Neuroendocrine responses to starvation and weight loss. *N Engl J Med* 1997; **336**: 1802–1811.

138. Kolaczynski JW, Considine RV, Ohannesian J, *et al.* Responses of leptin to short-term fasting and refeeding in humans: A link with ketogenesis but not ketones themselves. *Diabetes* 1996; **45**: 1511–1515.

139. Chehav F. The reproductive side of leptin. *Nat Med* 1997; **3**: 952–953.

140. Chehab F, Mounzih K, Lu R, Lim ME. Early onset of reproductive function in normal female mice treated with leptin. *Science* 1997; **275**: 88–90.

141. Chehab FF, Lim ME, Lu R. Correction of the sterility defect in homozygous obese female mice by treatment with human recombinant leptin. *Nat Genet* 1996; **12**: 318–320 (Letter).

25

Cardiovascular Disease

Antonio Tiengo and Angelo Avogaro
University of Padova, Padova, Italy

INTRODUCTION

Morbid obesity is linked to a higher mortality rate but the association between more modest overweight and mortality appears less clear (Figure 25.1) (1,2). Although data from more than four million subjects initially suggested a direct positive association between body weight and overall mortality, subsequent studies showed an increased mortality only above a certain threshold, but described J- or even U-shaped associations between weight and mortality (3,4). The relationship of indicators of obesity to all-cause mortality has been extensively analysed: univariate analysis concerning the body mass index (BMI) for various age groups, the two sexes, and variable periods of follow-up has almost invariably shown minimum levels of risk for BMI values of 27–29 (5,6).

However, the quantification of the excess mortality from all causes associated with obesity remains controversial. It has been recently shown in a large cohort of obese persons that morbid obesity (BMI $\geq 40\,\text{kg/m}^2$) was a strong predictor of premature death while moderate degrees of obesity (BMI 25–32 kg/m^2) were not significantly associated with excess mortality (7).

Much of the obesity-associated mortality is linked to the negative effect of excessive fat distribution on myocardial function and perfusion. As we will outline later in the chapter, much of the information on the relationship between obesity and heart disease derives from autopsy studies of massively obese patients dying of congestive heart failure without clinical evidence of hypertension or cardiac disease. In obesity major haemodynamic changes take place affecting cardiac output, cardiac index and left ventricular stroke work; this increased cardiac output is determined by a major increase in total body fat mass which requires increased blood flow to support metabolism (Table 25.1). It has been estimated that 2–3 mL of blood is necessary to perfuse every 100 g of adipose tissue at rest: in a patient with 100 kg of fat this would require up to a 3 L/min increase in blood flow. This increased workload leads to an increased ventricular mass and hypertrophy which predispose to an important imbalance between perfusion and metabolic demand (8). In the light of these observations obesity determines, at heart levels, structural alterations which make the myocardium and coronary vessels more prone to the atherosclerotic damage independently from the classic risk factors which are usually present in overweight people.

Undoubtedly, the negative effects of obesity appear closely linked to fat distribution. Central fat distribution is closely linked with a state of insulin resistance and the metabolic abnormalities associated with this syndrome; they all represent powerful risk factors for atherosclerotic cardiovascular disease (ACVD) (9). Nonetheless obesity irrespectively from fat distribution is associated with diabetes mellitus, hypertension and dyslipidaemia, which all predispose to ACVD (10).

ACVD is closely associated with adiposity as measured by either weight, BMI, or measures of central fat accumulation. This relationship is in part mediated by the other risk factors which co-segregate with obesity, in part by obesity itself. The rela-

International Textbook of Obesity. Edited by Per Björntorp.
© 2001 John Wiley & Sons, Ltd.

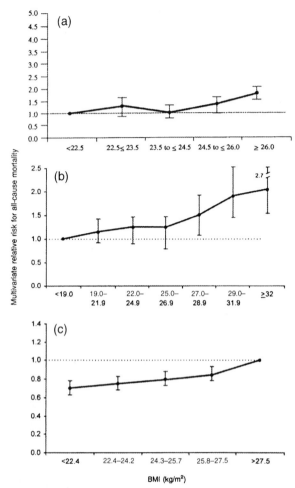

Table 25.1   Ventricular dysfunction reported in severely obese patients

1. Impaired ventricular function
2. Abnormal response to exercise
3. Depressed contractility related to ventricular mass
4. Reduced atrial dimension
5. Reduced ventricular wall and septal size

Adapted from Benotti *et al.* (8)

Figure 25.1   Relative risk from all-cause mortality according to BMI in three studies that minimized confounding by smoking and underlying diseases. (a) Harvard Alumni Study; (b) The Nurses Health Study population; (c) The Seventh Day Adventist Study. From Solomon and Manson (4)

cleotic cardiovascular disease (ACVD), obese people often present well-recognized coronary risk factors such as hypertension, lipid abnormalities, and type 2 diabetes (Table 25.2). There is now evidence that fat distribution rather than excess fatness is more commonly associated with these risk factors for ACVD. Abdominal fat deposition, which is principally observed in males and in postmenopausal females, is not only independently associated with ischaemic heart disease, but is a clinical condition in which the traditional risk factors for atherosclerosis are determined by the presence of insulin resistance which has likewise been associated with increased cardiovascular risk (11). The clinical aggregation of all these risk factors is also called the '(pluri)metabolic syndrome or syndrome X'. Regardless of these linguistic bagatelles, these patients will be exposed throughout their life to an excess risk for ACVD.

Obese people not only have an excess of traditional risk factors, they also have an excess presence of emerging risk factors such as a altered endothelial function and inappropriate production of cytokines, which are believed to play an important role in the development and progression of ACVD.

tionship between obesity and ACVD appears to be consistent for both coronary artery disease (CHD) and stroke (CVA), but doubtful for peripheral artery disease.

RISK FACTORS FOR ATHEROSCLEROTIC CARDIOVASCULAR DISEASE IN OBESITY

Although obesity has been established as an independent risk factor for the development of atheros-

Lipid Abnormalities

Lipid and lipoprotein abnormalities are commonly present in obese patients. Population studies have shown a linear relationship between body weight and lipoprotein levels in blood plasma (12). In patients of both sexes between the ages of 20 and 50 years there is a linear relationship between body weight, triglyceride and cholesterol concentrations. In people older than 50 years this relationship is no longer observed (13). Moreover, there is an inverse correlation between body weight and high density lipoprotein (HDL) cholesterol; this reciprocity is observed at all ages and in both sexes. Reduction in

Table 25.2 Atherogenic risk factors in obesity

Lipid and lipoprotein abnormalities	↑ Triglycerides
	↑ Cholesterol
	↑ Small dense LDL
	↓ HDL cholesterol
	↓ HDL_2/HDL_3 cholesterol
	↑ Postprandial free fatty acids
Hypertension	
Impaired glucose tolerance/type 2 diabetes	
Abnormalities of coagulation and fibrinolysis	↑ von Willebrand
	↑ Fibrinogen
	↑ PAI-1 antigen/activity
	↓ tPA
	↑ Factor VII
Abnormalities in acute phase reaction proteins	↑ C-reactive protein
	↑ TNFα
	↑ Interleukin-6
Endothelial dysfunction	↓ Endothelium-dependent vasodilation
	↓ Effect of insulin to augment endothelium-dependent vasodilation

LDL, low density lipoprotein; HDL, high density lipoprotein; PAI-1, plasminogen activator inhibitor 1; tPA, tissue plasminogen activator; TNFα, tumour necrosis factor α.

HDL cholesterol is a consistent finding in overweight patients (14). On the other hand, most patients with hypertriglyceridaemia and decreased HDL cholesterol are overweight.

Although the relationship between body weight and lipid abnormalities is weak and appreciable only in long-term prospective studies, the effects of obesity on lipoprotein metabolism are more profound than those predicted by the determination of their plasma levels. This concept is supported by kinetic studies which demonstrate that in obese people there is an increase of both production and clearance of very low density lipoprotein (VLDL) without significant alterations in their prevailing plasma concentrations (15).

In obese patients there is an increased hepatic synthesis of VLDL. However, a substantial fraction of these lipoproteins are removed from the circulation without being converted to LDL which are themselves removed faster than in non-obese subjects (16). The reduction of HDL-cholesterol in obese subjects is partly determined by the increased mass of triglyceride-rich lipoproteins (17).

More recently it has been shown that lipoprotein abnormalities are more profound in visceral than in subcutaneous adiposity (18). While excess fat does not appear to be significantly associated with lipid abnormalities, abdominal obesity is a better indicator of the lipoprotein abnormalities commonly used to quantify the risk for ACVD, particularly the LDL to HDL ratio (19).

In the general population, waist-to-hip ratio (WHR), an index of abdominal fat accumulation, correlates with VLDL triglyceride concentration and with HDL cholesterol. Furthermore, WHR has been reported to be negatively correlated with HDL_2 cholesterol, and positively with both the 'small dense' LDL and with the 'intermediate density lipoprotein' (20). In the light of these findings fat localization rather than total fat mass plays a major role in determining an atherogenic lipid profile. There exists much evidence suggesting a major role for the oxidized low density lipoprotein (LDL) and VLDL particles in the pathogenesis of atherosclerosis (21). In obese subjects there are not only quantitative but also qualitative alterations in circulating lipoproteins. Van Gaal et al. measured the oxidizability in vitro of lipoproteins in 21 obese premenopausal women and compared them to 18 age-matched non-obese controls (22). They found that TBARS, an index of lipid oxidation, measured every 30 minutes, increased in non-obese controls up to a maximum of 59.6 at 180 minutes in contrast to a maximum of 77.1 at 180 minutes ($P < 0.001$) in obese, but healthy, normocholesterolaemic subjects. At each measurement the TBARS were significantly higher ($P < 0.01$–0.001) in obese subjects. Also the lag-time (period from zero to the start of the particle oxidation process) was significantly lower in obese subjects, when compared to lean controls. BMI correlates significantly with TBARS formation. Thus *in vitro* oxidizability of non-HDL lipoproteins is significantly increased in obese, non-diabetic subjects and related to increased body weight (23). Thus patients present five main lipid abnormalities: (1) high triglycerides; (2) low HDL cholesterol; (3) reduced HDL$_2$ cholesterol; (4) increased proportion of small dense LDL; (5) increased susceptibility to oxidation of non-HDL lipoproteins.

Obesity and particularly abdominal obesity is associated with lipid and lipoprotein abnormalities not only in the fasting but also in postprandial state. In patients with visceral obesity there is an exaggerated postprandial free fatty acid (FFA) response which suggests that abdominal distribution of fat may contribute to both fasting and postprandial hypertryglyceridaemia by altering FFA metabolism in the postprandial state (16).

The negative effect of obesity on FFA metabolism appears to be determined by different components. First, insulin appears to have a blunted antilipolytic effect and this favours the delivery of FFA to the liver. Second, in viscerally obese women reduced post-heparin lipoprotein lipase activity has been observed. In viscerally obese patients, increased activity in another lipase, the hepatic lipase which operates on small triglyceride-rich lipoproteins, has also been observed (Figure 25.2) (24). This leads to an enrichment of LDL and HDL with triglycerides while VLDL become filled up with cholesterol esters. This process is the result of the action of plasma lipid transfer proteins which leads to increased levels of small dense LDL, a reduced HDL cholesterol (25,26).

Fasting hypertriglyceridaemia is a common feature of visceral obesity (27,28). This metabolic alteration is the result of an increased inflow of FFA to the liver. Several studies have shown that in obese subjects the lipolytic action of catecholamines in subcutaneous fat is reduced. This defect is caused by decreased expression and function of β_2-adrenoceptors, increased antilipolytic action of α_2-adrenoceptors and impaired ability of cyclic AMP to activate lipolysis (29). In contrast, visceral adipocytes show an enhanced lipolytic response to catecholamines due to an increased lipolytic activity of the β_2-adrenoceptors and to decreased antilipolytic activity of the α_2-adrenoceptors. Moreover, visceral adipocytes show an inappropriately elevated lipolytic activity which is poorly inhibited by insulin. This

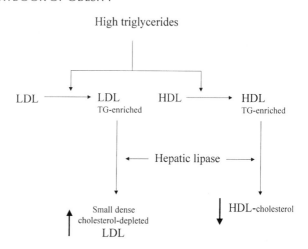

Figure 25.2 Potential mechanisms leading to the increased formation of small dense LDL and decreased levels of HDL. TG, triglyceride

metabolic abnormality results in increased FFA levels in both peripheral and portal circulation which leads to higher esterification of these substrates, to reduced degradation of apolipoprotein B, and to an increased synthesis and secretion of VLDL particles (15).

The association between abdominal obesity, hypertriglyceridaemia and small dense LDLs, which are more susceptible to oxidation, appears to be the most robust cluster in term of cardiovascular risk. However, this aggregation is liable to correction since it was shown that weight loss normalizes the physico-chemical properties of LDL. A hypocaloric diet and modest weight reduction induce a significant reduction of triglyceride concentrations within a few weeks (30). However, a longer period is necessary to bring about a reduction in total cholesterol and LDL cholesterol, and an increase in HDL cholesterol. When weight loss is achieved by a combination of diet and physical exercise, the improvement in lipid profile appears to be more consistent and stable (31).

Hypertension

The association between obesity and hypertension has been extensively documented by several studies and specifically from the Framingham Study and the National Health and Nutrition Examination

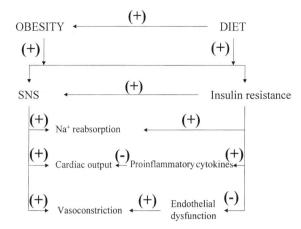

Figure 25.3 Relationship between obesity, diet, hypertension and endothelial dysfunction. SNS, sympathetic nervous system

Survey (32–35). In general, obesity and hypertension both are predictors of ACVD, obese people are more prone to hypertension, and most hypertensive patients are obese. Obesity and weight gain are predictors of hypertension independently from the age of onset of obesity; moreover, weight loss is associated with a reduction of blood pressure (36). Yet the pathophysiology of the relationship between obesity and hypertension has not been thoroughly clarified.

Obesity is characterized by an increased intravascular volume which appears to be a key factor in determining hypertension in these subjects. From a haemodynamic standpoint there is a resetting of pressor natriuresis in obesity, i.e. the maintenance of an expanded extracellular volume despite elevated blood pressure. This means that there must be an enhancement in tubular renal reabsorption (37). Some studies have claimed an important role for hyperinsulinaemia (Figure 25.3). Excessively elevated insulin would induce medullary vasoconstriction which plays an important part in forcing renal tubular reabsorption (38). Hyperinsulinaemia also stimulates the sympathetic nervous system (SNS), which in turn favours vasoconstriction of the deep medullary blood vessels which further increases sodium reabsorption (39,40). Insulin determines a dose-dependent increase of plasma noradrenaline (norepinephrine) concentration and of noradrenaline spillover from muscle. In obese patients there is also an exaggerated pressor response to noradrenaline, a reduced threshold to its pressor effect, and a reduced clearance of noradrenaline (41). In insulin-

resistant states the vasodilatory effect of insulin wanes and this phenomenon is closely related to the degree of insulin resistance. Hyperinsulinaemia stimulates the sodium/hydrogen countertransport. This leads to an intracellular accumulation of sodium and calcium which, in turn, increases the susceptibility of vascular smooth muscle cells to the hypertensive effect of noradrenaline and angiotensin (42).

In obese patients chronic hyperinsulinaemia may also lead to an inappropriate activation of the renin–angiotensin–aldosterone system and to an altered function of atrial natriuretic peptide (43).

Insulin also has the ability to increase intracellular calcium. Regulation of intracellular Ca^{2+} plays a key role in obesity, insulin resistance and hypertension, and disorder of $[Ca^{2+}]i$ may represent a factor linking these three conditions (44). In the insulin-resistant state, such as obesity, there is a lack of the insulin-mediated decrease in $[Ca^{2+}]i$; this leads to increased vascular resistance.

As well as the prominent effect of insulin on the aetiology of hypertension, other factors could mediate the increase in blood pressure observed in obese patients. Steroids could also play a role in the relationship between obesity and hypertension since these hormones may determine fat distribution and the type of obesity (45,46). Recently it has been hypothesized that central obesity may reflect a 'Cushing's disesase of the omentum'. Glucocorticoids not only regulate the differentiation of adipose stromal cells but they also affect the function of adipocytes. In fact adipose stromal cells from omentum can generate active cortisol through the expression of the 11β-hydroxysteroid dehydrogenase (47). *In vivo* such a mechanism would ensure a constant exposure of blood vessels to glucorticoid, thus aggravating the obesity-related hypertension. Furthermore, the excess of androgens observed in women with abdominal fat deposition and the increased response of cortisol to stress in men with reduced testosterone may contribute to the development of hypertension (48).

Thus in obese subjects both blood volume and cardiac output are increased but the peripheral vascular resistance is normal rather than decreased; this unexpectedly normal peripheral resistance is possibly determined by enhanced adrenergic tone; altered endothelial function, activation of renin–angiotensin systems, and possibly increased levels of neuropeptide Y (NPY), which has been shown to be a potent vasoconstrictor (49).

All these neurohumoral and haemodynamic alterations, as well as blood pressure levels, significantly improved after weight loss. This finding provides additional proof that they all play an important role in the development and progression of hypertension in obesity (50–52).

Haemostic and Endothelial Factors

Obesity predisposes to thrombosis by altering both the concentration and the activity of several factors involved in the coagulative and fibrinolytic processes. A closed and independent correlation between body mass index and fibrinogen levels has been observed (53,54). Fibrinogen was shown to correlate also with WHR and with the other components of the metabolic syndrome. Elevated fibrinogen levels are an independent risk factor for ACVD and it may partly explain the increased prevalence of cardiovascular mortality in the obese patients. A positive correlation was also shown between factor VII, von Willebrand and BMI (55). At variance, no change in the activity of antithrombin III was observed while protein C levels were increased.

A defect in fibrinolysis, usually observed in states of insulin resistance and in overweight patients, has been claimed as a key step in the development and progression of atherosclerotic lesions. This hypothesis has been supported by the finding of increased levels of plasminogen activator inhibitor (PAI)-1 antigen and decreased levels of tissue plasminogen activator (tPA) (56,57). A direct correlation between BMI and PAI-1 activity has been shown; furthermore, a correlation has been also observed between PAI-1, the degree of insulin resistance, and the degree of abdominal fat deposition. A defect in the fibrinolytic process is now considered as one of the most prominent in the metabolic syndrome. It has been recently shown that the adipose tissue is a site of active PAI-1 production which is a function of cell size and of their lipid content (58). Overproduction of PAI-1 is determined by an increased PAI-1 gene expression. Visceral rather than subcutaneous adipose tissue is a site of inappropriate PAI-1 production. This excessive PAI-1 production by visceral fat may partly explain its more pronounced atherogenic potential (59). It has been shown that insulin stimulates PAI-1 production, which may therefore be increased in state of insulin resistance. PAI-1 gene expression is stimulated by insulin both hepatocytes and endothelial cells (60). Recently, the potential role of VLDL and of its receptor in mediating VLDL-induced PAI-1 expression has also been demonstrated in in vitro studies (61,62). Therefore, in obesity several mechanisms such as elevated insulin levels, excessive visceral fat deposition, and increased VLDL contribute to the impaired fibrinolytic apparatus.

Platelet function was also shown to be impaired in the presence of insulin resistance (63). In this metabolic setting the altered insulin action on cyclic nucleotides is diminished; this leads to an increased inward calcium flux, enhanced platelet aggregation and hence to an increase thrombotic risk (64).

It has been recently hypothesized that the metabolic syndrome may represent an altered immunological response. In patients with visceral obesity an increase in acute phase proteins such as sialic acid, C-reactive protein, and the interleukin-6 (65). It has also been shown that tumour necrosis factor (TNFα) (also known as 'cachectin'), a pleiotropic cytokine involved in many metabolic responses in both normal and pathophysiological states, may also have a central role in obesity, modulating energy expenditure, fat deposition and insulin resistance (66). How TNFα-related insulin resistance is mediated is not fully clear, although phosphorylation of serine residues on insulin receptor substrate (IRS) 1 has previously been shown to be important (67). An approximately 2-fold increase in insulin-stimulated tyrosine phosphorylation of the insulin receptor in the muscle and adipose tissue of TNFα knockout mice was found, suggesting that insulin receptor signalling is an important target for TNFα (68).

The increase in inflammatory cytokines may contribute to impairment of the early steps in intracellular insulin signalling not only through a direct effect but also indirectly by altering endothelial function. Yudkin and colleagues have found a close relationship between cytokine levels and the amount of visceral fat deposition which is a site of active TNFα production (69). Yudkin's group also reported an increased secretion of interleukin-6 by subcutaneous adipose tissue (70). TNFα has been implicated as an inducer of the synthesis of PAI-1. Recent findings suggest that TNFα stimulation of PAI-1 is potentiated by insulin, and that adipocyte generation of reactive oxygen centred radicals mediates the induction of PAI-1 production by TNFα (71).

As a whole these data support the hypothesis that total fat mass determines a low chronic inflammatory state which may not only induce an insulin resistance state but could also favour the development and progression of atherosclerotic damage in the blood vessels.

Steinberg and colleagues have shown that in obese patients there is altered endothelial-mediated vasodilation and a reduced insulin haemodynamic response which is closely related to the degree of insulin resistance (72). A common link between the decreased insulin vascular and metabolic effects may be provided by altered intracellular phosphatidylinositol-3-kinase activity (73). On the other hand, obesity is characterized by increased levels of hypertension, increased oxidized LDL, increased FFA levels which all combine to alter endothelial function.

Recently it has been shown that in obese subjects acetylcholine-stimulated vasodilation is blunted and that the increase in forearm blood flow is inversely related to BMI, WHR, and insulin action (74).

Diabetes Mellitus

Impaired glucose tolerance and non-insulin-dependent diabetes mellitus represents the almost inevitable outcome in the natural history of obese subjects, in particular of those with abdominal fat accumulation (75). The evolution of obesity toward overt diabetes is characterized by the onset of peripheral insulin resistance, hyperglycaemia, and finally by reduced β-cell secretory capacity. Several mechanisms are involved in insulin resistance in subjects at risk for type 2 diabetes. Transport of insulin across the capillary endothelium is altered due to a reduced capillary permeability to insulin. The transport of insulin across the endothelial barrier not only limits the rate at which insulin stimulates glucose uptake by skeletal muscle, but appears also to determine the rate at which insulin suppresses liver glucose output. In addition, a strong correlation has been demonstrated between FFA and liver glucose output under a variety of experimental conditions (76). Moreover if FFAs are maintained at basal concentrations during insulin administration, glucose output fails to decline. Finally, if FFAs are reduced independent of insulin administration, glucose output is reduced. These points support the concept that insulin, by regulating adipocyte lipolysis, controls liver glucose production. Thus, the adipocyte appears to be a critical mediator between insulin and liver glucose output. Evidence that FFAs also suppress skeletal muscle glucose uptake and insulin secretion from the β-cell supports the overall central role of the adipocyte in the regulation of glycaemia. Insulin resistance at the fat cell may be an important component of the overall regulation of glycaemia because of the relationships between FFA and glucose production, glucose uptake and insulin release. It is possible that insulin resistance at the adipocyte itself can be a major cause of the dysregulation of carbohydrate metabolism in the prediabetic state (77).

Several prospective studies have conclusively shown that obesity is an important risk factor for the development of diabetes (78). The Framingham Study has shown that there is an increased incidence of impaired glucose tolerance in obese subjects (32). Once hyperglycaemia is established, this represents an independent risk factor for ACVD. Hyperglycaemia causes a direct negative effect on the vessel wall through an array of mechanisms, the most important being: (1) protein glycation, in particular the glycation of LDL: these modified lipoproteins have a prolonged half-life; (2) the accumulation of modified lipoproteins which can induce excessive cross-linking of collagen and other matrix proteins; (3) increased oxidative stress; (4) increased polyol pathway and the consequent increase of the NADH/NAD ratio; (5) activation of protein kinase C (PKC). This latter effect brings about the induction of cellular matrix and cytokines which eventually leads to vascular cell proliferation (79). Several studies have shown that hyperglycaemia is a risk factor for ACVD (80): a 1% increase in HbA1c results in a 10% increase in coronary events. High fasting plasma glucose predicts not only coronary events but also fatal and non-fatal stroke. The hyperinsulinaemia associated with insulin resistance, which is a common feature of non-insulin-dependent diabetes mellitus, appears to play a major role in the development and progression of ACVD in obese people with diabetes (81,82). This subject is described in detail in Chapter 24.

CARDIOVASCULAR DISEASE

Coronary Artery Disease

The Framingham Study showed in 2005 men and 2521 women that the 28-year age-adjusted rates (per 100) of CHD was 26.3 for a mean BMI of $21.6\,kg/m^2$ and 42.2 for a mean BMI of 31 in men, and 19.5 for a BMI of 20.4 and 28.8 for a BMI of 32.3 in women, respectively (82). The 28-year age-adjusted relative risks and their 95% confidence intervals for the highest quintile compared to the lowest were 1.9 (1.4–2.5) for CHD and 1.8 (1.4–2.4) for CHD excluding angina pectoris for men and 1.7 (1.3–2.3) and 1.6 (1.2–2.3) for women, respectively. The Gothenburg study, in a 12-year incidence period, showed in a multivariate analysis, that the WHR was the strongest predictor (84) of myocardial infarction in 1462 women. In 1990, the Nurses Health Study, during an 8-year observation, clearly showed in a population of 121 700 females that obesity is a determinant of CHD; after control for cigarette smoking, which is essential to assess the true effect of obesity, even mild-to-moderate overweight increased the risk of CHD (Figure 25.4) (85). This study showed a relative risk of 3.3 for a BMI of $\geq 29\,kg/m^2$ when compared to BMI < 21; a negative effect of obesity remained appreciable after a multivariate correction for hypertension, diabetes and high cholesterol levels. Similarly, the Honolulu Heart Program demonstrated over a 20-year observation period that a mean subscapular skinfold thickness of 27.2 mm increased the risk of developing CHD in Japanese American men aged 45–65 years by 1.5 when compared to a thickness of 8.1 mm (86). The Rochester Coronary Heart Disease project suggested that both weight and BMI are mildly associated with angina but not clearly with myocardial infarction or sudden unexpected death (87). This last event appears related to morbid obesity rather than to modest overweight. Duflou *et al.* showed in 22 patients with morbid obesity that dilated cardiomyopathy was the most frequent cause of sudden cardiac death followed by severe coronary atherosclerosis, left ventricular hypertrophy, pulmonary embolism and hypoplastic coronary arteries (Figure 25.5) (7). Recently the Paris Prospective Study has shown that increased BMI, along with resting heart rate, systolic or diastolic blood pressure, tobacco consumption, diabetes

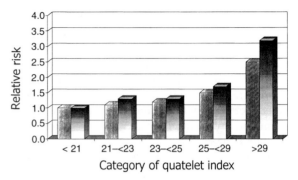

Figure 25.4 Relative risk of non-fatal myocardial infarction (left bars) and fatal coronary heart disease according to category of BMI in a cohort of US women 30 to 55 years of age in 1976. Adapted from Manson *et al.* (84)

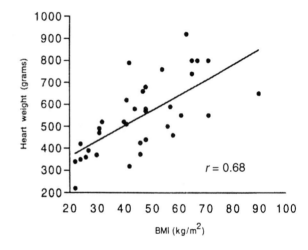

Figure 25.5 Linear regression comparing heart weight and BMI in people with massive obesity who died suddenly, of unnatural causes and who died from traumatic causes. From Duflou *et al.* (7)

status, serum cholesterol, and parental history of sudden death, was an independent predictor of sudden death during follow-up (23 years on average) (88,89).

The interaction between CHD and obesity has recently been confirmed by the PROCAM study, in which 16 288 men aged 40.6 ± 11.3 years and 7328 women aged 36.0 ± 12.3 years were enrolled between 1979 and 1991 (90). Among the 10 856 men aged 36–65 years at study entry, 313 deaths occurred within a follow-up period of 7.1 ± 2.4 years. Among these men, increased mortality was seen at high BMI in both smokers and non-smokers and was caused by coronary heart disease (CHD).

Increased mortality at low BMI was seen in smokers but not in non-smokers and was due to an increase in cancer deaths. However, in this study the BMI-associated increase in CHD death was completely accounted for by the factors contained in the risk algorithm, indicating that the effect of overweight and obesity on CHD is mediated via other risk factors.

The relationship between obesity per se and CHD therefore appears doubtful when the measure of adiposity is expressed with a classical anthropometric variable such as weight and BMI, which may be inadequate surrogates for adiposity itself. As previously mentioned, the association between obesity and CHD becomes more robust when the distribution of fat is considered. Although Gillum *et al.* (34) and Hodgson *et al.* (91) found that the increased risk for ACVD present in abdominal adiposity is indirectly mediated by the presence of the other classical risk factors, several subsequent papers confirmed that the abdominal distribution of fat is an independent risk for CHD. Clark *et al.* found that, at least in black women, the strongest predictor for CHD is WHR ≥ 0.85 followed by a family history of CHD and cigarette smoking (92). From forensic autopsy evaluations, Kortelainen and Sarkioja found that abdominal accumulation of fat is associated with the severity of coronary atherosclerosis and myocardial hypertrophy in women with no clinical evidence of cardiovascular disease (93,94). They also found that coronary lesions and myocardial hypertrophy are more advanced as WHR increases. Recently Gaudet *et al.* found that abdominal obesity is a powerful predictor of CHD in men, even in a group of patients with raised LDL cholesterol levels due to familial hypercholesterolaemia (95).

The relationship between obesity and CHD is operative not only in the elderly population but also in children and adolescents. Excessive body weight between 5 and 18 years is an independent predictor of future mortality in $> 13\,000$ person (96). Similarly, in the Harvard Growth Study, BMI between 13 and 18 years predicted CHD mortality: adolescents with a BMI above the 75th percentile have a relative risk of 2.3 as compared to those in the 25th percentile (97). These impressive data justify the notion that atherosclerosis may be considered a nutritional disease of childhood (98). The relationship between weight gain and CHD has been emphasized in a recent paper which demonstrated

in 6874 men aged 47 to 55 years at baseline and free of a history of myocardial infarction, followed for an average period of 19.7 years, that high BMI predicted death from CHD only at levels above $27.5 \, \text{kg/m}^2$ and that men with stable weight (defined as $\pm 4\%$ change from age 20) had the lowest death rate from CHD (99). The authors conclude that weight gain from age 20, even a very moderate increase, is strongly associated with an increased risk of CHD.

Cerebrovascular Disease

Obesity has been shown to be a risk factor also for cerebrovascular disease (CVD), although its negative role appears more clearly in women than in men. In the Framingham Study the 28-year age-adjusted relative risk for CVD was reported to be 1.4 (0.9–2.2) for men and 1.6 (1.1–2.4) for women in the upper quintile of BMI as compared to those in the lowest (83). Fatal stroke was also predicted by WHR in women in the Gothenburg Study and in US male army veterans (100). The relationship between obesity and stroke has not been confirmed in the Honolulu Heart Study where neither BMI nor central obesity was a predictor for such events (86). However, more recently publications from this group showed that elevated body mass was associated with an increased risk of thromboembolic stroke in non-smoking men in older middle age who were free from commonly observed conditions related to cardiovascular disease (101). In 1997 Rexrode *et al.* demonstrated in a prospective study that, during a 16-year follow-up, a BMI of $\geq 27 \, \text{kg/m}^2$ significantly increased the risk of ischaemic stroke, with relative risk of 2.37 (95% CI 1.60–3.50) for a BMI of $32 \, \text{kg/m}^2$ or more (102). No relationship was observed for haemorrhagic stroke. This study also showed that a weight gain of 20 kg or more was associated with a relative risk for ischaemic stroke of 2.52 (95% CI 1.80–3.52).

Folsom *et al.* for the ARIC (Atherosclerosis Risk In Communities Study) recently found that, in diabetic patients, the relative risk for ischaemic stroke was 1.74 (1.4–2.2) for a 0.11 increment of WHR, whereas the risk was not statistically related to BMI (103). This study further emphasizes the role of regional fat distribution, rather than total fat mass, as an important risk factor for CVD.

Peripheral Vascular Disease

Literature data on the effects of obesity on lower limb circulation are more contrasting than those regarding the coronary and cerebral circulaions. While the Framingham Study showed that the relative risk for intermittent claudication was 0.9 (0.5–1.4) for men and 1.1 (0.6–1.8) for women in the fifth quintile compared to the first quintile, a retrospective study in a small group of female patients (52–82 years) showed that obesity was a predictive risk factor for peripheral vascular disease (PVD) (83). This latter finding is supported by the data of the Swedish Obese Subjects Study which showed, in 1006 male and female subjects, that obesity was significantly associated with intermittent claudication (104).

While obesity per se does not appear to confer a significant risk for the development of PVD, the association of obesity and diabetes mellitus does contribute to an enhanced risk of lower limb problems. As thoroughly demonstrated in epidemiological studies, severe complications of PVD are very frequent in people with non-insulin-dependent diabetes, who have a 10- to 15-fold increased risk for lower extremity amputation and a 3.4- to 5.7-fold increased risk for caudication (80,105). This increased risk appears to be consistent in diabetics independently of total fat mass or fat distribution.

CONCLUSIONS

Obesity is a significant predictor of ACVD, this partly explains the increased risk of mortality in this group of patients. Obesity is not only a direct risk factor for ACVD but it also has a deleterious effect indirectly since this condition frequently co-segregate with other risk factors for ACVD such as diabetes, hypertension and hyperlipidaemia. The abdominal distribution of fat, and the consequent serious insulin resistance which accompanies this condition, further aggravates the negative impact of overweight on the development and progression of atherosclerotic lesion. Not only obesity as an established pathological condition but also weight gain may have a detrimental effect on ACVD, especially on the risk of stroke. Since childhood obesity is also an independent risk factor for ACVD, every effort must be made to avoid this condition,

by encouraging exercise and modifying dietary habits.

REFERENCES

1. Barrett-Connor EI. Obesity, atherosclerosis, and coronary artery disease. *Ann Inter Med* 1985; **103**: 1010–1019.
2. Manson JE, Stampfer MJ, Hennekens CH, Willett WC. Body weight and longevity. A reassessment. *JAMA* 1987; **257**: 353–358.
3. Waaler HT. Height, weight and mortality. The Norwegian experience. *Acta Med Scand Suppl* 1984; **679**: 1–56.
4. Solomon CG, Manson JE. Obesity and mortality: a review of the epidemiologic data. *Am J Clin Nutr* 1997; **66**: 1044S–1050S.
5. Menotti A, Descovich GC, Lanti M, Seccareccia F, Dormi A. [Obesity and mortality. Italian epidemiologic data]. *Recenti Prog Med* 1992; **83**: 121–126.
6. Lee IM, Manson JE, Hennekens CH, Paffenbarger RS. Jr. Body weight and mortality. A 27-year follow-up of middle-aged men [see comments]. *JAMA* 1993; **270**: 2823–2828.
7. Duflou J, Virmani R, Rabin I, Burke A, Farb A, Smialek J. Sudden death as a result of heart disease in morbid obesity. *Am Heart J* 1995; **130**: 306–313.
8. Benotti PN, Bistrain B, Benotti JR, Blackburn G, Forse RA. Heart disease and hypertension in severe obesity: the benefits of weight reduction. *Am J Clin Nutr* 1992; **55**: 586S–590S.
9. Björntorp P. Body fat distribution, insulin resistance, and metabolic diseases. *Nutrition* 1997; **13**: 795–803.
10. Wild RA. Obesity, lipids, cardiovascular risk, and androgen excess. *Am J Med* 1995; **98**: 27S–32S.
11. Despres JP. Abdominal obesity as important component of insulin-resistance syndrome. *Nutrition* 1993; **9**: 452–459.
12. Walton C, Lees B, Crook D, Worthington M, Godsland IF, Stevenson JC. Body fat distribution, rather than overall adiposity, influences serum lipids and lipoproteins in healthy men independently of age [see comments]. *Am J Med* 1995; **99**: 459–464.
13. Julien P, Vohl NC, Gaudet D, Cagne C, Levesque G, Despres JP, Cadelis F, Brun LD, Nadeau A, Ven Murthy MR. Hyperinsulinemia and abdominal obesity affect the expression of hypertriglyceridemia in hetrozygous familial lipoprotein lipase deficiency. *Diabetes* 1997; **46**: 2063–2068.
14. Glueck CJ, Taylor HL, Jacobs D, Morrison JA, Beaglehole R, Williams OD. Plasma high-density lipoprotein cholesterol: association with measurements of body mass. The Lipid Research Clinics Program Prevalence Study. *Circulation* 1980; **62**: IV-62–69.
15. Fisher RM, Coppack SW, Gibbons GF, Frayn KN. Postprandial VLDL subfraction metabolism in normal and obese subjects. *Int J Obes Relat Metab Disord* 1993; **17**: 263–269.
16. Couillard C, Bergeron N, Prud'homme D, Bergeron J, Tremblay A, Bouchard C, Mauriege P, Despres JP. Postprandial triglyceride response in visceral obesity in men. *Diabetes* 1998; **47**: 953–960.
17. Modan M, Halkin H, Lusky A, Segal P, Fuchs Z, Chetrit A. Hyperinsulinemia is characterized by jointly disturbed

plasma VLDL, LDL, and HDL levels. A population-based study. *Arteriosclerosis* 1988; **8**: 227–236.

18. Despres JP. Dyslipidaemia and obesity. *Bailliere's Clin Endocrinol Metab* 1994; **8**: 629–660.

19. Pouliot MC, Despres JP, Nadeau A, Moorjani S, Prud'Homme D, Lupien PJ, Tremblay A, Bouchard C. Visceral obesity in men. Associations with glucose tolerance, plasma insulin, and lipoprotein levels. *Diabetes* 1992; **41**: 826–834.

20. Terry RB, Wood PD, Haskell WL, Stefanick ML, Krauss RM. Regional adiposity patterns in relation to lipids, lipoprotein cholesterol, and lipoprotein subfraction mass in men. *J Clin Endocrinol Metab* 1989; **68**: 191–199.

21. Heinecke JW. Is lipid peroxidation relevant to atherogenesis? *J Clin Invest* 1999; **104**: 135–136.

22. Van Gaal LF, Vertommen J, De Leeuw IH. The in vitro oxidizability of lipoprotein particles in obese and non-obese subjects. *Atherosclerosis* 1998; **137**(Suppl): S39–44.

23. Cominacini L, Garbin U, Pastorino AM, Fratta Pasini A, Campagnola M, De Santis A, Davoli A, Lo Cascio V. Increased susceptibility of LDL to in vitro oxidation in patients with insulin-dependent and non-insulin-dependent diabetes mellitus. *Diabetes Res* 1994; **26**: 173–184.

24. Kobayashi J, Tashiro J, Murano S, Morisaki N, Saito Y. Lipoprotein lipase mass and activity in post-heparin plasma from subjects with intra-abdominal visceral fat accumulation. *Clin Endocrinol (Oxf)* 1998; **48**: 515–520.

25. Despres JP, Ferland M, Moorjani S, Nadeau A, Tremblay A, Lupien PJ, Theriault G, Bouchard C. Role of hepatic-triglyceride lipase activity in the association between intra-abdominal fat and plasma HDL cholesterol in obese women. *Arteriosclerosis* 1989; **9**: 485–492.

26. Despres JP. Lipoprotein metabolism in visceral obesity. *Int J Obes* 1991; **15**(Suppl 2): 45–52.

27. Björntorp P. Abdominal fat distribution and the metabolic syndrome. *J Cardiovasc Pharmacol* 1992; **20**: S26–28.

28. Kissebah AH, Hennes MM. Central obesity and free fatty acid metabolism. *Prostaglandins Leukot Essent Fatty Acids* 1995; **52**: 209–211.

29. Arner P. Catecholamine-induced lipolysis in obesity. *Int J Obest Relat Metab Disord* 1999; **23**(Suppl 1): 10–13.

30. Mingrone G, DeGaetano A, Greco AV, Capristo E, Benedetti G, Castagneto M, Gasbarrini G. Reversibility of insulin resistance in obese diabetic patients: role of plasma lipids. *Diabetologia* 1997; **40**: 599–605.

31. Katzel LI, Bleecker ER, Colman EG, Rogus EM, Sorkin JD, Goldberg AP. Effects of weight loss vs aerobic exercise training on risk factors for coronary disease in healthy, obese, middle-aged and older men. A randomized controlled trial [see comments]. *JAMA* 1995; **274**: 1915–1921.

32. Wilson PW. Established risk factors and coronary artery disease: the Framingham Study. *Am J Hypertens* 1994; **7**: 7S–12S.

33. Sundquist J, Winkleby MA. Cardiovascular risk factors in Mexican American adults: a transcultural analysis of NHANES III, 1988–1994. *Am J Public Health* 1999; **89**: 723–730.

34. Gillum RF, Mussolino ME, Madans JH. Body fat distribution and hypertension incidence in women and men. The NHANES I Epidemiologic Follow-up Study. *Int J Obes Relat Metab Disord* 1998; **22**: 127–134.

35. Ettinger WH, Davis MA, Neuhaus JM, Mallon KP. Long-term physical functioning in persons with knee osteoarthritis from NHANES. I: Effects of comorbid medical conditions. *J Clin Epidemiol* 1994; **47**: 809–815.

36. Modan M, Halkin H. Hyperinsulinemia or increased sympathetic drive as links for obesity and hypertension. *Diabetes Care* 1991; **14**: 470–487.

37. Kolanowski J. Obesity and hypertension: from pathophysiology to treatment. *Int J Obes Relat Metab Disord* 1999; **23**(Suppl 1): 42–46.

38. Hall JE. Louis K. Dahl Memorial Lecture. Renal and cardiovascular mechanisms of hypertension in obesity. *Hypertension* 1994; **23**: 381–394.

39. Brands MW, Hall JE, Van Vliet BN, Alonso-Galicia M, Herrera GA, Zappe D. Obesity and hypertension: roles of hyperinsulinemia, sympathetic nervous system and intrarenal mechanisms. *J Nutr* 1995; **125**: 1725S–1731S.

40. Daly PA, Landsberg L. Pathogenesis of hypertension in NIDDM: lessons from obesity. *J Hum Hypertens* 1991; **5**: 277–285.

41. Weidmann P, de Courten M, Boehlen L, Shaw S. The pathogenesis of hypertension in obese subjects. *Drugs* 1993; **46**: 197–208; discussion 208–209.

42. Doria A, Fioretto P, Avogaro A, Carraro A, Morocutti A, Trevisan R, Frigato F, Crapaldi G, Viberti G, Nosadini R. Insulin resistance is associated with high sodium-lithium countertransport in essential hypertension. *Am J Physiol* 1991; **261**: E684–691.

43. Dessi-Fulgheri P, Sarzani R, Rappelli A. The natriuretic peptide system in obesity-related hypertension: new pathophysiological aspects. *J Nephrol* 1998; **11**: 296–299.

44. Epstein M. Calcium channel blockers and hypertension: evolving perspective—1996. *Cardiovasc Drugs Ther* 1997; **10**(Suppl 3): 883–891.

45. Haffner SM, Karhapaa P, Mykkanen L, Laakso M. Insulin resistance, body fat distribution, and sex hormones in men. *Diabetes* 1994; **43**: 212–219.

46. Björntorp P. The regulation of adipose tissue distribution in humans. *Int J Obes Relat Metab Disord* 1996; **20**: 291–302.

47. Bujalska IJ, Kumar S, Stewart PM. Does central obesity reflect 'Cushing's disease of the omentum'? *Lancet* 1997; **349**: 1210–1213.

48. Björntorp P. Metabolic implications of body fat distribution. *Diabetes Car* 1991; **14**: 1132–1143.

49. Clarke J, Benjamin N, Larkin S, Webb D, Maseri A, Davies G. Interaction of neuropeptide Y and the sympathetic nervous system in vascular control in man. *Circulation* 1991; **83**: 774–777.

50. Cowan GS, Jr, Buffington CK. Significant changes in blood pressure, glucose, and lipids with gastric bypass surgery. *World J Surg* 1998; **22**: 987–992,

51. DasGupta P, Ramhanmdany E, Brigden G, Lahiri A, Baird IM, Raftery EB. Improvement in left ventricular function after rapid weight loss in obesity. *Eur Heart J* 1992; **13**: 1060–1066.

52. Despres JP, Tremblay A, Nadeau A, Bouchard C. Physical training and changes in regional adipose tissue distribution. *Acta Med Scand Suppl* 1988; **723**: 205–212.

53. Eliasson M, Evrin PE, Lundblad D. Fibrinogen and fibrinolytic variables in relation to anthropometry, lipids and

blood pressure. The Northern Sweden MONICA Study. *J Clin Epidemiol* 1994; **47**: 513–524.

54. Marckmann P, Toubro S, Astrup A. Sustained improvement in blood lipids, coagulation, and fibrinolysis after major weight loss in obese subjects. *Eur J Clin Nutr* 1998; **52**: 329–333.

55. Charles MA, Morange P, Eschwege E, Andre P, Vague P, Juhan-Vague I. Effect of weight change and metformin on fibrinolysis and the von Willebrand factor in obese non-diabetic subjects: the BIGPRO1 Study. Biguanides and the Prevention of the Risk of Obesity. *Diabetes Care* 1998; **21**: 1967–1972.

56. Scelles V, Raccah D, Alessi MC, Vialle JM, Juhan-Vague I, Vague P. Plasminogen activator inhibitor 1 and insulin levels in various insulin resistance states. *Diabete Metab* 1992; **18**: 38–42.

57. Vague P, Raccah D, Scelles V. Hypofibrinolysis and the insulin resistance syndrome. *Int J Obes Relat Metab Disord* 1995; **19**(Suppl 1): S11–15.

58. Shimomura I, Funahashi T, Takahashi M, Maeda K, Kotani K, Nakamura T, Yamashita S, Miura M, Fukuda Y, Takemura K, Tokunaga K, Matsuzawa Y. Enhanced expression of PAI-1 in visceral fat: possible contributor to vascular disease in obesity. *Nat Med* 1996; **2**: 800–803.

59. Janand-Delenne B, Chagnaud C, Raccah D, Alessi MC, Juhan-Vague I, Vague P. Visceral fat as a main determinant of plasminogen activator inhibitor 1 level in women. *In J Obes Relat Metab Disord* 1998; **22**: 312–317.

60. Latron Y, Alessi MC, George F, Anfosso F, Poncelet P, Juhan-Vague I. Characterization of epitheloid cells from human omentum: comparison with endothelial cells from umbilical veins. *Thromb Haemost* 1991; **66**: 361–367.

61. Heegaard CW, Simonsen AC, Oka K, Kjoller L, Christensen A, Madsen B, Ellgaard L, Chan L, Andreasen PA. Very low density lipoprotein receptor binds and mediates endocytosis of urokinase-type plasminogen activator-type-1 plasminogen activator inhibitor complex. *J Biol Chem* 1995; **270**: 20855–20861.

62. Willnow TE, Golstein JL, Orth K, Brown MS, Herz J. Low density lipoprotein receptor-related protein and gp330 bind similar ligands, including plasminogen activator-inhibitor complexes and lactoferrin, an inhibitor of chylomicron remnant clearance. *J Biol Chem* 1992; **267**: 26172–26180.

63. Corica F, Allegra A, Ientile R, Buemi M, Corsonello A, Bonanzinga S, Macoione S, Ceruso D. Changes in plasma, erythrocyte, and platelet magnesium levels in normotensive and hypertensive obese subjects during oral glucose tolerance test. *Am J Hypertens* 1999; **12**: 128–136.

64. Anfossi G, Mularoni EM, Burzacca S, Ponziani MC, Massucco P, Mattiello L, Cavalot F, Trovati M. Platelet resistance to nitrates in obesity and obese NIDDM, and normal platelet sensitivity to both insulin and nitrates in lean NIDDM. *Diabetes Care* 1998; **21**: 121–126.

65. McCarty MF. Interleukin-6 as a central mediator of cardiovascular risk associated with chronic inflammation, smoking, diabetes, and visceral obesity: down-regulation with essential fatty acids, ethanol and pentoxifylline [In Process Citation]. *Med Hypotheses* 1999; **52**: 465–477.

66. Hotamisligil GS. Mechanisms of TNF-alpha-induced insulin resistance [see comments]. *Exp Clin Endocrinol Diabetes* 1999; **107**: 119–125.

67. Hotamisligil GS. The role of TNFalpha and TNF receptors in obesity and insulin resistance. *J Intern Med* 1999; **245**: 621–625.

68. Le Marchand-Brustel Y. Molecular mechanisms of insulin action in normal and insulin-resistant states [see comments]. *Exp Clin Endocrinol Diabetes* 1999; **107**: 126–132.

69. Yudkin JS, Stehouwer CD, Emeis JJ, Coppack SW. C-reaction protein in healthy subjects: associations with obesity, insulin resistance, and endothelial dysfunction: a potential role for cytokines originating from adipose tissue? *Arterioscler Thromb Vasc Biol* 1999; **19**: 972–978.

70. Yudkin JS, Yajnik CS, Mohamed-Ali V, Bulmer K. High levels of circulating proinflammatory cytokines and leptin in urban, but not rural, Indians. A potential explanation for increased risk of diabetes and coronary heart disease [letter]. *Diabetes Care* 1999; **22**: 363–364.

71. Okada H, Woodcock-Mitchell J, Mitchell J, Sakamoto T, Marutsuka K, Sobel BE, Fujii S. Induction of plasminogen activator inhibitor type 1 and type 1 collagen expression in rat cardiac microvascular endothelial cells by interleukin-1 and its dependence on oxygen-centered free radicals. *Circulation* 1998; **97**: 2175–2182.

72. Steinberg HO, Chaker H, Leaming R, Johnson A, Brechtel G, Baron AD. Obesity/insulin resistance is associated with endothelial dysfunction. Implications for the syndrome of insulin resistance. *J Clin Invest* 1996; **97**: 2601–2610.

73. Zeng G, Quon MJ. Insulin-stimulated production of nitric oxide is inhibited by wortmannin. Direct measurement in vascular endothelial cells. *J Clin Invest* 1996; **98**: 894–898.

74. Perticone F, Ceravolo R, Candigliota M, Ventura G, Iacopino S, Sinopoli F, Mattioli PL. Obesity and body fat distribution induce endothelial dysfunction by oxidative stress: protective effect of vitamin C. *Diabetes* 2001; **50**: 159.

75. Edelstein SL, Knowler WC, Bain RP, Andres R, Barrett-Connor EL, Dowse GK, Haffner SM, Pettitt DJ, Sorkin JD, Muller DC, Collins VR, Hamman RF. Predictors of progression from impaired glucose tolerance to NBIDDM: an analysis of six prospective studies. *Diabetes* 1997; **46**: 701–710.

76. Bergman RN, Mittelman SD. Central role of the adipocyte in insulin resistance. *J Basic Clin Physiol Pharmacol* 1998; **9**: 205–221.

77. Turner NC, Clapham JC. Insulin resistance, impaired glucose tolerance and non-insulin-dependent diabetes, pathologic mechanisms and treatment: current status and therapeutic possibilities. *Prog Drug Res* 1998; **51**: 33–94.

78. Golay A, Felber JP. Evolution from obesity to diabetes. *Diabete Metab* 1994; **20**: 3–14.

79. Park JY, Ha SW, King GL. The role of protein kinase C activation in the pathogenesis of diabetic vascular complications. *Perit Dial Int* 1994; **19**: S222–227.

80. Laakso M. Hyperglycemia and cardiovascular disease in type 2 diabetes. *Diabetes* 1999; **48**: 937–942.

81. Fontbonne A, Thibult N, Eschwege E, Ducimetiere P. Body fat distribution and coronary heart disease mortality in subjects with impaired glucose tolerance or diabetes mellitus: the Paris Prospective Study, 15-year follow-up. *Diabetologia* 1992; **35**: 464–468.

82. Casassus P, Fontbonne A, Thibult N, Ducimetiere P, Richard JL, Claude JR, Warnet JM, Rosselin G, Eschwege

E. Upper-body fat distribution: a hyperinsulinemia-independent predictor of coronary heart disease mortality. The Paris Prospective Study. *Arterioscler Thromb* 1992; **12**: 1387–1392.

83. Higgins M, Kannel W, Garrison R, Pinsky J, Stokes JD. Hazards of obesity—the Framingham experience. *Acta Med Scand Suppl* 1988; **723**: 23–36.

84. Lapidus L, Bengtsson C, Hallstrom T, Björntorp P. Obesity, adipose tissue distribution and health in women—results from a population study in Gothenburg, Sweden. *Appetite* 1989; **13**: 25–35.

85. Manson JE, Colditz GA, Stampfer MJ, Willett WC, Rosner B, Monson RR, Speizer FE, Hennekens CH. A prospective study of obesity and risk of coronary heart disease in women [see comments]. *N Engl J Med* 1990; **322**: 882–889.

86. Curb JD, Marcus EB. Body fat, coronary heart disease, and stroke in Japanese men. *Am J Clin Nutr* 1991; **53**: 1612S–1615S.

87. Beard CM, Orencia A, Kottke T, Ballard DJ. Body mass index and the initial manifestation of coronary heart disease in women aged 40–59 years [published erratum appears in *Int J Epidemiol* 1992 Oct, **21**(5): 1037]. *Int J Epidemiol* 1992; **21**: 656–664.

88. Baljau B, Shipley M, Jarrett RJ, Pyorala K, Pyorala M, Forhan A, Eschwege E. High blood glucose concentration is a risk factor for mortality in middle-aged nondiabetic men. 20-year follow-up in the Whitehall Study, the Paris Prospective Study, and the Helsinki Policemen Study [see comments]. *Diabetes Care* 1998; **21**: 360–367.

89. Jouven X, Desnos M, Guerot C, Ducimetiere P. Predicting sudden death in the population: the Paris Prospective Study I. *Circulation* 1999; **99**: 1978–1983.

90. Schulte H, Cullen P, Assmann G. Obesity, mortality and cardiovascular disease in the Munster Heart Study (PROCAM). *Atherosclerosis* 1999; **144**: 199–209.

91. Hodgson JM, Wahlqvist ML, Balazs ND, Boxall JA. Coronary atherosclerosis in relation to body fatness and its distribution. *Int J Obes Relat Metab Disord* 1994; **18**: 41–46.

92. Clark LT, Karve MM, Rones KT, Chang-DeMoranville B, Atluri S, Feldman JG. Obesity, distribution of body fat and coronary heart disease in black women. *Am J Cardiol* 1994; **73**: 895–896.

93. Kortelainen ML. Association between cardiac pathology and fat tissue distribution in an autopsy series of men without premortem evidence of cardiovascular disease. *Int J Obes Relat Metab Disord* 1996; **20**: 245–252.

94. Kortelainen ML, Sarkioja T. Coronary atherosclerosis and myocardial hypertrophy in relation to body fat distribution in healthy women: an autopsy study on 33 violent deaths.

Int J Obes Relat Metab Disord 1997; **21**: 43–49.

95. Gaudet D, Vohl MC, Perron P, Tremblay G, Gagne C, Lesiege D, Bergeron J, Moorjani S, Despres JP. Relationships of abdominal obesity and hyperinsulinemia to angiographically assessed coronary artery disease in men with known mutations in the LDL receptor gene. *Circulation* 1998; **97**: 871–877.

96. Nieto FJ, Szklo M, Comstock GW. Childhood weight and growth rate as predictors of adult mortality [see comments]. *Am J Epidemiol* 1992; **136**: 201–213.

97. Must A, Jacques PF, Dallal GE, Bajerna CJ, Dietz WH. Long-term morbidity and mortality of overweight adolescents. A follow-up of the Harvard Growth Study of 1922 to 1935 [see comments]. *N Engl J Med* 1992; **327**: 1350–1355.

98. Berenson GS, Srinivasan SR, Nicklas TA. Atherosclerosis: a nutritional disease of childhood. *Am J Cardiol* 1998; **82**: 22T–29T.

99. Burke GL, Bild DE, Hilner JE, Folsom AR, Wagenknecht LE, Sidney S. Differences in weight gain in relation to race, gender, age and education in young adults: the CARDIA Study. Coronary Artery Risk Development in Young Adults. *Ethn Health* 1996; **1**: 327–335.

100. Lapidus L, Bengtsson C. Regional obesity as a health hazard in women—a prospective study. *Acta Med Scand Suppl* 1988; **723**: 53–59.

101. Abbott RD, Behrens GR, Sharp DS, Rodriguez BL, Burchfiel CM, Ross GW, Yano K, Curb JD. Body mass index and thromboembolic stroke in nonsmoking men in older middle age. The Honolulu Heart Program. *Stroke* 1994; **25**: 2370–2376.

102. Rexrode KM, Hennekens CH, Willett WC, Colditz GA, Stampfer MJ, Rich-Edwards JW, Speizer FE, Manson JE. A prospective study of body mass index, weight change, and risk of stroke in women. *JAMA* 1997; **277**: 1539–1545.

103. Folsom AR, Rasmussen ML, Chambless LE, Howard G, Cooper LS, Schmidt MI, Heiss G. Prospective associations of fasting insulin, body fat distribution, and diabetes with risk of ischemic stroke. The Atherosclerosis Risk in Communities (ARIC) Study Investigators. *Diabetes Care* 1999; **22**: 1077–1083.

104. Sjöström L, Larsson B, Backman L, Bengtsson C, Bouchard C, Dahlgren S, Hallgren P, Jonsson E, Karls-son J, Lapidus L *et al.* Swedish obese subjects (SOS). Recruitment for an intervention study and a selected description of the obese state. *Int J Obes Relat Metab Disord* 1992; **16**: 465–479.

105. Haffner SM, Mitchell BD, Stern MP Hazuda HP. Macrovascular complications in Mexican Americans with type II diabetes. *Diabetes Care* 1991; **14**: 665–671.

26

Obesity, Overweight and Human Cancer

Michael Hill

South Bank University, London, UK

INTRODUCTION

Overweight is a cultural concept that has changed steadily with time. In old pictures, the ideal weight was clearly very much higher than it is now. A high body weight was associated with social and economic success, and was a matter of pride. Then in the post World War II period, although the idealized female figure was less heavy than in previous decades, it was still of voluptuous proportions (e.g. Marilyn Monroe).

However, overweight is a medical reality that has clear health consequences including an increased risk of cancer at many sites of the body. This review summarizes the epidemiological data relating overweight to cancer risk. It discusses some of the proposed mechanisms for the relationship and reviews the measures that have been proposed to control this cancer risk.

EPIDEMIOLOGICAL EVIDENCE

The epidemiological evidence comes from a number of types of study. There have been large-scale population studies that have investigated the relationship between overweight and cancer at a range of sites. In addition, there have been studies of various types (cohort, case-control etc.) into the role of over-

weight in cancer at specific sites. Many of these studies are far from being unambiguous. Body wasting is a common symptom of cancer at many sites, particularly the lung, pancreas and the stomach. Loss of appetite and consequent loss of weight is a common response to the fear of cancer. By the time that a patient seeks medical advice and is diagnosed with cancer, underweight is a common feature. In consequence it is necessary to know the weight before the onset of symptoms. If the patient has been in regular contact with their general practitioner then the height and weight is likely be on the patient records. If not, then it would be necessary to use recall data, which are notoriously unreliable. For this reason, prospective studies of cohorts always give much more reliable information than can be obtained by using the case-control approach.

Large Population Studies

One of the early population cohort studies of note was the American Cancer Society 'One Million Study', in which the risk of cancer in relation to body weight was studied prospectively. This study showed (1) that there was an association between overweight and cancer of the colon, pancreas, stomach, kidney, gallbladder and prostate for men

International Textbook of Obesity. Edited by Per Björntorp.

Table 26.1 Relative risk of cancer at various sites in obese persons (BMI > 30 compared with 20–25) in three large cohort studies in the USA (1), Italy (3) and Denmark (4)

Cancer site		USA[a]	Italy	Denmark
Stomach	male	1.88		1.10
	female	1.03		1.10
Colorectum	male	1.73		1.30
	female	1.22		1.20
Pancreas	male	1.62		
Prostate	male	1.29	2.5	1.90
Breast	female	1.53	1.6	1.20
Endometrium	female	5.42	6.4	2.00
Kidney	male	1.91		
	female	2.03		2.00
Gallbladder	male			1.90
	Female			1.90

[1]Data for those $> 140\%$ of mean weight relative to mean weight.

(Table 26.1), and between overweight and cancer of the stomach, colon, kidney, gallbladder, breast, endometrium, ovary and cervix for women. This study had the advantage of being a prospective study of a very large cohort (though even then there were too few cases of gallbladder and renal carcinoma in men to give statistically significant results). The major disadvantage of the study was that it only considered weight and took no account of height. De Waard (2) highlighted the possibility of mutual confounding between these two measures in his study of risk factors in breast cancer. In more recent studies, therefore, the measure was of body mass index (BMI), This gave essentially similar results (3,4).

The prospective study of 8006 Japanese men aged 45–60 at recruitment (5) investigated the relation between BMI and risk of cancer at a range of sites. The results showed that weight gain after the age of 25 was correlated to colon cancer risk but not to that of other cancers (particularly prostate, gastric and lung cancer).

Case-control Studies

It is difficult to study the relation between body mass and cancer risk using the case-control approach because cancer at so many sites, particularly the digestive tract, leads to changes in the diet and consequent weight changes. There may be other body-wasting effects as well as loss of appetite, and it is notable that a number of cancers related to

overweight by Lew and Garfinkel (1) were also linked to neoplastic cachexia (3). These cancers include colorectal, pancreatic and ovarian cancers.

This is probably why the review of the literature for individual cancer sites carried out in the UK by the COMA panel (6) supported some, but not all, of the observations above (Table 26.2). Taking account of the evidence from case-control as well as from population studies, they found strong evidence that overweight was a risk factor for post-menopausal breast cancer (23/29 case-control and 12/13 cohort studies), colorectal cancer (4 of 7 case-control and 10 of 12 cohort studies in men; 2 of 5 case-control and 6 of 9 cohort studies in women) and endometrial cancer (14/14 case-control and 4/5 cohort studies). They found inconsistent evidence for a relation between overweight and prostate cancer (3/8 case-control and 5/8 prospective studies). They concluded that there was insufficient evidence to draw conclusions about cancer at other sites. La Vecchia and Negri (3) drew attention to the evidence from the cohort study of Whittemore et al. (7) as well as case-control studies such as that by Goodman et al. (8) supporting the role for excess body weight as a risk factor for renal cell adenocarcinoma. The COMA panel did not report on the relation between overweight and gallbladder cancer, but the evidence here is as consistent as that for endometrial cancer.

ENERGY INTAKE

Overweight and obesity is the inevitable result of an excess of energy intake over energy use. The question therefore arises as to which of these is the more important factor in relation to cancer risk. There is a formidable body of evidence from animal studies, built up over many decades, that excess energy intake is a major risk factor for cancer at many sites (9–11). All three groups showed that rodents fed *ad libitum* were fat, sedentary, had short lifespans and had a high rate of spontaneous or chemically induced cancers. In contrast, when the same species of rodents were fed calorie-restricted diets they were leaner, much more active, had longer lifespans and had a lower rate of spontaneous or chemically induced cancers. Many others have confirmed these results. Superficially the case for the association looks overwhelming.

Table 26.2 Data on energy balance and obesity and cancer from the COMA report (6)

Relationship		Observation
Physical exercise		Outside of the scope of the report
Energy intake		No relationship to colorectal cancer or to breast cancer (pre- or postmenopausal) but increased risk of endometrial cancer with high energy intake
Overweight/obesity		
Breast cancer	Premenopausal	9/25 found increased risk
		11/25 found decreased risk
	Post-menopausal	23/29 found increased risk
		6/29 found lower risk
Colorectal cancer	Men	4/7 case-control and 10/12 prospective studies showed increased risk
	Women	2/5 case control and 6/9 prospective studies showed increased risk
Prostate cancer	Case-control	3/8 show increased risk with overweight
	Prospective	5/8 show increased risk with overweight
Endometrial cancer		All case-control and all prospective studies showed increased risk with overweight

It has been a major disappointment that we have been unable to observe the same strength of association in human epidemiological studies. Indeed the COMA panel (6) failed to detect any relationship at all except for an increased risk of endometrial cancer. This may be because of the difficulty in getting a good measure of total energy intake in epidemiological studies, compared with the high level of precision seen in the animal model work. Alternatively it may be because energy intake is a surrogate measure of other things.

In the studies of Tucker (11) it was shown that rats fed *ad libitum* had a very high rate of spontaneous tumours. This high rate could be decreased by feeding the animals less food, but the identical effect on cancer risk could be obtained by feeding the animals the same amount of food but in meals instead of *ad libitum*. When the animals knew that the food hopper (which contained the amount of food eaten by the *ad libitum* fed animals) was to be taken away after a set time they concentrated on feeding. They ate until the hopper was empty, and so their intake was the same as that of animals fed *ad libitum*. However, between meals the animals were very active; as a consequence they were slimmer and lighter. In addition they lived longer than the *ad libitum* fed animals and had fewer cancers. In those studies, total energy intake would appear not to have been the risk factor whilst overweight and lack of physical activity were still associated with increased risk. This needs to be confirmed under a range of different circumstances. If true, perhaps this is the explanation for the lack of association between energy intake and cancer risk in human studies. High energy intake may only be a risk factor in the absence of high physical activity. The true risk factor may be overweight, or lack of physical activity.

PHYSICAL ACTIVITY

Physical activity is even less easy to measure objectively in epidemiological studies than is energy intake. Thune (12) reviewed more than 30 different methods of estimating both occupational and recreational physical activity before choosing the method to be used in the excellent Norwegian Cohort Study. Her results are summarized in Table 26.3. She observed a protective effect of recreational activity against cancers of the prostate, large bowel, lung and breast. There were interesting variations seen within sites. For example, in lung cancer the effect of physical activity was much less on the risk of squamous cell carcinoma than on small cell or adenocarcinoma. Within the large bowel the effect was greatest in the proximal colon and not apparent in the rectum. Within breast cancer cases the effect was greater in younger than in older women, and greater in premenopausal than in postmenopausal cases. The effects were independent of BMI, confirming that low physical activity in these studies was not simply a surrogate marker of overweight.

Because of the difficulties in measuring physical activity there have been many studies showing no relationship to cancer risk. However, the balance of

Table 26.3 The relationship between physical exercise and cancer risk in the Norwegian prospective study of Thune and Lund (13–15) and Thune *et al.* (16)

Cancer site	Effect of increased physical activity
Prostate cancer	Occupational—son-significant decrease
	Recreational—decreased risk of cancer
Testicular cancer	No effect of exercise on risk
Colon Female	Occupational—no effect
	Recreational—protective, particularly for proximal colon
Male	Occupational—protective
	Recreational—protective, particularly for proximal colon
Rectum	No effect of exercise in males or females
Lung Male	Protection by recreational but not occupational exercise
	Effect is on adenocarcinoma and small cell carcinoma but not on squamous cell carcinoma
Female	No effect of exercise on risk
Breast	Recreational and occupational activity protective. Effect is greater for pre- than for postmenopausal, and greater in younger than older women

the data, taking into account the developments in the methodology, are now strongly supporting a protective effect, and they have been reviewed recently by Moore *et al.* (17). However, most of these studies have not been controlled.

CONCLUSIONS

There is a clear association between obesity and increased risk of cancer at many sites including the large bowel and the hormone-related sites. Obesity is the result of a long-term excess of energy intake over energy expenditure. The observed relationship could therefore be an artefact, with the true relationship being with either of the other two related factors. There is, indeed, a strong relationship between lack of physical activity and cancer risk at the sites that correlate with overweight. This relationship is independent of overweight. The evidence available suggests, however, that there is a relationship between cancer risk and total energy intake.

The situation is, therefore, that there is a protective effect of physical activity that is independent of overweight. There is strong evidence of a correlation between overweight and risk of cancer at many sites; we do not know whether this is an independent relationship, or secondary to low physical activity.

REFERENCES

1. Lew EA, Garfinkel L. Variations in mortality by weight among 750 000 men and women. *J Chronic Dis* 1979; **32**: 563–576.
2. De Waard F. Breast cancer incidence and nutritional status with particular reference to body weight and height. *Cancer Res* 1975; **35**: 3351–3356.
3. La Vecchia C, Negri E. Public education on diet and cancer: Calories, weight and exercise. In: Benito E, Giacosa A, Hill M (eds). *Public Education on Diet and Cancer*. Dordrecht: Kluwer Academic Press, 1992: 91–100.
4. Moller H, Mellemgaard A, Ludvig K, Olsen JH. Obesity and cancer risk; a Danish record linkage study. *Eur J Cancer* 1994; **30A**: 344–350.
5. Nomura A, Heilbrun LK, Stemmerman GN. Body mass index as a predictor of cancer in men. *J Natl Cancer Inst* 1985; **74**: 319–323.
6. Department of Health. *RHSS 48; Nutritional Aspects of the Development of Cancer*. London: The Stationery Office, 1998.
7. Whittemore AS, Paffenbergher RS, Anderson K, Lee JE. Early precursers of site specific cancers in college men and women. *J Natl Cancer Inst* 1985; **74**: 43–51.
8. Goodman MT, Morgenstern H, Wynder EL. A case-control study of factors affecting the development of renal cell carcinoma. *Am J Epidemiol* 1986; **124**: 926–941.
9. Tannenbaum A. The dependence of tumour formation on the degree of caloric restriction. *Cancer Res* 1945; **5**: 609–615.
10. Klurfeld D, Weber MM, Kritchevsky D. Calories and chemical carcinogenesis. In: *Dietary Fiber; Basic and Clinical Aspects*. Vahouny G, Kritchevsky D (eds), New York: Plenum, 1986. 441–447.
11. Tucker MJ. The effect of long-term food restriction on tumours in animals. *Int J Cancer* 1979; **23**: 803–807.
12. Thune I. *Physical Activity and the Risk of Cancer*. Tromso: The Norwegian Cancer Society, 1997.
13. Thune I, Lund E. Physical activity and risk of prostate and testicular cancer; a cohort study of 53000 Norwegian men. *Cancer Causes Control* 1994; **5**: 549–556.

14. Thune I, Lund E. Physical activity and risk of colorectal cancer in men and women. *Br J Cancer* 1996; **73**: 1134–1140.

15. Thune I, Lund E. The influence of physical activity on lung cancer risk. A prospective study of 81516 men and women. *Int J Cancer* 1997; **70**: 57–62.

16. Thune I, Brenn T, Lund E, Gaard M. Physical activity and risk of breast cancer. *N Eng J Med* 1997; **336**: 1269–1275.

17. Moore MA, Park CB, Tsuda H. Physical exercise: a pillar for cancer prevention? *Eur J Cancer Prev* 1998; **7**: 177–194.

27

Pulmonary Diseases (Including Sleep Apnoea and Pickwickian Syndrome)

Tracey D. Robinson and Ronald R. Grunstein

Royal Prince Alfred Hospital, Sydney, New South Wales, Australia

INTRODUCTION

Obesity produces measurable reductions in pulmonary function and is strongly associated with breathing disorders in sleep, such as sleep apnoea and obesity–hypoventilation.

Moderate to severe degrees of obesity can lead to a restrictive abnormality in lung function due to the mechanical effects of central body fat. Similar fat deposition is linked to upper airway collapsibility in sleep and recent epidemiological data have identified obesity as a crucial risk factor in the development of obstructive sleep apnoea (OSA). Moreover, the combination of obesity-reduced pulmonary function and sleep apnoea can lead to progressive respiratory failure in sleep finally resulting in awake respiratory failure (obesity–hypoventilation syndrome).

Sleep-disordered breathing has a number of clinical consequences, including excess cardiovascular morbidity. Obesity is an important confounder of this association. Conservative measures such as weight reduction may reduce apnoea severity but long-term maintenance of weight reduction is a limiting factor. Treatment of sleep-breathing disorders has been advanced greatly by the use of positive airway pressure devices.

PULMONARY FUNCTION IN OBESITY

Pulmonary Function and Mechanics

Fat deposition in the neck, upper airway, chest wall and abdomen can impair the mechanical function of the respiratory system. In general, the effects of obesity alone are mild and are typically in proportion to the degree of obesity (1–3). Reduced lung volumes are seen, with falls in the expiratory reserve volume (ERV) and the functional residual capacity (FRC) the commonest findings. Reductions in vital capacity and total lung capacity are generally only seen when the body mass index (BMI) exceeds $40\,kg/m^2$. Reductions in lung volumes below 70% predicted are rarely due to obesity alone. Measurements of central obesity may correlate more closely than BMI with abnormalities of lung function (4,5). Patients with obesity–hypoventilation syndrome (OHS) tend to have more impaired respiratory function than patients without sleep-disordered breathing, despite identical degrees of obesity. The reasons for this are not clear.

In obese subjects, both airway and respiratory resistance are higher than normal and increase as BMI increases (2). The reduced lung volumes of obesity, in particular the low FRC, explain a large part of the increased resistance. Respiratory resistance increases further when obese subjects are supine (6). Despite this increased resistance, the FEV_1/FVC (forced expiratory volume in 1 second/ forced vital capacity) ratio is normal (1,2,7–9). Studies on total compliance of the respiratory system in obese subjects have found conflicting results, but lung compliance is probably reduced by around 25% (7). The reasons for this are unclear, but small airway closure and collapse may be responsible.

The fraction of total oxygen consumption dedicated to respiratory muscle work during quiet breathing can be up to 15% (i.e. five times normal) in patients with morbid obesity (10), suggesting significantly increased work of breathing. Respiratory muscle function, measured by maximal inspiratory and expiratory pressures, is normal in eucapnic obese subjects. In OHS, inspiratory muscles are weaker, possibly due to the effects of hypoxaemia and hypercapnia. There is little evidence of morphometric differences in respiratory muscles in obesity.

Gas Exchange

Hypoxaemia, with or without hypercapnia, is seen in many patients with morbid obesity but many patients with similar degrees of obesity have normal gas exchange (11–13). In obese hypoxaemic subjects, ventilation–perfusion mismatching has been demonstrated, with dependent well-perfused areas of lung relatively underventilated, probably due to partial airway collapse (14,15). The gas exchange abnormalities are usually greater when patients are supine.

More recently, the presence of sleep-disordered breathing has been found to impact significantly on gas exchange abnormalities and may explain some of the variation found in obese subjects. Obesity–hypoventilation syndrome (OHS) describes hypercapnic hypoxaemic respiratory failure in obese patients who have no significant lung disease. The respiratory failure is largely due to impaired ventilatory control secondary to sleep-disordered breathing, resulting in chronic awake alveolar hypoventilation. Patients with OHS can attain a normal $PaCO_2$ by voluntary hyperventilation (16). However the A–aPO_2 (alveolar–arterial oxygen gradient) is often increased in patients with OHS, suggesting the presence of increased ventilation–

perfusion mismatch in addition to hypoventilation. OSA without OHS can also contribute to awake gas exchange abnormalities. Laaban et al. (17) studied a group of 60 obese subjects (BMI around $50 \, kg/m^2$) and found that daytime hypoxaemia was significantly correlated with the presence of OSA. Similar findings have been reported by Gold et al. (13). This mild to moderate hypoxaemia with eucapnia seen in obese patients with OSA is probably attributable to abnormalities of ventilatory control causing mild hypoventilation: this group may represent an early form of OHS.

Interestingly, the single-breath diffusing capacity for carbon monoxide (DLCO), a measure of gas exchange capacity of the lung, is increased in obese subjects by about 10%, with increases in KCO (DLCO adjusted for lung volume) of around 25% (18). The cause is unclear, but may be related to increased pulmonary capillary blood volume.

Ventilatory Control

Assessment of ventilatory control, usually measured by responses to chemical stimuli such as hypercapnia and hypoxaemia, is complicated by the wide variation in normal responses. In most patients with simple obesity, ventilatory drive is normal. Reduced ventilatory responses to hypercapnia have been reported in patients with OSA (13). Patients with OHS often have blunted ventilatory responses to hypoxia and hypercapnia though typically there is a shift in CO_2 responsiveness, characterized by a normal slope of the ventilatory response to CO_2, albeit at a higher level of $PaCO_2$ (19). However, other findings have been mixed. The ability of patients with OHS to voluntarily hyperventilate their $PaCO_2$ to normal levels implies impaired control. Both familial factors and lifetime alcohol intake can influence ventilatory drive.

Respiratory Symptoms and Obesity

Some studies have reported an increased incidence of respiratory symptoms, in particular exertional breathlessness and chest discomfort in obese, otherwise healthy subjects (20,21). Interestingly when comparing subjects with similar degrees of obesity, those patients with OSA report more exertional dyspnoea than those without OSA (22). Weight loss following bariatric surgery results in significant relief of these symptoms (23), with an independent association between the reduction in sleep-disordered breathing and relief of breathlessness and chest pain. This suggests that OSA is implicated in the genesis of these symptoms in subjects with obesity, possibly through effects on respiratory control with relative daytime hypoventilation and resulting mild hypoxaemia. In the absence of weight loss, continuous positive airway pressure (CPAP) therapy can improve daytime gas exchange and respiratory control (24,25) in patients with OSA and so may also reduce the incidence of daytime respiratory symptoms in obese subjects with OSA.

There have been a number of recent studies describing an epidemiological association between obesity and asthma (26,27). However, the diagnosis of asthma in these studies was not confirmed with tests of bronchial hyperresponsiveness (BHR). A more recent study (28) showed an increased incidence of doctor-diagnosed asthma and asthma medication usage in obese subjects but found no increase in the incidence of BHR or atopy in obese subjects compared to normals. This suggests that asthma is over-diagnosed and over-treated in obese subjects, probably due to the respiratory symptoms associated with obesity alone. Weight loss, either by dietary means or by bariatric surgery, can result in a reduction in asthma symptoms and medication usage (29,30). However, these studies have not demonstrated changes in BHR. This suggests that the reduction in respiratory symptoms is due to the reduction in weight and improvement in obesity-associated conditions such as sleep-disordered breathing or gastro-oesophageal reflux, rather than to a change in the severity of asthma.

SLEEP-DISORDERED BREATHING—BACKGROUND

Physiology

Humans exist in three states—wakefulness, non-rapid eye movement (NREM) sleep and rapid eye movement (REM or dreaming) sleep. During sleep in normal subjects, there are falls in ventilation, pharyngeal muscle tone and chemosensitivity to chemical stimuli (e.g. hypoxia or hypercapnia).

These changes are most marked in REM sleep, when breathing irregularity and loss of postural muscle tone occur, leaving humans heavily reliant on the diaphragm for breathing. Patients with abnormal respiratory function when awake will have significantly impaired breathing during sleep, particularly REM sleep.

What is Sleep Apnoea?

Sleep-disordered breathing encompasses a spectrum of conditions ranging from snoring through to profound nocturnal hypoventilation and respiratory failure. Obstructive sleep apnoea (OSA) is characterized by repetitive cessation of airflow during sleep (apnoea), secondary to collapse of the upper airway at the level of the pharynx (31) (Figure 27.1). During apnoeas, respiratory efforts continue against the closed airway and hypoxaemia occurs, until the apnoea is terminated by arousal and upper airway patency is re-established. In the typical patient, after a few deep breaths (often loud snores), the cycle of events is repeated as often as 200–600 times per night. As a result of recurrent arousals, sleep is dramatically fragmented with loss of normal sleep architecture. This, in turn, results in loss of vigilance or even severe sleepiness during the day (32).

Clinically significant upper airway obstruction may occur in the absence of complete collapse of the upper airway. Partial obstruction (hypopnoea) may produce similar pathophysiological events (i.e. hypoxaemia and arousal). Even minor increases in airway resistance can be associated with repetitive arousal and excessive daytime sleepiness, the 'upper airway resistance' syndrome (33).

At the other end of the spectrum are patients with severe respiratory failure in sleep including patients with chronic lung disease, respiratory muscle failure due to neuromuscular disorders and the obesity–hypoventilation syndrome (OHS). These patients have prolonged periods of hypoxaemia usually due to reduced ventilation (lasting minutes) rather than apnoeas (lasting 10–60 seconds typically). The hypoventilation causes progressive hypercapnia in sleep, leading to resetting of central chemoreceptors and tolerance of higher awake carbon dioxide tensions. The prolonged exposure to hypoxaemia and hypercapnia can cause or worsen pulmonary hyper-

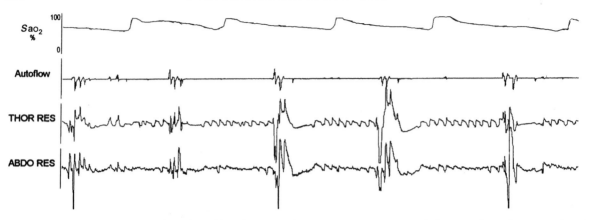

Figure 27.1   Five-minute tracing of a patient with typical severe sleep apnoea. The apnoeas are indicated by intermittent cessation of airflow and are obstructive in nature, as continued respiratory effort is seen when airflow is absent (THOR RES: thoracic movement or effort; ABDO RES: abdominal movement or effort). Repetitive falls in oxygen saturation (Sao_2) are seen following each apnoea

tension and right-sided heart failure, 'cor pulmonale'.

Pathogenesis of Sleep Apnoea

Collapse of the upper airway occurs when the negative (or suction) pressure applied to the upper airway during inspiration is greater than the dilating force applied by upper airway muscles, such as genioglossus (31,32). Any factors which reduce airway size, decrease muscle tone, increase upper airway compliance or lead to generation of a greater inspiratory pressure will predispose to OSA. Muscle tone and suction pressure are influenced by sleep stage and relative respiratory drive to the diaphragm versus the upper airway dilator muscles.

In general, obese sleep apnoea patients have larger tongues and smaller upper airway volumes than normal subjects (35). However, excess fat deposition around the airway is not a universal finding in obese OSA patients (36) and well-matched controls are often difficult to obtain. Neck fat deposition promotes mass loading and obstruction of the upper airway in sleep, leading to OSA (37) and in morbidly obese patients, neck size is a better predictor of sleep apnoea than other body anthropomorphic measures (22). In addition, abdominal obesity may reduce lung volumes and reflexly reduce pharyngeal cross-sectional area and increase pharyngeal resistance (38,39). Obesity may promote sleep apnoea through multiple mechanisms: in some patients,

subcutaneous neck fat may be the critical factor causing upper airway closure in sleep; in other patients, abdominal fat loading may be important.

Obesity–Hypoventilation Syndrome

When awake, the majority of patients with sleep apnoea have normal arterial carbon dioxide tensions. The original descriptions of OSA emphasized the minority of patients with awake respiratory failure who were labelled 'Pickwickian syndrome' (see Kryger (40) for review). The recognition that sleep apnoea was present in these patients and that relief of upper airway obstruction by tracheostomy effectively treated the respiratory failure altered the understanding of the evolution of OHS. Upper airway obstruction is clearly a crucial factor in the pathogenesis of OHS (34). However, since most OSA patients do not have hypercapnia when awake, upper airway obstruction alone is insufficient to cause OHS. Similarly, obesity is not a prerequisite to develop respiratory failure in OSA and obesity, per se, is associated with normal chemosensitivity. A number of recent studies have emphasized the multifactorial aetiology of awake respiratory failure in OSA. The key elements are a combination of obesity (increased upper airway loading and reduced lung volumes), airflow limitation, poor chemoreceptor function (particularly defective arousal responses to hypoxia) and possibly alcohol consumption (reducing upper airway tone and arousal responses to asphyxia) (34). It is important to stress that awake hypercapnia can occur in obese patients in the absence of any smoking history or lung disease (9).

Longitudinal studies demonstrating the development of OHS are lacking but almost certainly the severity of sleep-induced respiratory abnormalities is crucial in the development of OHS (9). During an apnoea, Paco$_2$ rises and Pao2 falls. When the apnoea is terminated by an arousal, ventilation increases and oxygen and carbon dioxide levels can return to normal. If arousal responses or ventilatory responses to either hypoxia or hypercapnia are depressed, the apnoeic periods will be longer, the degree of blood gas derangement greater and normalization of blood gases in the period following arousal compromised (34). In those patients able to increase ventilation between apnoeas, overall eucapnia will be maintained. In contrast, if the compensatory mechanisms are poor, ventilation will be inadequate during sleep. This will eventually allow the resetting of the chemoreceptors (19) and progression to daytime CO_2 retention. Arousal responses may further be impaired in patients prescribed sedatives/hypnotics to improve 'insomnia', opiate analgesics to ease musculoskeletal pain or by consumption of alcohol. This 'vicious cycle' will progress over time to cor pulmonale if left untreated. Alternatively there is a risk of sudden death due to an arrhythmia in sleep (41).

SLEEP-DISORDERED BREATHING—CLINICAL

Symptoms of Sleep-disordered Breathing

The dominant symptoms associated with OSA are heavy snoring and excessive daytime sleepiness (EDS). Witnessed apnoeas may be a relatively specific symptom in patients but is relatively insensitive. Other symptoms are listed in Table 27.1. Daytime symptoms include morning headaches, fatigue, poor memory and concentration, alteration in mood and impotence (32).

The nature of these symptoms emphasizes the importance of obtaining a history from the spouse, bed partner and other family members. Few patients are aware that they snore or stop breathing

Table 27.1 Symptoms of sleep-disordered breathing

Snoring
Choking in sleep
Disrupted sleep at night
Daytime sleepiness
Dry throat
Palpitations in sleep
Nocturia
Heartburn
Headaches (day or night)
Fatigue
Poor memory and concentration
Alteration in mood, irritability
Impotence

during sleep. Excessive sleepiness may be recognized by the patient, but often is either denied by the patient or considered to be 'normal'—again underlining the critical importance of confirmatory history from a family member, friend or workmate.

Examination of the upper airway may be important. The uvula and soft palate are often swollen and oedematous in patients with sleep apnoea due to the vibration of soft tissues with snoring.

Clinical Sequelae

PsychoSocial

Excessive daytime sleepiness (EDS) is characteristic but not pathognomonic of sleep apnoea. Sleepiness in OSA is predominantly related to the repetitive arousals and sleep fragmentation, but a direct effect of hypoxaemia is possible (42). There is a relatively poor correlation between severity of OSA and daytime sleepiness and no simple test accurately quantifies daytime sleepiness. Sleepiness may lead to both impaired work performance and impaired driving (43,44). Some studies have suggested sleep apnoea is a significant risk in commercial drivers. Treatment with nasal CPAP dramatically improves daytime sleepiness, quality of life and even driving simulator performance. A number of studies have found OSA patients perform poorly on psychometric tests compared to controls with a variable degree of improvement following nasal CPAP therapy (42,45). Data from the Swedish Obese Subjects (SOS) Study indicates that in equally obese men and women, a history of sleep apnoea is associated with impaired work performance, increased sick leave and a much higher divorce rate (46).

Cardiovascular Sequelae of Sleep Apnoea

Patients with sleep apnoea clearly have acute cardiovascular changes as an immediate consequence of their breathing disturbance. Obstructive apnoeas are accompanied by profound haemodynamic changes with increases in both systemic and pulmonary arterial blood pressure. With progressive apnoea, there is worsening hypoxaemia, increasing pleural pressure swings, bradycardia (and possibly bradyarrhythmias), increased sympathetic nerve activity and an overall rise in blood pressure. These marked changes in cardiorespiratory behaviour, together with reported changes in cerebral blood flow, provide an environment for increasing the risk of various vascular disease endpoints. Studies using a canine model of OSA have shown that sustained hypertension develops after 1–3 months of OSA (47). Similarly, studies with rats have found that intermittent hypoxia induces a persistent increase in diurnal blood pressure, possibly mediated through renal sympathetic nerve activity and the renin–angiotensin system (48).

Sleep apnoea is a common finding in hypertension clinic patients, but there are confounding factors such as central obesity and increasing age (49,50). A number of studies have strongly suggested that sleep apnoea is a risk factor for hypertension independent of obesity (22,50–53). Recently published cross-sectional data (54) from the Sleep Heart Health Study found a significant association between sleep-disordered breathing and hypertension after adjustment for BMI, neck circumference and waist-to-hip ratio. Similarly, prospective data from the Wisconsin Sleep Cohort Study (55) found a dose–response association between sleep-disordered breathing and hypertension, independent of measures of obesity. Studies using either intrarterial monitoring, automated daytime blood pressure readings or 24-hour ambulatory blood pressure have demonstrated a fall in blood pressure levels after CPAP treatment (56). Patients with OSA have increased left ventricular mass (measured using echocardiography) compared with non-OSA patients with similar daytime blood pressure values (57). Pulmonary hypertension is not uncommon in OSA (58). These observations in OSA have implications in analysis of data linking obesity and cardiac disease.

The advent of nasal CPAP has prevented large studies investigating the natural history of untreated OSA. He et al. (59) observed an increased cumulative mortality in untreated patients with an apnoea index (AI) > 20 compared to AI < 20. Tracheostomy or CPAP treatment but not uvulopalatopharyngoplasty (UPPP) reduced the mortality risk. A number of groups have reported an increased risk of myocardial infarction and stroke in sleep apnoea (60,61) and untreated OSA may be associated with an increased cardiovascular mortality in patients with coronary artery disease (62). Snoring is a strong risk factor for sleep-related strokes while sleep apnoea symptoms (snoring plus reported apnoeas or EDS) increase the risk of cerebral infarction (odds ratio of 8.0).

Endocrine Effects

Sleep apnoea patients are characterized by a neuroendocrine defect in growth hormone (GH) and testosterone secretion (63–66) that may be reversed by nasal CPAP treatment, without associated weight change. It is likely that GH impairment in sleep apnoea is additive to the low GH levels seen in obesity. In adults, impaired GH secretion leads to central adiposity and reduced muscle and bone mass. It is unknown whether these changes in GH and testosterone levels in adults with sleep apnoea are associated with measurable changes in body composition, body fat distribution, energy expenditure or bone density. Recently two reports have suggested that insulin levels are increased in patients with sleep apnoea independent of obesity (67) or visceral fat mass (22). Other data strongly suggest that reversal of sleep apnoea leads to increased insulin sensitivity in obese patients with type 2 (non-insulin-dependent) diabetes (68) and reduced visceral fat mass (69). More recently, leptin has been implicated in sleep-disordered breathing. In obese, leptin-deficient mice with OHS, leptin replacement increased both waking and sleeping minute ventilation and chemosensitivity to carbon dioxide during sleep (70). Leptin levels fell significantly in a group of 22 patients with OSA after 4 days of treatment with CPAP (69), possibly due to reduced sympathetic activity. OSA may well be a confounder in some of the hormonal associations observed in central obesity.

SLEEP-DISORDERED BREATHING—EPIDEMIOLOGY

Recognition of Sleep-disordered Breathing

Clinical impression has surprisingly poor specificity and sensitivity for detecting sleep apnoea (71). Symptoms such as sleepiness are common in the general community including obese patients (72) and may be secondary to lack of sleep, medications or other sleep disorders. Snoring may be underestimated. Physical examination generally has poor predictive value though obvious pharyngeal crowding and tonsillar hypertrophy suggest upper airway obstruction (73).

Breathing during sleep in obese children has attracted much less attention than in the adult population and no prevalence studies have been performed. It appears that obesity is not as dominant a factor in childhood apnoea as it is in adults (74,75).

Prevalence of Sleep-disordered Breathing—General

Results from the Wisconsin Sleep Cohort Study (76) indicate that 9% of female and 24% of male middle-aged public servants have an apnoea index $> 5/$ hour. Using a cut-off of 15 apnoeas per hour (a criterion which would satisfy most sleep researchers), 4% of women and 9% of men have sleep apnoea. Our group has found a similar prevalence of OSA in an Australian rural community using home monitoring of breathing (77).

Sleep Apnoea and Obesity—Epidemiology

All epidemiological investigations have consistently shown that obesity, especially central obesity, is strongly associated with adult sleep-disordered breathing (50,76,77). Measurements of central obesity such as waist or neck measurements are tightly linked to OSA in sleep clinic populations (50). In the Busselton Sleep Survey (77), there was a powerful effect of BMI in increasing the risk of sleep-disordered breathing in the community (Figure 27.2).

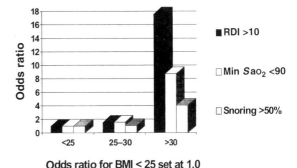

Odds ratio for BMI < 25 set at 1.0

Figure 27.2 Obesity (measured by BMI) is an important predictor of OSA. With the odds ratio for BMI < 25 set at 1.0, a BMI > 30 increased the odds ratio of either OSA (respiratory disturbance index RDI > 10), desaturation during the night (min Sa_2 < 90%) or heavy snoring (snoring for more than 50% of the night) by 5–18 times, depending on the variable

There are limited data on the prevalence of sleep apnoea in the obese population. Data from the SOS Study, which examined 3034 subjects with BMI > 35, found that over 50% of obese men and one-third of obese women reported habitual loud snoring (22). In the SOS Study, a history of frequent witnessed apnoeas (a sensitive marker of sleep apnoea in epidemiological studies), was reported by 33% of men and 12% of women. The exact prevalence of the spectrum of sleep-breathing disorders in the obese is unknown but it is clear that OSA and related conditions occur in a very high proportion of obese subjects.

Other Risk Factors for Sleep Apnoea

OSA increases in prevalence with age and is commonly recognized in the 5th to 7th decades. Some of the increase in prevalence with age is due to increased central fat deposition with age.

The male to female ratio in sleep apnoea is close to 2.5:1 (76,77). Sleep apnoea is rare in premenopausal women unless there is morbid obesity (78) or maxillo-facial abnormalities. The prevalence of OSA increases in women after the menopause, leading to speculation that female sex hormones are protective or male hormones may promote OSA. Alternatively, the increased prevalence in OSA after menopause may be secondary to changing body fat distribution in postmenopausal women.

Sleep apnoea aggregates in families and the risk

of having OSA increases progressively with increasing numbers of affected relatives (71). Such risk may be the result of similarities in facial structure affecting upper airway dynamics in sleep. Certain maxillo-facial appearances are linked with sleep apnoea. In obese patients, familial maxillo-mandibular structure will interact to increase the likelihood of sleep apnoea (79). This may explain why weight loss may not be enough to cure sleep apnoea in obese patients (80).

Apart from obesity, conditions causing narrowing of the upper airway will promote the development of sleep apnoea. These include fixed upper airway lesions (e.g. nasal obstruction, enlarged tonsils), macroglossia or neurological conditions impairing upper airway muscle tone (66).

Acute alcohol ingestion promotes apnoea development during later sleep. Lifetime alcohol consumption may be a risk factor for the development of OSA (81). Data from the Wisconsin Sleep Cohort suggests that smoking history may be a dose-dependent risk factor for OSA (82).

A number of endocrine and metabolic disorders apart from obesity are associated with an increased prevalence of OSA. Hypothyroidism may lead to sleep apnoea by reducing chemosensitivity, myxoedematous infiltration of the upper airway and upper airway myopathy (83). Over 50% of patients with acromegaly have sleep apnoea (84). Cushing's disease is also associated with sleep apnoea.

Cardiac failure (whatever the cause) is associated with a high incidence of sleep-disordered breathing. In a recent study of 450 patients with cardiac failure referred to a sleep laboratory (either with sleep symptoms or persistent dyspnoea), 72% had more than 10 apnoeas–hypopnoeas per hour (85). Patients had OSA or central sleep apnoea (Cheynes–Stokes respiration), with OSA more common in those patients with BMI > 35.

TREATMENT OF SLEEP APNOEA AND SNORING

The approach to treatment will vary according to severity of symptoms, severity of hypoxaemia during sleep and cost. In the absence of significant data showing a deleterious effect of asymptomatic sleep apnoea, treatment for prognosis alone is probably inappropriate. However, patient denial may produce an 'asymptomatic' patient, so if there is a highly positive diagnostic study in an 'asymptomatic' patient, it is advisable to check with relatives about any symptoms.

Weight Loss

A number of studies have demonstrated a reduction in sleep apnoea severity after weight loss, either through caloric restriction or bariatric surgery. However, it is important to reassess patients after weight loss and ensure there is little residual disordered breathing. Most published reports indicate that, although there is a reduction in apnoea index, a significant degree of apnoea persists, which in most cases warrants further treatment (86–88). Weight loss associated with apparently successful bariatric surgery may have limited efficacy in reducing sleep apnoea as many patients also have maxillo-facial abnormalities predisposing them to OSA (80). Recent data from the SOS Study show a marked reduction in sleep apnoea symptomatology in obese subjects 2 years after surgically induced weight loss compared with controls.

Lifestyle Factors

Some studies have suggested that reduction of smoking and alcohol consumption will lead to reduced self-reported snoring and reverse mild sleep apnoea (89). Sleep deprivation may reduce upper airway tone and chemosensitivity and should be avoided. Drugs such as benzodiazepines or opiates should be avoided at bedtime, particularly in patients with severe OSA or OHS.

Devices

Positive Airway Pressure

Until the early 1980s, tracheostomy was the only form of treatment available for sleep apnoea and was usually performed on patients with severe symptomatic disease. The advent of nasal CPAP revolutionized the management of OSA and allowed a wider range of patients to be treated (90,91). A CPAP machine delivers varying pressure to the upper airway through a nose or face mask, providing a 'pneumatic' splint which prevents upper airway closure. CPAP treatment leads to normalization of sleep architecture, decreased upper airway oedema and a reduction in daytime sleepiness (91,92). CPAP improves cognitive function and quality of life, as well as the associated symptoms listed in Table 27.1 for patients with all degrees of severity of OSA (93). CPAP is not a cure for sleep apnoea. Cessation of treatment will lead to a recurrence of sleep-disordered breathing and accompanying symptoms.

Nasal CPAP is an effective treatment, but compliance is variable (94,95), ranging between 40 and 80%. Problems affecting compliance with nasal CPAP include a sense of claustrophobia, mask air leaks, nasal congestion and dryness of the mouth and throat (usually associated with mask or mouth air leaks), and the inconvenience of using a machine. Patients with mild disease or those requiring high pressures are most likely to be non-compliant. Obese patients generally require higher CPAP pressures (96).

Devices that allow variation between the set inspiratory and expiratory pressures, known as bi-level positive airway pressure were originally introduced to improve compliance in CPAP users (97). Although not proven to improve compliance, this form of positive airway pressure therapy has been used increasingly in the management of severe respiratory failure and hypoventilation during sleep, such as OHS.

Mandibular Advancement Splints

The use of an orthodontic device designed to advance the mandible and thus increase the upper airway aperture has produced a major reduction in sleep apnoea severity in several studies (98) and is the subject of a large randomized clinical trial at present in Canada (A. Lowe, personal communication). The efficacy of these devices is likely to be reduced in the obese patient, as skeletal factors are less important in the genesis of upper airway obstruction. In general, these devices are less effective in patients with severe OSA (99). Data on compliance and the prevalence of side effects related to the temporomandibular joint are needed.

Surgery

Tracheostomy

Prior to the introduction of nasal CPAP as a treatment for OSA, tracheostomy was the major therapeutic modality. Tracheostomy is only currently indicated in patients with severe OSA who have been unable to comply with CPAP or related therapies. Tracheostomy can produce significant morbidity, particularly in the obese fat-necked individual and will be only partly effective in treating OHS. However with skilful minimalist surgery and close follow-up, tracheostomy may be a 'last-resort' therapeutic option in some patients.

Uvulopalatopharyngoplasty (UPPP) and Other Upper Airway Surgery

This operation was developed for the treatment of heavy snoring in the early 1950s and involves careful removal of the uvula and part of the soft palate. The introduction of UPPP for the treatment of OSA into North America occurred in 1981 (100) but despite early enthusiasm the operation has never lived up to its promise as a 'cure' for sleep apnoea (101). There are no preoperative tests that satisfactorily predict the response to surgery. There is a significant morbidity and even mortality (101). Excessive removal of palatal tissue will lead to velopharyngeal incompetence and nasal regurgitation and speech changes. Many studies report particularly poor results in obese patients. More recently UPPP has been performed with a surgical laser or high-frequency radio-waves ('somnoplasty'), aiming at stiffening palatal tissue rather than complete removal. Meaningful outcome data are lacking and, as in conventional UPPP, subjective reports of snoring improvement are not supported by objective benefit. There is clearly a 'placebo' effect in snoring surgery that has been demonstrated in other forms of surgical intervention, such as simple sternotomy for severe angina.

More complex maxillo-facial surgery, usually involving UPPP in combination with genioglossus advancement via a mandibular osteotomy and hyoid myotomy, has been used with some success in the treatment of OSA. However, this surgery is less effective in patients with severe disease (> 60 events per hour and desaturation to 70%) and in the morbidly obese (102).

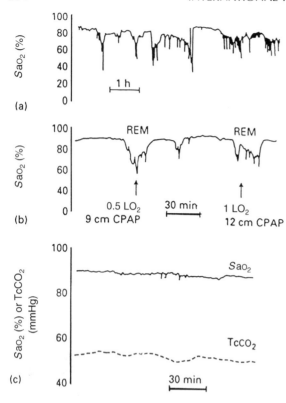

Figure 27.3 Efficacy of nasal ventilation in a patient with OHS. (a) Recordings of oxygen saturation show marked falls in oxygen level during sleep. (b) Addition of CPAP and low-flow oxygen results in normal oxygen saturation in NREM sleep but persisting hypoxaemia in REM sleep. (c) Use of nasal ventilation, either pressure support or volume cycled, will prevent oxygen desaturation and rises in CO_2 levels ($Tc\,CO_2$, transcutaneous CO_2) in REM sleep.

Management of Sleep Apnoea with Awake Respiratory Failure Including OHS

Many centres prefer to manage these patients in hospital, even for brief periods. While most patients starting CPAP require only one night of sleep monitoring to adequately determine required pressure, patients with sleep apnoea and awake respiratory failure require more detailed assessment. In these patients, oxygen alone should be used with caution and with close monitoring of hypercapnia. This is one group in whom sedation or use of hypnotics is contraindicated. Until recently, high CPAP pressures or CPAP plus added oxygen were

needed in the first weeks of treatment until blood gases improved (91,103) or, for the obtunded hypercapnic patient, a short period of intubation and ventilation may have been required. Currently, the bi-level positive airway pressure systems can deliver effective non-invasive pressure support ventilation to these patients and successfully treat hypercapnic respiratory failure (Figure 27.3). Home use of these devices is then prescribed with or without oxygen, depending on the degree of intrinsic lung disease.

ACKNOWLEDGEMENTS

The authors wish to thank Dr A. Piper for assistance in preparation of figures for this chapter.

REFERENCES

1. Ray CS, Sue DY, Bray G, *et al*. Effects of obesity on respiratory function. *Am Rev Respir Dis* 1983; **128**: 501–506.
2. Zerah F, Harf A, Perlemuter L, *et al*. Effects of obesity on respiratory resistance. *Chest* 1993; **103**: 1470–1476.
3. Jenkins SC, Moxham J. The effects of mild obesity on lung function. *Respir Med* 1991; **85**: 309–311.
4. Collins LC, Hoberty PD, Walker JF, *et al*. The effect of body fat distribution on pulmonary function tests. *Chest* 1995; **107**: 1298–1302.
5. Lazarus R, Sparrows D, Weiss ST. Effects of obesity and fat distribution on ventilatory function. *Chest* 1997; **111**: 891–898.
6. Yap JC, Watson RA, Gilbey S, Pride NB. Effects of posture on respiratory mechanics in obesity. *J Appl Physiol* 1995; **79**: 1199–1205.
7. Sharp JT, Henry JP, Sweaney SK *et al*. The total work of breathing in normal and obese men. *J Clin Invest* 1964; **43**: 728–739.
8. Lopata M, Onal E. Mass loading, sleep apnea, and the pathogenesis of obesity hypoventilation. *Am Rev Resp Dis* 1982; **126**: 640–645.
9. Leech J, Onal E, Baer P, Lopata M. Determinant of hypercapnia in occlusive sleep apnea syndrome. *Chest* 1987; **100**: 1334–1338.
10. Kress JP, Pohlman AS, Alverdy J, Hall JB. The impact of morbid obesity on oxygen cost of breathing at rest. *Am J Respir Crit Care Med* 1999; **160**: 883–886.
11. Barrera F, Hillyer P, Ascanio G, Bechteh J. The distribution of ventilation, diffusion and blood flow in obese patients with normal and abnormal blood gases. *Am Rev Respir Dis* 1973; **108**: 819–830.
12. Emirgil C, Sobol B. The effects of weight reduction on pulmonary function and the sensitivity of the respiratory center in obesity. *Am Rev Respir Dis* 1973; **108**: 831–842.
13. Gold AR, Schwartz AR, Wise RA, Smith PL. Pulmonary function and respiratory chemosensitivity in moderately obese patients with sleep apnoea. *Chest* 1993; **103**:

1325–1329.

14. Barrera F, Reidenberg MM, Winters WL, Hungspreugs S. Ventilation-perfusion relationship in the obese patient. *J Appl Physiol* 1969; **26**: 420–426.

15. Holley H, Milic-Emili J, Becklake M, *et al.* Regional distribution of pulmonary ventilation and perfusion in obesity. *J Clin Invest* 1967; **46**: 475–481.

16. Leech J, Onal E, Aronson R, Lopata M. Voluntary hyperventilation in obesity hypoventilation. *Chest* 1991; **100**: 1334–1338.

17. Laaban JP, Cassuto D, Orvoen-Frija E, *et al.* Cardiorespiratory consequences of sleep apnoea syndrome in patients with massive obesity. *Eur Respir J* 1997; **11**: 20–27.

18. Collard P, Wilputte J, Aubert G, *et al.* The single-breath diffusing capacity for carbon monoxide in obstructive sleep apnoea and obesity. *Chest* 1996; **110**: 1189–1193.

19. Berthon-Jones M, Sullivan CE. Time course of change in ventilatory response to CO_2 with long-term CPAP therapy for obstructive sleep apnea. *Am Rev Respir Dis* 1987; **35**: 144–147.

20. Sjöström L, Larsson B, Backman L, *et al.* Swedish Obese Subjects (SOS): recruitment for an intervention study and a selected description of the obese state. *Int J Obes Relat Metab Disord* 1992; **16**: 465–479.

21. Sahebjami H. Dyspnea in obese healthy men. *Chest* 1998; **114**: 1373–1377.

22. Grunstein RR, Stenlöf K, Hedner JA, Sjöström L. Impact of sleep apnea and sleepiness on metabolic and cardiovascular risk factors in the Swedish Obese Subjects (SOS) Study. *Int J Obes* 1995; **19**: 410–418.

23. Karason K, Lindross AK, Stenlöf K, Sjöström L. Relief of cardiorespiratory symptoms and increased physical activity after surgically induced weight loss. *Arch Intern Med* 2000; **160**: 1797–1802.

24. Sforza E, Krieger J, Wietzenblum E, *et al.* Long-term effects of treatment with nasal continuous positive airway pressure on daytime lung function and pulmonary haemodynamics in patients with obstructive sleep apnoea. *Am Rev Respir Dis* 1990; **141**: 866–870.

25. Leech JA, Onal E, Lopata M. Nasal continuous positive airway pressure continues to improve sleep-disordered breathing and daytime oxygenation over long-term follow-up of occlusive sleep apnea syndrome. *Chest* 1992; **102**: 1651–1656.

26. Shaheen SO, Sterne JA, Montgomery SM, Azima H. Birth weight, body mass index and asthma in young adults. *Thorax* 1999; **54**: 396–402.

27. Camargo CA, Weiss ST, Zhang S, *et al.* Prospective study of body mass index, weight change and risk of adult-onset asthma in women. *Arch Intern Med* 1999; **159**: 2582–2588.

28. Schachter LM, Salome CM, Peat JK, Woolcock AJ. Obesity is a risk factor for asthma and wheeze but not for airway responsiveness. *Thorax* 2001; **56**: 4–8.

29. Dixon JB, Chapman L, O'Brien P. Marked improvement in asthma after lap-band surgery for morbid obesity. *Obes Surg* 1999; **9**: 385–389.

30. Stenius-Aarniala B, Poussa T, Kvarnstrom J, *et al.* Immediate and long term effects of weight reduction in obese people with asthma: randomised controlled study. *BMJ* 2000; **320**: 827–832.

31. Remmers JE, De Groot WJ, Sauerland EK, *et al.* Pathogen-esis of upper airway occlusion during sleep. *J Appl Physiol* 1978; **44**: 931–939.

32. McNamara SG, Grunstein RR, Sullivan CE. Obstructive sleep apnoea. *Thorax* 1993; **48**: 754–764.

33. Guilleminault C, Stoohs R, Clerk A, *et al.* From obstructive sleep apnea syndrome to upper airway resistance syndrome: consistency of daytime sleepiness. *Sleep* 1992; **15**: 513–516.

34. Sullivan CE, Grunstein RR, Marrone O, Berthon-Jones M. Sleep apnea—pathophysiology: upper airway and control of breathing. In: Guilleminault C, M Partinnen (eds) *Obstructive Sleep Apnea Syndrome: Clinical Research and Treatment.* New York: Raven Press, 1990.

35. Fleetham JA. Upper airway imaging in relation to obstructive sleep apnoea. *Clin Chest Med* 1992; **13**: 399–416.

36. Schwab RJ, Gupta KB, Gefter WB, *et al.* Upper airway and soft tissue anatomy in normal subjects and patients with sleep-disordered breathing. Significance of the lateral pharyngeal walls. *Am J Respir Crit Care Med* 1995; **152**: 1673–1689.

37. Koenig JS, Thach BT. Effects of mass loading on the upper airway. *J Appl Physiol* 1988; **64**: 2294–2299.

38. Van de Graaf WB. Thoracic influence on upper airway patency *J Appl Physiol* 1988; **65**: 2124–2131.

39. Series F, Cormier Y, Lampron N, *et al.* Influence of passive changes of lung volume on upper airways. *J Appl Physiol* 1990; **68**: 2159–2164.

40. Kryger MH. Fat, sleep, and Charles Dickens: literary and medical contributions to the understanding of sleep apnea. *Clin Chest Med* 1985; **6**: 555–562.

41. Rössner S, Lagerstrand L, Persson HE, Sachs C. The sleep apnea syndrome of obesity: risk of sudden death. *J Intern Med* 1991; **230**: 135–142.

42. Montplaisir J, Bedard MA, Richer F, Rouleau I. Neurobehavioural manifestations of obstructive sleep apnea syndrome before and after treatment with continuous positive airway pressure. *Sleep* 1992; **15**: S17–19.

43. Findley L, Fabrizio M, Knight H, *et al.* Driving simulator performance in patients with sleep apnea. *Am Rev Resp Dis* 1989; **140**: 529–530.

44. Teran-Santos J, Jimenez-Gomez A, Cordero-Guevara A. The association between sleep apnea and the risk of traffic accidents. Cooperative Group Burgos-Santander. *N Engl J Med* 1999; **340**: 847–851.

45. Bearpark H, Grunstein RR, Touyz S, *et al.* Cognitive and psychological dysfunction in sleep apnea before and after treatment with CPAP. *Sleep Res* 1987; **17**: 303.

46. Grunstein RR, Stenlöf K, Hedner JA, Sjöström L. Impact of self reported sleep-breathing disturbances on psychosocial performance in the Swedish Obese Subjects (SOS) Study. *Sleep* 1995; **18**: 635–643.

47. Brooks D, Horner RI, Kozor KF, *et al.* Obstructive sleep apnoea as a cause of systemic hypertension. Evidence from a canine model. *J Clin Invest* 1997; **99**: 106–109.

48. Fletcher EC, Bao G, Li R. Renin activity and blood pressure in response to chronic episodic hypoxia. *Hypertension* 1999; **34**(2): 309–314.

49. Stradling JR, Crosby JH. Predictors and prevalence of obstructive sleep apnoea and snoring in 1001 middle aged men. *Thorax* 1991; **46**: 85–90.

50. Grunstein RR, Wilcox I, Yang TS, *et al.* Snoring and sleep

apnoea in men: association with central obesity and hypertension. *Int J Obes* 1993; **17**: 533–540.

51. Gislason T, Benediktsdottir B, Bjornsson JK, *et al.* Snoring, hypertension and the sleep apnea syndrome. An epidemiologic survey of middle aged women. *Chest* 1993; **103**: 1147–1151.

52. Carlson J, Hedner J, Carlson J, *et al.* High prevalence of hypertension in sleep apnea patients independent of obesity. *Am J Respir Crit Care Med* 1994; **150**: 72–77.

53. Hla KM, Young TB, Bidwell T, *et al.* Sleep apnea and hypertension. *Ann Intern Med* 1994; **120**: 382–388.

54. Nieto FJ, Young TB, Lind BK, *et al.* Association of sleep-disordered breathing, sleep apnea and hypertension in a large community-based study. *JAMA* 2000; **283**: 1829–1836.

55. Peppard PE, Young TB, Palta M, Skatrud J. Prospective study of the association between sleep-disordered breathing and hypertension. *N Engl J Med* 2000; **342**: 1378–1384.

56. Working Group on OSA and Hypertension. Obstructive sleep apnea and blood pressure—what is the relationship? *Blood Pressure* 1993; **2**: 166–682.

57. Hedner J, Ejnell H, Caidahl K. Left ventricular hypertrophy independent of hypertension in patients with obstructive sleep apnea. *J Hypertens* 1990; **8**: 941–946.

58. Laks L, Lehrhaft B, Grunstein RR, Sullivan CE. Pulmonary hypertension in obstructive sleep apnoea. *Eur Res J* 1995; **8**: 537–541.

59. He J, Kryger M, Zorick F, *et al.* Mortality and apnea index in obstructive sleep apnea. Experience in 385 patients. *Chest* 1988; **94**: 9–14.

60. Hung J, Whitford EG, Parsons RW, Hillman DR. Association of sleep apnoea and myocardial infarction in men. *Lancet* 1990; **336**: 261–264.

61. Palomaki H, Partinen M, Erkinjuntti T, Kaste M. Snoring, sleep apnoea syndrome, and stroke. *Neurology* 1992; **42**(Suppl 6): 75–81.

62. Peker Y, Hedner J, Kraiczi H, Loth S. Respiratory disturbance index—an independent predictor of mortality in coronary artery disease. *Am J Respir Crit Care Med* 2000; **162**: 81–86.

63. Grunstein RR, Handelsman DJ, Lawrence SJ, *et al.* Neuroendocrine dysfunction in sleep apnea. Reversal by continuous nasal positive airway pressure. *J Clin Endocrinol Metab* 1989; **68**: 352–358.

64. Grunstein RR, Stewart DA, Handelsman DJ, *et al.* Growth hormone and sex steroids in sleep apnea. In: Horne J (ed.) *Sleep 90.* Bochum: Pontenagel Press, 422–425, 1990.

65. Grunstein RR. Endocrine and metabolic disturbances in obstructive sleep apnea. In: Saunders NA, Sullivan CE (eds) *Sleep and Breathing*, 2nd edn. New York: Marcel Dekker, 1993.

66. Grunstein RR, Handelsman DJ, Stewart DA, Sullivan CE. Growth hormone secretion is increased by nasal CPAP treatment of sleep apnea. *Am Rev Respir Dis* 1993b; **47**: A686.

67. Strohl KP, Novak RD, Singer W, *et al.* Insulin levels, blood pressure and sleep apnea. *Sleep* 1994; **17**: 614–618.

68. Brooks D, Horner RL, Kozar LF, *et al.* Obstructive sleep apnoea as a cause of systemic hypertension Evidence from a canine model. *J Clin Invest* 1997; **99**(1); 106–109.

69. Chin K, Shimizu K, Nakamura T, *et al.* Changes in intra-abdominal visceral fat and leptin levels in patients with OSA syndrome following nasal CPAP. *Circulation* 1999; **100**(7): 706–712.

70. O'Donnell CP, Schaub CD, Berkowitz DE, *et al.* Leptin prevents respiratory depression in obesity. *Am J Respir Crit Care Med* 1999; **159**: 1477–1484.

71. Strohl KP, Redline S. Recognition of obstructive sleep apnea. *Am J Respir Crit Care Med* 1996; **154**: 279–289.

72. Vgontzas AN, Tan TL, Bixler EO, *et al.* Sleep apnea and sleep disruption in obese women. *Arch Intern Med* 1994; **154**: 1705–1711.

73. Hoffstein V, Szalai JP. Predictive value of clinical features in diagnosing obstructive sleep apnea. *Sleep* 1993; **16**: 118–122.

74. Mallory GB Jr, Fiser DH, Jackson R. Sleep-associated breathing disorders in morbidly obese children and adolescents. *J Pediatr* 1989; **115**(6): 892–897.

75. Leach J, Olson J, Hermann J, Manning S. Polysomnographic and clinical findings in children with obstructive sleep apnea. *Arch Otolaryngol Head Neck Surg* 1992; **118**: 741–744.

76. Young T, Palta M, Dempsey J, *et al.* Occurrence of sleep disordered breathing among middle-aged adults. *N Engl J Med* 1993; **328**: 1230–1235.

77. Bearpark H, Elliott L, Grunstein RR, *et al.* Snoring and sleep apnea; A population study in Australian men. *Am J Respir Crit Care Med* 1995; **151**: 1459–1465.

78. Guilleminault C, Quera-Selva MA, Partinen M, Jamieson A. Women and the obstructive sleep apnea syndrome. *Chest* 1988; **93**: 104–109.

79. Ferguson KA, Ono T, Lowe AA, *et al.* The relationship between obesity and cranio-facial structure in obstructive sleep apnea. *Chest* 1995; **108**: 375–381.

80. Pillar G, Peled R, Lavie P. Recurrence of sleep apnea without concomitant weight increase 7.5 years after weight reduction surgery. *Chest* 1994; **106**: 1702–1704.

81. Chan CS, Grunstein RR, Bye PTB, *et al.* Obstructive sleep apnea with severe chronic airflow limitation—Comparison of hypercapnic and eucapnic patients. *Am Rev Respir Dis* 1989; **140**: 1274–1278.

82. Wetter DW, Young TB, Bidwell TR, *et al.* Smoking as a risk factor for sleep-disordered breathing. *Arch Intern Med* 1994; **154**: 2219–2224.

83. Grunstein RR, Sullivan CE. Hypothyroidism and sleep apnea; mechanisms and management. *Am J Med* 1988; **85**: 775–779.

84. Grunstein RR, Ho KY, Sullivan CE. Sleep apnea and acromegaly. *Ann Intern Med* 1991; **115**: 527–532.

85. Sin DD, Fitzgerald F, Parker JD, *et al.* Risk factors for central and obstructive sleep apnoea in 450 men and women with congestive heart failure. *Am J Respir Crit Care Med* 1999; **160**: 1101–1106.

86. Smith PL, Gold AR, Meyers DA, *et al.* Weight loss in mildly to moderately obese patients with obstructive sleep apnea. *Ann Intern Med* 1985; **103**: 850–855.

87. Sugerman HJ. Long-term effects of gastric surgery for treating respiratory insufficiency of obesity. *Am J Clin Nutr* 1992; **55** (2 Suppl): 597S–601S.

88. Suratt PM, McTier RF, Findley; LJ, et al. Effect of very low calorie diets with weight loss on obstructive sleep apnea. *Am J Clin Nutr* 1992; **56**: 182S–184S.

89. Braver, HM, Block AJ, Perri MG. Treatment for snoring. Combined weight loss, sleeping on side, and nasal spray. *Chest* 1995; **107**: 1283–1288.

90. Sullivan CE, Issa FG, Berthon-Jones M, Eves L. Reversal of obstructive sleep apnoea by continuous positive airway pressure applied through the nares. *Lancet* 1981; **1**: 862–865.

91. Sullivan CE, Grunstein RR. Continuous positive airway pressure in sleep disordered breathing. In: Kryger MH, WC Dement, TP Roth (eds) *Principles and Practice of Sleep Disorders Medicine*.WB Saunders: Philadelphia, 1994: 559–570.

92. Jenkinson C, Davies RJ, Mullins R, Sradling JR. Comparison of therapeutic and subtherapeutic nasal continuous positive airway pressure for obstructive sleep apnoea: a randomised prospective parallel trial. *Lancet* 1999; **353**: 2100–2105.

93. Engleman HM, Kingshott RN, Wraith PK, *et al.* Randomized placebo-controlled crossover trial of CPAP for mild sleep apnoea-hypopnoea syndrome. *Am J Respir Crit Care Med* 1999; **159**: 461–467.

94. Grunstein RR. Sleep-related breathing disorders. 5. Nasal continuous positive airway pressure treatment for obstructive sleep apnoea. *Thorax* 1995; **50**: 1106–1113.

95. Pepin JL, Krieger J, Rodenstein D, *et al.* Effective compliance during the first 3 months of CPAP. *Am J Respir Crit Care Med* 1999; **160**: 1124–1129.

96. Miljeteig H, Hoffstein V. Determinants of continuous positive airway pressure level for treatment of obstructive sleep apnea. *Am Rev Respir Dis* 1993; **147**: 1526–1530.

97. Sanders MH, Kern N. Obstructive sleep apnea treated by independently adjusted inspiratory and expiratory positive airway pressures via nasal mask: physiological and clinical implications. *Chest* 1990; **98**: 317–324.

98. Clark GT, Arand D, Chung E, Tong D. Effect of anterior mandibular positioning on obstructive sleep apnea. *Am Rev Resp Dis* 1993; **147**: 624–629.

99. Millman RP, Rosenberg CL, Kramer NR. Oral appliances in the treatment of snoring and sleep apnoea. *Clin Chest Med* 1998; **19**(1): 69–75.

100. Fujita S, Conway W, Zorich F, Roth T. Surgical correction of anatomic abnormalities in obstructive sleep apnea syndrome: uvulopalato-pharyngoplasty. *Otolaryngol Head Neck Surg* 1981; **89**: 923–934.

101. Rodenstein DO. Assessment of uvulopalatopharyngoplasty for the treatment of sleep apnea syndrome. *Sleep* 1992; **15**(Suppl): S56–62.

102. Powell NB, Riley RW, Robinson A. Surgical management of OSA syndrome. *Clin Chest Med* 1998; **19**(1): 77–86.

103. Piper AJ, Sullivan CE. Effects of short-term NIPPV in the management of patients with severe obstructive sleep apnea and hypercapnia. *Chest* 1993; **105**: 434–440.

28

Obesity and Gallstones

S. Heshka and S. Heymsfield

St Luke's/Roosevelt Hospital Center, New York, USA

The formation of gallstones (cholelithiasis) has been identified as one of the risks associated with obesity. In this chapter, we:

- briefly describe the conditions and manner of gallstone formation,
- review the prevalence, incidence, or relative risk in various population samples,
- review some personal and dietary factors, known or suspected to affect gallstone formation and especially relevant to obesity,
- review some methods for prevention and treatment.

GALLSTONE FORMATION

There are two common types of gallstone in the USA and Europe. The most common, and the only type associated with obesity, is the cholesterol gallstone which consists mainly of accretions of cholesterol crystals around a nucleus. The other gallstone type, the pigment stone, is less frequently seen, contains larger amounts of calcium, and is usually associated with chronic hemolytic states and bacterial infections rather than with obesity (1).

Cholesterol gallstone formation is a process that requires the convergence of several conditions. First, in order for gallstones to form, the bile must be supersaturated with cholesterol. The degree of cholesterol saturation of bile is affected by many factors including the rate of cholesterol synthesis by the liver, the amount and composition of bile salts, the amount of phospholipids, and the rate of bile acid synthesis (2).

While bile supersaturation is a necessary condition for gallstone formation, it is not sufficient, as studies have identified many individuals with supersaturated bile and no sign of gallstones. An environment conducive to stone formation must also be present. This can take the form of conditions or contents in the gallbladder which promote nucleation and cholesterol crystallization, and provide binding materials to help form the stone-like accretions. Conditions which can make nucleation more or less likely have been identified and categorized as pronucleating (e.g. presence of mucin and other glucoproteins) or antinucleating factors (e.g. apolipoproteins A-I and A-II).

The lithogenicity of the gallbladder environment is also increased when the time that gallbladder contents are allowed to remain in stasis is lengthened. Thus, failure to have regular or complete gallbladder contractions to expel the gallbladder contents allows a longer time for nucleation and accretion to occur and can thereby contribute to the formation and growth of stones.

This outline of the conditions facilitating formation of stones will provide a framework for our subsequent discussion of the personal, environmental and behavioral factors affecting gallstone formation in obesity. However, we first look at some of the epidemiological evidence linking gallstones and obesity.

International Textbook of Obesity. Edited by Per Björntorp.
© 2001 John Wiley & Sons, Ltd.

EPIDEMIOLOGY

Gallbladder disease occurs frequently and is widespread. It is estimated that about 12% of adults in the USA have gallstones. Over 500 000 cholecystectomies occur annually in the USA (3,4).

A note about the research methods used to arrive at such figures is warranted. The prevalence of gallstones in various populations has been estimated using at least three different methods: surveys counting subject reports of cholecystectomies and symptoms; surveys using ultrasound screenings of population samples; and tabulations of autopsy results. In considering these data the following methodological observations should be kept in mind:

- About two-thirds of gallstones are asymptomatic and will not be detected unless radiology or ultrasonography is employed, and even with modern ultrasound instruments there is a small false-negative rate (about 4%) in severely obese subjects (5,6).
- Gallstones may be passed or evacuated without intervention, or may resolve spontaneously (7). Most cases remain asymptomatic and only a small proportion eventually require medical attention (5).
- Autopsy data provide only crude estimates of prevalence as autopsies are not performed on random or representative samples of the population.
- Estimates based on hospitalization and other forms of clinical diagnosis data are suspect even if the survey is on based on a representative sample of hospitalized cases because there may be unequal rates of diagnosis (ascertainment bias) or unequal access to medical facilities.

Thus, the adequacy of each survey method will depend on the uses to which the data are put. If the purpose is to estimate medical needs then surveys of self-reported cholecystectomies and symptoms may be adequate. On the other hand, if the interest is in risk factors and etiology, then ultrasound screening will provide better data.

A classic report of gallbladder disease epidemiology in the USA comes from the Framingham Study (3). A random sample of people (2336 men, 2873 women) aged 30 to 62 living in the town of Framingham, Massachusetts, was enrolled in a longitudinal study beginning in 1949. In this sample, over a 10-year period, there were 97 definite and 20 doubtful cases of gallbladder disease among the men and 330 definite and 96 doubtful cases among the women. Two hundred and one of these cases (31 men, 170 women) were found upon initial examination (prevalence: men 13/1000, women 59/1000), and 226 (66 men, 160 women) developed the disease during the 10-year follow-up. Women had a relative risk 2 or more times that of men.

Both initial prevalence and incidence of new gallstones during the 10-year period increased with increasing age and obesity. For obesity, as relative weight (a ratio of subject's weight to median weight for all individuals of same sex and height) increased from < 0.9 to > 1.2, relative risk increased from 0.55 to 1.25 in men, and from 0.85 to 1.77 in women.

While the Framingham Study was important because of its size and representative sample, it relied on self-report for its data and could not be used to estimate prevalence for asymptomatic gallstones. Jorgensen (8,9) reported on a study which used ultrasound screening on a cross-sectional, stratified random sample of 3608 Danish men and women, age 30, 40, 50 and 60, between 1982 and 1984. Rates ranged from a low of 1.8% in 30-year-old men, to 22.4% in 60-year-old women. The study also showed increasing prevalence of gallstones with increased body mass index (BMI, kg/m^2) in women but only a trend in men. In BMI categories < 20, 20–25, 25–29, 30 + , the mean prevalence was 5.5, 6.3, 5.3, 9.0% in men, and 7.5, 10.6, 13.0, 28.4% in women, pooling across age categories. These figures suggest that differences in BMI in the 20–30 range may be more important for women, while prevalence for men is less affected until BMI exceeds 30.

The Danish data show clearly that prevalence increases with both age and obesity. However, because persons tend to gain weight as they age, at least until around age 50, it is necessary to adjust the prevalence of gallstones for the age of the subjects if we want an estimate of the degree of association with BMI apart from its association with age.

One study that made such adjustments used data from 90 302 women in the Nurses Health Study (10). Aged 34 to 59 at baseline in 1980, an 8-year follow-up period identified 2122 cases of cholecystectomy, and in a 6-year period, 488 cases of newly diagnosed symptomatic but unremoved gallstones. The incidence of cholecystectomy or diagnosed gallstones was clearly related to BMI, rising in a monotonic fashion from 0.28 per 100 person/years at BMI

< 24, to around 1/100 person/years with BMI in the range of 30–35, and more than 2/100 for a BMI of 45 and greater. Multivariate adjustment for known or suspected confounding factors such as age attenuated only slightly the association of obesity and gallstone risk, indicating that most of the association is with BMI rather than age. Unfortunately, the sample is limited to women and data for a comparable sample of men are not available.

Acalovschi *et al.* (11) studied the rate of gallstone formation in a sample of 157 obese women hospital patients in Romania. The mean sample BMI ($\pm$ SD) was $31.4 \pm 3.6 \, kg/m^2$. Morbidly obese women (BMI > 40) and subjects with an abnormal initial ultrasound were excluded from the longitudinal study. These women were followed over a period of 2 to 6 years. Mean age at follow-up was 50.1 years. The cumulative incidence of gallstones, symptomatic and asymptomatic, was 2.6 cases per 100 women per year. Most of the cases were asymptomatic. Age, family history, early onset obesity and hyperlipoproteinemia type IV were associated with increased risk of gallstone formation.

A study of 2228 Japanese men, age 49 to 55, retiring from the Self-Defense Forces who had a retirement health examination including an ultrasound scan, failed to find an association of BMI with gallstones, although there was an association of BMI with having previously undergone cholecystectomy. The authors suggest that the power of the study may have been inadequate, but, in addition, the BMI of most of the men in the sample was low: 75% of the sample had a BMI below 25.4, and the BMI range is also limited. The authors observe that the overall prevalence rate of gallstone disease (gallstones or cholecystectomy) in their sample was 3.3%, much lower than among 50-year-old European men, which they cite as 24.5% in Norway, 6.7% in Denmark and 7.5% in Britain (12).

International comparisons are difficult to make because samples tend to be non-representative and methods of determining prevalence may differ. Thus the Japanese sample consisted of males retiring from the military, one US sample was female nurses, and the Romanian sample was selected from hospitalized women. Furthermore, there may be special subpopulations within a nation whose gene pool or risk factors may differ substantially from the majority population, which can greatly change the prevalence. For example, in the USA 70% of Pima Indian women over age 25 have been reported to have gallstones (4), and Mexican Americans are known to have elevated gallstone rates compared to persons of Caucasian descent (13).

Tables 28.1 and 28.2 summarize a large amount of epidemiological data.

Because obesity combines with variables such as sex, age and ethnicity in non-additive and non-linear ways to alter greatly the prevalence and incidence of gallstones, few general summary statements can be made: women have higher rates than men; rates increase with age; rates are greatest at highest levels of BMI.

FACTORS RELATED TO INCREASED GALLSTONE FORMATION IN THE OBESE

Why gallstones form in some persons and not in others, and in particular, why the obese are predisposed to the development of gallstones is an object of continued study. In this section we discuss some of the individual and environmental factors related to increased gallstone risk and the manner in which these factors may affect the mechanisms of gallstone formation.

Diet and Diet Composition

It has been suggested that high total caloric intake (after BMI is taken into account), meal spacing, fasting, caloric restriction and many other dietary variables can affect gallstone formation (14). We mention here some of the findings on diet composition most relevant to obesity.

Dietary Cholesterol

Surprisingly, there is little evidence that cholesterol intake or serum total cholesterol is related to risk for formation of cholesterol gallstones. It has been suggested that since obese people have higher bile saturation indices than the non-obese, perhaps because of increased hepatic secretion of cholesterol into the bile, that dietary cholesterol may make little additional difference for these individuals (3,14).

Table 28.1 Gallstone prevalence in men

Study[a]	Number of subjects	Age range (years)
North American studies		
Michigan (1959)[b]	1233	11.1% (≈30–50)
Hispanic Americans (1989)		
Mexican Americans	634	2.6% (30) · 9.7% (40–50) · 15.5% (60–70)
Cuban Americans	134	0.0% (30) · 5.1% (40–50) · 14.3% (60–70)
Puerto Ricans	200	2.0% (30) · 3.3% (40–50) · 11.1% (60–70)
European studies		
Austria (1984)	67	16% (≈55–60)
Denmark (1987)	1843	1.8% (30) · 1.5% (40) · 6.7% (50) · 12.9% (60)
Italy (1988)	1239	2.3% (20–30) · 2.0% (30) · 6.7% (40) · 14.7% (50) · 14.4% (60)
Italy (1987)	878	1.1% (20–30) · 4.4% (30) · 9.2% (40) · 11.0% (50–60)
Norway (1987)	637	4.9% (20–30) · 12.9% (30) · 18.2% (40) · 24.5% (50) · 37.0% (60–70)
Wales (1976)[b]	849	<6.0%> (40) · 5.0% (50) · 8.0% (60–70)

[a]Reference details for studies may be found in Diehl (4).
[b]Prevalence determined by oral cholecystography.
Reproduced from Diehl (4) by permission of W.B. Saunders Company.

Table 28.2 Gallstone prevalence in women

Study[a]	Number of subjects	Age range (years)						
		20	30	40	50	60	70	80
North American studies								
Nova Scotia (1980)[b]	133	←— 14.6% —→ 33.3%		←— 14.3% —→				
Hispanic Americans (1989)								
Mexican Americans	654		←— 13.8% —————————→		←— 26.4% —→		←— 44.1% —→	
Cuban Americans	189		←— 10.8% —————————→		←— 19.2% —→		←— 21.7% —→	
Puerto Ricans	382		←— 9.0% —————————→		←— 21.2% —→		←— 12.1% —→	
European studies								
Austria (1984)	86				←————— 32.5% —→			
Denmark (1987)	1765		4.8%	6.1%	14.4%	22.4%		
Sweden (1985)	424			17.4%	21.8%			
Sweden (1988)	109					< 25.0% >		50.5%
Italy (1984)	1081	←— 2.5% —→	←— 5.9% —→	←— 10.9% —→	←— 17.8% —→			
Italy (1987)	1033	←— 2.9% —→	←— 9.5% —→	←— 16.1% —→	←— 27.0% —→			
Norway (1987)	734	←— 6.0% —→	←— 15.3% —→	←— 24.8% —→	←— 29.2% —→	←— 41.3% —→		
Wales (1976)[b]	278			< 12.0% >	←— 14.1% —→	←— 10.1% —→		

[a]Reference details for studies may be found in Diehl (4).
[b]Prevalence determined by oral cholecystography.
Reproduced from Diehl (4) by permission of W.B. Saunders Company.

Dietary Fat

Of interest here are effects of low dietary fat content. Two separate effects need to be distinguished: ingestion of fats in the long-term regular diet versus fat content of diet during a weight loss program. With respect to the former, populations consuming a diet of regular foods with low fat content (animal fat in particular) are suspected to be at lower risk for gallstone formation and vegetarians have been found to have low gallstone rates (15). The situation with respect to fat ingestion during caloric restriction for weight loss appears to be quite different. Several studies which used very low calorie liquid diets (VLCD) with very low fat content to produce rapid weight loss showed strikingly elevated rates of gallstone formation.

For example, Liddle *et al.* (7) observed gallstone formation in 13 of 51 obese patients following 8 weeks on a 520 kcal (2177 kJ) diet during which patients lost a mean of 16.6 kg. In another study, Yang *et al.* (16) enrolled 457 adults in a hospital-based weight reduction program consisting of a 520 kcal diet (55 g protein, 79 g carbohydrates, 1 g fat). After 16 weeks 248 patients remained in the program and received a second ultrasound scan. Eleven of 58 men and 16 of 190 women developed gallstones during the interval. Univariate analysis comparing subjects who developed gallstones with those who did not identified three variables on which they differed significantly. These included larger initial BMI, greater BMI decrease during the intervention, and higher initial triglyceride levels. Subjects who showed greatest BMI change were most likely to develop gallstones, suggesting that rate of weight loss may be a factor in producing these elevated rates of gallstone formation.

However, both of the above studies used diets which were extremely low in fat content (< 2 g/day). Ingestion of fat promotes the release of cholecystokinin (CCK), a hormone secreted by the mucosa of the upper gastrointestinal tract which stimulates gallbladder contractions. The contractions expel the gallbladder contents thereby helping to prevent the accumulation of crystals and binding material which contribute to the growth of gallstone accretions. Suggestions that gallbladder stasis secondary to extremely low intake of dietary fat might be responsible for increased gallstone formation rates during rapid weight loss were put forward by Klawansky and Chalmers (17).

Stone *et al.* (18) showed that gallbladder functioning in individuals with elevated BMI was not impaired compared to normal weight individuals. A liquid meal containing less than 1 g of fat resulted in impaired emptying in both normal weight and obese subjects, whereas the addition of 10 or 20 g of fat to a liquid meal restored gallbladder emptying to maximal stimulus levels in both normal and obese individuals.

The effect of low fat content was initially difficult to separate from that of caloric restriction and rate of weight loss since all these variables were confounded. However, other, more recent studies have tended to clarify the important variables.

Gebhard *et al.* (19) attempted to separate the effects of rapid weight loss from those of very low fat content. They randomized obese men and women into a 520 kcal, less than 2 g fat/day diet group, and a 900 kcal (3769 kJ), 30 g fat/day diet group. The latter included one 10 g fat meal to stimulate gallbladder contraction. Over the 24 weeks of the study the subjects were gradually introduced to regular foods and by the end of the program subjects were on a 1200–1500 kcal/day (5025–6281 kJ/day) intake. Both groups lost similar amounts of weight (about 22% of initial weight) by the end of the 24-week period. Four subjects on the 2 g fat/day diet developed gallstones by the 12th week, whereas no one in the other group did ($P = 0.021$). The authors suggest that gallstone risk during rapid weight loss may be reduced by stimulating gallbladder emptying with adequate dietary fat.

Festi *et al.* (20) also investigated effects of two diets of different fat content on gallbladder emptying and gallstone formation in obese subjects. First, ultrasound evaluation in 32 subjects established their gallstone-free status, then, for 3 months they consumed either 3.0 g of fat/day on a 2.24 MJ (535 kcal) or 12.2 g fat in a 2.415 MJ (577 kcal) diet. After the first 3 months the same low calorie diet (LCD) was fed to both groups: 4.194 MJ (1002 kcal) for 3 more months. Eleven subjects in each group completed the study with significant weight loss. Asymptomatic gallstones developed in 6 of 11 subjects in the low fat group versus none in the high fat group. High fat always induced greater gallbladder emptying. This study effectively separates effects of low fat from those of caloric restriction and seems to conclude along with others that the low fat content is primarily responsible for the high gallstone rates seen in previous studies.

However, the protective role of dietary fat during weight loss is not always sufficient to prevent the formation of stones. Vezina *et al.* (6) studied a series of 272 obese subjects who began a 13-week 900 kcal/day (3769 kJ/day) liquid diet program with normal gallbladder ultrasonograms. Two diet formulations were used, one with 16 g fat/day, the other with 30 g fat/day, including at least one meal with 10 g of fat. In the first series with the low fat content, 16 of 94 (17%) subjects developed stones. In the second series with the higher fat content, 20 of 178 (11.2%) developed stones. Since other studies had shown that 10 g of fat per meal results in maximal gallbladder emptying they concluded that cholelithiasis which occurs during rapid weight loss may not be solely attributable to low fat content and gallbladder stasis. Unfortunately, the study was not a randomized trial and there were differences in mean BMI between the two groups of subjects upon entry and differences in the amount of weight lost during the study, and both of these differences could account in part for the high incidence of gallstone formation seen in the high fat group. However, other studies by Hoy *et al.* (21) and Moran *et al.* (22), described below, also suggest that low fat content does not entirely explain the elevated rates seen in rapid weight loss.

Dietary Fiber

Dietary fiber may induce bile acid synthesis, thereby reducing cholesterol saturation of bile. On this basis it has been suggested that fiber supplementation may have a beneficial effect in preventing gallstone development in obese patients on a calorically restricted diet (23).

The previously described study by Vezina *et al.* (6) varied fiber content (partially hydrogenated guar or cellulose) and amount in the diet. Among subjects consuming less than 1000 g of fiber, in 13 weeks 5 of 66 developed stones; among those consuming 1000–2000 g, in 13 weeks 8 of 88 developed stones. There was also no significant difference according to amount or type of fiber consumed.

Although there is some epidemiological evidence of a negative association of dietary fiber and gallstones, at this time evidence that fiber supplementation reduces the rate of gallstone formation in obese persons during rapid weight loss is lacking.

Weight Loss

Survey data suggest an association of weight loss and increased risk for gallstones. For example, the Nurses Health Study reported a relative risk of 1.97 for women who had lost 10 kg or more during the prior 2 years compared with women who had remained within 3.9 kg of initial weight. (10). However, most of this increased risk was associated with a higher initial BMI before weight loss occurred.

Rapid weight loss has been clearly associated with increased rates of gallstone formation in well-controlled trials. Weinsier *et al.* (24) summarized the results of nine different studies in an analysis which showed an increasing curvilinear relationship between incidence of gallstone formation and rate of weight loss. Risk of gallstone formation increased dramatically when weight loss exceeded 1.5 kg per week. Although all of the studies considered in that analysis which showed high incidence rates used diets with less than 2 g fat per day, there have been no subsequent studies which examined comparable weight loss rates with greater amounts of fat. Furthermore, the effect of fat on gallbladder function is inconclusive in some studies and does not produce the expected emptying. Studies which have attempted to match weight loss and only vary fat content between groups tended to employ less severe caloric restriction. Then, also, there are periodic reports of weight loss studies with what should be adequate amounts of fat which nevertheless show a clearly increased rate of gallstone formation. One study, by Vezina *et al.* (6), has been described above. Another study, by Hoy *et al.* (21) provided both more energy (800–840 kcal/day or 3350–3518 kJ/day) and a higher fat content (15 or 25 g/day) than the studies of Yang (16) or Liddle (7), but still found that two cases of gallstones developed over the 10-week intervention. Another study of 36 patients which only restricted caloric intake by approximately 500 kcal/day (2094 kJ/day) and provided about 25% of calories (48 g/day) from fat nevertheless observed three new gallstones after 8 weeks (22). Thus, there are probably aspects of rapid weight loss other than extreme fat restriction which promote gallstone formation. Potential mechanisms are the increased hepatic cholesterol secretion and the reduction in bile acid secretion which are known to occur during caloric restriction and which may increase bile supersaturation (25).

Finally, it is possible that even modest rates of weight loss for long periods of time might increase risk by means of the mechanisms mentioned above. These effects would be difficult to detect for several reasons. The low incidence of gallstone events means that very large samples are required to reach statistical significance. Furthermore, cross-sectional studies find that lower BMIs are associated with lower gallstone risk, thus the increased risk, if any, during weight loss may be offset by a decreased risk as BMI falls.

Weight Cycling

One study has reported an increased risk of cholecystectomy for women who intentionally lost weight and subsequently regained it (26). Compared to non-cyclers, and after adjusting for initial BMI, women who reported at least one episode of weight cycling during a 10-year period had relative risks of 1.31 (for moderate cycles of 10–19 lb (4.5–8.5 kg)) and 1.68 (for cycles of $\geq$ 20 lb (9 kg) loss or gain) of undergoing a cholecystectomy during a subsequent 6-year period. The rate of weight loss or regain during these cycles is not known and may be an important variable.

Inactivity

Obesity tends to be accompanied by low levels of physical activity. A recent prospective study using the Nurses Health Study sample examined correlations of recreational physical activity reported by questionnaires and incidence of cholecystectomy. The authors report relative risk in the most active quintile to be about 0.7 that of the least active quintile, and that a significant effect remained even after adjusting for BMI and recent weight changes (27). Similar results have been found for men (28). The results tend to show decreases in risk with increasing activity over the entire activity range, suggesting that even modest levels of activity might have some protective effect.

Fat Distribution

Surveys conducted as part of the San Antonio Heart Study investigated the occurrence of gall-bladder disease in samples of Mexican American and non-Hispanic white participants whose fat distribution was also assessed by skinfold thickness measurements (13). The subscapular/triceps ratio was used as an index of central fat deposits. The usual associations were found between gallbladder disease status and age and BMI in men, but women showed, in addition, an association of increased gallstone risk with central fat deposits, the association being especially strong in the Mexican American group.

Gallstone pathogenesis may be correlated with certain regional fat distribution patterns, these patterns being possible indicators of metabolic disturbances such as impaired glucose tolerance and lipid metabolism. Hendel *et al.* (29) investigated whether intra-abdominal fat and metabolic disturbances are related to known gallstone pathogenic factors such as gallbladder volume, lithogenic index of bile or gall bladder ejection fraction. They found that fasting gallbladder volume, while not correlated with total fat mass or percentage fat mass in their sample of 57 obese men and women, correlated positively with intra-abdominal fat mass as measured by computed tomography (CT) scan ($r = 0.51$), and also with impaired glucose tolerance ($r = 0.36$). The data also showed a trend for impaired glucose tolerance to be associated with intra-abdominal fat mass. The lithogenicity index of bile, however, was more strongly correlated with total fat mass ($r = 0.66$) than with intra-abdominal fat mass ($r = 0.22$).

Gastric Surgery

Many studies have reported gallstone occurrence in about 30% of cases following gastric restriction or bypass surgery (30,31). It is believed that this is most likely a consequence of the rapid weight loss which follows surgery rather than of any drastic alteration in gastrointestinal functioning. Because of the extremely high incidence, many of these surgery studies have looked at preventing or treating gallstones that form following the surgical procedure. Some of these studies are reviewed in the following section.

PREVENTION AND TREATMENT OF GALLSTONES

Because ursodeoxycholic acid (UDCA) acts to decrease bile saturation it was investigated as an agent to preventing lithogenic changes in bile during weight loss. Aspirin was also studied as an agent which might inhibit nucleation and thereby reduce gallstone risk. Broomfield et al. (32) randomized 68 obese patients into placebo, UDCA (1200 mg/day) and aspirin (1300 mg/day) treatment groups. All participants consumed a low-calorie powdered food supplement (55 g protein, 79 g carbohydrate, 1 g fat) amounting to 520 kcal/day (2177 kJ/day). Mean weight loss in the groups was between 21 and 25 kg over a period of 16 weeks. Follow-up ultrasound scans at 4 weeks and 19 weeks showed that UDCA successfully prevented formation of gallstones. The aspirin medication resulted in a lower but non-significant difference from placebo.

To investigate further the possible preventive effects of aspirin, Kurata et al. (33) examined data from 4524 patients in a randomized, controlled trial where half the patients received 1 g of aspirin per day. Hospitalization rates for gallstone disease were approximately equivalent to national rates and the usual associations of age, triglycerides, obesity and female gender were found. No effect was seen for aspirin medication. The authors conclude that a larger dose might be effective but because of aspirin's gastrointestinal side effects, its eventual utility is questionable.

In another study, Marks et al. (34) looked at effects of ursodiol or ibuprofen on gallbladder contractions and bile among obese patients during weight loss treatment. After a VLCD of 529 kcal/day (2215 kJ/day) for 12 weeks, reduced contraction of the gallbladder, increased cholesterol saturation and increased nucleation and growth of cholesterol crystals were noted. However, no gallstones formed in any group. Ibuprofen treatment showed some promise in that it prevented an increase in saturation and reduction in gallbladder contraction and showed a trend opposing the increase in nucleation and growth of crystals.

A double-blind study of effectiveness of UDCA in preventing gallstone development after vertical band gastroplasty in 29 morbidly obese patients is reported by Worobetz et al. (35). Three months after surgery patients had lost a mean of 17% of pre-operative weight. Six of 14 placebo patients versus none of 10 UDCA treated patients developed gallstones, suggesting that gallstone formation following gastroplasty can be prevented by UDCA therapy.

Sugerman et al. (31) investigated a 6-month regimen of prophylactic ursodiol to prevent development of gallstones after gastric bypass in patients with BMI of 40 or above before surgery. The study used three dose levels: placebo, and 300, 600 and 1200 mg daily. At 6 months, gallstone formation was noted in 32%, 13%, 2% and 6% respectively. The 600 and 1200 doses were significantly different from placebo. The authors conclude that a dose of 600 mg is an effective prophylactic in these patients.

In a multicenter, non-surgical study, Shiffman et al. (36) enrolled 1004 patients with BMI of 38 or greater into a 520 kcal/day (2177 kJ/day) liquid diet program. Subjects had ultrasound scans at the start and at 8 and 16 weeks. Again, subjects were randomized to placebo, 300, 600 or 1200 mg/day of ursodeoxycholic acid. Gallstones developed in 28%, 8%, 3% and 2% of subjects, respectively, and differences between groups remained even after long-term follow-up, showing that UDCA could be an effective prophylactic during well-defined, high-risk periods.

The use of UDCA for dissolution of existing gallstones has also been investigated, with mixed results. Administration of UDCA in a dose of 8–10 mg/kg/day leads to complete or partial gallstone dissolution in about 75% of cases. However, complications such as cystic duct obstruction and biliary pain may occur and only about 17% of cases achieved complete gallstone dissolution. (37).

Laparoscopic cholecystectomy is currently the preferred treatment for symptomatic gallbladder stones. Although it is more technically demanding in obese patients, the risks are comparable to those for non-obese patients and may be lower than with traditional surgical methods (38).

REFERENCES

1. Bilhartz LE, Horton JD. Gallstone disease and its complications. In Feldman M, Scharschmidt BF, Sleisenger MH, (eds) *Sleisenger and Fordtran's Gastrointestinal and Liver Disease*: Pathophysiology/ Diagnosis/ Management, 6th edn. Philadelphia, PA: WB Saunders, 1998: 948–973.
2. Strasberg SM. The pathogenesis of cholesterol gallstones: a

review. *J Gastrointest Surg* 1998; **2**: 109–125.

3. Friedman GD, Kannel WB, Dawber TR. The epidemiology of gallbladder disease: observations in the Framingham Study. *J Chron Dis* 1966; **19**: 273–292.

4. Diehl AK. Epidemiology and natural history of gallstone disease. *Gastroenterol Clin North Am* 1991; **20**: 1–9.

5. Egbert AM. Gallstone symptoms: myth and reality. *Postgrad Med* 1991; **90**: 119–126.

6. Vezina WC, Grace M, Hutton LC, Alfieri MH, Colby PR, Downey DB, Vanderwerf RJ, White NF, Ward RP. Similarity in gallstone formation from 900 kcal/day diets containing 16 g vs 30 g of daily fat. *Dig Dis Sci* 1998; **43**: 554–561.

7. Liddle RA, Goldstein RB, Saxton J. Gallstone formation during weight-reduction dieting. *Arch Intern Med* 1989; **149**: 1750–1753.

8. Jorgensen T. Prevalence of gallstones in a Danish population. *Am J Epidemiol* 1987; **126**: 912–921.

9. Jorgensen T. Gallstones in a Danish Population. *Gut* 1989; **30**: 528–534.

10. Stampfer MJ, Maclure MK, Colditz GA, Manson JE, Willett WC. Risk of symptomatic gallstones in women with severe obesity. *Am J Clin Nutr* 1992; **55**: 652–658.

11. Acalovschi MV, Blendea D, Pascu M, Georoceaunu A, Badea RI, Prelipceanu M. Risk of asymptomatic and symptomatic gallstones in moderately obese women: a longitudinal follow-up study. *Am J Gastroenterol* 1997; **92**: 127–131.

12. Kono S, Shinchi K, Todoroki I, Honjo S, Sakurai Y, Wakabayashi K, Imanishi K, Nishidawa H, Ogawa S, Katsurada M. Gallstone disease among Japanese men in relation to obesity, glucose intolerance, exercise, alcohol use, and smoking *Scand J Gastroenterol* 1995; **30**: 372–376. (Erratum in 1995; **30**: 1228.)

13. Haffner SM, Diehl AK, Stern MP, Hazuda HP. Central adiposity and gallbladder disease in Mexican Americans. *Am J Epidemiol* 1989; **129**: 587–595.

14. Bennion LJ, Grundy SM. Risk factors fot the development of cholelithiasis in man. *N Engl J Med* 1978; **299**: 1221–1227.

15. Pixley F, Wilson D, McPherson K, Mann J. Effect of vegetarianism on development of gall stones in women. *BMJ* 1985; **291**: 11–12.

16. Yang H, Petersen GM, Roth M, Schoenfield LJ, Marks JW. Risk factors for gallstone formation during rapid weight loss. *Dig Dis Sci* 1992; **37**: 912–918.

17. Klawansky S, Chalmers TC. Fat content of very low calorie diets and gallstone formation. *JAMA* 1992; **268**: 873 (Letter).

18. Stone BG, Ansel HJ, Peterson FJ, Gebhard RL. Gallbladder emptying stimuli in obese and normal-weight subjects. *Hepatology* 1992; **15**: 795–798.

19. Gebhard RL, Prigge WF, Ansel HJ, Schlasner L, Ketover SR, Sande D, Holtmeier K, Peterson FJ. The role of gallbladder emptying in gallstone formation during diet-induced rapid weight loss. *Hepatology* 1996; **24**: 544–548.

20. Festi D, Colecchia A, Orsini M, Sangermano A, Sottili S, Simoni P, Mazzella G, Villanova N, Bazzoli F, Lapenna D, Petroni ML, Pavesi S, Neri M, Roda E. Gallbladder motility and gallstone formation in obese patients following very low calorie diets. Use it (fat) to lose it (well). *Int J Obes Relat Metab Disord* 1998; **22**: 592–600.

21. Hoy KM, Heshka S, Allison DB, Grasset E, Blank R, Abiri M, Heymsfield SB. Reduced risk of liver-function-test abnormalities and new gallstone formation with weight loss on

3350 kJ (800 kcal) formula diets. *Am J Clin Nutr* 1994; **60**: 249–254.

22. Moran S, Milke P, Rodriguez-Leal G, Uribe M. Gallstone formation in obese subjects undergoing a weight reduction diet. *Int J Obes Relat Metab Disord* 1998; **22**: 282–283 (letter).

23. Moran S, Uribe M, Prado ME, de la Mora G, Munoz RM, Perez MF, Milke P, Blancas JM, Dehesa M. Effects of fiber administration in the prevention of gallstones in obese patients on a reducing diet. A clinical trial. [Spanish]. *Rev Gastroenterol Mex* 1997; **62**: 266–272.

24. Weinsier RL, Wilson LJ, Lee J. Medically safe rate of weight loss for the treatment of obesity: a guideline based on risk of gallstone formation. *Am J Med* 1995; **98**: 115–117.

25. Marks JW, Bonorris GG, Albers G, Schoenfeld LJ. The sequence of biliary events preceding the formation of gallstones in man. *Gastroenterology* 1992; **103**: 566–570.

26. Syngal S, Coakley EH, Willett WC, Byers T, Williamson DF, Colditz GA. Long-term weight patterns and risk for cholecystectomy in women. *Ann Intern Med* 1999; **130**: 471–477.

27. Leitzmann MF, Rimm EB, Willett WC, Spiegelman D, Grodstein F, Stampfer MJ, Colditz GA, Giovannucci E. Recreational physical activity and the risk of cholecystectomy in women. *N Engl J Med* 1999; **341**: 777–784.

28. Leitzmann MF, Giovannucci EL, Rimm EB, Stampfer MJ, Spiegelman D, Wing AL, Willett WC. The relation of physical activity to risk for symptomatic gallstone disease in men. *Ann Intern Med* 1998; **28**: 417–425.

29. Hendel HW, Hojgaard L, Andersen T, Pedersen BH, Paloheimo LI, Rehfeld JF, Gotfredsen A, Rasmussen, MH. Fasting gall bladder volume and lithogenicity in relation to glucose tolerance, total and intra-abdominal fat masses in obese non-diabetic subjects *Int J Obes Relat Metab Disord* 1998; **22**: 294–302.

30. Amaral JF, Thompson WR. Gallbladder disease in the morbidly obese. *Am J Surg* 1985; **149**: 551–557.

31. Sugerman HJ, Brewer WH, Shiffman ML, Brolin RE, Fobi MA, Linner JH, MacDonald KG, MacGregor AM, Martin LF. Oram-Smith JC, Schirmer BD. A multicenter, placebo-controlled, randomized, double-blind, prospective trial of prophylactic ursodiol for the prevention of gallstone formation following gastric-bypass-induced rapid weight loss. *Am J Surg* 1995; **169**: 91–96.

32. Broomfield PH, Chopra R, Sheinbaum RC, Bonorris GG, Silverman A, Schoenfield LJ, Marks JW. Effects of ursodeoxycholic acid and aspirin on the formation of lithogenic bile and gallstones during loss of weight. *N Engl J Med* 1988; **319**: 1567–1572.

33. Kurata JH, Marks J, Abbey D. One gram of aspirin per day does not reduce risk of hospitalization for gallstone disease. *Dig Dis Sci* 1991; **36**: 1110–1115.

34. Marks JW, Bonorris GG, Schoenfield LJ. Effects of ursodiol or ibuprofen on contraction of gallbladder and bile among obese patients during weight loss. *Dig Dis Sci* 1996; **41**: 242–249.

35. Worobetz LJ, Inglis FG, Shaffer EA. The effect of ursodeoxycholic acid therapy on gallstone formation in the morbidly obese during rapid weight loss. *Am J Gastroenterol* 1993; **88**: 1705–1710.

36. Shiffman ML, Kaplan GD, Brinkman-Kaplan V, Vickers

FF. Prophylaxis against gallstone formation with ursodeoxycholic acid in patients participating in a very-low-calorie-diet program. *Ann Intern Med* 1995; **122**: 899–905.

37. Gleeson D, Ruppin DC, Saunders A, Murphy GM, Dowling RH. Final outcome of ursodeoxycholic acid treatment in 126 patients with radiolucent gallstones. *Q J Med* 1990; **76**: 711–729.

38. Phillips EH, Carroll BJ, Fallas MJ, Pearlstein AR. Comparison of laparoscopic cholecystectomy in obese and non-obese patients. *Am Surg* 1994; **60**: 316–321.

Part VI

Management

29

Health Benefits and Risks of Weight Loss

Lalita Khaodhiar and George L. Blackburn

Beth Israel Deaconess Medical Center, Boston, Massachusetts, USA

Obese patients are at risk for developing a number of medical, psychological and behavioral problems. Medical conditions associated with obesity include insulin resistance and type 2 diabetes mellitus, hypertension, hyperlipidemia, cardiovascular disease, stroke, sleep apnea, gallbladder disease, hyperuricemia and gout, osteoarthritis, and certain types of cancer such as colon, rectum and prostate cancer in men, endometrial, breast and gallbladder cancer in women (1–6) (Table 29.1). Weight reduction results in an improvement or elimination of these obesity-related comorbid conditions (1,7–12). Weight loss as low as 5% has been shown to reduce health risks, while a greater degree of weight loss results in a better health outcome (13). Benefits maintain with the maintenance of weight loss. Generally, a calorie-reduced balanced diet and exercise that provide weight loss of 1–2 lb (0.45–91 kg) a week are very safe and effective. In patients who are unable to achieve weight loss goals, medical treatment such as a very low caloric diet (VLCD), medication, or gastric restrictive surgery may become necessary. The adverse effects of medical weight loss are usually mild, manageable, and do not outweigh the benefits. For example, gallstone formation and cholecystitis have been demonstrated with prolonged caloric restriction; however, they are successfully prevented by prophylactic use of ursodeoxycholic acid (8,14). Fluid, electrolyte abnormalities, and hyperuricemia may occur with VLCDs (8,15). A few years after gastric bypass surgery patients may develop digestive symptoms, vitamin and mineral deficiency (15). Certain preventive measures and close monitoring will significantly reduce these risks. In every case, with proper therapy, the benefit to risk should favor weight loss therapy (1). In particular, priority should focus on prevention of weight gain.

HEALTH BENEFITS OF WEIGHT LOSS IN SPECIFIC DISEASES

Hypertension

The prevalence of hypertension is significantly increased among obese subjects. Several cross-sectional studies have shown a linear relationship between blood pressure and body mass index (BMI) or body weight (16–18). For example, the data from the Third National Health and Examination Survey (NHANES III) showed the prevalence of hypertension among obese adults (BMI > 30) to be approximately two times that among normal weight adults (BMI < 25) (16). In the Swedish Obese Subjects Study, hypertension was present at baseline in 44–51% of subjects. In prospective longitudinal studies, a risk for a future development of high blood pressure is associated with weight changes, while weight gain increases and weight loss reduces the risks (19–21). Furthermore, in obese hypertensive persons, hypertension can improve with a reduction

International Textbook of Obesity. Edited by Per Björntorp.

Table 29.1 Relative risk of health problems associated with obesity

Greatley increased (relative Risk > 3)	Moderately increased (relative risk 2–3)	Slightly increased (relative risk 1–2)
Diabetes mellitus	Coronary heart disease	Cancer (breast cancer in postmenopausal women, endometrial cancer, colon cancer)
Insulin resistance	Osteoarthritis (knees)	Reproductive hormone abnormalities
Hypertension	Hyperuricemia and gout	Polycystic ovary syndrome
Dyslipidemia		Impaired fertility
Sleep apnea		Low back pain
Gallbladder disease		Increased anesthetic risk
		Fetal defects from maternal obesity

Reproduced with permission from Bray (3).

in weight (22–24). In the Nurses' Health Study, BMI at age 18 years and at mid-life were positively associated with the occurrence of hypertension (19). At age 18, for every 1 kg/m^2 increase in BMI, risk of hypertension increased 8%. After age 18, the risk for hypertension was reduced by 15% for a long-term (12–50 years) weight loss of 5.5 to 9.0 kg and by 26% for a long-term weight loss of 10 kg or more. In contrast, a five-fold increase in risk was noted in women who gained more than 25 kg after age 18 years. It was estimated that a 1 kg increase in weight was associated with a 5% increase in risk for hypertension. In the Framingham Study, a 15% decrease in weight was associated with a 10% decrease in systolic blood pressure (20).

Obesity and Hypertension: Pathophysiology

The pathophysiologic mechanisms underlying the association of obesity and hypertension are poorly understood. However, in obesity-related hypertension the cardiovascular abnormalities characterized by sodium retention, intravascular volume expansion, which induces an increase in venous return and cardiac output, and an increase in peripheral vascular resistance are well described (1,25,26). The maintenance of hypervolemia in hypertension implies a resetting of pressure natriuresis toward higher blood pressure (26). These changes in the cardiovascular system and the kidneys are believed to be related to insulin resistance, the enhancement in sympathetic nervous activity, and the activation of the renin–angiotensin system. In addition, interstitial cell proliferation and deposition of non-cellular matrix, histological changes seen within the renal medulla of obese persons, can lead to compression of tubules and vasa recta, and hence

increased sodium reabsorption (26). Weight loss is associated with a reduction in total circulating and cardiopulmonary blood volumes, cardiac output, and peripheral vascular resistance, an improvement in insulin resistance, and inhibition of sympathetic activity and of the renin–angiotensin system (27–29).

Effect of Different Modes of Weight Loss on Blood Pressure

1. Weight loss produced by lifestyle modification. Lifestyle modification, which includes diet intervention, physical activity, behavior therapy, or combination therapy, can cause a significant reduction in blood pressure in both hypertensive and non-hypertensive obese persons (1,30–44). The Trial of Antihypertensive Interventions and Management (TAIM) (30), a randomized, multicenter placebo-controlled trial of antihypertensive drug and diet treatment in 787 patients with mild hypertension, reported a mean drop in diastolic blood pressure of 11.6 mmHg at 6 months in patients who lost 4.5 kg or more. This was significantly greater than the drop in blood pressure in patients who lost less than 2.5 kg or were on placebo. This reduction in blood pressure was as effective as 25 mg chlorthalidone or 50 mg atenolol. Moreover, the effect of antihypertensive drugs was potentiated by weight loss (30). In phase II of this trial, 587 patients continued to be followed for a mean of 4.5 years. Of those receiving placebo, low dose diuretic, or beta blocker, the need for additional antihypertensive medications was reduced by 23% with a 2–3 kg weight loss (31). A meta-analysis by MacMahon (32), which covered five randomized controlled trials, supported the benefit of dietary intervention on blood pressure.

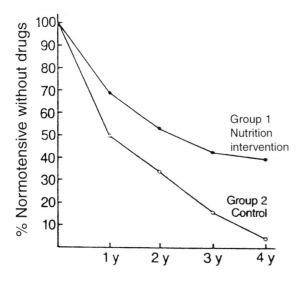

Figure 29.1 Percentage of patients remaining normotensive after withdrawal of antihypertensive drug therapy (group 1, nutrition intervention; group 2, control). Reproduced with permission from Stamler R *et al.* (34) (*JAMA* 1987; **257**: 1481–1491. Copyright 1987, American Medical Association)

Weight loss of 9.2 kg in hypertensive patients resulted in a reduction of 6.3 mmHg systolic and 3.1 mmHg diastolic blood pressure compared with controls (32).

In the Dietary Intervention Study in Hypertension (DISH) (33) and the Hypertension Control Program (HCP) (34), overweight patients with uncomplicated, well-controlled hypertension were withdrawn from drug treatment. Subsequent modest weight loss by diet therapy resulted in a significant reduction in the redevelopment of hypertension over 1 year (33,34) and 4 years (34) (Figure 29.1).

The reduction in blood pressure with weight loss is demonstrated regardless of sodium intake (28,35). One study showed greater benefit with weight loss than salt restriction for blood pressure reduction (36). In this study, the weight loss group lost an average of 6.9 kg with an 11.5 mmHg reduction in systolic and 7 mmHg reduction in diastolic blood pressure, whereas the salt restriction group lost no weight with only a 6.5 mmHg reduction in systolic and a 5 mmHg reduction in diastolic blood pressure.

For non-hypertensive obese persons, weight loss is a very effective way to prevent hypertension. Cutler reviewed four randomized controlled clinical trials in which 872 non-hypertensive subjected en-

gaged in weight loss programs, using dietary intervention and/or exercise (37). Three of these trials were conducted in adults (38–40) and one in adolescents (41). Weight loss of 1 kg in adults resulted in approximately 0.45 mmHg reduction in both systolic and diastolic blood pressure, while weight loss of 1 kg in adolescents, resulted in a 5 mmHg reduction in blood pressure. During one 5-year study, weight reduction (mean 2.7 kg) in conjunction with low salt and alcohol intake and increased physical activity reduced the incidence of hypertension by 52% (40). The Trial of Hypertension Prevention Phase I (TOHP I) (42) and Phase II (TOHP II) (43) are two large collaborative, randomized controlled trials designed to determine the efficacy of non-pharmacologic intervention in preventing an increase in blood pressure. In TOHP I, 664 overweight adults between 30–54 years of age with high normal diastolic blood pressure (80–89 mmHg) were recruited from 10 centers in the United States then followed for 18 months. Participants in weight loss intervention groups attended group meeting and received behavior therapy. At the conclusion of the study, the weight loss intervention group produced 3.9 kg weight loss, 2.3 mmHg diastolic, and 2.9 mmHg systolic blood pressure reduction compared with controls (42). In TOHP II, more patients (2382) were enrolled and followed for a longer period of time (up to 3–4 years). At 36 months, blood pressure decrease remained greater in the intervention group, even though they regained some weight (2 kg weight loss, 0.9 mmHg diastolic, and 1.3 mmHg systolic blood pressure reduction) (43). In addition, weight loss reduced the incidence of hypertension at 18 months by 20–50% (42) and at 3 years by 19% (43) (Figure 29.2).

Secondary analyses from phase I showed sex-related differences in blood pressure response (44). When compared with controls, the blood pressure reduction was significant for men but not for women. This was due to the smaller amount of weight loss by women which could be accounted for by the differences in baseline body weight. However, regression analyses showed a linear relationship between blood pressure reduction and weight loss in both sexes, and when men and women lost an equivalent amount of weight, they experienced a similar degree of blood pressure reduction (44). In this study, other factors, such as sodium intake, alcohol use and exercise frequency, were not found to predict changes in blood pressure.

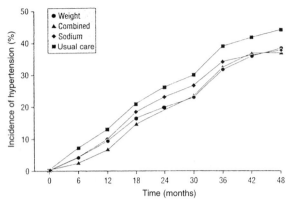

Figure 29.2 Plot of the incidence of hypertension for the respective randomized group (weight loss, salt restriction, combined weight loss and salt restriction, and usual care) through 48 months of follow-up, data from life table analysis in the Trials of Hypertension Prevent, Phase II. (From The Trials of Hypertension Prevention Collaborative Research Group (43) *Archives of Internal Medicine* 1997; **157**: 657–667)

2. Weight loss produced by medications. Most of the studies have shown that weight loss medications (except for those that act on the sympathetic nervous system), when combined with lifestyle modification, are associated with a reduction in blood pressure. Since these medications are usually used in conjunction with lifestyle modification, there is very little data on the effect of drug therapy alone on this cardiovascular risk. It appears likely that the beneficial effect on blood pressure is due to the weight loss itself, and is not a drug-related effect. Generally, serotoninergic drugs such as fenfluramine and dexfenfluramine (which have now been withdrawn from the market) produce similar or better weight loss than that seen in behavioral therapy alone (control) or placebo drug, and a similar or better reduction in blood pressure (1,45–47). In contrast, sibutramine, a serotonin and norepinephrine (noradrenaline) reuptake inhibitor, and other sympathomimetic drugs such as phentermine can be accompanied by an increase, decrease or no change in blood pressure as the action on the sympathetic nervous system would offset the effect of weight loss. A recent multicenter study showed an overall increase in blood pressure in patients on six different doses of sibutramine (1–30 mg), although the only statistically significant change was for diastolic blood pressure at the 20 mg dosage level (48). Individual variability of blood pressure response to medication was also noted, with some patients experiencing a decrease in diastolic blood

pressure of 18–26 mmHg while other patients experienced an increase of 26–40 mmHg.

3. Weight loss produced by surgery. Gastric restrictive surgery is the most effective treatment for morbid obesity. It is associated with both short-term and long-term weight loss and an improvement or resolution of obesity-related comorbidities (49,50). In one series of 289 patients followed for about 4 years after gastric surgery, 67 patients had preoperative hypertension. Of these, hypertension had resolved in 66% at the time of the last follow-up (51). In another study of 45 morbidly obese patients with diastolic hypertension who had undergone gastric surgery, 22 patients (54%) resolved, and 6 patients (15%) improved their hypertension at 12 months after surgery (52). The resolution of hypertension depended both on the severity of preoperative hypertension and on the amount of postoperative weight loss (51,52). Patients who required no antihypertensive medications preoperatively and patients who lost more weight tended to do better regardless of preoperative weight (51).

Dyslipidemia

The relationship between obesity and altered lipid metabolism is well established (53). In general, obese individuals tend to have elevated fasting plasma triglycerides and reduced plasma high density lipoprotein cholesterol (HDL-C) levels (7,8,53). Plasma cholesterol and low density lipoprotein cholesterol (LDL-C) levels are slightly elevated or normal, but the number of apo-B carrying lipoproteins is increased.

The low HDL-C and high LDL-C to HDL-C ratio put the patients at greater risk for atherosclerosis. In addition, abdominal obesity is associated with an increased proportion of small, dense atherogenic LDL particles in plasma, hypertriglyceridemia, and insulin resistance. This type of obesity is a significant risk factor for cardiovascular disease, type 2 diabetes, and their related mortality (54).

Obesity and Dyslipidemia: Pathophysiology

Central obesity and the hyperinsulinemia that accompanies insulin resistance are thought to cause an excess production of very low density lipoprotein (VLDL) which is triglyceride-rich in the liver (55). Since the lipolysis of visceral adipocytes appears to be insulin-resistant, this may cause an increased free fatty acid flux to the liver and stimulate VLDL secretion. Also, the lipoprotein lipase levels are decreased, resulting in a slower clearance of VLDL and a reduced production of HDL particles (53,55). In addition, alteration in VLDL metabolism can lead to production of smaller, denser LDL. With weight reduction, both free fatty acid levels and hyperinsulinemia decrease, resulting in decreased VLDL production and improvement of VLDL metabolism. Furthermore, weight loss improves lipoprotein lipase activity, greater triglyceride clearance and HDL production.

Effect of Different Modes of Weight Loss on Plasma Lipid Levels

1. Lifestyle modification. Modest weight loss induced either by dieting or by exercising is associated with an increase in HDL-C and a reduction in serum triglycerides. Serum total and LDL-C are also decreased (1,8). In 1992, a meta-analysis by Dattilo and Kris-Etherton showed that weight reduction was associated with significantly decreased LDL and VLDL cholesterol as well as triglycerides; during active weight loss, HDL increased by 0.007 mmol/L for every kilogram weight loss (56). Recently, National Insitutes of Health and National Heart, Lung, and Blood Institutes (1) have reviewed 14 randomized controlled trials conducted to evaluate the effect of weight loss induced by diet and/or physical activity on plasma lipid levels. The data demonstrated that the intervention group when compared with the control has a 5–13% weight loss accompanied by changes in total cholesterol of 0 to 18%, triglycerides of −2 to −44%, LDL cholesterol of −3 to −22%, and HDL cholesterol of −7 to +27%. Most of these trials lasted for about 4–12 months excluding the result of acute caloric deprivation. At longer durations, this beneficial effect of weight loss has been shown to continue; the study by Waki et al. (57) demonstrated a decrease in serum total, LDL cholesterol and triglycerides as well as an increase in the ratio of HDL to total cholesterol in healthy obese women who lost weight (mean 16.7 kg) at 17 months follow-up.

2. Weight loss medications. While weight loss induced by lifestyle modifications significantly improves plasma lipid levels, available data on weight loss induced by medications appear to show no consistent effects. Dexfenfluramine, for example, has been shown both to increase and decrease total cholesterol and triglyceride levels (45–47,58,59). HDL cholesterol was reported to be increased in one study (46). The trial on sibutramine showed statistically significant changes in serum lipids in patients who lost weight on medications; HDL cholesterol increased, LDL cholesterol and triglycerides decreased. In this study, however, the changes in serum lipids were similar for a given amount of weight loss whether weight loss was achieved on placebo or on sibutramine. Since sibutramine causes a greater weight loss than placebo, better lipid profiles were seen (48).

The effects of orlistat in obese patients with abnormal lipid profiles (LDL > 130 mg/dL, LDL/HDL > 3.5 or HDL < 35 mg/dL) have been evaluated in seven randomized controlled trials; 1-year treatment with orlistat showed a greater reduction in LDL cholesterol (−7.83% vs. +1.14%) and LDL/HDL ratio (−0.64 vs. −0.46) when compared to placebo, while HDL cholesterol increased in both groups (+18.8% vs. +20.1%) (60). Another short-term (12 weeks) study in obese patients without hyperlipidemia showed a small but significant decrease in serum total, LDL, and LDL/HDL ratio without significant changes in triglycerides or HDL cholesterol (61).

3. Surgery. Gleysteen et al. reported normalization of plasma triglycerides, an increase in plasma HDL cholesterol levels, and a reduction of total cholesterol/HDL ratio in 42 morbidly obese patients by 6 months after Roux-en-Y gastric bypass, with some further improvement occurring with additional weight loss at one year (mean weight loss of 61% of excess weight) (62,63). They also noted a sustained improvement in lipid profiles at 5–7 years postoperatively despite some weight regain. These data were similar to those reported by Brolin (64), Wolf (65), and Cowen (66): significant reduction in total triglycerides, total cholesterol, and increased HDL cholesterol levels within 6–12 months after gastric surgery.

Table 29.2   Age-adjusted relative risk for diabetes mellitus during 14 years of follow-up and weight change between age 18 years and 1976

Weight change (amount)	Cases, n^a	Person-years of follow-up	Age-adjusted relative risk	Relative risk adjusted for age and body mass index at age 18 years (95% CI)
Loss ($\geq$ 20.0 kg)	5	5921	1.9	0.13 (0.1 to 0.3)
Loss (11.0 to 19.9 kg)	17	22 493	1.8	0.23 (0.1 to 0.4)
Loss (5.0 to 10.9 kg)	43	73 645	1.4	0.54 (0.4 to 0.8)
Loss (4.9 to a gain of 4.9 kg)	197	464 001	1.0	1.0 (reference)
Gain (5.0 to 7.9 kg)	130	192 123	1.5	1.9 (1.5 to 2.3)
Gain (8.0 to 10.9 kg)	143	132 630	2.2	2.7 (2.1 to 3.3)
Gain (11.0 to 19.9 kg)	545	211 126	5.2	5.5 (4.7 to 6.3)
Gain ($\geq$ 20.0 kg)	724	93 840	15.1	12.3 (10.9 to 13.8)

^{a}Data missing on weight change from age 18 years to 1976 for 400 cases during 295 552 person-years of follow-up.
Reproduced from Colditz *et al.* (67) by permission of *Annals of Internal Medicine.*

Type 2 Diabetes Mellitus

A number of epidemiological studies have reported the increased risk of type 2 diabetes as body weight increases. The data from the Nurses' Health Study showed that the risk of diabetes increased with BMI as low as 22. Women with BMI in the average range (24.0–24.9) had a five-fold elevated risk compared to women with a BMI less than 22. At BMI of 31 or greater, the risk of type 2 diabetes increased to at least 40-fold. This relationship between BMI and diabetes was noted in both black and white women and in women as old as 69 years (67). In addition, this study also demonstrated that change in body weight was a strong predictor of risk for diabetes. When compared with women with stable weight (those who gained or lost less than 5 kg), women who gained 20 kg or more after age 18 had a 12-fold increased risk for type 2 diabetes; in contrast, for women who lost more than 20 kg during adulthood, the risk of diabetes reduced by 87% (64) (Table 29.2).

A similar relationship between body weight or weight change and the risk of type 2 diabetes was found in men in the Professionals Health Study, a study of 51 529 male health professionals aged 40–75 years in the United States. The relative risk of diabetes in men with a BMI of 35 kg/m² was 42 times higher than in men with a BMI <23 kg/m² while the corresponding number in men who gained 15 kg or more after age 21 was 34 times that of men who were within 2 kg of their weight at age 21 (Table 29.3) (68).

Table 29.3   (BMI) at age 21 and risk of diabetes among a cohort of 27 338 US men age 40–75 years in 1986 and followed for 5 years

Person-Range (kg/m²)	years	Cases	RR Age-adjusted (95% CI)	Multivariate RR (95% CI)
BMI at age 21				
< 21.0	29 085	69	1.0	1.0
21.0–22.9	36 891	50	0.6 (0.4–0.9)	1.0 (0.7–1.4)
23.0–24.9	33 649	55	0.8 (0.6–1.2)	1.5 (1.1–2.2)
25.0–26.9	17 775	44	1.2 (0.8–1.8)	2.5 (1.7–3.8)
27.0 +	8 357	48	2.9 (2.0–4.2)	6.4 (4.3–9.5)
Weight gain since age 21				
Loss 3 +	9 885	4	0.5 (0.2–1.5)	0.3 (0.1–0.8)
Loss 2–gain 2	26 261	19	1.0	1.0
Gain 3–5	22 787	14	0.8 (0.4–1.6)	0.9 (0.5–1.8)
Gain 6–7	12 987	17	1.7 (0.9–3.1)	1.9 (1.0–3.7)
Gain 8–9	11 621	29	3.0 (1.8–5.2)	3.5 (2.0–6.3)
Gain 10–14	20 964	48	2.6 (1.5–4.3)	3.4 (2.0–5.8)
Gain 15 +	24 019	141	6.5 (4.4–9.6)	8.9 (5.5–14.7)

Analysis includes 27 338 participants (266 cases) with complete information on BMI at age 21. Multivariate relative risk (RR) model for BMI at age 21 controls for age in 5-year intervals, family history, smoking status (never smoked, formerly smoked, or currently smoking < 15, 15–24, or $\geq$ 25 cigarettes/day), and seven categories of weight change since age 21. Multivariate RR model for weight gain since age 21 controls for age, family history, smoking status (never smoked, formerly smoked, or currently smoking < 15, 15–24, or $\geq$ 25 cigarettes/day), and quintiles of BMI at age 21.
Reproduced from Chan *et al.* (68) by permission of the American Diabetes Association.

Obesity and Type 2 Diabetes Mellitus: Pathophysiology

Obesity and type 2 diabetes both independently and synergistically result in insulin resistance with hyperinsulinemia, a state which is believed to play a primary role in the development of type 2 diabetes

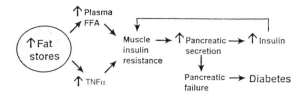

Figure 29.3 Pathophysiology of insulin resistance and diabetes in overweight individuals. Reproduced with permission from Bray (3)

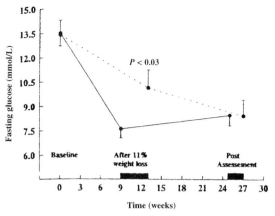

Figure 29.4 Fasting plasma glucose after an 11% reduction in body weight in subjects on a 400 kcal/day diet (solid line) vs. 1000 kcal/day diet (dashed line) and 15 weeks later when all subjeccts were consuming 1000 kcal/day. Reproduced from Wing *et al.* (76) by permission of the American Diabetes Association

(69–72). Although alterations in muscle fuel metabolism are central in insulin resistance related to obesity, all other major glucose-regulatory tissues including liver and adipocytes are affected. It is believed that obesity-induced insulin resistance is mediated in part by high levels of free fatty acid (FFA) and tumor necrosis factor α (TNFα) released by excess adipocytes (Figure 29.3). The elevation of FFA levels can inhibit muscle glucose utilization, increase hepatic glucose output, and stimulate insulin secretion from pancreatic β cells (69–72), causing hyperinsulinemia and, in genetically susceptible persons, overt hyperglycemia. Since insulin resistance is an adaptation of the obese state, any interventions that produce weight loss will improve insulin sensitivity. A reduction of fat mass that occurs with weight loss results in a reduction of lipid oxidation and an exhancement of glucose metabolism (73). Insulin secretion and plasma insulin concentrations have been shown to decrease significantly after weight loss. Furthermore, caloric restriction itself can deplete hepatic glycogen stores, thereby decreasing hepatic glucose output and improving fasting hyperglycemia. The effect of caloric restriction, however, will be maintained only if negative calorie balance leads to weight loss. Exercise, both aerobic and resistance, can also improve skeletal muscle glucose uptake and disposal (74).

Effects of Different Modes of Weight Loss on Type 2 diabetes Mellitus

1. Lifestyle modification.

Weight loss produced by diet and/or exercise has been proven to improve insulin sensitivity and reduce blood glucose levels in both obese diabetic and non-diabetic individuals. Frequently, hyperglycemia lessens upon initiating a hypocaloric diet, suggesting that the restriction in caloric intake has a beneficial effect independent of weight loss. In one study of a VLCD in obese patients with type 2 diabetes, 87% of the reduction in

plasma glucose levels was observed within the first 10 days of caloric restriction, while 60% of weight loss occurred between days 10 and 40 (75). In another study, 93 obese type 2 diabetic patients were assigned to receive either 1674 kJ/day (400 kcal) or 4185 kJ/day (1000 kcal) (76). At comparable degrees of weight loss (11% of initial body weight), subjects in the 1674 kJ/day (400 kcal) group had lower fasting glucose levels (7.61 vs. 10.13 mmol/L) and greater insulin sensitivity. When subjects who consumed 1674 kJ (400 kcal) changed to 4185 kJ (1000 kcal) 15 weeks later, glycemic control and insulin sensitivity worsened despite continued weight loss; whereas the group that consumed 4185 kJ (1000 kcal) from the beginning of the study had further improvement of glycemic control with further weight loss (76) (Figure 29.4).

In obese patients with type 2 diabetes, even moderate weight loss can significantly improve glycemic control, as shown by a reduction in glycosylated hemoglobin (HbA1C) levels, and in some patients, an ability to discontinue insulin or oral therapy. Such improvements can last many years based on the level of weight maintenance. In one randomized controlled study of diet and exercise in overweight Afrian Americans aged 55–79 years with type 2 diabetes, when compared to the control group, the intervention group lost 2.4 kg (3%) at 6 months and reduced HbA1C by 2.4% (77). In another study in newly diagnosed diabetes, patients who attended regular group education given by diabetes specialist

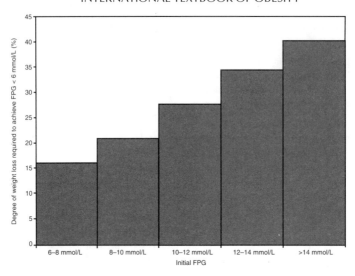

Figure 29.5   Initial fasting plasma glucose (FPG) levels determine degree of weight loss required to achieve normoglycemia (FPG < 6 mmol/L). Patients who began with a mildly elevated FPG of 6–8 mmol/L (108–144 mg/dL) had to lose 16% of initial body weight to achieve FBG < 6 mmol/L). Greater degree of weight loss were required with worse glycemic control, 21% for an initial FPG of 8–10 mmol/L, 35% for an initial FPG of 12–14 mmol/L, and 41% for an initial FPG > 12 mmol/L. Data from UKPDS Group (81)

nurses and dietitians lost 5 kg more weight than those who had no structured education, and had a lower HbA1C by 2% at 6 months (78). At 1 year (no further visits between 6 months and 1 year), the difference in weight loss was less (2.5 kg) and diabetic control was similar in both groups. For long-term effect of weight loss, Mancini *et al.* (79) have shown that patients who maintained losses of at least 5% of initial weight at 3 years had lasting improvement of glycemic control, whereas control worsened in those who had losses of less than 5%.

Although diet and exercise are mainstays of treatment in patients with type 2 diabetes, not all patients respond equally. The results of a 48-month retrospective study on 135 patients who were on diet therapy indicated that only 41% of patients who lost at least 9.1 kg had plasma glucose concentration below 10 mmol/L (80). Some of these individuals, however, decreased their plasma glucose levels after losing only 2.3 kg. It was noted that the improvement in glycemic control occurred early in the course of weight loss and patients who remained hyperglycemic after losses of 2.3 to 9.1 kg were unlikely to improve with additional weight reduction. These results might be explained by a relatively higher insulin resistance in patients who responded to diet therapy and a severe insulin deficiency in patients who did not do so. Other studies have shown that the initial fasting plasma glucose is a

strong predictor for a successful response to diet therapy. In the UK Prospective Diabetic Study (UKPDS), the amount of weight loss required to achieve a normal fasting plasma glucose below 6 mmol/L was 10 kg (16% of initial body weight) if patients had initial fasting blood glucose of 6 to 8 mmol/L (108–144 mg/dL) versus 26 kg (41%) if initial blood glucose was greater than 14 mmol/L (252 mg/dL) (Figure 29.5) (81).

Heilbronn *et al.* (82) have studied the effects of different diet composition on weight loss and blood glucose control. They found that regardless of carbohydrate and fat content in the diet, a similar amount of calorie restriction resulted in an equal degree of weight loss and reductions in fasting plasma glucose, insulin, and HbA1C. However, a high carbohydrate diet (10% fat, 4% saturated) and high monounsaturated (MUFA) (32% fat, 7% saturated) diets reduced LDL cholesterol by 10% and 17% respectively, while a high saturated fat diet (32% fat, 17% saturated) did not. HDL cholesterol was transiently reduced only on the high carbohydrate diet. It was recommended by the American Diabetes Association (ADA) that overweight type 2 diabetes patients restrict their caloric intake (250–500 kcal less than average daily intake as calculated from a food history) along with total fat, especially saturated fat, and increase their physical activity (83).

In overweight individuals without overt hyperglycemia, several randomized trials of lifestyle changes or behavioral therapy found improvement of fasting plasma glucose and insulin levels with weight loss (84,85). The incidence of frank diabetes in persons with impaired glucose tolerance was also reduced.

2. Weight loss medications.

Weight loss produced by weight loss medications has been shown to be no better than weight loss produced by lifestyle modification for lowering plasma glucose level in obese individuals with or without type 2 diabetes. Weight loss medications, however, may benefit those who have limited success with diet and exercise alone. One study of obese diabetes patients that used short-term treatment with dexfenfluramine in addition to conventional oral hypoglycemic drugs found a significant reduction in weight, BMI, and HbA1C at 3 months compared with the placebo (86). In another trial, 3 months treatment with dexfenfluramine was compared to behavioral therapy. Although, a greater weight loss was observed with medication at 3 months, there were no statistically significant differences in the improvement of HbA1C levels between the groups. At 1 year both groups regained some weight, resulting in similar total weight losses and HbA1C levels (87). A recent trial of fenfluramine and phentermine (88) showed that obese diabetic patients who were on active medication had significant reductions in body weight, BMI, and HbA1C between 2 and 6 months compared with patients on behavioral modification alone. At 6 months subjects taking active drug lost 9.6 kg and reduced HbA1C by 1.6%, while the corresponding figures for subjects taking placebo were 2.7 kg and 0.3% respectively. At 12 months, however, neither amount of weight loss nor reduction in HbA1C were significantly different between the two groups (Figure 29.6). It should be noted that only 16 of 44 subjects reached 12 months of treatment, when the study was terminated because of the withdrawal of fenfluramine.

A trial of sibutramine in 100 established type 2 diabetes with a mean baseline BMI of 31 kg/m^2 and mean HbA1C of 9.5% showed that subjects on medication and diet lost more weight at 2–12 weeks than subjects on diet alone (mean weight loss 2.4 kg vs. 0.1 kg). Although more patients treated with medication had a greater than 1% reduction in

HbA1C at 12 weeks (15 out of 45 patients vs. 2 out of 41 patients), the mean drop in HbA1C was not significantly different from the control group (0.4% vs. 0%) (89). Available data for orlistat in combination with diet therapy for the treatment of obese type 2 diabetes showed a fall in HbA1C and fasting plasma glucose (1).

3. Surgery.

It has been shown that gastric bypass operation can control type 2 diabetes in a majority of patients. In one large series from North Carolina (90,91), 608 morbidly obese patients underwent Roux-en-Y gastric bypass from 1980 to 1994; of these, 165 patients had type 2 diabetes and 165 had impaired glucose tolerance (IGT) prior to surgery. Adequate follow-up data was available for 90% of patients (146 of 165 with diabetes and 152 of 165 with IGT). Among patients who presented with diabetes, 121 of 146 patients (82.9%) maintained normal fasting blood glucose and HbA1C levels at the end of study, whereas 25 patients remained diabetic. Among patients who had IGT, only two progressed to overt disease. Normalization of blood glucose was observed as fast as a few days postoperatively before weight loss occurred, which is probably due to limitation of caloric intake, and by the end of first week, there were no longer requirements for insulin or oral hypoglycemic drugs in the majority of the patients. It was noted that diabetes patients who are older (48 vs. 40 years) or had diabetes of longer duration (4.6 vs. 1.6 years) were less likely to correct their hyperglycemia. In this series, mean BMI dropped from 50 kg/m^2 preoperatively to 31.5 kg/m^2 at 1 year after surgery and maintained at 34–35 kg/m^2 at 10 to 14 years.

Insulin Sensitizer in the Treatment of Type 2 Diabetes

Although dietary modification with subsequent weight loss can improve glycemic control, glycemic goals are usually not achieved by dietary restriction alone, and pharmacotherapy become necessary. Because obesity and insulin resistance are common in patients with type 2 diabetes, these patients often require high doses of insulin to control their hyperglycemia. However, insulin therapy is accompanied by weight gain, which would compromise the expected improvement of blood glucose levels. In such cases, addition of drugs that have different

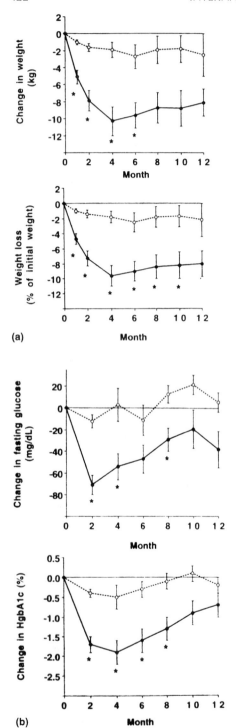

(a)

(b)

mechanism of actions such as sulfonylurea or bi-guanide can be complementary. Unlike a sul-fonylurea, which stimulates insulin secretion from the pancreas, a biguanide works by decreasing hepatic glucose output and improving peripheral insulin sensitivity (92,93). Metformin, a commonly used biguanide, has been shown to improve glycemic control in patients with type 2 diabetes when used either alone or in combination with sul-fonylurea or insulin. In addition, an improvement in hypertriglyceridemia and weight loss has been reported in many patients with metformin use (92–96). In the United Kingdom Prospective Dia-betes Study (UKPDS) (95), patients with subopti-mal glycemic control on maximal sulfonylurea ther-apy decreased their fasting blood glucose levels by mean of 0.47 mmol/L over 3 years after the addition of metformin, in contrast to an increase of 0.44 mmol/L in subjects continuing on sulfonylurea alone. Both groups also lost a small amount of weight. In one recent study, the addition of metfor-min in patients taking insulin resulted in HbA1C levels that were 10% lower than that achieved on insulin therapy alone and without significant weight gain (96). Because of its lipid-lowering and weight-loss-promoting effects, metformin is now recommended by many physicians as a first drug choice in obese type 2 diabetic patients (92,93).

Cardiovascular Disease

Obesity is a significant factor related to the develop-ment of cardiovascular disease. As mentioned pre-viously, obesity is strongly associated with hyper-tension, diabetes mellitus and dyslipidemia, classic

Figure 29.6 Mean ± SEM changes in weight from baseline and weight loss as a percentage of initial weight in placebo (○) and drug treatment group (●). Subjects in the fenfluramine/phentermine drug treatment group demonstrated rapid weight loss, which continued for the first 4–6 months and then reached a plateau. The control group showed a similar but quantitatively smaller, pattern of weight loss. * $P \leq 0.01$ vs. placebo group. Reproduced from Redmon *et al.* (88) by permission of the American Diabetes Association). (b) Mean ± SEM change in fasting plasma glucose and HbA1C from baseline in placebo (○) and drug treatment group (●). Both fasting and HbA1C declined rapidly in the drug treatment group. HbA1C was significantly lower with drug treatment at all time points through 6 months. * $P \leq 0.01$ vs. Placebo group. Reproduced from Redmon *et al.* (88) by permission of the American Diabetes Association

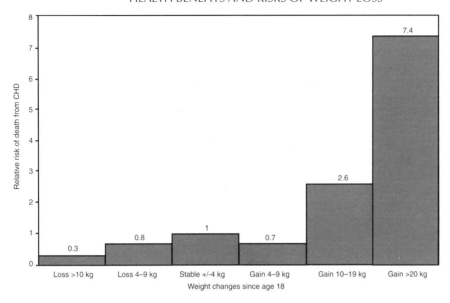

Figure 29.7 Weight changes since the age of 18 and relative risk of death from coronary heart disease among women who never smoked. Weight gain of 10 kg (22 lb) or more since the age of 18 was associated with increased mortality from coronary heart disease in middle adulthood. Data from Manson *et al.* (102)

cardiovascular risk factors. In addition, obstructive sleep apnoea and hemorheological abnormalities such as elevated plasma plasminogen activator inhibitor 1 (PAI-1) levels and high blood viscosity in obese persons may contribute to the pathogenesis of coronary atherosclerosis. High levels of PAI-1, produced by visceral fat, impair fibrinolytic activity and increase the extent of thrombosis (97,98). Obesity, especially abdominal obesity, is also associated with increased morbidity and mortality from cardiovascular disease (99).

Recent clinical studies have suggested an association between BMI and coronary events such as non-fatal myocardial infarction, angina pectoris, and death from coronary heart disease. In the Nurses' Health Study, after controlling for age, smoking, menopausal status, hormonal therapy, and family history, the risk of developing coronary heart disease (CHD) was increased 1.8-fold with a BMI of 25–29 and 3.3-fold with a BMI above 29, compared with a BMI of less than 21 (100,101). A weight gain of 20 kg or more during adulthood also increases mortality from CHD 7.4-fold when compared with women whose weight remained stable after 18 years of age (102) (Figure 29.7). Similar findings have been reported in men and many other populations. In British men, an increase of 1 BMI unit from BMI above 22 kg/m² is associated with a

10% increase in the incidence of CHD (103). Additional data suggest that the abnominal obesity may be a better predictor of cardiovascular disease than obesity per se (53).

Other cardiovascular diseases have been shown to be related to obesity including myocardial hypertrophy, cardiomyopathy, and congestive heart failure (104). These abnormalities are probably due to an elevation in cardiac workload to supply active metabolism of excess adipose tissue.

Effect of Weight Loss on Cardiovascular Disease

While the beneficial effects of weight loss on cardiovascular risk factors are well established, there is little information addressing the effect of weight loss on the progression of coronary artery disease. From available data, it appears that weight loss can help to reduce cardiovascular events and cardiovascular mortality (105). In the Lifestyle Heart Trial (106), patients with coronary artery disease were prescribed a lifetyle program including a low fat vegetarian diet, exercise, stress management training, stopping smoking, and group support. After one year, the treatment group had a mean weight loss of 10 kg, a significant reduction in total cholesterol and LDL-C, as well as a regression in coronary lesions assessed by computed tomography and quantitative angiography. In contrast, the control group showed no change in weight or lipid profiles, and a progression of the stenotic lesions (106). Although one cannot conclude that weight loss per se causes regression in coronary artery lesions, the study proves that lifestyle modifications can have an impact on CHD.

Weight loss also results in the reduction of PAI-1 levels. One study of 52 healthy, premenopausal women found a 54% decrease in PAI-1 antigen and 74% decrease in PAI activity after weight loss by hypocaloric diet (107). These changes in PAI-1 levels were associated with changes in both BMI and body fat. The decreased PAI-1 levels remained low in subjects who maintained their reduced weight, but increased in those who regained weight.

In addition to the effects on cardiovascular risks, weight loss produced by either diet or gastric surgery has been shown to improve cardiovascular structure and functions. After successful weight loss, heart weight decreases as well as intraventricular septal and wall thickness. Although, cardiac function may not revert to normal, some improvement has been observed (104,108).

Obstructive Sleep Apnea

Sleep-disordered breathing encompasses a number of clinical conditions in which a normal pattern of respiration in sleep was lost. Obstructive sleep apnea (OSA), the most common form of sleep-disordered breathing, is characterized by a repetitive cessation of airflow (apnea) during sleep caused by collapse of the upper airway. Frequent arousals and episodes of cyclic hypoxia and hypercapnia during sleep lead to excessive daytime sleepiness and other clinical sequelae including systemic hypertension, cardiac arrhythmias, myocardial ischemia, and obesity–hypoventilation syndrome (OHS), an extreme from of OSA associated with awake respiratory failure, pulmonary hypertension and a degree of heart failure (109–111).

There are several predisposing factors for sleep apnea, and obesity, especially central obesity, is one of the most important risk factors (112,113). An increase of one standard deviation in any standard measure of body habitus is related to a threefold increase in the occurrence of sleep apnea (112); 60 to

70% of sleep apnea sufferers are obese. One group of investigators has found that 50 to 200 (40%) obese men and 6 of 50 (3%) obese women (mean BMI 45.3 kg/m^2) without sleep complaints had sleep apnea severe enough for therapeutic intervention by a polysomnogram, compared with none of 128 non-obese age-matched control (114). Other risk factors for sleep apnea are male sex, age 40–65 years, family history, cigarette smoking and alcohol. In general, women have to be more obese than men for sleep apnea to be clinically apparent and at a similar degree of obesity, men tend to have more severe apnea (115). The difference in the severity of sleep apnea could be related to a man's propensity for central obesity and more upper airway fat deposition (116).

Obesity and Pathogenesis of Sleep Apnea

There are a number of potential mechanisms by which obesity may lead to sleep apnea. Excess adipose tissue in the neck may predispose the airway to narrowing and/or closure. Alteration in the upper airway size due to fat deposit around pharyngeal tissue has been demonstrated by magnetic resonance imaging (110). This volume of pharyngeal adipose tissue correlates well with the severity of sleep apnea documented by polysomnography. Clinically, a large neck circumference in both men and women who snore is a strong predictor for sleep apnea (117). Increased fat in the chest wall and abdomen can also reduce lung volume, alter respiratory pattern, and decrease compliance of the respiratory system. Total lung capacity and vital capacity are usually decreased, resulting in a reflex decreased in pharyngeal intraluminal dimension as well as increased in airway resistance. Furthermore, function of the muscle that maintains upper airway patency has been reported to be abnormal in obese patients with sleep apnea (109).

Physiology of Weight Loss

Weight loss improves both the function and structure of the upper airway. Both the propensity for pharyngeal collapsibility and pharyngeal adiposity decrease with successful weight loss (118,119). In addition, the loss of chest wall and abdominal fat results in an increase in lung volume and lung compliance, which in turn improves respiratory function. It has been observed that only a small amount

Table 29.4 Summary of studies examining the effects of weight loss in patients with sleep apnea

Study	Mode of weight loss	Weight[a]		Apnea index		Comment
		Before	After	Before	After	
Smith et al. (1985) (121)						
Diet	106 ± 7		97 ± 6	55 ± 7.5	29.2 ± 7.1	
Suratt et al. (1992) (122)	VLCDs	153 ± 37	132 ± 29	90 ± 32	62 ± 49	
Sugerman et al. (1992) (123)	Gastric bypass	166 ± 35	114 ± 28	64 ± 39	26 ± 26	Mean follow-up 4.5 ± 2.3 years after surgery
Charuzi et al. (1992) (124)	Gastric bypass	117 ± 36[b]	44 ± 35[b]	60 ± 35	8 ± 12	Mean follow-up 5 weeks to 2.5 years after surgery

[a]Weight in kilograms except the last study, which reported percentage excess body weight.
[b]Percent excess body weight.

of weight loss can result in an improvement or resolution of sleep apnea in obese patients. Similarly, the onset of clinically significant sleep apnea may be apparent after weight gain as small as 10 kg, particularly in patients with underlying anatomic abnormalities of the upper airway (116). Recent data have suggested a possible threshold effect that directly relates to the collapsibility of the airway; those with minimal airway collapsibility will achieve greater improvement for the same amount of weight loss (120).

Effects of Different Modes of Weight Loss on Sleep Apnea (Table 29.4)

1. Lifestyle modification.   Positive effects of weight loss induced by diet therapy on sleep apnea have been consistently demonstrated. An early study in a small number of moderately obese middle-aged patients (mean BMI 37 kg/m^2) found a significant improvement of sleep apnea as documented by a marked reduction in the frequency of apnea as well as an increase in arterial oxyhemoglobin saturation during remaining apneic events after only 9% weight loss (121). An increase in daytime alertness was also noted by patients and their spouses. Similarly, a study in eight morbidly obese patients (mean BMI of 54 kg/m^2) (122) showed a reduction in severity of sleep apnea after a successful weight loss produced by a 4-week course of VLCD; a decrease in the number of apnea + hypopneas per hour (respiratory disturbance index/ RDI) from 90 to 62 and in the number of desaturations/hour from 106 to 52. It was noted that the most obese subject with BMI 81, despite the most weight loss (47 kg), did not improve, nor did the subject who lost the least weight (7 kg). Although in both these studies weight loss improved sleep apnea in most patients, it did not eliminate it in any of them. In the new era of nasal continuous positive airway pressure (CPAP) as a primary treatment for sleep apnea, it is possible that the maintenance of weight loss will obviate the need for lifelong CPAP treatment. However, further sleep studies are needed to confirm this.

2. Surgery.   The results of gastric surgery on sleep apnea have been promising. In the largest series, 126 morbidly obese patients with sleep apnea and/or obesity–hypoventilation syndrome under-

went gastric bypass surgery between 1980 and 1990 (123). Fifty-seven of 110 patients with sleep apnea were evaluated at a mean of 4.5 years postoperatively, when they had lost a mean of 31% of their preoperative weight. Of these 57 patients, 66% were completely asymptomatic while 25% had mild persistent sleep apnea. Among 40 patients who had polysomnography before and after surgery, the sleep apnea index (number of apneas/hour of sleep) decreased from a mean of 64 to 26. In another study of 47 obese sleep apnea patients, polysomnography was performed before and at 1 and 7 years after gastric surgery (124). After 1 year, a dramatic reduction in weight and the apnea index were noted. Seventy-two percent of patients had the apnea index < 10, and 40% did not have any apnea. After 7 years, however, regaining of weight in some patients was associated with a recurrence of sleep apnea syndrome.

Liver Disease

Liver Abnormalities in Obesity

Morphological and functional changes in liver are not uncommon among obese individuals. Fatty change and inflammation of the liver are associated with obesity, and their severity is directly related to the degree of overweight. Almost 90% of morbidly obese patients have some degree of morphological abnormalities. In one study, 80% of morbidly obese patients were found to have a fatty change in the liver and in > 50% of these patients more than one-quarter of the liver was involved (125). An autopsy of 172 non-alcoholic obese patients found steatohepatitis (a concomitant of fatty liver and portal or parenchymal inflammation) in 18.5%, fibrosis in 13.8%, and cirrhosis in 1–3%, in contrast to 2.7% steatohepatitis in 121 non-obese subjects (126). Although non-alcoholic steatohepatitis (NASH) that occurs among obese subjects rarely progresses to hepatic fibrosis or cirrhosis, coexistent type 2 diabetes may increase this risk.

Effects of Weight Loss on the Liver

In 1970 Drenick reported a regression of fatty liver in a group of seven patients after VLCDs (127). Similarly, in 1991 Anderson et al. (128) observed a marked regression of fatty changes in 41 morbidly obese subjects without diabetes or history of alcohol use after a median weight loss of 34 kg produced by VLCDs. The regression of fatty change was significantly related to the degree of weight loss. However, some patients developed new lesions after weight loss, 10 patients developed slight degrees of portal inflammation, and five patients developed slight portal fibrosis. Of those who developed portal fibrosis, a large amount of weight loss occurred at a rapid rate. It was estimated that the risk for developing portal fibrosis during VLCD was 28% in patients with a mean weight loss greater than 230 g/day, in contrast to a 0% risk with a mean weight loss below this rate.

Effects of weight loss produced by gastric restrictive surgery on liver morphology have also been investigated. A liver biopsy of 91 patients performed 2 to 62 months after gastric bypass surgery showed a dramatic improvement of steatosis (129). In another study, 69 morbidly obese patients who received gastroplasty had a liver biopsy before and 27 ± 15 months after surgery when they had lost a mean weight of 32 ± 19 kg. Although almost 90% of preoperative biopsies showed pathological changes, 45% of the postoperative liver biopsies were considered normal. The incidence and the severity of fatty change were also significantly reduced. However, inflammatory lobular hepatitis was observed more often in postgastroplasty liver biopsy specimens (130).

Osteoarthritis

Osteoarthritis is one of the most common complications of obesity. The common sites of osteoarthritis in obese patients are the knee, carpometacarpal joint of the hand, and the hip. While osteoarthritis of the knee is contributed by mechanical trauma associated with excess body weight, the arthritis of non-weight-bearing joints is probably due to some systemic factors secreted in obese persons causing abnormalities of bone and cartilage metabolism (3,131). In a survey of more than 7000 Finnish people, BMI was closely related to the prevalence of osteoarthritis (132). The odds ratio for a BMI of 35, compared to a BMI of 25, was 2.8. In middle-aged women, it was estimated that for every kilogram increase in body weight, the risk of osteoarthritis of the knee and carpometacarpal joint of hand in-

creases by 9 to 13% (133). In addition, weight loss is associated with a reduced risk of osteoarthritis. In the Framingham Study (134), a decrease in BMI of 2 units or more (weight loss approximately 5.1 kg) over a 10-year period decreased the odds for developing osteoarthritis of the knee by more than 50% whereas weight gain was associated with a slightly increased risk. The benefit of weight loss was also demonstrated in high-risk patients whose baseline BMI was $> 25 \text{ kg/m}^2$ (134).

A prospective randomized controlled trial examined the effect of medication-induced weight loss on osteoarthritis. The group taking a course of phentermine had a mean weight loss of 12.6% over 6 months, in comparison to 9.2% in a control group. There was a significant clinical improvement in associated with weight loss, especially in patients with knee disease (135). One study from Japan (136) reported a better correlation between the percentage of fat loss and the symptomatic relief of knee osteoarthritis than percentage of weight loss per se. Similarly, a study of patients undergoing gastric bypass surgery showed a significant reduction in the prevalence of joint symptoms with a 45 kg weight loss at 1 year after surgery, although not all joint pains in this group were attributed to osteoarthritis (137).

Because osteoarthritis is very common among the elderly and accounts for much disability in lower extremities, prevention is very important, and one modifiable risk factor is overweight or obesity. It has been estimated that if men whose BMI was > 30 lost weight to BMI 26–29.9 and men whose BMI was 26–29.9 lost weight to BMI < 26, the rate of symptomatic knee osteoarthritis would decrease by 21.4%. In women, a similar degree of weight loss would decrease this rate by up to 33% (138).

Disorders of Female Reproductive Systems

Obesity, especially abdominal obesity, is a predisposing factor for polycystic ovary syndrome (PCOS). Up to 50% of patients with PCOS have BMIs $> 25 \text{ kg/m}^2$ (139). Patients usually present with chronic anovulation along with signs and symptoms of hyperandrogenemia such as hirsutism, acne, and/or androgen-dependent alopecia. Biochemically, testosterone levels may be slightly elevated as well as the ratio of luteinizing hormone and follicle-stimulating hormone (140). PCOS is associated with metabolic disturbance, i.e. hyperinsulinemia and insulin resistance, which may lead to coronary artery disease (139,140).

Besides an improvement in peripheral insulin sensitivity and a decrease in circulating insulin levels, weight loss can reduce serum testosterone levels and improve reproductive function in women with PCOS. Kiddy et al. (141) have examined the effect of weight loss on PCOS. Twenty-six obese women with PCOS (mean weight of 92 kg) were placed on a 1000 kcal low fat diet for 6–7 months; 13 patients who lost > 5% of their original weight had a decrease in free testosterone levels, and a decrease in insulin levels both fasting and in response to glucose load. Nine patients had return of normal menstrual cycle and four achieved pregnancy. Of those 13 patients who were unable to lose weight, only one had improved menstrual cycle.

Psychosocial Disorders

In Western society where people have negative attitudes toward the fatness, obese people usually suffer discrimination. This stigma is seen in many places including schools, the workplace, and health care. Obese people are less likely to be married or have high household income (3,142).

Depression and binge eating disorder are more common among obese subjects seeking weight loss programs than among the general population (142,143). Binger eating disorder (BED) is characterized by recurrent episodes of binge eating, eating a larger amount of food than most people would eat in a discrete time period (e.g. within 2 hours) with a sense of lack of control during the episodes (144). Generally, binge eaters do not engage in inappropriate compensatory behavior such as purging, dieting or laxative use like patients with bulimia nervosa. Compared to obese patients without BED, obese binge eaters tend to be heavier, are more likely to have a psychological illness (especially depression), or emotional distress.

Weight loss has been shown to improve mood, body image, self-esteem and interpersonal functioning. Obese patients who receive group support and behavioral therapy frequently report some improvements in mood after only a few treatment sessions even before 5% of their initial weight loss (142,143). They feel better as a result of their ability to take control of their eating, exercise habits, and their weight. Many patients enjoy a sense of well-being as their medical condition improves. Also an improvement or resolution of obesity-related comorbid conditions improves patients' mood. In obese binge eaters, symptoms of depression or emotional suffering can be ameliorated with successful weight reduction (10).

Other Benefits

While obese patients are more likely to require general surgical procedures, they are at a higher risk for perioperative complications; a 5–10% weight reduction and concomitant diuresis before surgery has been shown to shorten length of hospital stay and to reduce the incidence of postoperative complications (11).

HEALTH RISKS OF WEIGHT LOSS

Although there are substantial health benefits from weight loss, it is not without risks. Therefore the priority is for an incremental modest change in body weight for a period of time that has been established to be safe. In general, the reasonable initial goal of weight loss therapy is a reduction in body weight of 5 to 10% in 6 months with a rate that does not exceed 1–2 lb (0.45–91 kg) per week (1). Once this target is achieved, further weight loss may be considered. A combined therapy with a low calorie diet (800–1500 kcal/day), exercise, and behavior therapy can usually achieve this health risk reduction goal in a safe and effective fashion. In some patients for whom self-help and commercial programs are not successful in reaching this therapeutic goal, medical treatment may become necessary. In 10% of obese persons no comorbidity is identified; therefore medical treatment would not be indicated. These provider-conducted programs including VLCDs, weight loss medication, and gastric bypass surgery can be associated with some adverse side effects, but they are usually mild, well tolerated, and easily managed.

Table 29.5 Adverse side effects of very low calorie diet

Side effects	Treatment/prevention
Minor reactions	
Fatigue, weakness	Tend to be worse during the first 2 weeks and improve later
Dizziness	Increase fluid and sodium intake
Hunger	Tend to be worse during the first 2 weeks and improve later
Nausea	Tend to be worse during the first 2 weeks and improve later
Diarrhea	Antidiarrhea medication
Constipation	A bulk luxative and increase fluid intake
Hair loss	
Cold intolerance	Dress warmly
Edema	
Dry skin	Moisturizers
Significant reactions	
Gallstones	Prophylactic use of ursodeoxycholic acid
Hyperuricemia and gout	Unrestricted carbohydrate intake
Cardiac complications	Baseline echocardiogram; monitor serum electrolyte levels
Fluid and electrolytes imbalance	Monitor serum electrolyte levels

Adverse Effects of VLCD Therapy (Table 29.5)

The VLCDs are diets that provide fewer than 800 kcal/day, but greater than 400 kcal/day with complete protein, electrolytes, vitamin and mineral supplements. These diets have been shown to produce more weight loss in the first 3 months than general low calorie diets and exercise programs. VCLDs are more likely to cause adverse side effects than diet that provide more than 800 kcal/day due to metabolic consequences of semistarvation (8,145). They are, however, generally safe when administered to carefully selected patients under proper medical supervision. In patients with severe cardiac, renal or liver dysfunction, VLCDs should be avoided (146).

Minor Short-term Adverse Effects

The majority of patients using VLCDs experience some adverse health effects, but these are usually mild and well tolerated. The common complications are hunger, weakness, fatigue, dizziness, dry skin, hair loss, cold intolerance, nausea, diarrhea or constipation (146,147). These are usually transient, tend to improve with the time on diet, and rarely require modification of the program. When needed, symptomatic treatment is frequently adequate; constipation can be treated with a bulk laxative and increased fluid intake while diarrhea is easily con-trolled with over-the-counter antidiarrhea medication.

Significant Short-term Adverse Effects

Gallstone formation.   Obesity itself is an important risk factor for gallstone formation in both men and women. In the Nurses' Health Study (148), women with a BMI $> 45 \, kg/m^2$ had a seven-fold increased risk compared with those with a BMI $< 24 \, kg/m^2$. The incidence of gallstones was $> 1\%$ per year in women whose BMI $> 30 \, kg/m^2$, and up to 2% per year in women with a BMI equal to or greater than $45 \, kg/m^2$. The high incidence of gallstone formation in obese individuals is due to an elevation of biliary cholesterol excretion, the presence of nucleating factors, and gallbladder hypomotility (125).

Prior to the prophylactic use of ursodeoxycholic acid, there was evidence of an increased risk of gallstones with a hypocaloric diet (126). One large prospective study of 648 obese subjects without gallbladder disease demonstrated an 11% incidence of gallstones after 16 weeks of VLCDs (149). Similarly, Liddle *et al.* (14) reported that 25% of their patients developed gallstones detected on abdominal ultrasonography following 8 weeks of VLCDs (26 kg weight loss) and another 6% developed biliary sludge, while the control group remained free of disease. Importantly, 6% of these patients developed symptoms severe enough to require a cholecys-tectomy. In one study, patients who developed gall-stones were significantly heavier (BMI 43 kg/m^2), stayed in an active weight loss program longer and lost more weight, compared to those who did not develop disease (150). A meta-analysis by Weinsier *et al.* (151) indicated a linear relationship between rates of weight loss and incidence of gallstone for-mation. Among patients who lost more than 1.5 kg per week, the incidence of gallstone formation was at least 0.5% per week, and when weight loss was greater than 3 kg per week, the rate went up to 3% per week. Interestingly, gallstone formation related to VLCDs may occur during active treatment or after solid foods have been reintroduced and some may disappear without any treatment (14).

The composition of biliary sludge and gallstones associated with dieting and rapid weight loss is primarily of cholesterol (152). The combination of caloric restriction and low fat intake increases cho-lesterol saturation in the bile as well as decreasing gallbladder contractility. This may be in part ex-plained by inadequate diet stimulated cholecys-tokinin (125,126).

A controlled trial of 22 obese patients defined the importance of fat intake in maintaining adequate gallbladder emptying (153). Eleven patients assig-ned to VLCDs high in fat content (12.2 g of fat/day) did not have gallstone on ultrasonogram at 6-month follow-up, in contrst to 6 of 11 (54.5%) in a group receiving low fat VLCDs (3 g of fat/day) des-pite the same amount of weight loss. Gallbladder emptying was also greater with the high fat meals (154). In addition, ursodeoxycholic acid (UDCA) has been used successfully to reduce the risk of gallstone formation during VLCDs (125). It works by reducing the bile saturation of cholesterol and inhibiting prostaglandin-mediated gallbladder se-cretion of glycoprotein, a promoter of gallstone nucleation.

Hyperuricemia and gout.

Plasma uric acid levels may increase transiently at the onset of VLCDs, but the levels rarely exceed 590 μmol/L (10 mg/dL) (146) nor is treatment required. This elevation is caused in part by cell breakdown and in part by ketone competition for tubular reabsorption of urate at the kidney tubule (8). Although patients with a history of gout may develop an acute gouty attack while on VLCDs, the development of symptoms is uncom-mon in patients without prior disease (146,147,153). When the symptoms occur, unrestricted carbohy-drate intake will often normalize the levels.

Cardiac complications.

Cardiac dysrhythmias and sudden death were reported with the earlier use of VLCDs in the 1970s (154,155). This VLCD (called liquid protein diet) consisted of low quality protein from hydrolyzed gelatin and collagen was not routinely supplemented with vitamins and min-erals. In some of these patients, dysrhythmias were refractory to antiarrhythmic drugs and patients subsequently died. It is believed that myocardial protein depletion and electrolyte abnormalities may be responsible for the development of these dysrhythmias, although the actual causes have never been proven (146). More recent use of VLCDs containing protein of high biological quality with appropriate electrolyte supplementation for 16 weeks or less have not been found to increase the risk of cardiac conduction disturbance (155–157). Moreover, the mortality rate has been reported to be lower in patients receiving VLCDs with high quality protein than in similarly obese persons not dieting. Nonetheless, every patient who considers VLCDs should have a baseline echocardiogram done. Any patients with unstable angina, recent myocardial infarction, malignant arrhythmia, or prolonged QTc syndrome should not be placed on VLCDs, and asymptomatic patients with QTc in-terval prolongation, i.e. greater than 0.44 ms, should be evaluated by a cardiologist before starting a diet (146). It is recommended that all patients on VLCDs are examined by a physician and have their serum electrolyte levels checked on a regular basis during both the active weight loss and refeeding states (155).

Fluid and electrolyte abnormalities.

Weight loss results in substantial loss of water and electrolytes including sodium, potassium, magnesium, calcium, and phosphorus in the urine (8). These minerals must be replaced accordingly to maintain normal serum and tissue levels. Without proper replace-ment, deficiency states can occur leading to abnor-mal cardiac, respiratory, neuromuscular, and other organ functions.

Adverse Effects of Weight Loss Medications

Medications for the treatment of obesity may include drugs that reduce energy intake, drugs that increase energy expenditure, and drugs that block nutrient absorption from the gastrointestinal tract (158). Although all of these medications can help obese patients lose weight, they also have some limitations. Fenfluramine and desfenfluramine have been reported to be associated with pulmonary hypertension (159) and valvular heart disease (160), leading to the withdrawal of these drugs in 1997. The adverse side effects of the newer drugs are usually mild and self-limiting, and in carefully selected patients, pharmacotherapy should not be excluded.

Drugs that Reduce Food Intake (Anorectic Drugs)

By decreasing appetite, drugs in this group can reduce food intake, which leads to weight reduction.

Noradrenergic drugs.   Noradrenergic drugs release norepinephrine (noradrenaline) or blocks its reuptake into neurons of the hypothelamus. Amphetamine, methamphetamine, and phenmetrazine are no longer recommended for treatment of obesity due to their strong central nervous system stimulation and high potential for abuse (161,162). Newer drugs such as diethlpropion, phentermine, phenylpropanolamine, and mazindol are less stimulant and less addictive, but retain anorectic properties. Some patients, however, may experience adverse side effects related to central nervous system stimulation including insomnia, irritability, agitation, nervousness, and anxiety, which may require discontinuation of the drugs. Other side effects are abdominal pain, nausea, diarrhea, and constipation. Severe hypertension, severe headache, atrioventricular blocks, and bowel infarction has been reported with phenylpropanolamine, but they rarely occur (163). Recently, pulmonary hypertension and valcular heart disease have been described especially, with combined use of phentermine and fenfluramine.

Serotoninergic drugs.   Fenfluramine and dexfenfluramine work at the neurons by stimulating serotonin release and at the receptors as serotonin agonists. In addition, dexfenfluramine can inhibit reuptake of serotonin into the neuron (158). Both medications were withdrawn from the world market in September 1997 after several reports of pulmonary hypertension (159) and cardiac valvular heart abnormalities causing significant insufficiency of the valve (160). The incidence of pulmonary hypertension is low with short-term use of anorexiants, but increases significantly with use of more than 3 months. The Center for Disease Control and Prevention recommends that all people who have taken fenfluramine or dexfenfluramine have a complete physical examination to determine any possible heart or lung disease (164). If cardiac abnormalities are suspected, an echocardiogram should be performed to identify possible valvular heart disease. This is especially important in patients before undergoing medical or dental procedures for which the American Heart Association recommend prophylactic antibiotic therapy to prevent bacterial endocarditis.

Drugs that affect both norepinephrine and serotonin.
Sibutramine blocks the reuptake of both serotonin and norepinephrine, but has no effect on their release. Although there is no association between sibutramine and valvular heart disease, this drug may cause an increase in blood pressure and heart rate in some individuals (48,165). It should not be used in patients with hypertension, coronary artery disease, and those who take certain medications such as monoamine-oxidase inhibitors, tricyclic antidepressants, and decongestants (162). In addition, patients on sibutramine should have blood pressure checked regularly. Other minor side effects include insomnia, dry mouth, headache, irritability, anorexia, and constipation (165).

Drugs that Increase Energy Expenditure

Ephedrine stimulates norepinephrine secretion, which in turn increase thermogenesis. In high doses, it can increase heart rate, blood pressure, plasma glucose levels, and cause tremor (158). Currently, none of the drugs in this group is approved by the Food and Drug Administration (FDA) for weight reduction.

Drugs that Reduce Absorption of Nutrients from the Gastrointestinal Tract

Tetrahydrolipstatin (orlistat), a selective gastric and pancreatic lipase inhibitor, blocks systemic absorption of dietary fat. Its main adverse effects are gastrointestinal, such as soft or liquid stool, oily spotting, fatty and oily stool, flatus with discharge, fecal urgency, increased defecation, and fecal incontinence (60). The incidence of these side effects appear to be dose-related, and gastrointestinal tolerability is also inversely related to the amount of dietary fat intake. In addition, orlistat can reduce the absorption of some fat-soluble vitamins and β-carotene. Patients taking orlistat should be instructed to consume less than 30% of dietary fat and take a multivitamin supplement.

Complications of Gastric Restrictive Surgery (Table 29.6)

The original operation introduced in the mid 1950s was jejuno-ileal bypass, which was designed to create a controlled malabsorption. This operation is not currently used due to significant late sequelae including liver failure, protein malnutrition, vitamin and mineral deficiency, urinary calculi, and arthritis. Liver disease was reported in about 29% of patients and frank cirrhosis in up to 7%, leading to a 12% mortality rate at 15 years (120,160,161). In addition, 25% of patients developed severe diarrhea, dehydration, abdominal pain, and vomiting which required hospitalization within the first 2 years. Most of these problems were caused by either nutrient malabsorption or bacterial overgrowth in the bypass intestinal segment (166,167).

The current gastric restrictive procedures, gastroplasty, gastric bypass, and gastric banding, are associated with low postoperative complication rates. Mortality has been reported to be less than 1% (166). Perioperative complications include anastomotic leaks, peritonitis, wound infection, thromboembolic disease, pulmonary and cardiac events, or even death. Older and heavier patients are at higher risk for severe complications (50).

Late complications can also occur, particularly when patients are not compliant with vitamin and mineral supplements or do not consume a healthy diet. Once complications occur, they are often easy to manage. These complications include macronut-

Table 29.6 Complications of gastric restrictive surgery

Early complications
Wound infection
Anastomotic leaks
Peritonitis
Subphrenic abscess
Deep venous thrombosis
Pulmonary embolism

Late complications
Macronutrients deficiency
Micronutrient deficiency—Iron, folate, vitamin B_{12}
Persistent vomiting and maladaptive eating behavior
Dumping syndrome
Gallstones

rient and micronutrient deficiencies, dehydration, persistent nausea, dumping syndrome, and gallstones. As in VLCD treatment, surgical weight reduction also increases risks for nutrient deficiencies, especially with gastric bypass procedure due to gastroduodenal discontinuity. Low blood levels of iron and vitamin B_{12} occur in up to 70% of patients, while low levels of folate occur in 30–45%. About 12–25% of patients develop actual clinical deficiency states (50), such as iron deficiency anemia, megaloblastic anemia, peripheral neuropathy, and encephalopathy. Although hematological syndrome is not uncommon, neurological syndrome is rare and tends to occur in patients with protracted vomiting and maladaptive eating behavior. With routine use of oral vitamin and mineral supplements, these micronutrient deficiencies and caloric malnutrition are seen less commonly. However, lifelong period assessment of complete blood count, iron, folate, vitamin B_{12}, calcium, and phosphorus levels is necessary (15).

Persistent vomiting and maladaptive eating behavior may occur in as many as 20–30% of patients (15). This is a complex problem usually related to inappropriate eating behavior and psychological instability, but structural failure from surgery may also be responsible. These patients should be managed by the multidisciplinary team assisting in eating behavior, lifestyle changes, and stress management.

Fluoroscopic or endoscopic examination of the surgical area is essential in patients with persistent vomiting or other digestive symptoms after gastric restrictive surgery. Occasionally, revision surgery may be required to treat structural abnormalities occurring during the late postoperative period (50).

The incidence of gallstone formation also increases with rapid weight loss after gastric restrictive surgery. Shiffman *et al.* (168) found that 36% of their patients developed gallstones and another 13% developed gallbladder sludge 6 to 18 months after gastric bypass surgery (168). Of those who developed gallstones 40% became symptomatic, and 28% underwent elective cholecystectomy. As with gallstone associated with VLCDs, gallstones occurring after surgical weight reduction are composed primarily of cholesterol (152) and prophylactic use of UDCA (600 mg/day) has also been shown to be effective (169).

Weight Loss and Mortality

Several epidemiologic studies of weight loss and mortality have been published (1,7,170,171). Most, but not all, of these studies have suggested that weight loss is associated with increased mortality risk. For example, data from the NHANES I Epidemiologic Follow-up Study (170), a longitudinal study of 2140 men and 2550 women aged 45–74 years who participated in the NHANES I (1971–1975), show an increased risk of death with increasing weight loss among men and women whose baseline BMI was 26 to 29 kg/m^2. Subjects who lost 15% or more of their maximum weight had more than twice the mortality risk of those who lost less than 5%, after adjustment for age, race, smoking, parity, preexisting illness, and maximum BMI. At a BMI of 29 or higher, mortality risk increased with the degree of weight loss in women, but weight loss of 5–15% appeared to decrease the risk in men (170).

These observational studies, however, have several methodological problems and some limitations. Hardly any studies have examined the cause of weight loss or differentiated between intentional and unintentional weight loss, and it is possible that weight loss, especially unintentional weight loss, is an indicator for subclinical disease.

Two studies of factors related to weight loss intention have been conducted in the general population (172,173). The results suggested that both intentional and unintentional weight losses occur at similar frequency in the US population. Older populations, however, have a higher incidence of unintentional weight loss and lower incidence of intentional weight loss, and unintentional weight loss often occurs in patients who have poor health status, who use medications for chronic diseases, and who smoke.

To date, very few studies have examined the association between intentional weight loss and mortality. In the Iowa Women's Health Study (174), a prospective cohort study of health risk factors in postmenopausal women showed that one or more intentional weight loss episodes of 9.1 or more kilograms (20 lb) during adulthood was not associated with higher total or cardiovascular disease mortality risk, compared with never losing more than 9.1 kg. On the other hand, one or more unintentional weight loss episodes of at least 9.1 kg was associated with a 26–57% higher total mortality risk and a 51–114% higher cardiovascular mortality risk, compared with never losing more than 9.1 kg. The increased mortality risk with unintentional weight loss were seen mostly in women with prevalent disease, hypertension, or diabetes (174).

In premenopausal women, Williamson *et al.* (175) have reported a 12-year prospective observation study of intentional weight loss and mortality in 43 457 overweight, non-smoking, white women aged 40 to 64 years. In women with obesity-related comorbid conditions, intentional weight loss of any amount was associated with a 20% reduction in all cause mortality, compared to women who had stable weight (175); this is primarily due to a 40–50% reduction in mortality from obesity-related cancer and 30–40% reduction in mortality from diabetes. In women without comorbidities, intentional weight loss was generally not related to mortality. However, a loss of at least 9 kg (20 lb) in the previous year was associated with small to moderate increases in mortality. This suggested that the association between weight loss and mortality may be influenced by health status. One study of diet and exercise in diabetic patients (176) showed that a modest weight loss decreased the 5-year mortality in diabetic patients to lower than the mean for the general population (3.2% vs. 3.7%). In contrast, diabetic patients who did not lose weight had a mortality of 11.9% (176).

GUIDELINES ON THE EVALUATION AND TREATMENT OF OBESITY (1,177)

Treatment of overweight and obesity consists of two processes: assessment and management (1). Assessment requires the determination of the degree of obesity and absolute risk status. Management involves not only weight loss and weight maintenance at a lower weight, but also the measures to control other risk factors. Persons at increased risk for obesity-related morbidity and mortality include those with BMI $> 30 \text{kg/m}^2$, those with upper body fat distribution (waist circumference > 40 inches (102 cm) in men, > 35 inches (89 cm) in women), and those who have obesity-related diseases or psychological disorders.

Depending on the severity of obesity and associated risk factors, management of obesity can be done at four different levels of care, from self-help, a certified commercial weight loss clinic, a primary care physician to a nutrition medicine clinic. Patients at high risk should be managed more aggressively by obesity specialists.

Step one: self-help. All overweight or obese individuals should incorporate healthy lifestyle changes including a reduction of caloric intake by 500–1000 kcal/day and an increase in physical activity. The minimal goal in this step is to stop weight gain and to achieve weight loss of 5–10% in 3 to 6 months.

Step two: a commercial weight loss clinic. Patients are screened by their primary physicians and referred to a certified commercial weight loss clinic to assist in achieving weight loss goals.

Step three: primary physician care. Patients are monitored and supervised by their primary physicians; intervention can be carried out by a commercial weight loss clinic or by patients themselves.

Step four: a nutrition medicine clinic. Patients are referred to an obesity treatment clinic for aggressive intervention which includes use of VLCDs, medication, or surgery. The goal of treatment is a 30–50% reduction of excess body fat and improvement of overall metabolic fitness.

In general, low calorie diet, exercise, and behavior therapy are safe and effective. Patients should be instructed to modify their diets to a lower calorie intake. Individually planned diets should help to create a deficit of 500–1000 kcal/day and aim to achieve weight loss of 1–2 lb (0.45–91 kg) per week. Alternatively, an energy controlled, nutrient dense meal replacement can be used, as it is viable, practical, safe and also effective (178). Medical treatment

of obesity, when conducted by a physician specializing in obesity treatment, is associated with mild and tolerable side effects.

CONCLUSIONS

Overall, there is ample evidence that weight loss improves obesity-related comorbid conditions, including hypertension, hyperlipidemia, type 2 diabetes, cardiovascular disease, sleep apnea, and osteoarthritis. Although the data on the relationship of weight loss and cardiovascular or overall mortality are limited, available evidence also suggests a beneficial effect of intentional weight loss. Safe and effective diet, exercise and lifestyle modifications are available to most patients. Adverse effects of weight loss are not uncommon with medical treatment of obesity such as VLCDs, medications, or gastric bypass surgery. However, they can usually be prevented or effectively treated and do not contraindicate weight loss.

REFERENCES

1. National Institutes of Health, National Heart, Lung, and Blood Institute. *Clinical Guideline on the Identification, Evaluation, and Treatment of Overweight and Obesity in Adults: The Evidence Report*, Bethesda, MD: National Institutes of Health, 1998.
2. Pi-Sunyer FX. Medical hazards of obesity. *Ann Intern Med* 1993; **119**: 655–660.
3. Bray GA. Health hazards associated with overweight. In: Bray GA (ed.) *Contemporary Diagnosis and Management of Obesity*. Newtown, PA: Handbooks in Health Care, 1998: 68–103.
4. Lean ME, Han TS, Seidell JC. Impairment of health and quality of life using new US federal guidelines for the identification of obesity. *Arch Intern Med* 1999; **159**: 837–843.
5. Sjöström LV. Morbidity of severely obese patients. *Am J Clin Nutr* 1992; **55**: 508S–515S.
6. Stunkard AJ. Current views on obesity. *Am J Med* 1996; **100**: 230–236.
7. Committee to Develop Criteria for Evaluating the Outcomes of Approaches to Prevent and Treat Obesity. Food and Nutrition Board. The nature and problem of obesity. In: Thomas PR (ed.) *Weighing the Options: Criteria for Evaluating Weight-Management Programs*. Washington DC: National Academy Press, 1995: 37–63.
8. Pi-Sunyer FX. Short-term medical benefits and adverse effects of weight loss. *Ann Intern Med* 1993; **119**: 722–726.
9. Higgins M, D'Agostino R, Kannel W, Cobb J. Benefits and adverse effects of weight loss. Observations from the Framingham study. *Ann Intern Med* 1993; **119**: 758–763.

10. Blackburn G. Effect of degree of weight loss on health benefits. *Obes Res* 1995; **3**: 211S–216S.

11. Blackburn G. How much weight loss? In: Angel A, Anderson H, Bouchard C, Lau D, Leiter L, Mendelson R (eds) *Progress in Obesity Research*. 7th International Congress on Obesity. London: John Libbey, 1996: 621–625.

12. Goldstein DJ. Beneficial health effects of modest weight loss. *Int J Obes* 1992; **16**: 397–415.

13. Kanders BS, Peterson FJ, Lavin PT, Norton DE, Istfan NW, Blackburn GL. Long-term health effects associated with significant weight loss: a study of the dose–response effect. In: Blackburn GL, Kanders BS (eds) *Obesity: Pathophysiology, Psychology and Treatment*. New York: Chapman & Hall, 1994: 167–181.

14. Liddle RA, Goldstein RB, Saxton J. Gallstone formation during weight-reduction dieting. *Arch Intern Med* 1989; **149**: 1750–1753.

15. Blackburn G, Ishikawa M. Intensive diet and surgical management of obesity. *Curr Opin Endocrinol Diabetes* 1996; **3**: 66–73.

16. Ernst ND, Obarzanek E, Clark MB, Briefel RR, Brown CD, Donato K. Cardiovascular health risks related to overweight. *J Am Diet Assoc* 1997; **97**(7 Suppl): 547–551.

17. Dyer AR, Elliott P. The INTERSALT study: relations of body mass index to blood pressure. INTERSALT Co-operative Research Group. *J Hum Hypertens* 1989; **3**: 299–308.

18. Havlik RJ, Hubert HB, Fabsitz RR, Feinleib M. Weight and hypertension. *Ann Intern Med* 1983; **98**: 855–859.

19. Huang Z, Willett WC, Manson JE *et al.* Body weight, weight change, and risk for hypertension in women. *Ann Intern Med* 1998; **128**: 81–88.

20. Kannel WB, Brand N, Skinner JJ Jr, Dawbwe TR, McNamara PM. The relation of adiposity to blood pressure and development of hypertension. The Framingham study. *Ann Intern Med* 1967; **67**: 48–59.

21. Sonne-Holm S, Sorensen T, Jensen G, Schnohr P. Independent effects of weight change and attained body weight on prevalence of arterial hypertension in obese and non-obese men. *BMJ* 1989; **299**: 767–770.

22. Corrigan SA, Raczynski JM, Swencionis C, Jennings SG. Weight reduction in the prevention and treatment of hypertension: a review of representative clinical trials. *Am J Health Promot* 1991; **5**: 208–214.

23. Reisin E. Nonpharmacologic approaches to hypertension: Weight, sodium, alcohol, exercise, and tobacco considerations. *Med Clin North Am* 1997; **81**: 1289–1303.

24. Leiter LA, Abbott D, Campbell NR, Mendelson R, Ogilvie RI, Chockalingam A. Lifestyle modifications to prevent and control hypertension. 2. Recommendations on obesity and weight loss. Canadian Hypertension Society, Canadian Coalition for High Blood Pressure Prevention and Control, Laboratory Center for Disease Control at Health Canada, Heart and Stroke Foundation of Canada. *Can Med Assoc J* 1999; **160**: 7S–12S.

25. Kolanowski J. Obesity and hypertension: from pathophysiology to treatment. *Int J Obes Relat Metab Disord* 1999; **23**: 42S–46S.

26. Hall JE. Renal and cardiovascular mechanisms of obesity. *Hypertension* 1994; **23**: 381–394.

27. Reisin E. Weight reduction in the management of hypertension: epidemiologic and mechanistic evidence. *Can J Physiol Pharmacol* 1986; **64**: 818–824.

28. Tuck ML, Sowers J, Dornfeld L, Kledzik G, Maxwell M. The effect of weight reduction on blood pressure, plasma renin activity, and plasma aldosterone levels in obese patients. *N Engl J Med* 1981; **16**: 930–933.

29. Reisin E, Frohlich ED, Messerli FH, *et al.* Cardiovascular changes after weight reduction in obesity hypertension. *Ann Intern Med* 1983; **98**: 315–319.

30. Wassertheil-Smoller S, Blaufox D, Oberman A, Langford H, Davis B, Wylie-Rosett J. The Trial of Antihypertensive Interventios and Management (TAIM) Study: Adequate weight loss, alone and combined with drug therapy in the treatment of mild hypertension. *Arch Intern Med* 1992; **152**: 131–136.

31. Davis B, Blaufox D, Oberman A, *et al.* Reduction in long-term antihypertensive medication requirements: Effect of weight reduction by dietary intervention in overweight persons with mild hypertension. *Arch Intern Med* 1993; **153**: 1773–1782.

32. MacMahon S, Cutler J, Brittain E, Higgins M. Obesity and hypertension: epidemiological and clinical issues. *Eur Heart J* 1987; **8**(Suppl B): 57S–70S.

33. Langford HG, Blaufox MD, Oberman A, *et al.* Dietary therapy slows the return of hypertension after stopping prolonged medication. *JAMA* 1985; **253**: 657–664.

34. Stamler R, Stamler J, Grimm R, *et al.* Nutritional therapy for high blood pressure: final report of the four-year randomized controlled trial: The Hypertension Control Program. *JAMA* 1987; **257**: 1484–1491.

35. Maxwell MH, Kushiro T, Dornfield LP, Tuck ML, Waks AU. Blood pressure changes in obese hypertensive subjects during rapid weight loss: comparison of restricted versus unchanged salt intake. *Arch Intern Med* 1984; **144**: 1581–1584.

36. Rissanen A, Pietinen P, Siljamaki-Ojansuu U, Piirainen H, Reissel P. Treatment of hypertension in obese patients: efficacy and feasibility of weight and salt reduction programs. *Acta Med Scand* 1985; **218**: 149–156.

37. Cutler JA. Randomized clinical trials of weight reduction in nonhypertensive persons. *Ann Epidemiol* 1991; **1**: 363–370.

38. Fortmann SP, Haskell WL, Wood PD. Effects of weight loss on clinic and ambulatory blood pressure in normotensive men. *Am J Cardiol* 1988; **62**: 89–93.

39. Hypertension Prevention Trial Research Group. The Hypertension Prevention Trial: three year effects of dietary changes in blood pressure. *Arch Intern Med* 1990; **150**: 153–162.

40. Stamler R, Stamler J, Gosch FC, *et al.* Primary prevention of hypertension by nutritional hygienic means. Final report of a randomized controlled trial. *JAMA* 1989; **262**: 1801–1807.

41. Rocchini AP, Katch V, Schork A, Kelch RP. Insulin and blood pressure during weight loss in obese adolescents. *Hypertension* 1987; **10**: 267–273.

42. The Trials of Hypertension Prevention Collaborative Research Group. The effects of nonpharmacologic interventions on blood pressure of persons with high normal levels. Results of the Trials of Hypertension Prevention, Phase I. *JAMA* 1992; **267**: 1213–1220.

43. The Trials of Hypertension Prevention Collaborative Research Group. Effects of weight loss and sodium reduction

intervention on blood pressure and hypertension incidence in overweight people with high-normal blood pressure: The Trials of Hypertension Prevention, Phase II. *Arch Intern Med* 1997; **157**: 657–667.

44. Steven VJ, Corrigan SA, Obarzzanek E, *et al.* Weight loss intervention in phase 1 of the Trials of Hypertension Prevention. The TOHP Collaborative Research Group. *Arch Intern Med* 1993; **153**: 849–858.

45. Holdaway IM, Wallace E, Westbrooke L, Gamble G. Effect of dexfenfluramine on body weight, blood pressure, insulin resistance and serum cholesterol in obese individuals. *Int J Obes Relat Metab Disord* 1995; **19**: 749–751.

46. Bremer JM, Scott RS, Lincott CJ. Dexfenfluramine reduces cardiovascular risk factors. *Int J Obes Relat Metab Disord* 1994; **18**: 199–205.

47. Mathus-vliegen EM, van de Voorde K, Kok AM, Res AM. Dexfenfluramine in the treatment of severe obesity: a placebo-controlled investigation of the effects on weight loss, cardiovascular risk factors, food intake and eating behavior. *J Intern Med* 1992; **232**: 119–127.

48. Bray G, Blackburn G, Ferguson J, *et al.* Sibutramine produces dose-related weight loss. *Obes Res* 1999; **7**: 189–198.

49. Consensus Development Conference Panel. Gastrointestinal surgery for severe obesity. *Ann Intern Med* 1991; **115**: 956–961.

50. Benotti P, Forse A. The role of gastric surgery in the multidisciplinary management of severe obesity. *Am J Surg* 1995; **169**: 361–367.

51. Foley EF, Benotti PN, Borlase B, Hollingshead J, Blackburn G. Impact of gastric restrictive surgery on hypertension in morbidly obese. *Am J Surg* 1992; **163**: 294–297.

52. Carson JL, Ruddy ME, Duff AE, Holmes NJ, Cody RP, Brolin RE. The effect of gastric bypass surgery on hypertension in morbidly obese patients. *Arch Intern Med* 1994; **154**: 193–200.

53. Despres JP. Dyslipidemia and obesity. *Baillière's Clin Endocrinol Metab* 1994; **8**: 629–659.

54. Despres JP. Abominal obesity as important component of insulin-resistance syndrome. *Nutrition* 1993; **9**: 452–459.

55. Howard BV. Insulin resistance and lipid metabolism. *Am J Cardiol* 1999; **84**: 28J–32J.

56. Dattilo AM, Kris-Etherton PM. Effect of weight reduction on blood lipids and lipoproteins: a meta-analysis. *Am J Clin Nutr* 1992; **56**: 320–328.

57. Waki M, Heshka S, Heymsfield SB. Long-term serum lipid lowering, behavior modification, and weight loss in obese women. *Nutrition* 1993; **9**: 23–28.

58. Mathus-Vliegen EM. Prolonged surveillance of dexfenfluramine in severe obesity. *Neth J Med* 1993; **43**: 246–253.

59. Swinburn BA, Carmichael HE, Wilson MR. Dexfenfluramine as an adjunct to a reduced fat, ad libitum diet: effects on body composition, nutrient intake and cardiovascular risk factors. *Int J Obes Relat Metab Disord* 1996; **20**: 1033–1040.

60. Product Information: Xenical, Orlistat. Roche Pharmaceuticals, Nutley, New Jersey, 1999.

61. Drent ML, Larsson I, William-Olsson T, *et al.* Orlistat (Ro 18-0647), a lipase inhibitor, in the treatment of human obesity: a multiple dose study. *Int J Obes Relat Metab Disord* 1995; **19**: 221–226.

62. Gleysteen J, Barboriak J, Sasse E. Sustained coronary-risk-factor reduction after gastric bypass for morbid obesity. *Am J Clin Nutr* 1990; **5**: 774–778.

63. Gleysteen J. Results of surgery: long term effects on hyperlipidemia. *Am J Clin Nutr* 1992; **55**: 591S–593S.

64. Brolin RE, Kenler HA, Wilson AC, Kuo PT, Cody RP. Serum lipids after gastric bypass surgery for morbid obesity. In *J Obes Relat Metab Disord* 1990; **14**: 939–950.

65. Wolf AM, Beisiegel U, Kortner B, Kuhlmann HW. Does gastric restriction surgery reduce the risks of metabolic diseases? *Obes Surg* 1998; **8**: 9–13.

66. Cowen GS Jr, Buffington CK. Significant changes in blood pressure, glucose, and lipids with gastric bypass surgery. *World J Surg* 1998; **22**: 987–992.

67. Colditz GA, Willett WC, Rotnitzky A, Manson JE. Weight gain as a risk factor for clinical diabetes mellitus in women. *Ann Intern Med* 1995; **122**: 481–486.

68. Chan J, Rimm E, Colditz G, Stampfer M, Willett W. Obesity, fat distribution, and weight gain as risk factors for clinical diabetes in men. *Diabetes Care* 1994; **17**: 961–969.

69. Shulman GI. Cellular mechanisms of insulin resistance in humans. *Am J Cardiol* 1999; **84**: 3J–10J.

70. Bray G. Health hazards associated with obesity. *UpToDate* (CD ROM), vol. 7.1. UpToDate Inc., 1999.

71. Flier J, Foster D. Eating disorders: obesity, anorexia nervosa, and bulimia nervosa. In: Wilson J, Foster D, Kronenberg H, Larsen P (eds) *Williams Textbook of Endocrinology.* Philadelphia, PA: WB Saunders, 1998: 1061–1097.

72. Unger R, Foster D. Diabetes mellitus. In: Wilson J, Foster D, Kronenberg H, Larsen P (eds) *Williams Textbook of Endocrinology.* Philadelphia, PA: WB Saunders, 1998: 973–1059.

73. Franssila-Kallunki A, Rissanen A, Ekstrand A, Ollus A, Groop L. Weight loss by very-low calorie diets: effects on substrate oxidation, energy expenditure, and insulin sensitivity in obese subjects. *Am J Clin Nutr* 1992; **56**: 247S–248S.

74. van Baak M, Borghouts L. Relationships between physical activity and insulin resistance. In: *ILSI North America Project Committee on Insulin Resistance. Program and abstracts. Contributing factors to insulin resistance.* Washington DC, 1998.

75. Henry RR, Scheaffer L, Olefsky JM. Glycemic effects of intensive caloric restriction and isocaloric feeding in non-insulin-dependent diabetes mellitus. *J Clin Endocrinol Metab* 1985; **61**: 917–925.

76. Wing RR, Blair EH, Bononi P, Marcus MD, Watanabe R, Bergman RN. Caloric restriction per se is a significant factor in improvements in glycemic control and insulin sensitivity during weight loss in obese NIDDM patients. *Diabetes Care* 1994; **17**: 30–36.

77. Agurs-Collins TD, Have TR, Kumanyika SK, Adams-Campbell LL. A randomized controlled trial of weight reduction and exercise for diabetes management in older African-American subjects. *Diabetes Care* 1997; **20**: 1503–1511.

78. Heller SR, Clarke P, Daly H, Davis I, McCulloch DK, Allison SP, Tattersall RB. Group education for obese patients with type 2 diabetes: greater success at less cost. *Diabet Med* 1998; **5**: 552–556.

79. Mancini M, Di Biase G, Contaldo F, Fischetti A, Grasso L, Mattiolli P. Medical complications of severe obesity: im-

portance of treatment by very-low calorie diets. Intermediate and long-term effects. *Int J Obes Relat Metab Disord* 1981; **5**: 341–352.

80. Watt NB, Spanheimer RG, DiGirolamo M, *et al.* Prediction of glucose response to weight loss in patients with non-insulin dependent diabetes mellitus. *Arch Intern Med* 1990; **150**: 803–806.

81. UKPDS Group. UK Prospective Diabetes Study 7: response of fasting plasma glucose to diet therapy in newly presenting type II diabetic patients. *Metabolism* 1990; **39**: 905–912.

82. Heilbronn L, Noakes M, Clifton P. Effects of energy restriction, weight loss and diet composition on plasma lipids and glucose in patients with type 2 diabetes. *Diabetes Care* 1999; **22**: 889–895.

83. American Diabetes Association. Nutrition recommendations and principles for people with diabetes mellitus. *Diabetes Care* 1998; **21**: 32S–35S.

84. Nilsson PM, Lindholm LH, Schersten BF. Lifestyle changes improve insulin resistance in hyperinsulinemic subjects: a one-year intervention study of hypertensives and normotensives in Delby. *J Hypertens* 1992; **10**: 1071–1078.

85. Simkin-Silverman L, Wing RR, Hansen DH, *et al.* Prevention of cardiovascular risk factor elevations in healthy premenopausal women. *Prev Med* 1995; **24**: 509–517.

86. Willey KA, Molneaux LM. Overland JE, Yue DK. The effects of dexfenfluramine on blood glucose control in patients with type 2 diabetes. *Diabet Med* 1992; **9**: 341–343.

87. Manning RM, Jung RT, Leese GP, Newton RW. The comparison of four weight reduction strategies aimed at overweight diabetic patients. *Diabet Med* 1995; **12**: 409–415.

88. Redmon JB, Raatz SK, Kwong CA, Swanson JE, Thomas W, Bantle JP. Pharmacologic induction of weight loss to treat type 2 diabetes. *Diabetes Care* 1999; **22**: 896–903.

89. Lean MEJ. Sibutramine—a review of clinical efficacy. *Int J Obes Relat Metab Disord* 1997; **21**: 30S–36S.

90. Pories WJ, Macdonald KG. Morgan EJ, *et al.* Surgical treatment of obesity and its effect on diabetes: 10-y follow-up. *Am J Clin Nutr* 1992; **55**: 582S–585S.

91. Pories WJ, Swanson MS, MacDonald KG, *et al.* Who would have thought it? An operation proves to be the most effective therapy for adult-onset diabetes mellitus. *Ann Surg* 1995; **3**: 339–352.

92. Consoli A. Metformin. In: DeFronzo RA (ed.) *Current Management of Diabetes Mellitus*. St Louis, MO: Mosby-Year Book, 1998: 102–104.

93. Blonde L, Guthrie RD Jr, Sandberg. Metformin: An effective and safe agent for initial monotherapy in patients with non-insulin-dependent diabetes mellitus. *Endocrinologist* 1996; **6**: 431–438.

94. United Kingdom Prospective Diabetes Study Group. United Kingdom Prospective Diabetes Study 24: A 6-year randomized, controlled trial comparing sulfonylurea, insulin, and metformin therapy in patients with newly diagnosed type 2 diabetes that could not be controlled with diet therapy. *Ann Intern Med* 1998; **128**: 165–175.

95. United Kingdom Prospective Diabetes Study Group. UKPDS 28: A randomized trial of efficacy of early addition of metformin in sulfonylurea-treated type 2 diabetes. *Diabetes Care* 1998; **21**: 87–92.

96. Aviles-Santa L, Sinding J, Raskin P. Effects of metformin in patients with poorly controlled insulin-treated type 2 diabetes mellitus. A randomized, double blind, placebo-controlled trial. *Ann Intern Med* 1999; **131**: 182–188.

97. Alessi MC, Peiretti F, Morange P, Henry M, Nelbone G, Juhan-Vague I. Production of plasminogen activator inhibitor 1 by human adipose tissue: possible link between visceral fat accumulation and vascular disease. *Diabetes* 1997; **46**: 860–887.

98. Eriksson P, Reynisdottir S, Lonnqvist F, Stemme V, Hamsten A, Arner P. Adipose tissue secretion of plasminogen activator inhibitor-1 in non-obese and obese individuals. *Diabetologia* 1998; **41**: 65–71.

99. Health implications of obesity. National Institutes of Health Consensus Development Conference Statement. *Ann Intern Med* 1985; **103**: 1073–1077.

100. Manson JE, Colditz GA, Stampfer MJ, *et al.* A prospective study of obesity and risk of coronary heart disease in women. *N Engl J Med* 1990; **322**: 882–889.

101. Willett WC, Manson JE, Stmpfer MJ, *et al.* Weight, weight change, and coronary heart disease in women. Risk within the 'normal' weight range. *JAMA* 1995; **273**: 461–465.

102. Manson JE, Willett WC, Stampfer MJ, *et al.* Body weight and mortality among women. *N Engl J Med* 1995; **333**: 677–685.

103. Shaper AG, Wannamethee SG, Walker M. Body weight: implications for the prevention of coronary heart disease, stroke, and diabetes mellitus in a cohort study of middle aged men. *BMJ* 1997; **314**: 1311–1317.

104. Benotti PN, Bistrian BR, Benotti JR, Blackburn G, Forse RA. Heart disease and hypertension in severe obesity: the benefits of weight reduction. *Am J Clin Nutr* 1992; **55**: 586S–590S.

105. Van Gaal LF, Wauters MA, De Leeuw IH. The beneficial effects of modest weight loss on cardiovascular risk factors. *Int J Obes Relat Metab Disord* 1997; **21**: S5–S9.

106. Ornish D, Brown SE, Scherwitz LW, *et al.* Can lifestyle changes reverse coronary heart disease? The Lifestyle Heart Trial. *Lancet* 1990; **336**: 129–133.

107. Mavri A, Stegnar M, Krebs M, Sentocnik JT, Geiger M, Binder BR. Impact of adipose tissue on plasma plasminogen activitor inhibitor-1 in dieting obese women. *Arterioscler Thromb Vasc Biol* 1999; **6**: 1582–1587.

108. Fisler JS. Cardiac effects of starvation and semistarvation diets: safety and mechanisms of action. *Am J Clin Nutr* 1992; **56**: 230S–234S.

109. Grunstein RR, Wilcox I. Sleep-disordered breathing and obesity. *Baillière's Clin Endocrinol Metab* 1994; **8**: 601–628.

110. Strollo PJ, Rogers RM. Obstructive sleep apnea. *N Engl J Med* 1996; **334**: 99–104.

111. Strohl KP, Redline S. Recognition of obstructive sleep apnea. *Am J Respir Crit Care Med* 1996; **154**: 279–289.

112. Young T, Palta M, Dempsey J, Skatrud J, Weber S, Badr S. The occurrence of sleep-disorder breathing among middle-aged adults. *N Engl J Med* 1993; **328**: 1230–1235.

113. Partinen M, Telakivi T. Epidemiology of obstructive sleep apnea syndrome. *Sleep* 1992; **15**: S1–S4.

114. Vgontzas AN, Tan TL, Bixler B, Martin LF, Shubert D, Kales A. Sleep apnea and sleep disruption in obese patients. *Arch Intern Med* 1994; **154**: 1705–1711.

115. van Boxem TJ, de Groot GH. Prevalence and severity of

sleep disordered breathing in a group of morbidity obese patients. *Neth J Med* 1999; **54**: 202–206.

116. Loube MI, Loube AA, Mitler MM. Weight loss for obstructive sleep apnea: the optimal therapy for obese patients. *J Am Diet Assoc* 1994; **94**: 1291–1295.

117. Davies RJ, Stradling JR. The relationship between neck circumference, radiographic pharyngeal anatomy, and the obstructive sleep apnoea syndrome. *Eur Respir J* 1990; **3**: 509–514.

118. Rubinstein I, Colapinto N, Rotstein E, Brown IG, Hoffstein N. Improvement in upper airway function after weight loss in patients with obstructive sleep apnea. *Am Rev Respir Dis* 1988; **138**: 1192–1195.

119. Shelton KE, Woodson H, Gay S, Suratt PM. Pharyngeal fat in obstructive sleep apnea. *Am Rev Respir Dis* 1993; **148**: 462–468.

120. Schwartz AR, Gold AR, Schubert N, *et al.* Effect of weight loss on upper airway collapsibility in obstructive sleep apnea. *Am Rev Respir Dis* 1991; **144**: 494–498.

121. Smith PL, Gold AR, Meyers DA, Naponik EF, Bleecker ER. Weight loss in mildly to moderately obese patients with obstructive sleep apnea. *Ann Intern Med* 1985; **103**: 850–855.

122. Suratt PM, McTier RF, Findley LJ, Pohl SL, Wilhoit SC. Effect of very-low-calorie diets with weight loss on obstructive sleep apnea. *Am J Clin Nutr* 1992; **56**: 182S–184S.

123. Sugerman HJ, Fairman RP, Sood RK, Engle K, Wolfe L, Kellum JM. Long-term effects of gastric surgery for treating respiratory insufficiency of obesity. *Am J Clin Nutr* 1992; **55**: 597S–601S.

124. Charuzi I, Lavie P, Peiser J, Peled R. Bariatric surgery in morbidly obese sleep-apnea patients: short- and long-term follow-up. *Am J Clin Nutr* 1992; **55**: 594S–596S.

125. Anderson T. Liver and gallbladder disease before and after very-low-calorie diets. *Am J Clin Nutr* 1992; **56**: 235S–239S.

126. Halsted CH, Newton J, Phinney SD. Obesity and its health risks. *Curr Opin Gastroenterol* 1996; **12**: 204–209.

127. Drenick EJ, Simmons F, Murphy JF. Effect on hepatic morphology of treatment of obesity by fasting, reducing diets and small bowel bypass. *N Engl J Med* 1970; **282**: 829–834.

128. Anderson T, Gluud C, Franzmann M-B, Christoffersen P. Hepatic effects of dietary weight loss in morbidly obese subjects. *J Hepatol* 1991; **12**: 224–229.

129. Silverman EM, Sapala JA, Appelman HD. Regression of hepatic steatohepatitis in morbidly obese persons after gastric bypass. *Am J Clin Pathol* 1995; **104**: 23–31.

130. Luyckx FH, Desaive C, Thiry A, *et al.* Liver abnormalities in severely obese subjects: effect of drastic weight loss after gastroplasty. *Int J Obes Relat Metab Disord* 1998; **22**: 222–226.

131. Felson DT. Weight and osteoarthritis. *J Rheumatol* 1995; **43**: 7–9.

132. Heliovaara M, Makela M, Impivaara O, Knekt P, Aromaa A, Sievers K. Association of overweight, trauma and workload with coxarthrosis. A health survey of 7,217 persons. *Acta Orthop Scand* 1993; **64**: 513–518.

133. Cicuttini FM, Baker JR, Spector TD. The association of obesity with osteoarthritis of the hand and knee in women: a twin study. *J Rheumatol* 1996; **23**: 1221–1226.

134. Felson DT, Zhang Y, Anthony JM, Naimark A, Anderson.

Weight loss reduces the risk for symptomatic knee osteoarthritis in women. The Framingham Study. *Ann Intern Med* 1992; **116**: 535–539.

135. Wiliam RA, Foulsham BM. Weight reduction in osteoarthritis using phentermine. *Practitioner* 1981; **225**: 231–232.

136. Toda Y, Toda T, Takemura S, Wada T, Morimoto T, Ogawa R. Change in body fat, but not body weight or metabolic correlates of obesity, is related to symptomatic relief of obese patients with knee osteoarthritis after a weight control program. *J Rheumatol* 1998; **25**: 2181–2186.

137. McGoey BV, Deitel M, Saplys RJF, Kliman ME. Effect of weight loss on musculoskeletal pain in morbidly obese. *J bone Joint Surg* 1990; **72B**: 322–323.

138. Felson DT. Weight and osteoarthritis. *Am J Clin Nutr* 1996; **63**: 430S–432S.

139. Soulez B, Dewailly D, Rosenfield RL. Polycystic ovary syndrome: a multidisciplinary challenge. *Endocrinologist* 1996; **6**: 19–29.

140. Franks S. Polycystic ovary syndrome. *N Engl J Med* 1995; **333**: 853–860.

141. Kiddy DS, Hamilton-Fairley D, Bush A, *et al.* Improvement in endocrine and ovarian function during dietary treatment of obese women with polycystic ovary syndrome. *Clin Endocrinol* 1992; **36**: 105–111.

142. Foster GD, Wadden TA. The psychology of obesity, weight loss, and weight regain: research and clinical findings. In: Blackburn GL, Kanders BS (eds) *Obesity: Pathophysiology, Pscyhology and Treatment*. New York: Chapman & Hall, 1994: 140–166.

143. Wadden TA, Steen SN, Wingate BJ, Foster GD. Psychosocial consequences of weight reduction: how much weight loss is enough? *Am J Clin Nutr* 1996; **63**: 461S–465S.

144. Fairburn CG, Wilson GT. Binge eating: definition and classification. In: Fairburn CG, Wilson GT (eds) *Binge Eating*. New York: Guilford Press, 1993: 3–13.

145. Blackburn GL. Comparison of medically supervised and unsupervised approaches to weight loss and control. *Ann Intern Med* 1993; **119**: 714–718.

146. National Task Force on the Prevention and Treatment of Obesity. Very-low calorie diets. *JAMA* 1993; **270**: 967–974.

147. Kanders BS, Blackburn GL. Very-low calorie diets for the treatment of obesity. In: Blackburn GL, Kanders BS (eds) *Obesity: Pathophysiology, Psychology and Treatment*. New York: Chapman & Hall, 1994: 197–216.

148. Stampfer MJ, Maclure KM, Colditz GA, Manson JE, Willett WC. Risk of symptomatic gallstones in women with severe obesity. *Am J Clin Nutr* 1992; **55**: 652–658.

149. Yang H, Peterson GM, Roth M-P, Schoenfield LJ, Marks JW. Risk factors for gallstones formation during rapid loss of weight. *Dig Dis Sci* 1992; **37**: 912–918.

150. Kanders BS, Blackburn GL, Lavin P, Norton D. Weight loss outcome and health benefits associated with the Optifast program in the treatment of obesity. *Int J Obes Relat Metab Disord* 1989; **13**: S131–134.

151. Weinsier RL, Wilson LJ, Lee J. Medically safe rate of weight loss for the treatment of obesity: a guideline based on risk of gallstone formation. *Am J Med* 1995; **98**: 115–117.

152. Ko CW, Sekijima JH, Lee SP. Biliary sludge. *Ann Intern Med* 1999; **130**: 301–311.

153. Festi D, Colecchia A, Orsini M, *et al.* Gallbladder motility and gallstone formation in obese patients following very

low calorie diets. Use it (fat) or lose it (well). *Int J Obes Relat Metab Disord* 1998; **22**: 592–600.

154. Anderson JW, Hamilton CC, Brinkman-Kaplan V. Benefits and risks of intensive very-low-calorie diet program for severe obesity. *Am J Gastroentol* 1992; **87**: 6–15.

155. Wadden TA, Van Itallie TB, Blackburn GL. Responsible and Irresponsible use of very-low-calorie diets in the treatment of obesity. *JAMA* 1990; **263**: 83–85.

156. Phinney SD, Bistrian BR, Kosinski E, *et al.* Normal cardiac rhythm during hypocaloric diets varying carbohydrate conttent. *Arch Intern Med* 1983; **143**: 2258–2261.

157. Amatruda JM, Biddle TL, Patton ML, Lockwood DH. Vigorous supplementation of hypocaloric diet prevents cardiac arrhythmias and mineral depletion. *Am J Med* 1983; **74**: 1016–1022.

158. Scheen AJ, Lefebvre PJ. Pharmacological treatment of obesity: present status. *Int J Obes Relat Metab Disord* 1999; **23**: S47–53.

159. Abenhaim L, Moride Y, Brenot F, *et al.* Appetite-suppressant drugs and the risk of primary pulmonary hypertension. *N Engl J Med* 1996; **335**: 609–616.

160. Connolly HM, Crary JL, McGoon MD, *et al.* Valvular heart disease associated with fenfluramine-phentermine. *N Engl J Med* 1997; **337**: 581–588.

161. National Task Force on the Prevention and Treatment of Obesity. Long-term pharmacotherapy in the management of obesity. *JAMA* 1996; **276**: 1907–1915.

162. Bray GA. Use and abuse of appetite-suppressant drugs in the treatment of obesity. *Ann Intern Med* 1993; **119**: 707–713.

163. Elks ML. Appetite suppressants as adjuncts in the treatment of obesity. *J Fam Pract* 1996; **42**: 287–292.

164. Massachusetts Medical Society. Committee on Nutrition. *Obesity Treatment Using Drug Therapy*. Massachusetts Medical Society, 1998: 1–8.

165. Product Information. Meridia ®, Sibutramine hydrochloride monohydrate. Knoll Pharmaceutical Company, Mount Olive, NJ, 1997.

166. Shikora SA, Benetti PN, Forse RA. Surgical treatment of obesity. In: Blackburn GL, Kander BS (eds) *Obesity: Pathophysiology, Psychology and Treatment*. New York: Chapman & Hall, 1994: 264–282.

167. Brolin RE. Surgery for morbid obesity: current perspective. *Curr Pract Surg* 1991; **3**: 48–56.

168. Shiffman ML, Sugerman HJ, Kellum JM, Brewer WH, Moore EW. Gallstone formation after rapid weight loss: a prospective study in patients undergoing gastric bypass surgery for treatment of morbid obesity. *Am J Gastroenterol* 1991; **86**: 1000–1005.

169. Sugerman HJ, Brewer WH, Shiffman ML, *et al.* A multicenter, placebo-controlled, randomized, double-blind, prospective trial of prophylactic ursodiol for the prevention of gallstone formation following gastric-bypass-induced rapid weight loss. *Am J Surg* 1995; **169**: 91–96.

170. Pamuk ER, Williamson DF, Madans J, Serdula MK, Kleinman JC, Byers T. Weight loss and mortality in a national cohort of adults, 1971–1987. *Am J Epidemiol* 1992; **136**: 686–697.

171. Pamuk ER, Williamson DF, Madans J, Serdula MK, Madans J, Byers. Weight loss and subsequent death in a cohort of US adults. *Ann Intern Med* 1993; **119**: 744–748.

172. French SA, Jeffery RW, Folsom AR, Williamson DF, Byers T. History of intentional and unintentional weight loss in a population-based sample of women aged 55 to 69 years. *Obes Res* 1995; **3**: 163–170.

173. Meltzer AA, Everhart JE, Unintentional weight loss in the United States. *Am J Epidemiol* 1995; **142**: 1039–1046.

174. French SA, Folsom AR, Jeffery RW, Williamson DF. prospective study of intentionality of weight loss and mortality in older women: the Iowa Women's Health Study. *Am J Epidemiol* 1999; **149**: 504–514.

175. Williamson DF, Pamuk E, Thun M, Flanders D, Byers T, Heath C. Prospective study of intentional weight loss and mortality in never-smoking overweight US white women aged 40–64 years. *Am J Epidemiol* 1995; **141**: 1128–1141.

176. eriksson KF, Lindgarde F. Prevention of type 2 (non-insulin-dependent) diabetes mellitus by diet and physical exercise: the 6 year Malmo feasibility study. *Diabetologia* 1991; **34**: 891–898.

177. Academy Advisory Group; National Academy of Sciences. *Institute of Medicine, AdHoc Advisory Group on Preventive Services, Preventive Services for a Well Population*. Washington DC: National Academy of Sciences, 1978.

178. Ditschuneit HH, Flechtner-Mors M, Johnson TD, Adler G. Metabolic and weight loss effects of a long term dietary intervention in obese patients. *Am J Clin Nutr* 1999; **69**: 198–204.

30

Treatment: Diet

Stephan Rössner

Huddinge University Hospital, Huddinge, Sweden

DIETARY ASSESSMENT

Although diets for obesity treatment may vary according to financial, personal, cultural, religious and social beliefs, it is essential before any such diet is prescribed that a background describing the patient's habitual eating habits is obtained. Dietary habits can be assessed by numerous techniques. In specialist clinics where dieticians are available sophisticated methods can be used and also evaluated. In a primary health care setting where specialists may not be available to interpret a diet, simpler techniques may have to be relied upon.

Specialists are well aware of the numerous pitfalls associated with the interpretation of dietary records. For many patients, the suggestion to keep a diet record in itself is provocative and may cause even violent reactions and questioning. For others, the records may actually serve as a helpful and constructive tool to identify eating habits, of which the subject was actually unaware until a record was kept. For others again, the diet record may be a frustrating and painstaking process leading to conscious or unconscious omission of important dietary items.

Several studies have demonstrated that many obese patients report considerably less than what is estimated from predicted equations for such obese persons in energy balance (1). This could be explained in several different ways. It is possible that these patients underreport at the time of the diary period and especially that they underreport food items which they are aware that they should avoid. However, as stated above, it is also possible that the recording period in itself will lead to a diet period during the recording process, in which case the dietary record actually reflects a true energy intake, but only for a period which is not representative of the general eating pattern of the patient.

There is general agreement that dietary assessments are worthwhile and should be compared to the energy intake from predictive equations to allow a realistic dietary prescription. As pointed out by Frost, it is not uncommon that the dietary advice will contain more energy than what is reported by the obese person, and surprisingly such a paradoxical recommendation may work well (2).

DIETING AS A CHANGE BEHAVIOUR

Dieting is part of a complex process of changing behaviour. Prochaska has described the various steps which a person takes in contemplating a possible change in behaviour before such change is actually implemented and hopefully also maintained during later phases (3). For such changes to take place, realistic goals must be available. Foster *et al.* have described that most patients joining an obesity clinic have goals which are clearly unrealistic and which may lead to frustration, early drop-out and relapse (4). For practical reasons, goals can be divided into an overall long-term goal (where a 10% maintained weight loss is realistic) and short-term goals (which are helpful to cope with everyday problems). These goals may be changed at short notice in relation to everyday life problems. The point is to make the obese patient in dietary

International Textbook of Obesity. Edited by Per Björntorp.

Table 30.1 Characteristics of macronutrients (modified after Blundell (5))

	Fat	Protein	Carbohydrate	Alcohol
Ability to bring eating to an end	Low	High	Intermediate	Stimulates appetite
Ability to suppress hunger	Low	High	High	Stimulates appetite
Contribution to daily energy intake	High	Low	High	Varies
Energy density	High	Low	Low	High
Storage capacity in body	High	None	Low	None
Metabolic pathway to transfer excess intake to another compartment	No	Yes	Yes	Yes
Autoregulation (ability to stimulate own oxidation on intake)	Poor	Good	Good	Poor
Calories per gram	9	4	4	7

treatment aware of the fact that the goals should target the eating behaviour and not other extrinsic factors (4). In emergency situations a realistic goal may even be to limit weight increase during, for example, a high-risk holiday season to a certain number of kilograms.

SATIATING PROPERTIES OF MACRONUTRIENTS

In contrast to popular belief an overall nutritional goal in dietary treatment of obesity is to increase the proportion of carbohydrates in the diet since carbohydrate rich foods have high satiating properties, especially when compared to fat. Numerous studies have demonstrated that fat not only is the most energy dense macronutrient but also has weak satiating properties (5). Table 30.1 summarizes the characteristics of macronutrients in their ability to regulate daily dietary food intake. A key issue in dietary treatment strategies for obesity has thus been not only to reduce the daily energy intake but also in particular to cut fat to 30% or less of total energy intake. Carbohydrates generally appear in starchy and fibre-rich natural products, which means that a diet rich in natural carbohydrates will have a low energy density and thus enhance satiety. If fat intake is reduced, the protein proportion of the daily food intake will increase. The role of the protein in a diet for weight control will be discussed below.

DIETARY RECOMMENDATION

In comparing dietary advice from different textbooks it becomes obvious that national and even regional variations exist to such an extent that diets developed in one region are not applicable elsewhere. In the Summerbell chapter on dietary treatment of obesity, a diet for an Englishman is described which would not be well understood in a Scandinavian setting, where items such as a 'Cornish pastie' are not even recognized (6). During the production of a Nordic textbook on obesity it became clear that the Finnish dietary recommendations containing several milk and cereal products were not recognized in Denmark (7). Thus, in this context it seems more practical to concentrate on the general principles of these diets than to list specific items which always tend to be nationally, culturally and socially specific.

An extremely simple but helpful general principle is the recommendation from the Stockholm County Council Nutritional Board: substitute fat with fibre. This is a message in only four words, which does not include calorie counting and has a positive message in that it suggests substitution and not reduction.

Basic dietary principles are shown in Tables 30.2 and 30.3.

EFFICACY OF DIETARY TREATMENT

In the Clinical Guidelines, published by the National Institutes of Health and National Heart, Lung and Blood Institute 1998, an extensive analysis of the efficacy of various treatments for obesity is given (8). In this report, 86 randomized clinical trial publications were evaluated. These diets included ordinary low calorie diets, very low calorie diets (VLCDs), vegetarian, American Heart Association Guidelines and the National Cholesterol Education Program Step 1 Diet, as well as other low fat regimens with varying combinations of macronutrients.

Table 30.2 Basic principles for weight-reducing diets

Reduce fat intake
- Eliminate fat when possible (no fat on bread, lean meat products, control of hidden fat sources such as desserts, pastries, confectionery, sausages, patés etc.)
- Substitute (use low fat products when possible)
- Introduce low fat cooking methods (instead of frying use grilling, broiling, fat spray use etc.)

Reduce certain carbohydrates
- Eliminate sugar, sweet and soft drinks, confectionery, puddings, ice-cream etc.
- Limit alcohol consumption
- Substitute sugar with artificial sweeteners when possible
- Increase the consumption of high fibre vegetables such as beans, lentils, wholemeal, bread, cabbage etc.

A problem in interpreting the outcome of these trials is related to the fact that many of these programmes also include physical activity and behaviour modification to some, often unspecified extent, which makes evaluation of the true impact of the diet in itself more difficult. The Guidelines conclude that low calorie diets can reduce total body weight by an average of 8% over 3–12 months, for which there is solid scientific evidence. In the four studies that included also a long-term weight loss and maintenance intervention lasting 3–4.5 years, an average weight loss of 4% was reported over the long term (9–12). In addition to weight loss achieved by such diets, there is also strong evidence for a decrease in abdominal fat. Interestingly, cardiovascular fitness does not seem to be improved by

weight loss unless physical activity is increased simultaneously (13).

VLCDs will produce greater initial weight losses than low calorie diets (LCDs), due to the more pronounced initial caloric restriction, but the long-term outcome after one year or more is not different from that of low calorie diets only (14).

The Clinical Guidelines conclude that although lower fat diets without target caloric reduction help promote weight loss by producing a reduced caloric intake, lower fat diets coupled with total caloric reduction produced greater weight loss than lower fat diets alone (15–17). Furthermore, the Clinical Guidelines conclude that lower fat diets produce their weight loss primarily by decreasing caloric intake.

The overall recommendations in the Clinical Guidelines are summarized as follows: LCDs are recommended for weight loss in overweight and obese persons. Reducing fat as part of an LCD is a practical way to reduce calories.

MEAL PATTERNS

Dietary treatment of obesity not only focuses on the total energy intake over the day but also addresses the distribution of energy into meals. It is a common clinical experience that obese individuals tend to skip meals in the hope that they will in doing so reduce their total energy intake over the day (18). Often this is fallacious reasoning, since an eating

Table 30.3 Characteristics of a balanced low calorie diet for long-term use (in part based on the NHBLI guidelines (8)

Nutrient	Recommended intake
Calorie[a]	Approximately 500 to 1000 kcal/day reduction from usual intake
Total fat[b]	30% or less of total calories
Saturated fatty acids	8–10% of total calories
Monounsaturated fatty acids	Up to 15% of total calories
Polyunsaturated fatty acids	Up to 10% of total calories
Cholesterol[c]	< 300 mg/day
Protein[d]	Approximately 15% of total calories
Carbohydrate[e]	55% or more of total calories
Fibre	20–30 g/day
Vitamins, minerals and trace elements[f]	From natural sources according to recommended national daily intake

[a]A reduction in energy of 500–1000 kcal/day will help achieve a weight loss of 1–2 lb/week (0.45–0.91 kg/week).
[b]Fat-modified foods may provide a helpful strategy for lowering total fat intake but will only be effective if they are also low in calories and if there is no compensation of calories (such as sugar) from other foods.
[c]Patients with high blood cholesterol levels may need to restrict cholesterol intake even further.
[d]Proteins should be derived from plant sources and lean sources of animal protein.
[e]Complex carbohydrates from different vegetables, fruits, and whole grains are also sources of vitamins, minerals and fibre. A diet high in all types of fibre may also aid in weight management by promoting satiety at lower levels of calorie and fat intake.
[f]During weight loss, attention should be given to maintaining an adequate intake of vitamins, minerals and trace elements.

behaviour of this kind often results in overeating in the later part of the day when resistance to good intentions is weakened by increasing hunger sensations. Thus there is general agreement that obese persons should consume three main meals per day with two balanced snacks in between. By eating at regular intervals these patients should always be satiated, without hunger sensations which make them lose control and overeat. The Swedish Dietary Guidelines recommend 20–25% of the daily intake at breakfast, 30–35% at lunch and 30–35% at dinner, with the remaining allowance spread between two snacks of similar size (19).

In an obesity unit many patients report a marked shift of the total energy intake towards the later part of the day, the so-called night-eating syndrome (20,21). The identification of such specific eating behaviours clearly has implications for the design of an effective dietary programme.

BEHAVIOURAL TECHNIQUES

Most dietary treatment programmes use behavioural techniques as part of the overall 'package'. Behavioural therapy of obesity does not address underlying causes of overeating but works under the assumption that eating patterns are learned behaviours which can be modified and that the environment, including daily exposure to foods, must be changed to achieve long-term success. Some techniques directly associated with the eating situation and the diet itself are summarized in Table 30.4.

PRACTICAL APPLICATION

The basic principles for dietary treatment of obesity are thus extremely simple: when energy expenditure exceeds energy intake, weight loss follows. This weight loss will continue until a new equilibrium has been obtained. Dietary treatment remains a simple, easily available, cheap and safe way to treat overweight and obesity. In spite of this, the results are surprisingly unimpressive.

The easiest way to construct a diet that functions for a long time is to reduce the most energy dense component of the diet, which is fat, and to increase the portion size by using food components rich in

Table 30.4 Behavioural techniques to improve effects of dietary treatment for obesity. Examples of advice

- Plan cooking so that there are no leftovers
- Serve meals on small size plates
- Never eat out of kitchen utensils
- Always eat at the same place
- Concentrate on food, avoid external distractions
- Chew each bite at least 20 times
- Put down knife and fork between each bite
- Let each meal last at least 20 minutes
- Remove leftovers out of sight immediately after meal
- Cover food with invisible plastic cover or aluminium foil to avoid eating cues
- Never shop on empty stomach
- Always make a shopping list
- Shop with others, to control spontaneous purchases of unintended items

dietary fibre to enhance satiety. In most weight-reducing diets, the protein percentage of the diet will be slightly increased, since this part of the diet is not altered. With a reduction of total energy intake, protein will form a larger percentage of the total daily energy intake. Since protein in itself has a higher satiating effect than fat, this also has the beneficial effect of controlling food intake during a meal (22).

The qualities of an acceptable long-term dietary weight-reducing programme can in principle be summarized (23):

- Energy intake is lower than energy expenditure.
- The dietary composition is adequate with regard to essential components such as proteins, vitamins, minerals and essential fatty acids.
- The diet has a satiating effect.
- The diet is socially acceptable, for everyday use and can be adapted into a long-term lifestyle without major complications.
- The diet satisfies taste and habits of the individual.

Murphree recently described the practical aspects of running a weight loss clinic and indicated that theoretically adequate recommendations from the therapist will not result in sustained weight loss unless very practical problems are addressed, such as arrangements for child care during sessions (24). Patients are unwilling to give up their old eating habits and so a change in diet should be directed towards a modification of the currently used recipes of these patients. Murphree also underscores that the dietary modification should address food taste and texture, not only energy content, to be acceptable for long-term use.

OTHER DIETARY TREATMENT PROGRAMMES

Starvation

Dietary treatment of obesity can vary between total starvation to diets which are only slightly hypocaloric. The most extreme form of diet is total starvation which means that no energy is given, whereas losses of water, electrolytes, vitamins and trace elements are compensated. Starvation obviously results in fast initial weight loss but requires medical supervision. Lethal complications have been described, probably because of cardiac arrhythmias (25). Starvation has the disadvantage of leading to considerable loss of lean body mass. Since most of the combustion takes place in such tissues, an increased breakdown of muscle in particular will result in a disproportionate reduction of the basic metabolic rate.

Most studies demonstrate that the long-term results of starvation programmes are not satisfactory. Rebound generally occurs and sustained weight loss is rare (26). An often held argument that starvation 'cleans the body' is not scientifically supported.

Very Low Calorie Diets

Modern VLCD products are composed of high quality proteins with adequate addition of electrolytes, vitamins and trace elements (27). Previously, the VLCDs were considered dangerous, an opinion that to a great extent seems to be based on the results of early treatment with the so-called liquid protein diet (28), an incomplete VLCD preparation, which resulted in several deaths. Today there is agreement that VLCDs can be used without medical supervision for 2 weeks and under medical supervision generally up to 26 weeks. However, almost continuous VLCD treatment for up to one year without serious side-effects has been reported (29).

Most VLCD products contain 400–800 kcal per day. During treatment with VLCD ketonaemia develops within a few days. Generally an anorectic effect is observed, and most patients on VLCD

programmes do not complain of hunger as long as they adhere to the diet. The advantage of the VLCD is that it safely makes it possible to avoid the food cues and the temptations associated with food cues. Many patients experience a euphoric sensation, at least during the initial phase of the treatment programme.

During VLCD the initial weight loss is several kilograms during the first week of treatmnt. The energy deficit results in initial breakdown of liver and muscle glycogen. Since glycogen in these stores binds its weight in water almost three times, there is an initial phase of diuresis explaining early losses. Towards the end of the first week the hypocaloric situation stabilizes and weight loss generally is about 2 kg/week, consisting of 60–70% of fat, the rest being lean body mass (30).

VLCD treatment may also be used in place of an ordinary meal. However, since most patients substitute the lunch meal, which often is not the most energy containing meal of the day, the effects of this strategy are generally modest. Probably, a dietary programme substituting dinner for VLCD would exhibit more marked long-term results.

VLCDs should not be used in patients with unstable metabolic conditions (such as renal or hepatic insufficiency), in patients with eating disorders, infections, or other acute catabolic conditions such as renal failure, severe liver disease etc. When VLCDs were introduced, several medical precautions were taken and patients kept under strict medical supervision. Later experience has demonstrated that after an initial metabolic screening, laboratory tests and safety control can be kept to a minimum.

Recently low calorie diets (LCD) have been introduced, generally consisting of 800–1200 kcal/day and based on the same components as VLCDs. Whereas these seem to result in safe weight losses, rather similar to those achieved with VLCDs, they may not induce ketonaemia and so may be more dificult to adhere to (31). Diets with an energy content in this range can also be composed of regular low caloric food products.

Vegetarian Diet

Vegetarian diets have often been promoted as healthy and suitable for weight reduction programmes. Several studies suggest that vegetarians weigh less and have fewer obesity-associated comorbidities. However, this may not only depend on the diet but could be explained by self-selection. Studies lasting for 1 year indicate that a lacto-vegetarian diet, hypocaloric diet and a complete diet containing animal products with the same energy content results in the same weight loss (32).

Diet acceptance for long-term use is probably the most important component in making patients comply with dietary restrictions.

Special Diets

Numerous special diets are described in the literature, often marketed as 'different' or 'magic'. The principles are described by Summerbell in her review (6). As long as obese subjects attend to them and they result in energy deficiency, weight loss will follow. In reality few of them have been found to have any sustained effects on body weight and invariably the 'scientific advance' they are supposed to represent illustrates a commercial rather than scentific breakthrough.

DIETARY FIBRE

The effects of dietary fibre on weight control can be summarized as follows: Few controlled clinical studies have been carried out showing that supplementation with dietary fibre improves weight loss. In one study, patients were asked to maintain their dietary habits, while receiving 10 g guar gum twice daily for 8 weeks; average weight fell from 95.6 to 91.3 kg, but this was difficult to evaluate, since no control group was included (33). In further studies patients were given a reduced diet of 1000 kcal/day, which in one group was supplemented with 24 g of fibre as oat bran biscuit, for 8 weeks (34). Weight loss in the fibre group was reported as high as 5.1 ± 1.7 kg/week, compared with 3.8 ± 1.8 kg in the control group. This study was, however, not blind, as the authors themselves also point out.

A few studies with adequate designs have been published that demonstrate that dietary fibre supplementation improves weight loss. Tuomilehto et al. (35) demonstrated that in a 16-week study period 15 g of guar gum daily resulted in a signifi-

cant weight loss compared with placebo, in normal weight subjects. Walsh et al. (36) treated 20 obese women with 3 g of purified glucomannan or placebo for 8 weeks. Patients on fibre lost a mean of 2.5 kg, whereas in the placebo group surprisingly a weight increase of 0.7 kg was seen during the corresponding time.

The most systematic approach to evaluating the role of dietary fibre supplementation on weight loss and weight maintenance seems to be the data summarized by Ryttig et al. (Table 30.5). In these studies, tablets consisting of combinations of 10–20% soluble (citrus) and 80–90% insoluble (grain) fibres were used (37). The studies were double-blind, randomized and placebo-controlled. A 1600 kcal diet was given for 12 weeks and this design resulted in similar weight losses in both groups. As indicated in Table 30.5, the other six Ryttig studies demonstrated that fibre supplementation significantly improved weight loss compared with placebo. These studies comprised 45 to 97 patients, who were mildly to moderately obese. The fibre supplementation was up to 7 g/day, the hypocaloric diets up to about 1800 kcal/day, the treatment period ranging from 8 to 52 weeks. Overall, fibre improved the weight loss obtained by the diet by about 40%. In these studies hunger feelings in fibre groups decreased with time, in contrast to ratings in controls, and the number of withdrawals was significantly lower in fibre-treated patients than in controls.

These studies were performed with fibre-supplemented diets. No studies performed with diets varying in fibre content have tested the effect of dietary manipulation with fibre. The overall effects of dietary fibre on obesity treatment are summarized in Table 30.6.

FAT AND WEIGHT LOSS

The question whether the percentage of dietary fat in the diet plays an important role in the rising prevalence of overweight and its treatment has been repeatedly debated in recent years. It has been argued that obesity can rarely develop in a diet which is not rich in fat, but recently this assumption has been refuted by Willett (43). Although there is agreement that total energy intake is a main determinant of body weight, if energy expenditure is controlled for, the interpretations of the epi-

Table 30.5 Effects of dietary fibre on weight reduction

Reference	Energy intake (kJ/day)	Added fibre (g/day)	Number of patients	Duration (weeks)	Initial BMI (kg/m^2)	Mean weight reduction (kg)	
						Fibre	Placebo
Ryttig et al. (1985) (37)	5000	7	89	11	29.0	6.3	4.2
Solum et al. (1987) (38)	5000	6	60	12	26.8	8.5	6.4
Ryttig et al. (1989) (39)	5000/6700/ad lib	7/6/6	97	11/26/52	27.4	3.8	2.8
Ryttig (1990) (40)	5000	6/4	53	24	27.5	8.0	5.8
Rigaud et al. (1990) (41)	7376/7544	7	52	24	29.3	5.3	2.9
Rössner et al. (1987) (42)	5880/4550	5	60	8	36.3	7.0	6.0
Rössner et al. (1987) (42)	6720	7	45	12	35.9	6.2	4,1

Table 30.6 Effects of dietary fibre in obesity treatment

- Dietary fibre increases food volume, reduces energy density and exerts a displacement effect
- Dietary fibre increases chewing work and prolongs mealtime
- Dietary fibre-rich food retains satiety more than diets poor in dietary fibre
- Dietary fibre (soluble) maintains glucose homeostasis in the circulation for longer periods
- Dietary fibre (soluble) may reduce low density lipoprotein cholesterol levels
- Dietary fibre (non-soluble) improves gastrointestinal function and prevents constipation

demiological data on fat and body have differed. Willett has argued that there is no evidence that energy density has an important effect on long-term weight control and thus that the importance of fat restrictions in dietary treatment is unproven. On the other hand, Bray and Popkin suggest, in a meta-analysis from 28 clinical trials, that a reduction of 10% in the proportion of energy from fat would be associated with the reduction in weight of 16 g per day (44).

HIGH VERSUS LOW PROTEIN HYPOCALORIC DIETS

Rosenvinge Skov has studied the effects of different diet types on body weight, body composition and blood lipids in obese subjects by comparing diets which varied in protein energy (e) percentage (high protein group 25 E% protein, low protein group 12 E% protein) (45). The diet itself was an *ad libitum* low fat diet and all food was provided by self-selection in a 'special store', where the food the patients selected, consumed or returned could be adequately assessed. Weight loss after 6 months was 5.1 kg in the low protein group vs. 8.9 kg in the high protein group ($P < 0.001$). No negative side effects with the high protein diet were observed; in particular, kidney function remained unaffected. The authors conclude that replacement of some dietary carbohydrates by protein in the *ad libitum* fat-reduced diet improved weight loss without any adverse effects. These effects could be explained by satiating signals of the protein or the increased diet-induced thermogenesis of the high protein diet. It has been suggested that the inhibition of energy intake caused by the high protein diet may be due to other mechanisms than energy density, such as release of cholecystokinin (46), insulin/glucagon effects (47) in the liver or a direct effect in the central nervous system of certain amino acids (48).

ALCOHOL

The role of alcohol in weight control is still controversial. Although alcohol, containing 7 kcal/g, has the highest energy density after fat, it is still unclear whether alcohol intake is of importance in body weight regulation. Alcohol may either be added to the diet or substitute for other energy containing food components. Whereas alcoholics who are lean have often experienced the wasting long-term consequences of high alcohol intake with anorexia, vomiting etc., other alcohol consumers experience an appetite enhancing effect of alcohol.

LONG-TERM RESULTS OF DIETING

Weight loss after dieting generally is 6–12 kg, most of which occurs during the first 6 months of treatment. Treatment results will be improved if dietary treatment is combined with exercise and behaviour modification. Although many programmes reported in the literature (8) are unimpressive, long-term studies showing excellent results have been described, such as the Finnish programme by Karvetti and Hakala demonstrating that a dietary programme for 1 year resulted in sustained weight loss for both men and women during a follow-up period of up to 7 years (49). We also demonstrated sustained weight loss and acceptable adherence with a combined dietary–behavioural modification programme after 10–12 years of monitoring (50).

During recent years it has become obvious that weight loss and weight maintenance after such weight loss represent two different components of the treatment strategy. Numerous programmes have shown considerable weight loss whereas weight maintenance after initial weight loss is rare. Thus the dietary composition during the initial weight loss may be of less importance during a phase when the weight loss is more driven by the energy deficiency than by the dietary composition in itself. As long as adequate protein supplies are available, preventing unnecessary breakdown of lean body mass with an ensuing reduction in basic metabolic rate, the composition of the diet during this phase may not be of major importance. However, when the weight-losing phase is over, generally after 6 months, the composition of the diet with regard to macronutrients may be crucial (51).

REFERENCES

1. Goldberg GR, Black AE, Jebb SA, *et al.* Critical evaluation of energy intake data using fundamental principles of energy physiology, 1: derivation of cut-off limits to identify under-recording. *Eur J Clin Nutr* 1991; **45**: 569–581.
2. Frost G, Masters K, King C, *et al.* A new method of energy prescription to improve weight loss. *J Hum Nutr Diet* 1991; **4**: 369–373.
3. Prochaska JO, Norcross JC, Diclemente CC. *Changing for Good.* New York: Avon Brooks, 1995.
4. Foster GD, Wadden TA, Vogt RA, Brewer G. What is a reasonable weight loss? Patients' expectations and evaluations of obesity treatment outcomes. *J Consult Clin Psychol* 1997; **65**: 79–85.
5. Blundell JE, Burley VJ, Cotton JR, Lawton CL. Dietary fat and the control of energy intake: Evaluating the effects of fat on meal size and post-meal satiety. *Am J Clin Nutr* 1993; **57**: 772S–778S.
6. Sommerbell CD. Dietary treatment of obesity. In: Kopelman PG, Stock MJ (eds). *Clinical Obesity.* Oxford: Blackwell Science, 1998: 377–408.
7. Hakala P, Kostterapi. In: Andersen T, Rissanen A, Rössner S (eds). *Fetma/fedme—en Nordisk Lärobok.* Lund; Studentlitteratur, 1998: 234–248.
8. National Institutes of Health, National Heart Lung, and Blood Institute. Clinical guidelines on the identification, evaluation, and treatment of overweight and obesity in adults—the evience report. *Obes Res* 1998; **6**: Suppl 2.
9. Davis BR, Blaufox MD, Oberman A, *et al.* Reduction in long-term antihypertension medication requirements. Effects of weight reduction by dietary intervention in overweight persons with mild hypertension. *Arch Intern Med* 1992; **153**: 1773–1782.
10. Stamler R, Stamler J, Grimm R, *et al.* Nutritional therapy for high blood pressure. Final report of a 4-year randomized controlled trial—the Hypertension Control Program. *JAMA* 1987; **257**: 1484–1491.
11. Hypertension Prevention Trial Research Group. The Hypertension Prevention Trial: three-year effects of dietary changes on blood pressure. *Arch Intern Med* 1990; **150**: 153–162.
12. The Trials of Hypertension Prevention Collaborative Research Group. Effects of weight loss and sodium reduction intervention on blood pressure and hypertension incidence in overweight people with high-normal blood pressure. The Trials of Hypertension Prevention, phase II. Effects of weight loss and sodium reduction intervention on blood pressure and hypertension incidence in overweight people with high-normal blood pressure. The Trials of Hypertension Prevention, phase II. *Arch Intern Med* 1997; **157**: 657–667.
13. Stefanick ML, Mackey S, Sheehan M, Ellsworth N, Haskell WL, Wood PD. Effects of the NCEP Step 2 diet and exercise on lipoprotein in postmenopausal women and men with low HDL-cholesterol and high LDL-cholesterol. *N Engl J Med* 1998; **329**: 12–20.
14. Ryttig KR, Flaten H, Rössner S. Long-term effects of a very low calorie diet (Nutrilett®) in obesity treatment. A prospective, randomized, comparison between VLCD and a hypocaloric diet + behavior modification and their combination. *Int J Obes* 1997; **21**: 674–679.
15. Singh RB, Rastogi SS, Verma R, *et al.* Randomised controlled trial of cardioprotective diet in patients with recent acute myocardial infarction: results of 1-year follow up. *BMJ* 1992; **304**: 1015–1019.
16. Jeffery RW, Hellerstedt WL, French SA, Baxter JE. A randomized trial of counseling for fat restriction versus calorie restriction in the treatment of obesity. *Int J Obes Relat Metab Disord* 1995; **19**: 132–137.
17. Sheppard L, Kristal AR, Kushi LH. Weight loss in women participating in a randomized trial of low-fat diets. *Am J Clin Nutr* 1991; **54**: 821–828.
18. Hill AJ, Rogers PJ. Food intake and eating behaviour in humans. In: Kopelman PG, Stock MJ (eds). *Clinical Obesity.* Oxford: Blackwell Science, 1998: 86–111.

19. National Board of Health and Welfare. *Diet, Exercise and Health* (in Swedish). Stockholm: Liber, 1992.

20. Stunkard AJ, Grace WJ, Wolff HG. The night-eating syndrome. A pattern of food intake among certain obese patients. *Am J Med* 1955; **19**: 78–86.

21. Birketvedt GS, Florholmen J, Sundsfjord J, *et al.* Behavioral and neuroendocrine characteristics of the night-eating syndrome. *JAMA* 1999; **282**: 657–663.

22. Barkeling B, Rössner S, Björvell H. Effects of a high-protein meal (meat) and a high-carbohydrate meal (vegetarian) on satiety measured by automated computerized monitoring of subsequent food intake, motivation to eat and food preferences. *Int J Obes* 1990; **14**: 743–751.

23. Garrow JS. *Obesity and Related Disease*. Edinburgh: Churchill Livingstone, 1988.

24. Murphree D. Patient attitude toward physician treatment of obesity. *J Fam Pract* 1994; **38**: 45–48.

25. Garnett ES, Bernard DL, Ford J, Goodbody RA, Woodhouse MA. Gross fragmentation of starvation for obesity. *Lancet* 1969; **i**: 14–16.

26. Drenick EJ, Smith R. Weight reduction by starvation. *Postgrad Med* 1964; A-95–A-100.

27. Wadden TA, Stunkard AJ, Brownell KD. Very low calorie diets: Their efficacy, safety, and future. *Ann Intern Med* 1983; **99**: 675–684.

28. Linn R, Stuart SL. *The Last Chance Diet*. Secaucus, NJ: Lyle Stuart, 1976.

29. Rössner S. Effect of 46 weeks of very-low-calorie-diet treatment on weight loss and cardiac function—a case report. *Obes Res* 1998; **6**: 462–463.

30. Ryttig K, Rössner S. Weight maintenance after a very low calorie diet (VLCD) weight reduction period and the effects of VLCD supplementation. A prospective, randomized, comparative, controlled longterm trial. *J Intern Med* 1995; **238**: 299–306.

31. Rössner S, Flaten H. VLCD versus LCD in long-term treatment of obesity. *Int J Obes* 1997; **21**: 22–26.

32. Summerbell CD, Watts C, Higgins JP, Garrow JS. Randomised controlled trial of novel, simple, and well supervised weight loss in outpatients. *BMJ* 1998; **317**: 1487–1498.

33. Krotkiewski M. Effect of guar-gum on body weight, hunger ratings and metabolism in obese subjects. *Br J Nutr* 1984; **52**: 97–105.

34. Krotkiewski M, Smith U. Dietary fiber in obesity. In: Leeds AR, Avenell A (eds). *Dietary Fibre Perspectives—Reviews and Bibliography, 1*. London: John Libbey, 1985: 61–67.

35. Tuomilehto J, Voutilainen E, Huttonen J, Vinni S, Homan K. Effect of guar gum on body weight and serum lipids in hypercholesterolaemic females. *Acta Med Scand* 1980; **208**: 45–48.

36. Walsh DE, Yaghoubian V, Behforooz A. Effect of glucomannan on obese patients. A clinical study. *Int J Obes* 1984; **8**: 289–293.

37. Ryttig KR, Larsen S, Haegh L. Treatment of slightly to moderately overweight persons. A double-blind placebo-controlled investigation with diet and fiber tablets (Dumovital). In: Björntorp P, Vahouny GV, Kritchevsky A (eds). *Dietary Fiber and Obesity*. New York: Alan R Liss, 1985: 77–84.

38. Solum TT, Ryttig KR, Solum E, Larsen S. The influence of a high-fibre diet on body weight, serum lipids and blood pressure in slightly overweight persons. A randomized, double-blind, placebo-controlled investigation with diet and fibre tablets (Dumovital). *Int J Obes* 1987; **11** (Suppl 1): 67–71.

39. Ryttig KR, Tellnes G, Haegh L, Böe E, Fagerthun H. A dietary fibre supplement and weight maintenance after weight reduction. A randomized double-blind, placebo-controlled study. *Int J Obes* 1989; **13**: 165–171.

40. Ryttig KR. Clinical effects of dietary fibre supplements in overweight and in hypertension. Thesis. Stockholm: Karolinska Institute, 1990.

41. Rigaud D, Ryttig KR, Angel LA, Apfelbaum M. Overweight treated with energy restriction and a dietary fibre supplement: a 6-month randomized, double-blind, placebo-controlled trial. *Int J Obes* 1990; **14**: 763–770.

42. Rössner S, van Zweigberg D, Öhlin A, Ryttig KR. Weight reduction with dietary fibre supplements. Results of two double-blind randomized studies. *Acta Med Scand* 1987; **222**: 83–88.

43. Willett WC. Dietary fat and obesity: an unconvincing relation. *Am J Clin Nutr* 1998; **68**: 1149–1150.

44. Bray GA, Popkin BM. Dietary fat intake does affect obesity. *Am J Clin Nutr* 1998; **68**: 1157–1173.

45. Rosenvinge Skov A. Low-fat diets: high-vs. low-protein. Thesis. The Royal Veterinary and Agricultural University, Frederiksberg, Denmark, 1998.

46. Butler RN. The effects of preloads of amino acid on short-term satiety. *Am J Clin Nutr* 1981; **34**: 2045–2047.

47. Eisenstein AB, Strack I, Steiner A. Glucagon stimulation of hepatic gluconeogenesis in rats fed a high-protein, carbohydrate free diet. *Metabolism* 1974; **23**: 15–23.

48. Hill AJ, Blundell JE. Role of amino acids in appetite control in man. In: Huether G (ed.). *Amino Acid Availability and Brain Function in Health and Disease*. Berlin, Heidelberg: Springer-Verlag, 1988: 239–248.

49. Karvetti R-L, Hakala P. A seven-year follow-up of a weight reduction programme in Finnish primary health care. *Eur J Clin Nutr* 1992; **46**: 743–752.

50. Björvell H, Rössner S. Short communication: A ten-year follow-up of weight change in severely obese subjects treated in a combined behavioural modification programme. *Int J Obes* 1992; **16**: 623–625.

51. Hill JO, Drougas H, Peters JC. Obesity treatment: Can diet composition play a role? *Ann Intern Med* 1993; **119**: 694–697.

31

Recent and Future Drugs for the Treatment of Obesity

Luc F. Van Gaal, Ilse L. Mertens and Ivo H. De Leeuw

University Hospital Antwerp, Belgium

INTRODUCTION

Obesity is becoming increasingly common and is recognized as a major public health problem worldwide (1). The prevalence of obesity continues to increase in the majority of affluent societies. In most European countries, the prevalence of obesity (body mass index (BMI) $> 30\,kg/m^2$) is roughly between 10 and 20% among middle-aged people, and over the last 10–15 years the overweight and obese population has increased by almost 15%, mainly in young adults and adolescents.

There is, in addition, growing evidence that obesity—central adiposity in particular—has an important impact on predisposing risk factors for coronary heart disease, namely dyslipidaemia, glucose intolerance, insulin resistance and elevated blood pressure. Reversal of these 'obesity associated' metabolic abnormalities is one of the most important targets in the current clinical management of obesity (2,3).

The aetiology of obesity is multifactorial and is the result of a complex interaction between genetic, environmental (predominantly dietary) and psychosocial factors. Due to this complexity, obesity is difficult to treat and comprehensive treatment programmes combine diet, exercise and behavioural therapy.

Although dietary approaches and lifestyle adaptation remain the cornerstones of obesity therapy (4,5), long-term success is extremely disappointing, despite the variety of dietary manipulations that have been proposed, ranging from scientifically studied diet plans (calorie restriction, fat restriction only, very low calorie diet (VLCD)) to the most ridiculous approaches, the long-term maintenance of clinically significant weight loss (5–10% of initial body weight) remains rare (4). In recent years a lot of attention has been paid to the role of pharmacotherapy as an additional treatment option with new drugs being marketed and exploration of new biochemical pathways and new pharmacological intervention potentials.

New clinical guidelines for the management of obesity have been published by different organizations such as the North American Association for the Study of Obesity (6), the Institute of Medicine (7), the US National Institutes of Health (8), the Scottish Intercollegiate Guidelines Network (9) and the Royal College of Physicians of London (10). In these documents a modest weight loss (5–10% of initial weight) and weight maintenance is recommended, rather than targeting on ideal weight.

It has previously been shown that an intentional modest weight reduction may lead to a marked improvement in cardiovascular risk factors and a substantial reduction—up to 20–25%—in comorbidity (11,12) (Table 31.1). Large-scale 1- and 2-year placebo-controlled studies with orlistat, sibutramine and dexfenfluramine have shown that a mean weight loss of 10% can be reached with these compounds (13). Weight loss is not the only goal of

International Textbook of Obesity. Edited by Per Björntorp.

Table 31.1 Risk factors that can be reduced by at least 10% by drug-induced weight changes

- Hypertension
- Glucose intolerance
- Hypercholesterolaemia
- Hypertriglyceridaemia
- Low HDL cholesterol levels
- Haemostatic/fibrinolytic parameters (FVII, PAI-1)

HDL, high density lipoprotein; FVII, haemostatic factor VII; PAI-1, plasminogen activator inhibitor 1.

Table 31.2 Characteristics of an ideal anti-obesity agent

- Produce weight (fat) reduction in a dose-dependent manner
- Proven to be safe without major side effects
- Effects should be long lasting
- By preference be active via oral administration
- May not show any addictive properties and/or toxicity
- By preference reduce the amount of visceral fat
- Inexpensive

obesity treatment: improvement in comorbidities, such as diabetes, hypertension and dyslipidaemia, is an important second endpoint in these studies. Some anti-obesity agents have even proven to have a positive effect on these comorbidities independent of weight loss. Dexfenfluramine, a serotoninergic compound, seems to have a blood pressure lowering effect, independent of weight loss, which is probably mediated through a decrease in noradrenergic activity (14,15). Orlistat, a selective inhibitor of gastric and pancreatic lipase, has been shown to produce a significant decrease in lipids that is greater than can be expected from weight loss alone (16).

For morbid obesity, however, the 10% weight loss option may be inappropriate and larger weight loss may be necessary. The results of the large, prospective, Swedish Obese Subjects (SOS) Study on surgical intervention will most probably give more insights and answers to this question (17). The place and appropriateness of surgery will be reviewed in detail in Chapter 34.

For several decades pharmacological treatment of obesity had a negative reputation most likely due to the abuse of thyroid hormones, amphetamines, digitalis and diuretics. In 1997, fenfluramine and dexfenfluramine were withdrawn from the market due to reports of pulmonary hypertension (18) and valvular heart disease (19) in patients treated with fenfluramine and phentermine. These events led some people to suggest that drugs are not appropriate for the treatment of obesity. Recently, however,

obesity has been recognized as a chronic disease (8) for which no cure is available yet (20). This implies that short-term treatment is not enough for most obese patients and that obesity should be treated as any other chronic disease—such as type 2 diabetes and hypertension—requiring lifelong treatment in which pharmacological agents could play an important role (21). The search for anti-obesity drugs which are effective and safe for chronic use is an important challenge.

GENERAL PHARMACOLOGICAL ASPECTS

Large-scale, long-term (up to 2 years) studies have demonstrated that pharmacological agents (dexfenfluramine previously, more recently orlistat and sibutramine) are able to induce significant weight loss in conjunction with dietary approaches, and important reduction of comorbidities as well. The majority of these drugs allow maintenance of the reduced body weight for at least 1–2 years. The weight loss that can be attributed to these drugs is in general modest, in accordance with the 10% weight loss option, but will be accompanied by a reduction of around 25% of most of the well-known comorbid conditions.

Although the ideal weight loss drug does not exist yet, a series of characteristics should be considered in qualifying a molecule for human use (Table 31.2). It is important that drugs are effective in reducing body fat, visceral fat in preference, without displaying any major health risks (13,22). In addition, the effect of the drug should be long lasting. In this context, the effect of the drug on the maintenance of achieved weight loss is as important as the initiation of weight loss. It is not the case that a drug designed for weight loss does not have any effect once a phase of weight stabilization after weight loss has been reached. In this situation, discontinuation of the drug treatment will most probably result in weight regain (23).

Overweight and obesity are a consequence of an energy imbalance between energy intake and expenditure: the human body is as an interface of environmental and biological factors, influenced by this energy balance. The components—both environmental and biological—that may interfere with this balance, should be modulated during obesity management.

Table 31.3 Classification of drugs according to their effect on energy balance

---

- Drugs involved in appetite behaviour (nutrient intake), mainly appetite suppression and satiety enhancement
- Drugs involved in increasing energy expenditure, mainly thermogenic properties
- Drugs affecting metabolism or nutrient partitioning

Anti-obesity drugs can be classified according to their mechanism of action on energy balance (2,24). Considering these components involved in the regulation of body weight, three different mechanisms may be used to classify pharmacological treatment of obesity (Table 31.3).

Contrary to previous reviews on drug therapy, dealing with a classification based on these mechanisms of action, this chapter will follow the experience with drug therapy that has been accumulated in the past, that is happening at present and that will come in the following years. Only drugs that reduce food intake and influence nutrient partitioning are currently available; drugs that stimulate energy expenditure, such as β_3 agonists, are still under development (25).

WHO SHOULD BE MANAGED PHARMACOLOGICALLY?

The decision concerning who to treat should be based on an individual assessment of all available factors and the appropriate indications for treatment need to be carefully considered. The inherent risk of the disease must be assessed in relation to the risks of treatment (26).

It is clear that classical weight loss techniques do not produce a satisfactory long-term outcome for most obese patients (27). Pharmacotherapy could be valuable in addition to classical weight loss therapy both in achieving initial weight loss and in maintaining weight loss.

The Clinical Guidelines for evaluation and treatment of obesity, released by the National Institutes of Health (8), recommend that weight loss drugs should only be used as part of a comprehensive programme which includes dietary adaptation, physical activity and behavioural and psychological support. Recent data have shown that regular scheduled visits including dietetic and physical activity advice add a significant additional weight reduction to that obtained with drug therapy combined with a calorie restricted diet (28). This shows that the specific approach to the non-pharmacological components of the weight loss programme plays an important role in the final outcome of the programme. To be considered for pharmacotherapy, candidates should have a BMI ≥ 30 without risk factors, or a BMI of ≥ 27 associated with the well-known—mostly metabolic—obesity-related health and risk problems. Risk factors and diseases considered important enough to warrant pharmacotherapy for patients with a BMI of 27 to 29.9 include hypertension, dyslipidaemia, coronary heart disease, type 2 diabetes, and sleep apnoea (8). Only patients that have failed to lose weight on a regular weight loss programme of diet, exercise and behaviour therapy can be considered for drug therapy. However, although not endorsed by American and European drug agencies, subjects with a recent onset of obesity and a rather sudden weight gain of 10–15 kg, might qualify for safe pharmacological treatment as well.

Patients selected for drug therapy should be given complete information about the drug, the potential adverse effects, and long-term efficacy (29). Patients should know that not all will respond to drug therapy and that it is important to visit the doctor and dietician on a regular basis. Close medical monitoring for adverse effects while using the medications is important. Understanding the risks and benefits of anti-obesity medications is critical in the development of effective approaches for weight management and obesity prevention.

Recently much attention has been paid to the identification of factors predicting the outcome of weight loss programmes. Different papers have described the impact of biological, psychological and behavioural characteristics such as sex (30), race (30), pre-treatment weight (30,31), initial weight loss (31), 24-hour energy expenditure, % fat oxidation, plasma dihydrotestosterone, postprandial noradrenaline concentration (32), binge eating disorder (33) and previous weight loss attempts (30,34).

In clinical trials evaluating drug therapy the initial weight of the patients, weight loss achieved during the run-in phase of the study and/or first month of the study, fat distribution and genetic factors could play a role in the determination of the final outcome for the individual patient. Genetic polymorphisms linked to the mechanism of action of the drug could play an additional role. In a study with dexfenfluramine high compliance with the drug regimen and a positive family history of obesity were predictive of final weight loss. Previous failure to lose weight did not have any effect on treatment outcome (35). In a 24-week trial including 1047 patients treated with sibutramine, weight loss achieved at week 4 was predictive for weight loss achieved after 24 weeks of treatment (36). An analysis of pooled data from two European multicentre trials with orlistat revealed that, in orlistat-treated patients, mean weight loss was greater after 1 year in patients who lost $\geq 5\%$ of body weight after 12 weeks of treatment than in those who lost $< 5\%$ (37).

From a clinical point of view, identifying the characteristics of those patients most likely to benefit from therapy will make it easier to match the individual patient to the most effective treatment for this patient and prevent unnecessary drug prescription. The Clinical Guidelines from the National Institutes of Health (8) advise discontinuing drug therapy if the patient fails to lose $\geq 2\,kg$ after 4 weeks of treatment. The Royal College of Physicians of London (10) has recommended 5% weight loss after 12 weeks of treatment as the goal for continued treatment.

PREVIOUS EXPERIENCE WITH ANTI-OBESITY DRUGS (Table 31.4)

Drugs Affecting Energy Intake

Use of anorectic drugs usually results in a reduction of nutrient intake, leading to a loss in body weight and fat mass in particular; this effect is usually obtained by a decrease in appetite. Anorectic drugs can play a useful role in an overall weight reduction programme, but should only be prescribed as part of such a programme, including dietary and behavioural advice.

Catecholaminergic Anorectics

Most of the previously available appetite-suppressing drugs, except mazindol, are derivatives of phenylethylamine (amphetamine, phenmetrazine, amfepramone or diethylpropion, phentermine, phenylpropanolamine). Noradrenergic drugs re-

Table 31.4 Drugs that have been used in the treatment of obesity

Catecholaminergic drugs	Serotoninergic drugs	Other
Amphetamine	Fenfluramine	Thyroid hormones
Phenmetrazine	Dexfenfluramine	Diuretics
Diethylpropion	(Fluoxetine)	Ephedrine–caffeine
Phentermine		
Phenylpropanolamine		
Mazindol		

lease noradrenaline (norepinephrine) or block its reuptake into neurons of the hypothalamus (21,24).

Among the catecholaminergic anorectics, amphetamine and phenmetrazine are no longer recommended because of their strong stimulatory properties and addictive potential. Side effects of a sympathomimetic nature may occur in some subjects. These drugs should be used carefully because of the risk of drug abuse and addiction. Recently, more serious side effects such as pulmonary hypertension and valvular heart disease have been described but most cases were observed when these noradrenergic drugs (essentially phentermine) were associated with serotoninergic drugs such as dexfenfluramine (18,19).

Fenfluramine and Dexfenfluramine

The serotoninergic drugs fenfluramine and dexfenfluramine are metabolized to d-norfenfluramine, which enhances serotonin release from the neurons and acts as an agonist for serotonin (5-HT) receptors. In addition, dexfenfluramine acts also by inhibiting reuptake of serotonin into the neurons (24). The clinical efficacy of fenfluramine and dexfenfluramine ($2 \times 15\,mg/day$) has been demonstrated in trials of short and long duration conducted over the past 30 years (38). In contrast to catecholaminergic drugs, serotoninergic compounds should be used continuously and do not exert stimulant or sympathomimetic activities or induce tolerance.

However, several reports of pulmonary hypertension and, more recently, of cardiac valvular abnormalities have been published (18,19). In 1996, a case-control study conducted by the International Primary Pulmonary Hypertension Study Group (18) showed that the use of fenfluramine derivates for 3 months or more was associated with a 23-fold increase in the risk of primary pulmonary hypertension, a rare but often fatal disorder. One year later, in 1997, a paper by Connolly *et al.* (19) reported on the association between treatment with the fenfluramine–phentermine combination and valvular heart disease. These observations led to a worldwide withdrawal of both fenfluramine and dexfenfluramine. Since this first publication by Connolly *et al.* (19), new studies have been published on the association between appetite suppressants and valvular heart disease (39–41). Weissman *et al.* (41) performed echocardiography after 72 days of treatment with dexfenfluramine and found cardiac valve abnormalities in 6.9% of treated patients compared to 4.5% in the placebo groups. Jick *et al.* (39) performed a population-based follow-up study over 4 years of patients treated with dexfenfluramine ($n = 6532$), fenfluramine ($n = 2371$) and phentermine ($n = 862$) and found five new cases of valvular disease in the dexfenfluramine group and six new cases treated with fenfluramine. Finally, Kahn *et al.* (40) studied the prevalence of cardiac valve insufficiency in patients taking dexfenfluramine (13%), dexfenfluramine and phentermine (23%), or fenfluramine and phentermine (25%). The results from these studies seem to confirm the earlier findings of Connolly *et al.* (19). However, the studies show differences in the magnitude of the risk that may influence the subsequent clinical significance. The difference in results could be due to methodological differences such as the type of anorectic used or lack of baseline echocardiographic studies, duration of treatment and the method of diagnoses (42). The precise mechanism linking the use of fenfluramine derivates to valvular heart disease is not yet completely understood. One of the hypotheses relates to the serotonin-releasing effect of the drugs. Serotonin could have an effect on the cardiac valves, as seen in the carcinoid syndrome which is associated with high serotonin levels due to a serotonin-secreting neoplasm (43).

Fluoxetine

Fluoxetine is a well-known antidepressant drug which acts by inhibiting the reuptake of serotonin. In contrast to fenfluramine, fluoxetine does not stimulate serotonin release and enhances synaptic serotonin concentration by blocking its reuptake (44). This characteristic may explain why no cases of pulmonary hypertension or cardiac valvular abnormalities have been described so far with this compound despite its very wide utilization as an antidepressant drug. Fluoxetine is an effective anorectic agent promoting weight loss: this has been confirmed in obese subjects, even in the absence of depression. This effect was also seen in obese diabetic subjects, as shown in a multicentre study (45). However, the dose effective to reduce body weight is higher (60 mg/day) than that generally used in the treatment of depression and the effect may be transient as a significant weight regain has been reported after 6–12 months of treatment (45).

Drugs Affecting Energy Expenditure

Much less experience exists in the field of clinical obesity with drugs that increase energy expenditure, thermogenesis in particular. Pharmacological stimulation of thermogenesis would be a rational target for anti-obesity action, however (46). The largest experience exists with the ephedrine–caffeine combination therapy, which may increase metabolic rate and delay noredrenaline degradation (47). Cardiovascular side effects, often seen with high doses of ephedrine, have limited the widespread use of this kind of approach. Also the clinical application of the β_3-adrenergic receptor agonists, an interesting category of drugs involved in increasing thermogenesis and metabolic rate, has been very disappointing and mostly unsuccessful in clinical trials until now, despite their promising and sometimes even spectacular results in rodents (48).

RECENT NEW EXPERIENCE WITH ANTI-OBESITY DRUGS

Centrally Active Drugs: Sibutramine

Sibutramine (Figure 31.1) is a centrally acting agent that dose-dependently inhibits serotonin and noradrenaline reuptake (49). Sibutramine's action in inhibiting the reuptake of serotonin enhances satiety and thus decreases energy intake (50). By inhibiting noradrenaline reuptake, sibutramine enhances sympathetic outflow, including to brown adipose tissue, leading to increased thermogenesis and thus increased energy expenditure.

Sibutramine

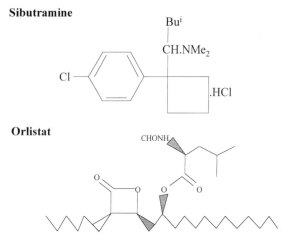

Orlistat

Figure 31.1 Structure of sibutramine and orlistat, two recent drugs developed for the treatment of obesity

The sibutramine parent molecule is efficiently absorbed from the gastrointestinal tract and undergoes an extensive first-pass metabolism. Hepatic metabolism of the parent molecule by the cytochrome P450 enzyme system leads to the formation of two active metabolites, termed metabolite 1 and metabolite 2 (51). Metabolite 1 is a secondary amine and metabolite 2 is a primary amine. These two metabolites mediate the pharmacological activity of the sibutramine molecule. Further metabolism yields inactive glucoronidases, which are excreted in the urine. As metabolites 1 and 2 have half-lives of 14 h and 16 h, respectively, sibutramine can be given as a once-daily dose (51).

The pharmacological activity of sibutramine does not appear to be a result of increased serotonin release; this differentiates it from the actions of dexfenfluramine, a predominantly serotonin-releasing compound, and dexamphetamine, which predominantly releases dopamine and noradrenaline. This might explain why sibutramine has not been associated with cardiac valve insufficiency. This was illustrated in a study of 210 obese patients with late-onset diabetes treated with sibutramine or placebo, in which the rate of valve problems was 2.3% in the sibutramine group and 2.6% in the placebo group (52). In *in vitro* studies as well as trials conducted in animals and humans, sibutramine and its metabolites also showed no significant potential for inducing dopamine release, unlike dexamphetamine. This may account for the lack of abuse potential with sibutramine.

Given the role of the liver in sibutramine metabolism, administration of sibutramine to patients with severe hepatic disease is inadvisable, at least until further information becomes available. It would also seem wise to exercise caution regarding the use of sibutramine in conjunction with other drugs requiring the cytochrome P450 enzyme system (53).

Both pre- and postsynaptic α_2-adrenoceptors in brain tissue appear to be rapidly downregulated by sibutramine. The effect of sibutramine on clonidine-induced hypoactivity and mydriasis was used in mice to measure the activity of the drug at, respectively, pre- and postsynaptic α_2-adrenoceptors (54). Sibutramine significantly reduced these activities after 3 days ($P < 0.01$ vs. placebo) with a greater effect on post- than presynaptic α_2-adrenoceptors (42 vs. 15% reduction after 14 days' sibutramine administration) (55). Daily administration of sibutramine (3 mg/kg) reduced the total number of β-adrenoceptors in rat cortex by 23% after 3 days and by 38% after 10 days; this was exclusively via reduction of the β_1-adrenoceptor subset (56). Data regarding the effects of sibutramine on food behaviour via a variety of α- and β-adrenergic receptors seems conflicting. Studies of the hypophagic effects of sibutramine support an α-adrenergic and β_1-adrenergic but not β_2-adrenergic effect of the drug. There are few published primary data on the effects of sibutramine on β_3-adrenoceptors (55,57).

Sibutramine has no effect on the binding affinity or number of dopamine D_1 (58,59) or dopamine D_2 receptors (60) in rat striatal membranes. Sibutramine's weight-reducing efficacy is comparable with that of earlier appetite-suppressant noradrenergic and serotonergic compounds (55).

Most clinical trials in obese patients combined sibutramine administration with a reduction in calorie intake, an increase in daily physical activity and advice on eating behaviour (61,62). Indeed, the drug should be administered in conjunction with a reduced calorie intake. Most clinical trials investigating the effects of sibutramine followed a similar protocol: a 1- to 3-week single-blind placebo run-in period followed by a double-blind placebo-controlled treatment period. The single-blind run-in period observed the effects of diet and/or behavioural changes. The treatment phase lasted 8–52 weeks and was commonly followed by a second single-blind placebo period to assess weight change after drug discontinuation (55).

A report of a 24-week dose-ranging study, recent-

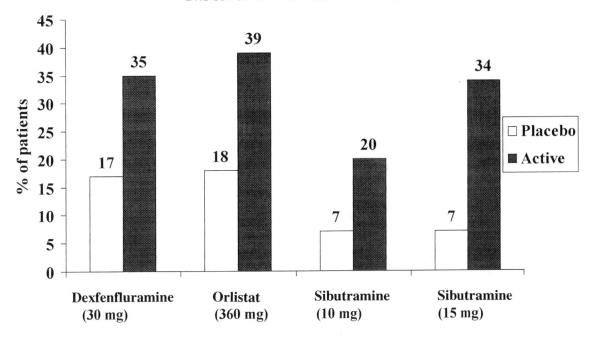

Figure 31.2   Percentage of patients obtaining a weight loss of 10% or more of baseline weight in clinical trials after 1 year of treatment with dexfenfluramine (63), orlistat (64) and sibutramine (65). Adapted from Scheen and Lefèbvre (13)

ly published, indicated that sibutramine administered once daily for 24 weeks in the weight loss phase of treatment for uncomplicated obesity produced dose-related weight loss and was well tolerated (36), leading to a mean weight loss of up to 9–10% from baseline weight. With 10 mg sibutramine, almost 60% of patients could obtain 5% weight loss and 17.2% reached the clinically important 10% weight loss (36) (see also Figure 31.2).

Long-term clinical trials indicate that sibutramine given for 6 months induces a significant dosage-dependent reduction in body weight, which for dosages ranging from 10 to 20 mg/day was 3 to 5 kg greater than the loss of body weight with placebo.

Following a very low calorie diet, sibutramine-treated patients lost more weight than placebo-treated patients during the subsequent 12 months. A substantial tendency to regain weight was observed in the placebo group, compared with additional weight loss in the sibutramine group (66). This time-course of weight loss is similar to that observed in the 20 long-term weight-reduction studies reviewed by Goldstein and Potvin (67). Sibut-

ramine helped greater proportions of patients to maintain $\geq 100\%$, $\geq 50\%$, or 25% of weight loss following a very low calorie diet and was associated with decreases in waist circumference (66).

The STORM trial, a 2-year sibutramine trial of obesity reduction and maintenance, and presented at the most recent European Congress (68), assessed the usefulness of the drug in maintaining substantial weight loss in a randomized controlled double-blind trial. Over 600 obese individuals were studied in eight European centres for a 6-month period of weight loss with sibutramine, combined with an individualized 600 kcal deficit programme based on measured basal metabolic rates. Seventy-seven per cent of patients with > 5% weight loss after 6 months were randomized 3:1 to sibutramine (10 mg/day) and placebo groups to study weight maintenance over a further 18 months. Sibutramine was increased up to 20 mg/day if weight regain occurred. Initially weight loss progressed to a total of − 11.3 kg after 6 months. After randomization the placebo group regained weight to − 4.7 ± 7.2 kg at 2 years; the sibutramine group only showed slight weight regain to − 10.2 kg ± 9.3 kg at 2 years (Fig-

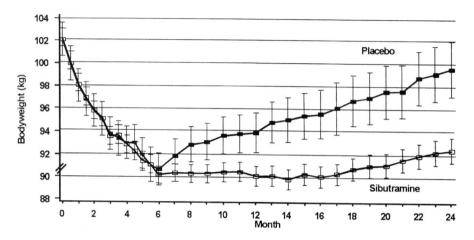

Figure 31.3 The Sibutramine Trial of Obesity Reduction and Maintenance (STORM) (68). Mean weight changes during the 6-month weight loss phase under open drug therapy and the 18-month double-blind placebo-controlled weight maintenance phase

ure 31.3). Marked and sustained falls occurred with sibutramine over the first 6 months in cardiovascular risk factors such as triglycerides, very low density lipoprotein (VLDL), insulin, C-peptide and uric acid. An important finding was the rise in high density lipoprotein (HDL) cholesterol in the second year with overall increases of 20.7% (sibutramine) and 11.7% (placebo). Adverse events were modest: only 20 (3%) patients were withdrawn with blood pressure problems (68).

Sibutramine is, in some preliminary studies at least, also able to stimulate thermogenesis (69) and to reduce significantly the amount of visceral fat (70). Energy expenditure was significantly increased during the 5-hour period after administration of sibutramine 30 mg compared with placebo in healthy volunteers (71). Energy expenditure, as measured by indirect calorimetry, was increased during the fasted and the fed states by 152 and 34% versus placebo, respectively. These sibutramine-induced increases were accompanied by increases in plasma catecholamines and glucose concentrations, heart rate and diastolic blood pressure. Resting energy expenditure was decreased from baseline values by about half as much with sibutramine 10 mg as with placebo (by 5.3 vs. 9.4%; not statistically significantly different) in obese female patients (55,72). It is thought that this smaller decrease in resting energy expenditure may contribute to the long-term maintenance of weight seen with sibutramine (55).

As reported previously, sibutramine (10 mg), is

associated with an increase in heart rate (3 to 6 beats/min) and systolic blood pressure (2 mmHg). This effect of sibutramine is in keeping with its noradrenergic action. This effect seems to be attenuated the more (visceral) fat is lost. The most frequently reported adverse events included dry mouth, anorexia, constipation, insomnia, dizziness and nausea.

Pre-absorptive Nutrient Partitioning: Orlistat

Due to their high energy content and low potential for inducing satiety, high fat diets are very conducive to weight gain, particularly in individuals who are relatively inactive. Indeed, humans are much more likely to become obese through the excessive consumption of dietary fat than by excess consumption of carbohydrate (73). It is rational, therefore, to decrease the proportion of fat, as well as the total number of calories. By reducing fat absorption after ingestion, a continued calorie deficit may be maintained more easily over the long term than by dieting alone.

Orlistat, the first of a new class of agents specifically designed for the long-term management of obesity, is a chemically synthesized derivative of lipstatin (a natural product of *Streptomyces toxytricini*). Orlistat is an inhibitor of gastric and pancreatic lipases, which are instrumental in the digestion and absorption of fat from the gastrointestinal tract. Inhibition of lipase activity has the effect of decreasing fat absorption by 30%, independent of the amount of fat intake, and increasing the excretion of triglycerides in the faeces (74,75).

In vitro studies showed that the concentration of orlistat required to produce 50% inhibition of lipases present in human duodenal juice was low (76). The actual pharmacodynamic interaction between lipase and orlistat is complex (77). The extent of enzyme inhibition by the drug is time and concentration dependent (76). Orlistat is highly lipophilic and distributes into the lipid phase of an aqueous/oil partition model. *In vitro* experiments suggest that inhibition of pancreatic lipase by orlistat is practically irreversible (76). The effects of orlistat on hydrolases other than lipases have been investigated *in vitro*. The drug had no effect on other enzymes such as phospholipase or amylase and a minimal effect on trypsin (16,76).

The systemic absorption of orlistat is minimal. After oral administration of a single dose of 360 mg ^{14}C-labelled orlistat to healthy or obese volunteers, peak plasma radioactivity levels were reached approximately 6 to 8 hours after the dose (78,79). Plasma concentrations of intact orlistat were small, indicating negligible systemic absorption of the drug (79). Pooled data from five long-term (6 months to 2 years) clinical trials with orlistat 180 to 720 mg/day in obese patients indicated that there was a dose-related increase in plasma concentrations of orlistat in several clinical studies. However, these plasma concentrations were generally below the level of assay detection (16).

No pharmacodynamic or pharmacokinetic interactions were observed with orlistat 360 mg/day and warfarin (80) or glyburide (81) in healthy volunteers or with pravastatin in patients with mild hypercholesterolaemia (82). No pharmacokinetic interactions were reported with orlistat and digoxin (83), nifedipine (84) or phenytoin (85). Orlistat did not interfere with oral contraceptive medication in healthy women (86). Orlistat had no clinically significant effects on the pharmacokinetics of captopril, nifedipine, atenolol or fruscmide in healthy volunteers (85). Short-term treatment with orlistat had no effect on ethanol pharmacokinetics, nor did ethanol interfere with the ability of orlistat to inhibit dietary fat absorption in healthy male volunteers (16,87).

A number of short-term trials have revealed that orlistat promotes weight loss and improves hypercholesterolaemia in obese patients. The weight-reducing effect of orlistat was initially shown in a short-term multiple dose study involving almost 200 healthy, obese subjects. Weight reduction was statistically significant in those subjects receiving orlistat 120 mg three times daily (tid) compared to those dieting alone (74,88). Initial studies on healthy volunteers have shown that the maximum amount of fat excreted in the faeces following doses of orlistat at 400 mg/day is approximately 32% of fat ingested. Orlistat (10–20 mg tid) has also been shown to improve the lipid profile of non-obese and obese patients with primary hyperlipidaemia.

A European dose-ranging study, conducted by our own research group, indicated that among 676 obese male and female subjects orlistat treatment resulted in a dose-dependent reduction in body weight, with orlistat 120 mg tid representing the optimal dosage regimen (89).

The efficacy of orlistat has meanwhile been evaluated in obese patients aged 18 to 78 years in seven randomized, double-blind, placebo-controlled multicentre US and European trials of 12 weeks to 2 years duration. Generally, patients were obese but otherwise healthy although one trial evaluated the efficacy of orlistat in obese patients with type 2 diabetes mellitus (90). Obesity was classified according to BMI; mean BMI values were 31 to 36 kg/m^2. Patients were also prescribed a hypocaloric weight loss diet (500 to 800 kcal/day deficit) consisting of 30% of calories as fat, 50% as carbohydrate, 20% as protein, and a maximum of 300 mg per day of cholesterol (16).

In the 2-year randomized double-blind placebo-controlled trial with orlistat conducted recently by Sjöström and colleagues, 38.8% of patients treated with orlistat lost > 10% of their initial body weight versus 17.7% in the placebo group (64) (Figure 31.4). This indicates that orlistat can be considered as a valuable adjunct to dietary therapy in patients on weight maintenance.

However, as emphasized by the authors, 'the use of orlistat beyond 2 years needs careful monitoring with respect to efficacy and adverse events' (64).

A comparable 2-year orlistat trial, conducted in 18 US research centres, confirmed the Sjöström data: orlistat treatment in addition to dietary approaches promotes significant weight loss, decreases weight regain and improves some obesity-related disease risk factors. During the first year

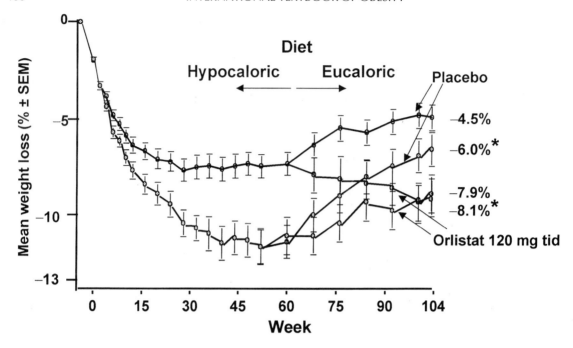

Figure 31.4 Mean percentage change in body weight in a 2-year trial with orlistat studying weight loss and prevention of weight regain in obese patients. In the first year patients were assigned double-blind to treatment with orlistat 120 mg tid or placebo together with a 600 kcal deficit diet. In the second year patients were reassigned to orlistat or placebo with a eucaloric diet. * Chi-square $P < 0.05$ (vs. placebo). Adapted from Sjöström *et al.* (64)

obesity treated subjects lost approximately 3 kg more weight than did placebo subjects (91). Also in subjects with type 2 diabetes, a beneficial effect of orlistat has been proven, despite the usually very limited successes with weight loss in diabetics (90). The results showed a weight loss superior in diabetics compared to placebo, improvement of metabolic control and a decrease in the concomitant ongoing anti-diabetic therapy (90).

The most reported adverse effects consisted of abdominal pain, liquid stools, faecal incontinence with oily stools, nausea, vomiting and flatulence, but these symptoms were in general mild and transient. There was also some trend towards a decrease in lipid-soluble vitamin levels, but only the decrease in vitamin E levels was statistically significant, while remaining within normal ranges.

Post-absorptive Nutrient Partitioning: Testosterone and Growth Hormone

Another potential target for drug treatment is modulation of metabolic processes. Although not yet tested in large clinical trials, testosterone and growth hormone therapy have been shown to have positive effects on body fat and body fat distribution. Studies evaluating the effect of growth hormone replacement therapy in multiple pituitary hormone deficiencies (92,93) or isolated growth hormone deficiency (94,95) show that growth hormone is an important regulator of intra-abdominal fat mass. Recently two studies showed that growth hormone treatment reduces the size of total abdominal fat (95) subcutaneous fat (94), as well as intra-abdominal fat mass (94,95). Mårin *et al.* (96) treated 23 middle-aged abdominally obese men with oral testosterone supplements for 8 months. Visceral fat mass, measured by computerised tomography, decreased significantly without a change in body mass, subcutaneous fat mass or lean body mass.

EFFECTS OF PHARMACOLOGICAL TREATMENT ON WEIGHT MAINTENANCE (Table 31.5)

Long-term results of weight loss programmes are often disappointing. This was shown by the work of

Table 31.5 Long-lasting effects of drug therapy on weight: 1- and 2-year trials

Study	Duration (years)	Dose (mg/day)	Subjects (n) Drug/Placebo	Weight change (kg) Drug/Placebo	Weight change (%) Drug/Placebo	Remarks
Desfenfluramine						
Guy-Grand et al. (63)	1	30	404/418	−9.8/−7.1	−10.3/−7.2	INDEX trial; Diet dependent on usual practice of each centre
Andersen et al. (99)	1	30	21/21	−10/−9	−10.8/−8.4	Part of INDEX trial; Diet: VLCD
Mathus-Vliegen et al. (100)	1	30	36/39	−10.7/−8.0	−9.6/−7.3	Part of INDEX trial
Pfohl et al. (101)	1	30	24/24	−10.9/−9.6	−11.2/−9.1	Part of INDEX trial
Sibutramine						
Jones et al. (65)	1	10	161/163	−6.2/−2.2	−7.1/−2.5	
		15	161/163	−6.9/−2.2	−7.9/−2.5	Weight maintenance after 4 weeks of VLCD treatment. Maintenance phase: dose could be increased up to 20 mg/day; % weight loss calculated from overall start weight; Diet: 600 kcal/day deficit
Apfelbaum et al. (66)	1	10	82/78	−5.2/+0.5	−5.4/+0.5	
James et al. (68)	2	10	206/57	−10.2/−4.7	−9.6/−4.6	
Orlistat						
James et al. (102)	1	360	23/23	−8.4/−2.6	−8.4/−2.6	Diet: 600 kcal/day deficit
Finer et al. (103)	1	360	108/110	−8.3/−5.3	−8.5/−5.4	Diet: 600 kcal/day deficit
Sjöström et al. (64)	1	360	343/340	−10.3/−6.1	−10.2/−6.1	Weight reduction phase; Diet: 600 kcal/day deficit
Hollander et al. (90)	1	360	162/159	−6.2/−4.3	−6.2/−4.3	Type 2 diabetics. Diet: 500 kcal/day deficit
Davidson et al. (91)	1	360	657/223	−8.8/−5.8	−8.7/−5.8	Weight reduction phase; Diet: 600 kcal/day deficit
Hill et al. (97)	1	90	187/188	−5.1/−5.9	−5.9/−6.4	Weight maintenance (eucaloric diet) after 6 months of conventional dieting (1000 kcal/day deficit)
		180	173/188	−6.2/−5.9	−6.7/−6.4	
		360	181/188	−7.2/−5.9	−8.2/−6.4	
Rössner S et al. (98)	2	180	239/237	−8.5/−6.4	−8.6/−6.6	Diet: 1st year 600 kcal/day deficit; 2nd year weight maintenance diet
		360	242/237	−9.4/−6.4	−9.7/−6.6	

Toubro and Astrup (27). After a marked weight loss in obese patients using traditional energy restriction supported by an anorectic/thermogenic compound, the subjects entered a 1-year weight maintenance programme and were randomized to careful instruction in either calorie counting with a fixed energy intake, or to an *ad libitum* low-fat high-carbohydrate diet. Both groups were seen as outpatients and had regular reinforced advice during booster sessions. At the end of the programme 1 year later, patients were seen for follow-up. It is clear that even in the hands of a specialized team, a considerable number of patients could not maintain their weight loss. These results show that continuous pharmacological treatment should be considered in patients who have lost weight, but are unable to maintain this reduced weight in the long term. Efficient pharmacotherapy should be considered for weight maintenance purposes as recently shown in a number of clinical trials (66,68,97,98).

Very low calorie diets (VLCDs) are often used to achieve a rapid and substantial weight loss. However, long-term maintenance of this weight loss has been shown to be difficult (104). Pharmacotherapy could be useful to maintain or even improve the initial weight loss with VLCDs. Finer *et al.* (105) evaluated the efficacy of dexfenfluramine treatment for 6 months in obese patients who had lost weight by means of VLCDs. Patients continued on a hypocaloric diet and either placebo or 15 mg dexfenfluramine twice daily. Patients treated with dexfenfluramine lost an additional 5.8 kg to the weight lost during VLCD; placebo-treated patients, however, regained 2.9 kg of the weight lost during VLCD. The recent study by Apfelbaum *et al.* (66) showed similar results for treatment with sibutramine after VLCD: the sibutramine-treated group lost an additional 5.2 kg compared to a weight gain of 0.5 kg in the placebo treated group.

The STORM trial (68) showed the effects of sibutramine on weight maintenance after an initial weight loss period with sibutramine 10 mg and a hypocaloric diet calculated from measured basal metabolic rate. In a study by Hill *et al.* (97), a 24-week period of a hypoenergetic diet, calculated from estimated energy expenditure, was followed by 1-year treatment with orlistat 30 mg tid, 60 mg tid or 120 mg tid or placebo treatment. After 1 year, subjects treated with 120 mg orlistat regained less weight than placebo-treated patients (32.8% versus 58.7%). Another recent 2-year trial (98) studying the effect of orlistat 60 or 120 mg on weight loss and weight maintenance demonstrated that, after an initial weight loss phase with orlistat (60 or 120 mg tid) combined with a hypocaloric diet, orlistat 60 or 120 mg tid combined with a weight maintenance diet was associated with less weight regain compared to placebo.

EFFECTS OF PHARMACOLOGICAL TREATMENT ON ABDOMINAL FAT DISTRIBUTION

Numerous studies have shown that the health risk associated with obesity is more closely related to visceral fat (3) than to a more peripheral fat distribution. Weight loss, independent of the therapy used, is associated with loss of visceral fat (106). As stated in Table 31.2 the ideal anti-obesity drug preferentially reduces abdominal fat mass.

Visser *et al.* (107) investigated the effect of fluoxetine on visceral fat reduction, but could not demonstrate any significant effect. In a study by Marks *et al.* (108) treatment with dexfenfluramine in obese type 2 diabetic subjects resulted in a selective reduction of visceral fat area, measured by magnetic resonance imaging. Meta-analysis of four long-term studies with sibutramine showed a significantly greater decrease in waist circumference, as an indicator of visceral fat mass, in sibutramine-treated subjects compared with those receiving placebo (53). The same paper reported on the preliminary data on absolute changes in visceral fat, measured by computed tomography (CT) scan, after 6 months of treatment with sibutramine, as part of the STORM trial. In these patients visceral fat decreased by 22%, which was associated with significant decreases in associated risk factors such as fasting glucose and insulin and serum triglycerides. Reduction in blood pressure was most significant in subjects with the largest visceral fat reduction (53). However, studies comparing the effect of caloric restriction with that of pharmacotherapy without caloric restriction are needed to determine the role of pharmacotherapy in reducing visceral fat (106).

FUTURE PROSPECTS WITH PROMISING MOLECULES

Recent years have been very exciting for researchers

working in the field of obesity. The discovery of the *ob* gene and its product leptin (109) has stimulated research in the field of genetics and molecular biology, with rapid advances being made in the understanding of weight-regulating mechanisms. This has led to the identification of a series of potential new targets for the treatment of obesity. However, experience has shown that it is not easy to translate this knowledge into clinically safe and effective pharmacological compounds. An important reason is that results found in laboratory animals are not always reproducible in human subjects. We will focus on a few of these newly identified targets and the corresponding compounds in development, which can be divided into those acting on energy intake and those acting on energy expenditure (110).

Drugs Altering Energy Intake

Appetite and food intake are modulated by several hormones and neurotransmitters acting in a complex interaction. Two major systems can be identified: the short-term regulation of food intake with cholecystokinin (CCK) and glucagon-like-peptide 1 (GLP-1) as major representatives and the long-term regulation of food intake through the leptin system. Recent data seem to suggest an interaction between these two weight-regulating systems (111–113).

Cholecystokin and Glucagon-like Peptide 1

Cholecystokinin and GLP-1 are both gastrointestinal hormones secreted by the duodenum in the presence of food. Cholecystokinin inhibits gastric emptying, contracts the pyloric sphincter and stimulates gallbladder contraction and pancreatic exocrine secretion (114). Intravenous infusion of cholecystokinin or GLP-1 has a satiety effect in both lean (115,116) and obese subjects (115,117). The satiety effect of cholecystokinin is mediated through its type A receptor found in the periphery and the central nervous system (118). Cholecystokinin agonists could be useful in the treatment of obesity but should be orally active, selective for the CCK-A receptor and should have a long biological half-life (119).

Glucagon-like peptide is an incretin hormone, stimulating the pancreatic secretion of insulin after

food intake (120). In this context, GLP-1 has been extensively studied as an anti-diabetic agent and could be particularly useful for the obese type 2 diabetic patient through its action on both hyperglycaemia and food intake (121). However, GLP-1 is metabolized very quickly by the dipeptidyl-peptidase IV (DPP-IV) enzyme (122), making it difficult to turn GLP-1 into a clinical useful therapeutic agent. Recently, considerable effort has been put into the development of DPP-IV resistant analogues of GLP-1 (123), DPP-IV inhibitors (124) and GLP-1 receptor agonists such as exendin-4 (125).

The Leptin System

Since the discovery of leptin in 1994 (109), extensive research has shown that is more than just a simple mediator of energy intake and expenditure and that it plays a role in different physiological processes such as reproduction and insulin secretion (126).

Leptin was first discovered through the *ob/ob* mouse, where due to a mutation in the *ob* gene, no leptin is secreted (109). In these animals, treatment with leptin resulted in reduction of body weight (109). Obese humans, however, appear to have elevated leptin levels correlating with the amount of body fat (127). In a few cases mutations in the obese gene (128,129) or the leptin receptor gene (130) have been described. Treatment of a 9-year-old girl with a congenital leptin deficiency with recombinant leptin resulted in an important reduction of body weight, predominantly body fat (131).

The use of leptin as an anti-obesity agent is limited by the fact that it has to be given subcutaneously and in very high doses, which could result in inflammatory reactions at the injection site. More promising perspectives will probably come from leptin analogues and leptin receptor agonists.

Leptin exerts its action through different neurotransmitters such as neuropeptide Y (NPY), glucagon-like peptide 1 (GLP-1), α-melanocyte-stimulating hormone (α-MSH), corticotrophin-releasing hormone (CRH) and cocaine and amphetamine regulated transcript (132,133). Extensive research has been done on the role of these peptides in the regulation of food intake in both animals and humans.

Two major pathways of post-receptor leptin signalling effects can be described: the NPY pathway leading to a decrease in food intake and the pro-opiomelanocortin pathway with an opposite effect.

NPY is one of the most potent stimulators of food intake (134) and six different receptor subtypes have been cloned. The type 1 and type 5 receptors appear to be most important receptors in the regulation of food intake (135,136). Several NPY receptor antagonists are now in different stages of preclinical and clinical development.

Melanocortins are peptides cleaved from its precursor pro-opiomelanocortin, with α-MSH being the most important melanocortin in the regulation of food intake (137). It binds to the melanocortin receptors MC3-R and MC4-R, resulting in a decrease in food intake (138). The agouti-related protein (AGRP) selectively antagonises MC3-R and MC4-R (139). Recently, melanin-concentrating hormone (MCH) was identified as another functional antagonist of α-MSH acting on a separate G-protein-coupled receptor, somatostatin-like receptor 1 SLC-1 (140).

The most recently discovered families of hypothalamic peptides involved in the regulation of food intake are the cocaine and amphetamine regulated transcript peptides (CART) (141) and the orexins (142) or hypocretins (143), confirming the complex neuroendocrine system of weight regulation.

Drugs Altering Energy Expenditure

The β_3-Adrenergic Receptor

The β_3 adrenergic receptor, first discovered in the early 1980s (144), is mainly located in adipose tissue and plays an important role in adrenergic stimulation of lipolysis and thermogenesis in white and brown adipose tissue. Several pharmaceutical companies have developed β_3-agonists. Early compounds yielded positive results in animals but showed rather disappointing results in humans (145,146), which could in part be explained by the substantial differences between the animal and human receptor (144,147). After the cloning of the human receptor in 1989 (148), new highly selective compounds were developed (147). However, the effectiveness of β_3-adrenergic receptor agonists remains questionable since the amount of brown adipose tissue in humans is very small (147).

Uncoupling Proteins

Uncoupling proteins (UCPs) are mitochondrial proteins that uncouple adenosine triphosphate (ATP) production from mitochondrial respiration, producing heat leading to a net increase in energy utilization (149). UCP1 was identified in the 1980s and is mainly located in brown adipose tissue (150). Recently two new uncoupling proteins were identified: UCP2 is widely expressed in human tissues (151) and UCP3 (152) is found predominantly in skeletal muscle. Many papers have focused on the expression of UCP1 (153–155), UCP2 (156) and UCP3 (157) in obesity and type 2 diabetes, yielding conflicting results.

CONCLUSION

Despite the extensive research performed with dexfenfluramine, this drug was withdrawn from the market because of its association with cardiac valvulopathy. New drugs such as sibutramine and orlistat are replacing dexfenfluramine.

Both sibutramine and orlistat have been shown to be efficacious, with a mean weight loss of approximately 10% of baseline body weight. This is in line with recent recommendations that a modest weight reduction up to 10% has important beneficial health effects. In clinical trials, however, the net benefit above placebo results seems less spectacular. However, it should be kept in mind that these results have been obtained under strictly controlled conditions, also for the placebo groups. The future will show whether these effects will be as positive and as long-lasting in daily life conditions.

It is important to acknowledge that on an individual basis the clinician's decision to treat an obese patient with weight loss medication may be a reasonable one, despite the uncertainties about the long-term benefits of pharmacotherapy in the population. We learned that from the dexfenfluramine experience. For some obese patients, who respond well to these drugs and can tolerate the adverse effects, pharmacotherapy is undoubtedly beneficial, as stated recently by Williamson in an editorial comment (158).

The benefit risk ratio of the new anti-obesity drugs is not yet possible to determine because of the lack of long-term evaluation of their safety. Obesity is now recognized as a serious health problem and given the lack of long-term success of non-surgical and non-pharmacological treatments for obesity, there is clearly a need for efficient weight-reducing drugs (159). Since 10% weight loss may not be enough for seriously obese subjects, the search is on for even more effective compounds. The development of such new compounds, acting on different mechanisms, is urgently required: they include leptin analogues, NPY antagonists, orexins, glucagon-like peptide and other promising compounds.

REFERENCES

1. WHO *Obesity: Preventing and Managing the Global Epidemic: Report of a WHO Consultation on Obesity.* Geneva, June 3–5, 1997. Geneva: World Health Organization.

2. Després JP, Lemieux S, Lamarche B. The insulin resistance-dyslipidemic syndrome: contribution to visceral obesity and therapeutic implications. *Int J Obes Relat Metab Disord* 1995; **19**: S76–S86.

3. Van Gaal LF, Mertens IL. Effects of obesity on cardiovascular system and blood pressure control, digestive disease and cancer. In: Kopelman P, Stock M (eds) *Clinical Obesity*, Oxford: Blackwell Science, 1998, 205–225.

4. Van Gaal LF. Dietary treatment of obesity. In: Bray GA, Bouchard C, James WPT (eds) *Handbook of Obesity*, New York: Marcel Dekker, 1998, 875–890.

5. Vansant G, Muls E. New directions in public health approach to obesity management. *Acta Clin Belg* 1999; **54**: 151–153.

6. North American Association for the Study of Obesity. Guidelines for the approval and use of drugs to treat obesity. *Obes Res* 1995; **3**: 473–478.

7. Institute of Medicine. *Weighing the Options. Criteria for Evaluating Weight Management Programs.* Washington DC: National Acadamy Press, 1995: 1–282.

8. National Institutes of Health, National Heart, Lung and Blood Institute. Clinical guidelines on the identification, evaluation, and treatment of overweight and obesity in adults. Bethesda, MD: Department of Health and Human Services, 1998.

9. Scottish Intercollegiate Guidelines Network (SIGN). *Obesity in Scotland. Integrating Prevention with Weight Management.* Edinburgh: HMSO, 1996.

10. Royal College of Physicians. *Clinical Management of Overweight and Obese Patients with Particular Reference to the Use of Drugs.* The Royal College Physicians of London, December 1998.

11. Goldstein D. Beneficial health effects of modest weight loss. *Int J Obes Relat Metab Disord* 1992; **16**: 397–415.

12. Van Gaal L, Wauters M, De Leeuw I. The beneficial effects of modest weight loss on cardiovascular risk factors. *Int J Obes Relat Metab Disord* 1997; **21**(Suppl 1): S5–S9.

13. Scheen AJ, Lefèbvre PJ. Pharmacological treatment of obesity: present status. *Int J Obes Relat Metab Disord* 1999; **23**(Suppl 1): 47–53.

14. Flechtner-Mors M, Ditschuneit HH, Yip I, Adler G. Blood pressure and plasma norepinephrine responses to dexfenfluramine in obese postmenopausal women. *Am J Clin Nutr* 1998; **67**: 611–615.

15. Kolanowski J, Younis LT, Vanbutsele R, Detry JM. Effect of dexfenfluramine treatment on body weight, blood pressure and noradrenergic activity in obese hypertensive patients. *Eur J Clin Pharmacol* 1992; **42**: 599–606.

16. Hvizdos KM, Markham A. Orlistat. A review of its use in the management of obesity. *Drugs* 1999; **58**: 743–760.

17. Sjöström L, Larsson B, Backman L, *et al.* Swedish Obese Subjects (SOS): recruitment for an intervention study and a selected description of the obese state. *Int J Obes Relat Metab Disord* 1992; **16**: 465–479.

18. Abenhaim L, Moride Y, Brenot F, Rich S, Benichou J, Kurz X, Higenbottam T, Oakley C, Wouters E, Aubier M, Simonneau G, Bégaud B for the International Primary Pulmonary Hypertension Study Group. Appetite-suppressant drugs and the risk of pulmonary hypertension. *N Engl J Med* 1996; **335**: 609–616.

19. Connolly HM, Crary JL, McGoon MD, Hensrud DD, Edwards BS, Edwards WD, Schaff HV. Valvular heart disease associated with fenfluramine-phentermine. *N Engl J Med* 1997; **337**: 581–588.

20. Bray G. Drug treatment of obesity: don't throw the baby out with the bath water. *Am J Clin Nutr* 1998; **67**: 1–2.

21. Atkinson RL. Use of drugs in the treatment of obesity. *Ann Rev Nutr* 1997; **17**: 383–403.

22. Bray GA. Evaluation of drugs for treating obesity. *Obes Res* 1995; **3**(Suppl 4): 425S–434S.

23. Finer N. Present and future pharmaceutical approaches. *Bri Med Bull* 1997; **53**: 409–432.

24. Bray GA, Ryan DH. Drugs used in the treatment of obesity. *Diabetes Rev* 1997; **5**: 83–103.

25. Arch JRS, Wilson S. Prospects for β3-adrenoceptor agonists in the treatment of obesity and diabetes. *Int J Obes Relat Metab Disord* 1996; **20**: 191–199.

26. Astrup A, Lundsgaard C. What do pharmacological approaches to obesity management offer? *Exp Clin Endocrinol Diabetes* 1998; **106**(Suppl 2): 29–34.

27. Toubro S, Astrup A. Randomised comparison of diets for maintaining obese subjects' weight after major weight loss: ad lib, low fat, high carbohydrate diet vs fixed energy intake. *Br Med J* 1997; **314**: 29–34.

28. Finer N, James WPT, Kopelman PG, Lean MEJ, Williams G. One-year treatment of obesity: a randomised, double-blind, placebo-controlled, multicentre study of orlistat, a gastrointestinal lipase inhibitor. *Int J Obes* 2000; **24**: 306–313.

29. National Task Force on Obesity. Long-term pharmacotherapy in the management of obesity. *JAMA* 1996; **276**: 1907–1915.

30. Bild DE, Sholinsky P, Smith DE, Lewis CE, Hardin JM, Burke GL. Correlates and predictors of weight loss in young adults: the CARDIA study. *Int J Obes Relat Metab Disord* 1996; **20**: 47–55.

31. Wadden TA, Foster GD, Wang J, Pierson RN, Yang MU, Moreland K, Stunkard AJ, VanItallie TB. Clinical correlates of short- and long-term weight loss. *Am J Clin Nutr* 1992; **27**: 1S–4S.

32. Astrup A, Buemann B, Gluud C, Bennett P, Tjur T, Christensen N. Prognostic markers for diet-induced weight loss in obese women *Int J Obes Relat Metab Disord* 1995; **19**: 275–278.

33. Sherwood NE, Jeffery RW, Wing RR. Binge eating status as a predictor of weight loss outcome. *Int J Obes Relat Metab Disord* 1999; **23**: 485–493.

34. Pasman WJ, Saris WHM, Westerterp-Plantenga MS. Predictors of weight maintenance. *Obes Res* 1999; **7**: 43–50.

35. Toornvliet AC, Pijl H, Hopman E, Westendorp RG, Meinders AE. Predictors of weight loss during treatment with d-fenfluramine. *J Intern Med* 1997; **241**: 401–406.

36. Bray GA, Blackburn GL, Ferguson JM, Greenway FL, Jain AK, Mendel CM, Mendels J, Ryan DH, Schwartz SL, Scheinbaum ML, Seaton TB. Sibutramine produces dose-related weight loss. *Obes Res* 1999; **7**: 189–198.

37. Rissanen A, Sjöström L, Rössner S. Early weight loss with orlistat as a predictor of long-term success in obesity treatment (Abstract). *Int J Obes Relat Metab Disord* 1999; **23**(Suppl 5): S174.

38. Guy-Grand B. Clinical studies with dexfenfluramine: from past to future. *Obes Res* 1995; **3**(Suppl 4): 491S–496S.

39. Jick H, Vasilakis C, Weinrauch LA, Meier CR, Jick SS, Derby LE. A population-based study of appetite-suppressant drugs and the risk of cardiac-valve regurgation. *N Engl J Med* 1998; **325**: 719–724.

40. Kahn MA, Herzog CA, St Peter JV, Hartley GG, Madlon-Kay R, Dick CC, Asinger RW, Vessey JT. The prevalence of cardiac valvular insufficiency assessed by transthoracic echocardiography in obese patients treated with appetite-supressant drugs. *N Engl J Med* 1998; **339**: 713–718.

41. Weissman NJ, Tighe JF, Gottdiener JS, Gwynne JT, for the Sustained-Release Dexfenfluramine Study Group. An assessment of heart-valve abnormalities in obese patients taking dexfenfluramine, sustained-release dexfenfluramine, or placebo. *N Engl J Med* 1998; **325**: 725–732.

42. Devereux RB. Appetite suppressants and valvular heart disease. *N Engl J Med* 1998; **339**: 765–767.

43. Robiolio PA, Rigolin VH, Wilson JS, Harrison JK, Sanders LL, Bashore TM, Feldman JM. Correlation of high serotonin levels with valvular abnormalities detected by cardiac catheterization and echocardiography. *Circulation* 1995; **92**: 790–795.

44. Fuller RW, Wong DT. Fluoxetine: a serotonergic appetite suppressant drug. *Drug Devel Res* 1988; **17**: 1–15.

45. Daubresse J, Kolanowski J, Krzentowski M, Kutnowski M, Scheen A, Van Gaal L. Usefulness of fluoxetine in obese non-insulin dependent diabetics. A multicenter study. *Obes Res* 1996; **4**: 391–396.

46. Dulloo AG (ed.). Ephedrine, xanthines, aspirin and other thermogenic drugs to assist the dietary management of obesity. *Int J Obes Relat Metab Disord* 1993; **17**(Suppl 1): S1–S83.

47. Astrup A, Breum L, Toubro S. Pharmacological and clinical studies of ephedrine and other thermogenic agonists. *Obes Res* 1995; **3**(Suppl 4): 537S–540S.

48. Liu YL, Toubro S, Astrup A, Stock MJ. Contribution of beta3-adrenoceptor activation to ephedrine-induced thermogenesis in humans. *Int J Obes Relat Metab Disord* 1995; **19**: 678–685.

49. Bucket WR, Thomas PC, Luscombe GP. The pharmacology of sibutramine hydrochloride, a new anti-depressant which induces rapid nor-adrenergic down regulation. *Prog Neuropsychopharmacol Biol Psychiatry* 1988; **12**: 575–584.

50. Lean ME. Sibutramine: a review of clinical efficacy. *Int J*

51. Cheetham SC, Viggers JA, Slater NA, Heal DJ, Buckett WR. [3H]Paroxetine binding in rat frontal cortex strongly correlates with 5HT uptake: effect of administration of various anti-depressant treatments. *Neuropharmacology* 1993; **32**: 737–743.

52. Bach DS, Rissanen AM, Mendel CM, Shepherd G, Weinstein SP, Kelly F, Seaton TB, Patel B, Pekkarinen TA, Armstrong WF. Absence of cardiac valve dysfunction in obese patients treated with sibutramine (Abstract). *Int J Obes Relat Metab Disord* 1998; **22**(Suppl 3): S76.

53. Van Gaal LF, Wauters MA, De Leeuw IH. Anti-obesity drugs: what does sibutramine offer? An analysis of its potential contribution to obesity treatment. *Exp Clin Endocrinol Diabetes* 1998; **106**(Suppl 2): 35–39.

54. Heal DJ, Prow MR, Gosden J, Luscombe GP, Buckett WR. A comparison of various antidepressant drugs demonstrates rapid desensitisation of alpha2-adrenoceptors exclusively by sibutramine hydrochloride. *Psychopharmacology* 1992; **107**: 497–502.

55. McNeely W, Goa KL. Sibutramine. A review of its contribution to the management of obesity. *Drugs* 1998; **56**: 1093–1124.

56. Heal DJ, Butler SA, Hurst EM, Buckett WR. Antidepressant treatments, including sibutramine hydrochloride and electroconvulsive shock, decrease beta-1- but not beta-2-adrenoceptors in rat cortex. *J Neurochem* 1989; **53**: 1019–1025.

57. Stock MJ. Sibutramine: a review of the pharmacology of a novel anti-obesity agent. *Int J Obes Relat Metab Disord* 1997; **21**(Suppl 1): S25–S29.

58. Cheetham SC, Kettle CJ, Martin KF, Heal DJ. D1 receptor binding in rat striatum: modification by various D1 and D2 antagonists, but not by sibutramine hydrochloride, antidepressants or treatments which enhance central dopaminergic function. *J Neural Transm Gen Sect* 1995; **102**: 35–46.

59. Martin KF, Needham PL, Atkinson J, Cowan A, Heal DJ, Buckett WR. Rat striatal and mesolimbic D1 receptor binding is not altered by antidepressant treatments including ECS and sibutramine HCL (Abstract). *Br J Pharmacol* 1988; **95**: 896P.

60. Martin KF, Philips I, Cheetham SC, Heal DJ. Dopamine D-2 receptors: a potential pharmacological target for nomifense and tranylcypromine but not other antidepressant treatments. *Pharmacol Biochem Behav* 1995; **51**: 565–569.

61. Bray GA, Ryan DH, Gordon D, Heidingsfelder S, Cerise F, Wilson K. A double-blind randomized placebo-controlled trial of sibutramine. *Obes Res* 1996; **4**: 263–270.

62. Weintraub M, Rubio A, Golik A, Byrne L. Sibutramine in weight control: a dose-ranging, efficacy study. *Clin Pharmacol Ther* 1991; **50**: 330–337.

63. Guy-Grand B, Crepaldi G, Lefebvre P, Apfelbaum M, Gries A, Turner P. International trial of long-term dexfenfluramine in obesity. *Lancet* 1989; **ii**: 1142–1145.

64. Sjöström L, Rissanen A, Andersen T, Boldrin M, Golay A, Koppeschaar HPF, Krempf M, for the European Multicentre Orlistat Study Group. Randomized placebo-controlled trial of orlistat for weight loss and prevention of weight regain in obese patients. *Lancet* 1998; **352**: 167–173.

65. Jones SP, Smith IG, Kelly F, Gray JA. Long-term weight

Obes Relat Metabolic Disord 1997; **21**(Suppl 1): 30–36.

loss with sibutramine (Abstract). *Int J Obes Relat Metab Disord* 1995; **19**(Suppl 2): 41.

66. Apfelbaum M, Vague P, Ziegler O, Hanotin C, Thomas F, Leutenegger E. Long-term maintenance of weight loss after a VLCD diet: a randomized blinded trial of the efficacy and tolerability of sibutramine. *Am J Med* 1999; **106**: 179–184.

67. Goldstein DJ, Potvin JH. Long-term weight loss: the effect of pharmacologic agents. *Am J Clin Nut* 1994; **60**: 647–657.

68. James WPT, Astrup A, Finer N, Hilsted J, Kopelman P, Rössner S, Saris WHM, Van Gaal LF, for the STORM Study Group. Effect of sibutramine on weight maintenance after weight loss: a randomised trial. *Lancet* 2000; **356**: 2119–2125.

69. Astrup A, Hansen D, Lundsgaard C, Toubro S. Sibutramine and energy balance. *Int J Obes Relat Metab Disord* 1998; **22**(Suppl 1), S30–S35.

70. Van Gaal L, Wauters M, Peiffer FW, De Leeuw IH. Sibutramine and fat distribution: is there a role for pharmacotherapy in abdominal/visceral fat reduction. *Int J Obes Relat Metab Disord* 1998; **22**(Suppl 1): S38–S40.

71. Stock MJ, Hansen L, Toubro S, Macdonald I, Astrup A. Sibutramine targets both sides of the energy balance in humans (Abstract). *Int J Obes Relat Metab Disord* 1998; **22**(Suppl 3): S269.

72. Walsh K, Lean MEJ. The effects of sibutramine on resting energy expenditure and adrenaline-induced thermogenesis in obese females with dyslipidaemia (Abstract). *Int J Obes Relat Metab Disord* 1998; **22**(Suppl 3): S269.

73. Lissner L, Heitmann B. Dietary fat and obesity: evidence from epidemiology. *Eur J Clin Nutr* 1995; **49**: 79–90.

74. Drent ML, van der Veen EA. Lipase inhibition: a novel concept in the treatment of obesity. *Int J Obes Relat Metab Disord* 1993; **17**: 241–244.

75. Hauptman JB, Jeunet FS, Hartmann D. Initial studies in humans with the novel gastrointestinal lipase inhibitor Ro18-0647 (tetrahydrolipstatin). *Am J Clin Nutr* 1992; **55**: 309S–313S.

76. Hadvary P, Lengsfeld H, Wolfer H. Inhibition of pancreatic lipase in vitro by the covalent inhibitor tetrahydrolipstatin. *Biochem J* 1988; **256**: 357–361.

77. Borgström B. Mode of action of tetrahydrolipstatin: a derivative of the naturally occurring lipase inhibitor lipstatin. *Biochim Biophys Acta* 1988; **962**: 308–316.

78. Zhi J, Melia AT, Eggers H, Joly R, Patel IH. Review of limited systemic absorption of orlistat, a lipase inhibitor, in healthy human volunteers. *J Clin Pharmacol* 1995; **35**: 1103–1108.

79. Zhi J, Melia AT, Funk C, Viger-Chougnet A, Hopfgartner G, Lausecker B, Wang K, Fulton JS, Gabriel L, Mulligan TE. Metabolic profiles of minimally absorbed orlistat in obese/overweight volunteers. *J Clin Pharmacol* 1996; **36**: 1006–1011.

80. Zhi J, Melia AT, Guerciolini R, Koss-Twardy SG, Passe SM, Rakhit A, Sadowski JA. The effect of tetrahydrolipstatin on the pharmacokinetics and pharmacodynamics of warfarin in healthy volunteers. *J Clin Pharmacol* 1996; + **36**: 659–666.

81. Zhi J, Melia AT, Koss-Twardy SG, Min B, Guerciolini R, Freundlich NL, Milla G, Patel IH. The influence of orlistat on the pharmacokinetics and pharmacodynamics of glyburide in healthy volunteers. *J Clin Pharmacol* 1995; **35**: 521–525.

82. Oo CY, Akbari B, Lee S. Effect of orlistat, a novel anti-obesity agent, on the pharmacokinetics and pharmacodynamics of pravastatin in patients with mild hypercholesterolaemia. *Clin Drug Invest* 1999; **17**: 217–223.

83. Melia AT, Zhi J, Koss-Twardy SG, Min Bh, Smith BL, Freundlich NL, Arora S, Passe SM. The influence of reduced dietary fat absorption induced by orlistat on the pharmacokinetics of digoxin in healthy volunteers. *J Clin Pharmacol* 1995; **35**: 840–843.

84. Melia AT, Mulligan TE, Zhi J. Lack of effect of orlistat on the bioavailability of a single dose of nifedipine extended-release tablets (Procardia XL) in healthy volunteers. *J Clin Pharmacol* 1996; **36**: 352–355.

85. Melia AT, Mulligan TE, Zhi J. The effect of orlistat on the pharmacokinetics of phenytoin in healthy volunteers. *J Clin Pharmacol* 1996; **36**: 654–658.

86. Hartmann D, Güzelhan C, Zuiderwijk PBM. Lack of interaction between orlistat and oral contraceptives. *Eur J Clin Pharmacol* 1996; **50**: 421–424.

87. Melia AT, Zhi J, Zelasko R, Hartmann D, Guzelhan C, Guerciolini R, Odink J. The interaction of the lipase inhibitor orlistat with ethanol in healthy volunteers. *Eur J Clin Pharmacol* 1998; **54**: 773–777.

88. Drent ML, Larsson I, Williams-Olssen T. Orlistat (RO 18-0647), a lipase inhibitor, in the treatment of human obesity: a multiple dose study. *Int J Obes Relat Metab Disord* 1995; **19**: 221–226.

89. Van Gaal LF, Broom J, Enzi G, Toplak H. The orlistat dose-ranging study group. Efficacy and tolerability of orlistat in the treatment of obesity: a 6 month dose ranging study. *Eur J Clin Pharmacol* 1998; **54**: 125–132.

90. Hollander PA, Elbein SC, Hirsch IB, Kelley D, McGill J, Taylor T, Weiss SR, Crockett SE, Kaplan RA, Comstock J, Lucas CP, Lodewick PA, Canovatchel W, Chung J, Hauptman J. Role of orlistat in the treatment of obese patients with type 2 diabetes. *Diabetes Care* 1998; **21**: 1288–1294.

91. Davidson MH, Hauptman J, DiGirolamo M, Foreyt JP, Halsted CH, Heber D, Heimburger DC, Lucas CP, Robbins DC, Chung J, Heymsfield SB. Weight control and risk factor reduction in obese subjects treated for 2 years with orlistat. *JAMA* 1999; **281**: 235–242.

92. Bengtsson BA, Edén S, Lönn L, Kvist H, Stokland A, Lindstedt G, Bosaeus I, Tölli J, Sjöström L, Isaksson OGP. Treatment of adults with growth hormone (GH) deficiency with recombinant human growth hormone. *J Clin Endocrinol Metab* 1993; **76**: 309–317.

93. Snel YEM, Brummer RJM, Doerga ME, Zelissen PMJ, Bakker AJG, Hendriks MJ, Koppeschaar HPF. Adipose tissue assessed by magnetic imaging in growth hormone-deficient adults: the effect of growth hormone replacement and a comparison with control subjects. *Am J Clin Nutr* 1995; **61**: 1290–1294.

94. de Boer H, Blok GJ, Voerman B, Derriks P, van der Veen E. Changes in subcutaneous and visceral fat mass during growth hormone replacement therapy in adult men. *Int J Obes Relat Metab Disord* 1996; **20**: 580–587.

95. Johansson G, Marin P, Lönn L, Ottosson M, Stenlöf K, Björntorp P, Sjöström L, Bengtsson B. Growth hormone treatment of abdominally obese men, reduces abdominal fat mass, improves glucose and lipoprotein metabolism and

reduces diastolic blood pressure. *J Clin Endocrinol Metab* 1997; **82**: 727–734.

96. Mårin P, Holmäng, Jönsson L, Sjöström L, Kvist H, Holm G, Lindstedt G, Björntorp P. The effects of testosterone treatment on body composition and metabolism in middle-aged obese men. *Int J Obes Relat Metab Disord* 1992; **16**: 991–997.

97. Hill JO, Hauptmann J, Anderson JW, Fujioka K, O'Neil PM, Smith DK, Zavoral JH, Aronne LJ. Orlistat, a lipase inhibitor, for weight maintenance after conventional dieting: a 1-y study. *Am J Clin Nutr* 1999; **69**: 1108–1116.

98. Rössner S, Sjöström L, Noack R, Meinders AE, Noseda G, on behalf of the European Orlistat Obesity Study Group. Weight loss, weight maintenance, and improved cardiovascular risk factors after 2 years treatment with orlistat for obesity. *Obes Res* 2000; **8**: 49–61.

99. Andersen T, Astrup A, Quaade F. Dexfenfluramine as adjuvant to low-calorie formula diet in the treatment of obesity: a randomized clinical trial. *Int J Obes Relat Metab Disord* 1992; **16**: 35–40.

100. Mathus-Vliegen EMH, Van De Voorde K, Kok AME, Res AMA. Dexfenfluramine in the treatment of severe obesity: a placebo-controlled investigation of the effects on weight loss, cardiovascular risk factors, food intake and eating behaviour. *J Intern Med* 1992; **232**: 119–127.

101. Pfohl M, Luft D, Blomberg I, Schmülling RM. Long term changes of body weight and cardiovascular risk factors after weight reduction with group therapy and dexfenfluramine. *Int J Obes Relat Metab Disord* 1994; **18**: 391–395.

102. James WP, Avenell A, Broom J, Whitehead J. A one-year trial to assess the value of orlistat in the management of obesity. *Int J Obes Relat Metab Disord* 1997; **21**(Suppl 3): S24–30.

103. Finer N, for the UK Orlistat Group Weight reduction with orlistat and effects on risk factors: a 1-year UK study (Abstract). *Int J Obes Relat Metab Disord* 1997; **21**(Suppl 2): S31.

104. Wadden TA. Treatment of obesity by moderate and severe caloric restriction. Results of clinical research trials. *Ann Intern Med* 1993; **119**: 688–693.

105. Finer N, Finer S, Naoumova RP. Drug therapy after very-low-calorie diets. *Am J Clin Nutr* 1992; **56**: 195S–198S.

106. Smith SR, Zachwieja JJ. Visceral adipose tissue: a critical review of intervention strategies. *Int J Obes Relat Metab Disord* 1999; **23**: 329–335.

107. Visser M, Seidell JC, Koppeschaar HP, Smits P. The effect of fluoxetine on body weight, body composition and visceral fat accumulation. *Int J Obes* 1993; **17**: 247–253.

108. Marks SJ, Moore NR, Clark ML, Strauss BJG, Hockaday TDR. Reduction of visceral adipose tissue and improvement of metabolic indices: effect of dexfenfluramine in NIDDM. *Obes Res* 1996; **4**: 1–7.

109. Zhang Y, Proenca R, Maffei M, Barone M, Leopold L, Friedman JM. Positional cloning of the mouse obese gene and its human homolog. *Nature* 1994; **372**: 425–432.

110. Mertens IL, Van Gaal LF. Promising new approaches to the management of obesity. *Drugs* 2000; **60**: 1–9.

111. Barrachina MD, Martinez V, Wang L, Wei JY, Taché Y. Synergistic interaction between leptin and cholecystokinin to reduce short-term food intake in lean mice. *Proc Nat*

Acad Sci USA 1997; **94**: 10455–10460.

112. Matson CA, Ritter RC. Long-term CCK-leptin synergy suggests a role for CCK in the regulation of body weight. *Am J Physiol* 1999; **45**: 1038–1045.

113. Goldstone AP, Mercer JG, Gunn I, *et al.* Leptin interacts with glucagon-like peptide-1 neurons to reduce food intake and body weight in rodents. *FEBS Lett* 1997; **415**: 134–138.

114. Fink H, Rex A, Voits M, Voigt JP. Major biological actions of CCK—a critical evaluation of research findings. *Exp Brain Res* 1998; **123**: 77–83.

115. Lieverse RJ, Jansen JBMJ, Masclee AAM, Lamers CBHW. Satiety effects of cholecystokinin in humans. *Gastroenterology* 1994; **106**: 1451–1454.

116. Flint A, Raben A, Astrup A, Holst JJ. Glucagon-like peptide 1 promotes satiety and suppresses energy intake in humans. *J Clin Invest* 1998; **101**: 515–520.

117. Näslund E, Gutniak M, Skogar S, Rössner S, Hellström PM. Glucagon-like peptide 1 increases the period of postprandial satiety and slows gastric emptying in obese men. *Am J Clin Nutr* 1998; **68**: 525–530.

118. Moran TH, Ameglio Pj, Peyton HJ, Schwartz GJ, McHugh PR. Blockade of type A, but not type B, CCK receptors postpones satiety in rhesus monkeys. *Am J Physiol* 1993; **265**: R620–R624.

119. Blundell JE, Halford CG. Pharmacological aspects of obesity treatment: towards the 21st century. *Int J Obes Relat Metab Disord* 1995; **19**(Suppl 3): S51–S55.

120. Creutzfeldt W. The incretin concept today. *Diabetologia* 1979; **16**: 75–85.

121. Holst JJ. Treatment of type 2 diabetes with glucagonlike peptide 1. *Curr Opin Endocrinol Diabetes* 1998; **5**: 108–115.

122. Deacon CF, Johnsen AH, Holst JJ. Degradation of glucagon-like peptide-1 by human plasma in vitro yields an N-terminally truncated peptide that is a major endogenous metabolite in vivo. *J Clin Endocrinol Metab* 1995; **80**: 952–957.

123. Burcelin R, Dolci W, Thorens B. Long-lasting antidiabetic effect of a dipeptidyl peptidase IV-resistant analogue of glucagon-like peptide 1. *Metabolism* 1999; **48**: 252–258.

124. Pauly RP, Demuth HU, Rosche F. Improved glucose tolerance in rats treated with the dipeptidyl peptidase IV (CD26) inhibitor in Ile-Thiazolidide. *Metabolism* 1999; **48**: 385–389.

125. Kolterman O, Fineman M, Gottlieb A, Petrella E, Pricket K, Young A. AC2993 (synthetic exendin-4) lowered postprandial plasma glucose concentrations in people with type 2 diabetes (Abstract). *Diabetologia* 1999; **42**(Suppl 1): A41.

126. Van Gaal LF, Wauters MA, Mertens IL, Considine RV, De Leeuw IH. Clinical endocrinology of human leptin. *Int J Obes Relat Metab Disord* 1999; **23**(Suppl 1): 29–36.

127. Considine RV, Sinha MK, Heiman ML, Kriauciunas A, Stephens TW, Nyce MR, Ohannesian JP, Marco CC, McKee LJ, Bauer TL, Caro JF. Serum immunoreactive-leptin concentrations in normal-weight and obese humans. *N Engl J Med* 1996; **334**: 292–295.

128. Montague CT, Farooqi IS, Whitehead JP, Soos MA, Rau H, Wareham NJ, Sewter CP, Digby JE, Mohammaed SN, Hurst JA, Cheetham CH, Early AR, Barnett AH, Prins AH, O'Rahilly S. Congenital leptin deficiency is associated with severe early-onset obesity in humans. *Nature* 1997; **387**: 903–907.

129. Strobel A, Issad T, Camoin L, Ozata M, Strosberg AD. A

leptin missense mutation associated with hypogonadism and morbid obesity. *Nat Genet* 1998; **18**: 213–215.

130. Clément K, Vaisse C, Lahlou N, Cabrol S, Pelloux V, Cassuto D, Gourmelen M, Dina C, Chambaz J, Lacorte JM, Basdevant A. A mutation in the human leptin receptor gene causes obesity and pituitary dysfunction. *Nature* 1998; **392**: 398–401.

131. Farooqi IS, Jebb SA, Langmack G, Lawrence E, Cheetham CH, Prentice AM, Hughes IA, McCamish MA, O'Rahilly S. Effects of recombinant leptin therapy in a child with congenital leptin deficiency. *N Engl J Med* 1999; **341**: 879–884.

132. Campfield LA, Smith FJ, Burn P. Strategies and potential molecular targets for obesity treatment. *Science* 1998; **280**: 1383–1387.

133. Trayhurn P, Hoggard N, Mercer JG, Rayner DV. Leptin: fundamental aspects. *Int J Obes Relat Metab Disord* 1999; **23**(Suppl 1): 22–28.

134. Clark JT, Kalra PS, Crowley WR, Kalra SP. Neuropeptide Y and human pancreatic polypeptide stimulate feeding behavior in rats. *Endocrinology* 1984; **115**: 427–429.

135. Gerald C, Walker MW, Criscione L, *et al.* A receptor subtype involved in neuropeptide-Y induced food intake. *Nature* 1996; **11**: 168–171.

136. Inui A. Neuropeptide Y feeding receptors: are multiple subtypes involved? *Trends Pharmacol Sci* 1999; **20**: 43–46.

137. Woods SC, Seeley RJ, Porte D, Schwartz MW. Signals that regulate food intake and energy homeostasis. *Science* 1998; **280**: 1378–1383.

138. Schioth HB, Muceniece R, Larsson M, Wikberg JE. The melanocortin 1,3,4 or 5 receptors do not have binding epitope for ACTH beyond the sequence of alpha-MSH. *J Endocrinol* 1997; **155**: 73–78.

139. Ollmann MM, Wilson BD, Yang YK, Kerns JA, Chen Y, Grantz I, Barsh GS. Antagonism of central melancortin receptors in vitro and in vivo by agouti-related protein. *Science* 1997; **278**: 135–138.

140. Chambers J, Ames RS, Bergsma D, Muir A, Fitzgerald LR, Hervieu G, Dytko GM, Foley JJ, Martin J, Liu WD, Park J, Ellis C, Ganguly S, Konchar S, Cluderay J, Leslie R, Wilson S, Sarau HM. Melanin-concentrating hormone is the cognate ligand for the orphan G-protein-coupled receptor SLC-1. *Nature* 1999; **400**: 261–265.

141. Kristensen P, Judge ME, Thim L, Ribel U, Christjansen Kn, Wulff BS, Clausen JT, Jensen PB, Madsen OD, Vrang N, Larsen PJ, Hastrup S. Hypothalamic CART is a new anorectic peptide regulated by leptin. *Nature* 1998; **393**: 72–76.

142. Sakurai T, Amemiya A, Ishii M, *et al.* Orexins and orexin receptors: a family of hypothalamic neuropeptides and G protein-coupled receptors that regulate feeding behavior. *Cell* 1998; **92**: 573–585.

143. De Lecea L, Kilduff TS, Peyron C, Gao XB, Foye PE, Danielson PE, Fukuhara C, Battenberg ELF, Gautvik VT, Bartlett FS, Frankel WN, van den Pol AN, Bloom FE, Gautvik KM, Sutcliffe JG. The hypocretins: hypothalamic-specific peptide with neuroexicitatory activity. *Proc Nat*

Acad Sci USA 1998; **95**: 322–327.

144. Arch JRS, Ainsworth AT. Thermogenic and antiobesity activity of a novel β-adrenoceptor agonist (BRL 26830A) in mice and rats. *Am J Clin Nutr* 1983; **38**: 549–558.

145. Fisher MH, Amend AM, Bach TJ, *et al.* A selective human β₃ adrenergic receptor agonist increases metabolic rate in rhesus monkeys. *J Clin Invest* 1998; **101**: 2387–2393.

146. Holloway BR, Howe R, Rao BS, Stribling D. ICI D7114: a novel selective adrenoceptor agonist of brown fat and thermogenesis. *Am J Clin Nutr* 1992; **55**: 262S–264S.

147. Weyer C, Gautier JF, Danforth E. Development of beta₃-adrenoceptor agonists for the treatment of obesity and diabetes—an update. *Diabetes Metab* 1999; **25**: 11–21.

148. Arch JRS. The brown adipocyte β-adrenoceptor. *Proc Nutr Soc* 1989; **48**: 215–223.

149. Schrauwen P, Walder K, Ravussin E. Human uncoupling proteins and obesity. *Obes Res* 1999; **7**: 97–105.

150. Nicholls DG, Locke RM. Thermogenic mechanisms in brown fat. *Physiol Rev* 1984; **64**: 1–64.

151. Fleury C, Neverova M, Collins S, Raimbault S, Champigny O, Levi-Meyrueis C, Bouillaud F, Seldin MF, Surwit RS, Ricquier D, Warden CH. Uncoupling protein-2: a novel gene linked to obesity and hyperinsulinemia. *Nat Genet* 1997; **15**: 269–270.

152. Boss O, Samec S, Paoloni-Giacobino A, Rossier C, Dulloo A, Seydoux J, Muzzin P, Giacobino JP. Uncoupling protein-3: a new member of the mitochondrial carrier family with tissue-specific distribution. *FEBS Lett* 1997; **408**: 39–42.

153. Gagnon J, Lago F, Chagnon YC, Pérusse L, Näslund I, Lissner L, Sjöström L, Bouchard C. DNA polymorphism in the uncoupling protein 1 (UCP1) gene has no effect on obesity related phenotypes in the Swedish Obese Subjects cohorts. *Int J Obes Relat Metab Disord* 1998; **22**: 500–505.

154. Luyckx FH, Scheen AJ, Proenza AM, Strosberg AD, Lefèbvre PJ, Gielen JE. Influence of the A → G (-3826) uncoupling protein-1 gene (UCP1) variant on the dynamics of body weight before and after gastroplasty in morbidly obese subjects. *Int J Obes Relat Metab Disord* 1998; **22**: 1244–1245.

155. Oppert JM, Vohl MC, Chagnon M, Dionne FT, Cassard-Doulcier AM, Ricquier D, Pérusse L, Bouchard C. DNA polymorphism in the uncoupling protein (UCP) gene and human body fat. *Int J Obes Relat Metab Disord* 1994; **18**: 526–531.

156. Bouchard C, Pérusse L, Chagnon YC, Warden C, Ricquier D. Linkage between markers in the vinicity of the uncoupling protein 2 gene and resting metabolic rate in humans. *Hum Mol Genet* 1997; **6**: 1187–1189.

157. Schrauwen P, Xia J, Bogardus C, Pratley RE, Ravussin E. Skeletal muscle UCP3 expression is a determinant of energy expenditure in Pima Indians. *Diabetes* 1999b; **48**: 146–149.

158. Williamson D. Pharmacotherapy for obesity (editorial). *JAMA* 1999; **281**: 278–280.

159. Kolanowski J. A risk-benefit assessment of anti-obesity drugs. *Drugs Safety* 1999; **20**: 119–131.

32

Treatment: Hormones

Björn Andersson, Gudmundur Johannsson and Bengt-Åke Bengtsson

Sahlgrenska University Hospital, Göteborg, Sweden

INTRODUCTION

Recent years have clearly shown that sex steroid hormones and growth hormone (GH) are involved in the syndrome of visceral obesity. Increased levels of free testosterone in women and low testosterone values in men are endocrine aberrations associated with central obesity as well as a blunted GH secretion.

These endocrine perturbations may independently, or in concert with visceral obesity, increase the risk for cardiovascular disease and non-insulin-dependent diabetes mellitus (NIDDM: type 2 diabetes). With this background there are, however, potential possibilities of hormone treatment of visceral obesity which will be further analysed in this chapter.

TESTOSTERONE

Background

Several studies have shown that abdominal body fat distribution in men is associated with low testosterone and low sex hormone-binding globulin (SHBG) levels (1,2) and recent evidence also suggests that deficiency of testosterone is related to insulin resistance (1,3) (Table 32.1). Men with NIDDM seem to have lower levels of endogenous sex hormones (4,5) and Haffner *et al.* (6) have recently reported an inverse association between SHBG concentrations at baseline and the subsequent development of diabetes.

In women the relationship between androgens and body fat distribution seems to be the opposite (Table 32.1). It has been previously demonstrated that in women abdominal body fat distribution is associated with increased free testosterone and decreased SHBG levels (7). SHBG is a major determinant of the ratio of free to bound plasma testosterone and other androgens and low levels are thought to reflect increased androgenicity. Furthermore, a low SHBG level has also been shown to be associated with insulin resistance and an increased risk of developing NIDDM in women (8–10).

Thus, there are several pieces of evidence that underline the importance of testosterone in obesity and the close association between testosterone and visceral adiposity both in men and women. *Hyperandrogenicity* in women and *hypoandrogenicity* in men may work in concert with the visceral fat mass to further increase the risk for cardiovascular disease and NIDDM.

Hyperandrogenicity and Insulin Resistance in Women

The direction of causality between testosterone and insulin resistance is not fully clarified. The hypothesis that has gained most support is that hyperinsulinaemia increases androgen output from the ovary and may suppress SHBG production in the liver, shown both *in vitro* and *in vivo* (11,12) (Figure 32.1).

Conversely, previous studies of anabolic steroids (13), women with polycystic ovaries (14), androgen

International Textbook of Obesity. Edited by Per Björntorp.

Table 32.1 Testosterone levels in visceral obesity

Sex	Testosterone	SHBG	Consequences
Male	Low	Low	Visceral obesity Insulin resistance
Female	Increased (free testosterone)	Low	Visceral obesity Insulin resistance

SHBG, Sex hormone-binding globulin.

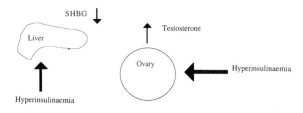

Figure 32.1 Insulin-mediated increase in testosterone and decrease in sex hormone-binding blobulin (SHBG)

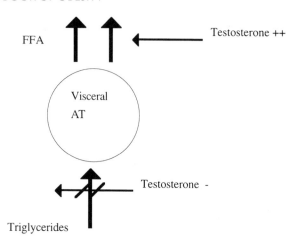

Figure 32.2 The effects of testosterone on visceral adipose tissue (AT). Lipid uptake is inhibited and mobilization is stimulated with an increased release of free fatty acids (FFA)

treatment of female to male transsexuals (15) and studies of the effect of testosterone on insulin sensitivity in female rats (16) have suggested that hyperandrogenicity may also induce muscular and systemic insulin resistance. This might partly be due to a diminished insulin binding to a contracted bed of capillary endothelium, and subsequent diminished blood flow and insufficient delivery of insulin to its site of action on the muscle cell (16). Postreceptor perturbations may also be involved.

Whatever the cause–effect sequence it is clear that hyperandrogenicity in women is closely associated with insulin resistance. Furthermore, this is not a rare condition and it is estimated that about 20% of middle-aged women of a non-selected population may be hyperandrogenic with SHBG values in the lower range (17). The increased risk of disease therefore is a problem of considerable quantitative importance.

Hypoandrogenicity and Insulin Resistance in Men

In men, data on the direction of causality between testosterone and insulin resistance are more scarce. Previous findings of a positive correlation between insulin sensitivity and SHBG levels in men with type 2 diabetes (18), and increased SHBG concentration and reduced testosterone levels after insulin

suppression by diazoxide (19), are in accordance with the concept that insulin inhibits SHBG synthesis and stimulates testosterone production.

However, since obese men usually have a lowered baseline testosterone concentration these findings do not fully explain the cause–effect sequence. Therefore, probably other mechanisms are also involved. Recently, Vermeulen (20) suggested that hypogonadism in obese men has a central, hypothalamo-pituitary origin since a group of obese men had decreased luteinizing hormone (LH) pulse amplitude and decreased free testosterone concentration, but a normal response of the Leydig cells to chorion gonadotrophin stimulation.

Consequently, it may be hypothesized that the hypogonadism in obese men may be at least partly of neuroendocrine origin, but other factors, such as the insulin-mediated suppression of SHBG synthesis, play an additional role.

Testosterone and Adipose Tissue

Previous works (21,22) on lipid transport to and mobilization from adipose tissue measured *in vivo* in men have shown that lipid uptake and mobilization are higher in intra-abdominal adipose tissue than in subcutaneous (s.c.) ones. After testosterone treatment, lipid uptake is markedly inhibited, apparently more in s.c. abdominal fat than in s.c. femoral fat and particularly in intra-abdominal adi-

Table 32.2 Effects of testosterone treatment in men

Study	Duration of treatment	Body composition	Metabolic variables
Mårin et al. (28)	8 months	↓ Visceral fat	↑ Glucose tolerance ↑ Insulin sensitivity ↓ Cholesterol
Friedl et al. (32)	6 weeks	→ WHR	→ glucose tolerance → Insulin
Lovejoy et al. (33)	9 months	↑ Visceral fat	↓ Cholesterol
Tenover JS (34)	3 months	→ WHR → Body fat	↓ Cholesterol

WHR, waist-to-hip ratio; tol, tolerance.

pose tissues (23). Lipid mobilization is stimulated in abdominal, but not in femoral, fat and evidence from rats (24) suggests that this might be more pronounced in visceral than in s.c. adipose tissue.

The total effects of testosterone on intra-abdominal tissue may, therefore, be to inhibit uptake and increase the mobilization of triglycerides in intra-abdominal adipose tissue depots (Figure 32.2). Low testosterone values would then presumably result in lipid accumulation in the visceral fat region, a phenomenon frequently seen in men with abdominal distribution of adipose tissue.

The effects of testosterone on adipose tissue metabolism are probably mediated via a specific androgen receptor that in the rat shows marked regional differences in density, being higher in visceral than in s.c. adipose tissue (25). Therefore, it is suggested that the regional different effects of testosterone may be explained by differences in androgen receptor density.

Treatment with Testosterone

Although the primary treatment of obesity is to induce a negative energy balance the prognosis of dietary treatment is poor with a high rate of relapse (26). Furthermore, there is currently no specific treatment of visceral obesity except surgery, which shows some promising results (27) but so far is only offered to the most obese subjects. Since aberrations in the sex steroid hormonres seem to be of major importance in the pathogenesis of visceral obesity several studies have recently been focused on the effect of hormone treatment.

Mårin (28) treated abdominally obese men with low baseline testosterone values with two types of

androgens, testosterone and dihydrotestosterone (DHT) for 8 months. Testosterone substitution was followed by a decrease in visceral fat mass, cholesterol, systolic and diastolic blood pressure, blood glucose and an increase in insulin sensitivity, whereas DHT treatment resulted in no such beneficial effects (Table 32.2). On the contrary, there was even an increase in visceral fat mass with DHT substitution. The rationale for testing DHT was that this androgen is generally considered to be the hormone acting on target tissues.

The explanation for these different results is presently unclear, but an obvious hypothesis is that testosterone has other important physiological functions in the body than to act only as a sex steroid on its target organs. It may be hypothesized that the specific regulatory effect of testosterone on the visceral adipose tissue is a more important background mechanism for the improvement in metabolic risk factors, than the sex steroid effect on different target tissues. This hypothesis is supported by recent identification of both testosterone and dihydrotestosterone receptors in intra-abdominal adipose tissue in man (29).

It is also possible that an increase of insulin sensitivity is the primary event followed by amelioration of metabolic risk variables and blood pressure, which are all closely dependent on insulin resistance. Supporting this hypothesis are the findings in male rats, where normalization of insulin sensitivity after castration was seen already after 48 hours of testosterone treatment (30).

Testosterone can be transformed to oestrogens by aromatization, particularly in the adipose tissue (31), but there was no evidence of increased oestradiol concentration in these studies, so obviously the observed effects of testosterone administration were those of testosterone alone.

However, there are also conflicting data on the beneficial effect of testosterone administration. Friedl *et al.* (32) observed no effect of short-term treatment with testosterone on glucose homeostasis in non-obese men (Table 32.2) and Lovejoy *et al.* (33) have recently reported that long-term treatment with testosterone in middle-aged obese males was followed by an increase in visceral fat, but a decrease in s.c. abdominal fat, whereas treatment with an anabolic steroid produced a decrease in visceral fat (table 32.2). The latter observation is inconsistent with previous findings of diminished glucose tolerance and insulin resistance in powerlifters ingesting anabolic steroids (13).

In the ageing male testosterone supplementation seems, though, to have positive effects on lipid profile but not on body fat (34) (Table 32.2).

There is no obvious explanation to the different outcome between these studies, but it may depend on difference in age, study population or the obese state *per se*. Because of this inconsistency further studies are warranted before testosterone treatment can be recommended to obese, hypogonadal men.

Testosterone Supplementation in Women

Previous studies have demonstrated that testosterone administration to women significantly increases the visceral fat depot and induces insulin resistance (15,35). However, in spite of these adverse effects there is currently considerable interest in the use of testosterone as a component of hormone replacement therapy for postmenopausal women (36).

Testosterone enhances sexuality and acts as an antiresorptive agent on bone, thus limiting bone loss (36), but testosterone should only be administered to women who are concurrently taking oestrogen replacement since otherwise the likelihood of adverse effects on lipids and insulin sensitivity is increased.

Conclusions

In men testosterone concentrations in the lower range are associated with accumulation of visceral fat and hyperinsulinaemia. Testosterone treatment may be followed by a decrease of insulin resistance and other metabolic risk factors, as well as, a specific decrease of the visceral adipose tissue mass, mediated by an inhibition of triglyceride assimilation and an enhanced turnover.

In women *hyperandrogenicity* is associated with enlarged visceral fat depots and insulin resistance leading to an increased risk of developing NIDDM and cardiovascular disease.

FEMALE SEX STEROID HORMONES

Oestrogen, Progesterone and Adipose Tissue

Previous works have clearly demonstrated that female sex hormones influence adipose tissue metabolism differently in various fat depots (37). The typical female adipose tissue in the femoral-gluteal region in premenopausal women tends to accumulate fat, particularly during pregnancy, which can then be mobilized efficiently during lactation. These findings suggest a specific female function for this depot, to provide a reserve of energy for lactation purpose. In contrast, lipolytic responsiveness and sensitivity are higher in subcutaneous abdominal adipocytes.

The disappearance of this typical metabolic pattern with menopause and its reappearance with hormonal substitution indicate that sex steroid hormones exert an important influence here (38). The specific role of oestrogen and progesterone is, however, not fully clarified.

Furthermore, current data are from *in vitro* studies and there is no evidence relating to the effect of female sex hormones on adipose tissue *in vivo*, as there is in men.

Female Sex Hormones and Body Composition

Previous studies have demonstrated that increasing androgenicity in women, as reflected by low SHBG concentration, or an increase in the percentage of free testosterone, is associated with visceral obesity (7,39). Menopause seems to be associated with increasing body fat and with an increasing proportion of abdominal body fat distribution (40). It may be conceivable that these changes in body fat and its distribution are related to the marked decrease in oestrogen and progesterone levels associated with menopause. Consequently, it may therefore be hy-

Table 32.3 The effects of hormone replacement therapy on body composition

Study	Body composition (vs. baseline)	Effect compared vs. placebo
Haarbo et al. (41)	→ Visceral fat	
	→ Body fat	↓ Visceral fat
	→ Lean body mass	
PEPI trial (42)	→ Body weight	↓ Body weight
	→ Waist circumference	↓ Waist circumference
Kritz-Silverstein et al. (43)	→ BMI	→ BMI
	→ WHR	→ WHR
	→ Body fat	→ Body fat
Hassager et al. (44)	→ Body weight	→ Body weight
	→ Fat mass	↓ Fat mass
Jensen et al. (46)	→ Body weight	→ Body weight
	→ Muscle mass	↑ Muscle mass

BMI, body mass index; WHR, waist-to-hip ratio.

pothesized that hormone replacement therapy (HRT) would be beneficial.

The effect of HRT on body composition is, however, controversial. Haarbo et al. (41) reported that combined oestrogen–progestogen therapy prevented the increase in abdominal fat after menopause, but did not reduce the existing visceral fat depot (Table 32.3). These data have recently been confirmed in the large PEPI (Postmenopausal Estrogen/Progestin Interventions) trial (42), where 875 women were randomized to four different hormone regims for 3 years. Compared to placebo there was less weight gain in women assigned to hormone treatment and smaller changes in waist circumference, although the differences were very small (Table 32.3).

These findings are consistent with other studies that reported little or no effect (43–45) (Table 32.3). Jensen et al. (46) have, however, reported that high doses of HRT increased muscle mass and subsequently reduced body fat (Table 32.3). The inconsistency may depend on number of subjects and different methods of determining body fat and muscle mass.

In conclusion, the age- and menopause-related increase in body fat and waist-to-hip ratio seem at least partially to be prevented by HRT. The effects are, however, moderate.

Treatment of Hyperandrogenicity

Postmenopausal women with visceral obesity are, as mentioned earlier, at high risk for developing NIDDM and cardiovascular disease. Clearly, visceral obesity is a pre-diabetic condition where the clock for cardiovascular disease starts ticking before the onset of clinical diabetes (47). NIDDM is preceded by a long period of hyperinsulinaemia and insulin resistance, which may contribute to development of hyperlipidaemia, hypertension and atherosclerosis in the arterial wall.

Most of these women are also hyperandrogenic with SHBG concentrations in the lower range, which is known to be associated with insulin resistance and impaired glucose homeostasis (8).

Body weight reduction improves most metabolic risk factors and may defer the onset of clinical diabetes, but as previously mentioned the long-term prognosis for weight reduction is poor. It may be hypothesized that allieviating hyperandrogenicity in women may be followed by reduced insulin resistance and an improvement in blood lipids. Recent studies have, however, presented conflicting results.

Dunaif et al. (48) have reported that suppression of androgens into normal levels did not result in improvement in insulin resistance. In contrast Moghetti et al. (49) and Shoupe (50) have demonstrated recently that anti-androgen treatment resulted in partly reversed insulin resistance. Furthermore, Diamanti-Kandarakis et al. (51) have demonstrated that treatment with a pure anti-androgenreceptor blocker markedly improved lipid profile in women with polycystic ovary syndrome (PCOS).

HRT and Cardiovascular Disease

Previously several studies (52–56) (Table 32.4) have shown a reduced risk by 30–40% for myocardial

Table 38.4 Hormone replacement therapy and cardiovascular disease and mortality

Study	RR AMI	RR stroke	RR mortality
Falkeborn *et al.* (52)			
0.69	n.e.	n.e.	
Falkeborn *et al.* (53)	n.e.	Any stroke 0.72	n.e.
		Acute stroke 0.61	
Grodstein *et al.* (54)	n.e.	n.e.	0.63
Heckbert *et al.* (55)	0.91 < 2 years HRT	n.e.	n.e.
	0.55 > 8 years of HRT		
Grodstein *et al.* (56)	0.39	1.09	n.e.
Hulley *et al.* (57)	0.99	n.e.	n.e.

RR, relative risk (odds ratio); AMI, acute myocardial infarction; HRT, hormone replacement therapy; n.e., not examined.

infarction, stroke and mortality in women taking unopposed oestrogen or oestrogen combined with progestogen. All of these studies have, however, been observational studies with the consequent risk of bias.

Conflicting evidence has recently been reported by Hulley *et al.* (57), who showed in the first large randomized trial that treatment with oestrogen plus progestin failed to reduced the overall rate of coronary heart disease (CHD) events in postmenopausal women with known coronary disease, despite lower low density lipoprotein (LDL) levels and higher high density lipoprotein (HDL) levels in the hormone group.

Before any firm conclusion may be drawn on the effect of HRT on CHD, further placebo-controlled, randomized studies are needed. It is probable that the seemingly protective effect of oestrogens on CHD is partly mediated through a favourable change in the lipoprotein pattern, as well as a direct vasodilatory effect in the coronary arteries (58) and a suppression of fibrinogen and plasminogen activator inhibitor 1 (PAI-1) levels (59,60).

HRT and Insulin Resistance

The effect of HRT on insulin resistance is controversial, but most observations suggest that unopposed oestradiol replacement is associated with improved insulin sensitivity both in muscle and in adipose tissue (61), while the addition of progestogens seems to worsen insulin sensitivity. In women with an intact uterus, the addition of progestogens is, however, necessary for endometrial protection. In combined HRT, depending on the type of progestogen used, insulin sensitivity may be unchanged or deteriorated.

In accordance with these findings, we and others (62,63) have recently shown that short-term unopposed oestradiol replacement therapy decreased hyperandrogenicity and improved glucose tolerance and blood lipids in postmenopausal obese women with NIDDM.

The route of administration seems to be important, since transdermal oestradiol replacement therapy in postmenopausal women with NIDDM was not followed by any beneficial changes in glucose tolerance, lipid profile or SHBG concentrations (64,65). A plausible explanation is that transdermal application of oestradiol bypasses the liver and, consequently, affects the liver and its production of lipoproteins and SHBG to a much lower degree. These observations may underline the importance of hyperandrogenicity as a predisposing factor for attenuated glucose homeostasis and insulin resistance.

There are several possible background mechanisms to the oestrogen-induced improvements in glucose homeostatis. In addition to alleviating androgen effects on skeletal muscle, oestrogens alone may have direct effects on skeletal muscle. Oestrogens regulate insulin-induced transport (66) via translocation of glucose transporter 4 (67), and oestrogens may also enhance basal and insulin-mediated suppression of hepatic glucose output (68).

Conclusion

Overall, hormone treatment in postmenopausal women seems to be beneficial by reducing the risk for CHD and stroke and by improving lipid profile even though there is no change in visceral fat depots. The effect on insulin resistance is more controversial, but at least in diabetic women glucose tolerance seems to be improved by short-term treatment with unopposed oestradiol.

Whether HRT has any long-term effect on glucose homeostasis and insulin resistance in diabetic and in pre-diabetic women with visceral obesity and a relative hyperandrogenicity is currently not known. It must, however, be considered of potential interest, given the large population of post-menopausal obese women at risk for disease.

GROWTH HORMONE AND ABDOMINAL OBESITY

Secretion of Growth Hormone in Abdominal Obesity

With increased adiposity, GH secretion is blunted with a decrease in the mass of GH secreted per burst but without any major impact on GH secretory burst frequency (69). Moreover, the metabolic clearance rate of GH is accelerated (70). The serum insulin-like growth factor I (IGF-I) concentration is primarily GH dependent and influences GH secretion though a negative feedback system (71). The serum levels of IGF-I are inversely related to the percentage of body fat (69). In addition, the low serum IGF-I concentration in obesity is predominantly related to the amount of visceral adipose tissue and not to the amount of subcutaneous fat mass (72). Serum free IGF-I concentration may, on the other hand, be increased in abdominal obesity (73) possibly as an effect of the concomitant insulin-induced suppression of serum IGF binding protein-1 levels.

The relationship between regional fat distribution and GH secretion has only recently been considered. No significant correlation was found between the waist-to-hip ratio and 24-hour GH secretion rates in a study of 21 healthy men (74). However, in healthy non-obese men and women intra-abdominal fat mass had a strong negative exponential relationship with mean 24-hour serum GH concentrations which was independent of age, gender and physical fitness (75). This indicates that, for each increment in intra-abdominal fat mass, there is a more than linear reduction in mean 24-hour GH concentration.

Striking similarities exist between the metabolic syndrome and untreated GH deficiency in adults (76). The central findings in both these syndromes are abdominal/visceral obesity and insulin resistance. Other features common to both conditions are high triglyceride and HDL cholesterol concentrations, an increased prevalence of hypertension, elevated levels of PAI-1 activity, premature atherosclerosis and increased mortality from cardiovascular diseases (77). Due to the similarities between two syndromes, undetectable and low levels of GH may be of importance for the metabolic aberrations observed in both these conditions.

Low levels of GH may be of importance for the metabolic consequences and the maintenance of the obese condition. One trial has demonstrated near normalization of 24-hour GH secretion and serum IGF-I in nine obese subjects after massive weight loss (78) whereas others have not found a normalization of the GH response to provocative testing in response to weight loss (79,80). Amount of intra-abdominal fat was, however, not considered in these studies.

There is now considerable evidence that the metabolic syndrome might be considered to be a consequence of perturbations in the hypothalamo-pituitary-adrenocortical (HPA) axis due to environmental pressure which are expressed in individuals with molecular genetic susceptibility in the feedback, inhibitory mechanism exerted by central glucocorticoid receptors (GRs). This together with attenuating activity of the gonadotrophic and GH axis may be responsible for the development of the metabolic syndrome with visceral obesity, insulin resistance, dyslipoproteinaemia and hypertension. Attenuated GH secretion is therefore an important component of this cascade of events. Interestingly, the metabolic syndrome may apparently also develop with only low GH secretion (reduced serum IGF-I concentration), i.e. without involvement of the HPA axis inhibition. This condition seems to have a prevalence of 5% in middle-aged Swedish men (81).

Visceral Fat Mass

Patients with acromegaly have reduced adipose tissue mass. After successful treatment which normalizes their GH secretion they demonstrate an increase of predominantly visceral adipose tissue mass (82). The reverse scenario is seen in adults with hypopituitarism and untreated GH deficiency who have increased body fat mass with adbominal preponderance; after GH administration there is a profound reduction of visceral adipose tissue and less marked effects on other adipose tissue depots (83,84). These observations indicate that GH has profoundly effects on adipose tissue mass and distribution.

Insulin Resistance

Insulin resistance is a common conditions and can be seen, for example, in type 2 diabetes, obesity and hypertension. The interrelationship between insulin resistance and these conditions, as well as the exact mechanisms for insulin resistance, have not yet been fully clarified. It recently became clear that even adults with GH deficiency have insulin resistance in peripheral tissues as measured using the hyperinsulinaemic euglycemic clamp technique (85,86). The glucose disposal rate (GDR) in GH-deficient adults is found to be less than half that of controls, both when calculated according to body weight and when corrected for amount of body fat. The decreased lean body mass and the increased abdominal obesity in GH deficiency may be of importance for this finding as the association between increased body fat mass and insulin resistance is stronger in the presence of abdominal obesity (87). The attenuated GDR seen in abdominal obesity has in some studies been quantitatively similar to that seen in overtly hyperglycaemic type 2 diabetes (88). Low levels of serum IGF-I may also contribute to insulin resistance as IGF-I stimulates glucose transport in skeletal muscle. Other factors such as different composition of skeletal muscle fibres with a decrease in the slow-twitch, insulin-sensitive type I fibres and an increase in the fast-twitch, type Ib fibres, the degree of capillary rarefaction and decreased physical activity in adults with GH deficiency may be of importance just as it is in healthy adults (89,90).

Dyslipoproteinaemia

GH has important effects on lipoprotein metabolism. For example, hypophysectomy in the rat changes the lipoprotein pattern from being predominantly HDL to a pattern with a predominately LDL peak, suggesting that the presence of GH is essential for maintaining a normal lipoprotein profile. Moreover, in response to GH the serum LDL cholesterol and apolipoprotein B concentrations decrease (91,92), probably as a result of the increased clearance of these lipoproteins through increased hepatic LDL receptor activity (93).

A common finding in both GH deficiency and the metabolic syndrome is high levels of serum triglycerides and low HDL cholesterol concentrations. This may be associated with increased adbominal adiposity and insulin resistance in both conditions. However, although a dramatic reduction in visceral adipose tissue occurs in response to GH treatment in adults with GH deficiency, serum triglyceride concentration is not reduced while the concentration of HDL cholesterol is increased (92).

This may be an effect of the lipolytic action of GH treatment which may increase the flux of FFA to the liver which in turn may increase the synthesis and secretion of VLDL from the liver. The LPL activity in adipose tissue is attenuated and the post-heparin plasma LPL is not affected by GH treatment (94). As serum triglyceride concentrations do not increase under conditions of increased VLDL secretion the peripheral catabolism must be enhanced. Increased LPL activity in other tissues such as muscle is therefore likely (94). Furthermore, the strong association between glucose/insulin homeostasis and VLDL metabolism (95) might be reflected in the response to GH. The unaffected triglyceride levels might thus be explained by essentially unchanged insulin sensitivity during more prolonged GH treatment in GH-deficient adults.

Blood Pressure

Both GH deficiency in adults and the metabolic syndrome are associated with increased prevalence of hypertension. The insulin resistance in the metabolic syndrome syndrome X) has been linked with hypertension through increased activity of the sympathetic nervous system (96). Direct evidence for this assumption is provided by an apparent parallel activation of hypothalamic centres regulating the sympathetic nervous sysem and the HPA axis, a 'hypohalamic arousal syndrome' (97). Central arousal of the sympathetic nervous system is considered to be a main pathogenic pathway for essential hypertension (98).

In adults with hypopituitarism and untreated GH deficiency augmented activity of the sympathetic nervous system has been demonstrated by direct intraneural recordings (99) linking this condition to increased prevalence of hypertension. In addition, GH deficiency has been found to be associated with low levels of nitric oxide (NO), a paracrine vasodilator produced in endothelial cells, which normalizes in response to GH treatment (100).

Growth Hormone Treatment in Abdominal Obesity

We have learned that GH treatment can improve several of the aberrations that GH deficiency has in common with the metabolic syndrome. Thus, in adults with GH deficiency the lipolytic effects of GH result in a preferential reduction in visceral adipose tissue (83). Furthermore, GH reduces diastolic blood pressure, total cholesterol, LDL cholesterol and increases HDL cholesterol concentrations (91,101,102). Long-term GH treatment does not impair insulin sensitivity (103). Against this background we have, in a 9-month randomized double-blind placebod-controlled trial, studied the effects of GH on the metabolic, circulatory and anthropometric aberrations associated with abdominal/visceral obesity and the metabolic syndrome (104).

The men who were studied were moderately obese with a prepondernace of abdominal localization of body fat. As a group, they had slight to moderate metabolic changes known to be associated with abdominal/visceral obesity. Nine months of GH treatment in these middle-aged men with abdominal/visceral obesity reduced their total body fat and resulted in a specific and marked decrease in both abdominal subcutaneous and visceral adipose tissue. Moreover, insulin sensitivity improved and serum concentrations of total cholesterol and triglyceride decreased. Diastolic blood pressure decreased while plasma fibrinogen increased slightly.

GH exerts direct insulin-antagonistic effects even after the administration of physiologic doses of GH. GH has been considered to be the principal factor in the decrease in insulin sensitivity observed in the early morning, the so-called 'dawn phenomenon' and the insulin resistance following hypoglycaemia. Thus, our observation of increased insulin sensitivity during prolonged GH treatment could be explained by the decrease in visceral adipose tissue mass induced by GH, followed by a decrease in free fatty acid (FFA) exposure to the liver counteracting the insulin-antagonistic effects of GH. Alternatively, as the major site of glucose disposal is in the skeletal muscle, the improvement in GDR in response to more prolonged GH treatment might also be an effect of increased glucose transport in the skeletal muscle. This might be mediated hrough the IGF-I receptor and/or be an effect of an increased proportion of insulin-sensitive type I muscle fibres in response to the treatment.

This is the first trial clearly to demonstrate favourable effects of GH on the multiple perturbations associated with abdominal/visceral obesity. We therefore suggest that a blunted GH secretion could be an important factor in the development of the metabolic and circulatory consequences of abdominal/visceral obesity.

The abnormal activity of the HPA axis, low levels of sex steroids and attenuated GH secretion in abdominal obesity suggest a central neuroendocrine dysregulation. The finding that replacement therapy with testosterone and GH in men with abdominal obesity is able to diminish the negative metabolic consequences of visceral obesity suggests that the low levels of these hormones are of importance for the metabolic aberrations associated with visceral/abdominal obesity.

SUMMARY

Several pieces of evidence now clearly indicate that aberrations in sex hormones, together with blunted GH secretion, are important factors in the development of metabolic and circulatory consequences of visceral obesity. Replacement therapy with testosterone and GH in abdominally obese men has been shown to reduce visceral adipose tissue and accordingly decrease several risk factors for cardiovascular disease and NIDDM. In postmenopausal women, oestrogen and progestogens seem to prevent age-related increase in visceral fat mass and significantly reduce the risk of cardiovascular disease.

Hormone replacement therapy therefore seems to be a valuable adjunct to conventional obesity treatment, but further knowledge of the association between the metabolic and the neuroendocrine aberrations in abdominal obesity is needed before we fully understand the place of hormonal treatment in subjects with visceral obesity.

REFERENCES

1. Seidell JC, Björntorp P, Sjöström L, Kvist H, Sannerstedt R. Visceral fat accumulation in men is positively associated with insulin, glucose and c-peptide levels, but negatively with testosterone levels. *Metabolism* 1990; **39**: 897–901.

2. Khaw K-T, Chir MBB, Barrett-Connor E. Lower endogenous androgens predict central adiposity in men. *Ann Epidemiol* 1991; **2**: 675–682.

3. Simon D, Charles M-A, Nahoul K, Orsaud G, Kremski J, Hully V, et al. Association between plasma total testosterone and cardiovascular risk factors in healthy adult men: The Telecom Study. *J Clin Endocrinol Metab* 1997; **82**: 682–685.

4. Barrett-Connor E, Khaw K-T, Yen SSC. Endogenous sex hormone levels in older adult men with diabetes mellitus. *Am J Epidemiol* 1990; **132**: 895–901.

5. Andersson B, Mårin P, Lissner L, Vermeulen A, Björntorp P. Testosterone concentrations in women and men with NIDDM. *Diabetes Care* 1994; **17**: 405–411.

6. Haffner SM, Shaten J, Stern MP, Smith GD, Kuller L. Low levels of sex hormone-binding globulin and testosterone predict the development of non-insulin-dependent diabetes mellitus in men. *Am J Epidemiol* 1996; **143**: 889–897.

7. Evans DJ, Hoffman RG, Kalkhoff RK, Kissebah AH. Relationship of androgenic activity to body fat topography, fat cell morphology, and metabolic aberrations in premenopausal women. *J Clin Endocrinol Metab* 1983; **57**: 304–310.

8. Haffner SM, Dunn JF, Katz MS, Relationship of sex-hormone-binding globulin to lipid, lipoprotein, glucose and insulin concentrations in postmenopausal women. *Metabolism* 1992; **41**: 278–284.

9. Lindstedt G, Lundberg P-A, Lapidus L, Lundgren H, Bengtsson C, björntorp P. Low sex-hormone-binding globulin concentration as independent risk factor for development of NIDDM. *Diabetes* 1991; **40**: 123–128,

10. Haffner SM, Valdez RA, Morales PA, Hazuda HP, Stern MP. Decreased sex-hormone-binding globulin predicts non-insulin-dependent diabetes mellitus in women but not in men. *J Clin Endocrinol Metab* 1993; **77**: 56–60.

11. Plymate SR, Matej LA, Jones RE, Friedl KE. Inhibition of sex hormone-binding globulin production in the human hepatoma (Hep G2) cell line by insulin and prolactin. *J Clin Endocrinol Metab* 1988; **67**: 460–464.

12. Nestler JE, Powers LP, Matt DW, Steingold KA, Plymate SR, Rittmaster RS, et al. A direct effect of hyperinsulinemia on serum sex hormone-binding globulin levels in obese women with the polycystic ovary syndrome. *J Clin Endocrinol Metab* 1991; **72**: 83–89.

13. Cohen J, Hickman R. Insulin resistance and diminished glucose tolerance in powerlifters ingesting anabolic steroids. *J Clin Endocrinol Metab* 1987; **64**: 960–963.

14. Burghen GA, Givens JR, Kitabachi AE. Correlation of hyperandrogenism with hyperinsulinism in polycystic ovarian disease. *J Clin Endocrinol Metab* 1980; **50**: 113–116.

15. Polderman KH, Gooren LJG, Asscheman H, Bakker A, Heine RJ. Induction of insulin resistance by androgens and estrogens. *J Clin Endocrinol Metab* 1994; **79**: 265–271.

16. Holmäng A, Svedberg J, Jennische E, Björntorp P. Effects of testosterone on muscle insulin sensitivity and morphology in female rats. *Am J Physiol* 1990; **259**: 555–560.

17. Björntorp P. The android woman—a risky condition. *J Intern Med* 1996; **239**: 105–10.

18. Birkjeland KI, Hanssen KF, Torjesen PA, Vaaler S. Level of sex hormone-binding globulin is positively correlated with insulin sensitivity in men with type 2 diabetes. *J Clin Endocrinol Metab* 1993; **76**: 275–278.

19. Pasquali R, Casimirri F, De Iaso R, Mesini P, Boschi S, Chierici R, et al. Insulin regulates testosterone and sex hormone-binding globulin concentrations in adult normal weight and obese men. *J Clin Endocrinol Metab* 1995; **80**: 654–658.

20. Vermeulen A. Decreased androgen levels and obesity in men. *Ann Med* 1996; **28**: 13–15.

21. Mårin P, Andersson B, Ottosson M, Olbe L, Chowdbury B, Kvist H, et al. The morphology and metabolism of intraabdominal adipose tissue in men. *Metabolism* 1992; **41**: 1242–1248.

22. Rebuffé-Scrive M, Mårin P, Björntorp P. Effect of testosterone on abdominal adipose tissue in men. *Int J Obes* 1991; **15**: 791–795.

23. Mårin P, Lönn L, Andersson B, Odén B, Olbe L, Bengtsson B-Å, et al. Assimilation of triglycerides in subcutaneous and intraabdominal adipose tissue in vivo in men: Effects of testosterone. *J Clin Endocrinol Metab* 1996; **81**: 1018–1022.

24. Min L, Björntorp P. Effects of testosterone on triglyceride uptake and mobilization in different adipose tissues of male rats *in vivo*. *Obes Res* 1995; **3**: 113–119.

25. Sjögren J, Li M, Björntorp P. Androgen hormone binding to adipose tissue. *Biochim Biophys Acta* 1995; **1244**: 117–120.

26. Dwyer JT. Treatment of obesity: conventional programs and fad diets. *Obesity*. Philadelphia: JB Lippincott, 1992: 662–675.

27. Näslund I, Hallgren P, Sjöström L. Fat cell weight and number before and after gastric surgery for morbid obesity in women. *Int J Obes* 1988; **12**: 191–197.

28. Mårin P. Effects of androgens in men with the metabolic syndrome. *The Aging Male* 1998; **1**: 129–136.

29. Boumediene A, Pecquery R, Dieudonné M-N, Leneveu M-C. Androgen receptors in human adipocytes and preadipocytes: *in vitro* effects of androgens and adipogenesis. *Int J Obes* 1997; **21**(Suppl 2): S8.

30. Holmäng A, Björntorp P. The effects of testosterone on insulin sensitivity in male rats. *Acta Physiol Scand* 1992; **146**: 505–510.

31. Mooradian AD, Morley JE, Korenman SG. Biological effects of androgens. *Endocr Rev* 1987; **8**: 1–27.

32. Friedl KE, Jones RE, Hannan CJ, Plymate SR. The administration of pharmacological doses of testosterone or 19-

nortestosterone to normal men is not associated with increased insulin secretion or impaired glucose tolerance. *J Clin Endocrinol Metab* 1989; **68**: 971–975.

33. Lovejoy JC, Bray GA, Greeson CS, Klemperer M, Morris J, Partington C, *et al.* Oral anabolic steroid treatment, but not parenteral androgen treatment, decreases visceral, abdominal fat in obese, older men. *Int J Obes* 1995; **19**: 614–624.

34. Tenover JS. Effects of testosterone supplementation in the aging male. *J Clin Endocrinol Metab* 1992; **75**: 1092–1098.

35. Elbers JMH, Asscheman H, Seidell JC, Megens JAJ, Gooren LJG. Long-term testosterone administration increases visceral fat in female to male transsexuals. *J Clin Endocrinol Metab* 1997; **82**: 2044–2047.

36. Davis SR, Burger HG. Androgens and the postmenopausal women. *J Clin Endocrinol Metab* 1996; **81**: 2759–2763.

37. Rebuffé-Scrive M, Enk L, Crona N, Lönnroth P, Abrahamsson L, Smith U, Björntorp P. Fat cell metabolism in different regions in women. Effect of menstrual cycle, pregnancy and lactation. *J Clin Invest* 1985; **75**: 1973–1976.

38. Rebuffé-Scrive M, Lönnroth P, Mårin P, Wesslau C, Björntorp P, Smith U. Regional adipose tissue in men and postmenopausal women. *Int J Obes* 1987; **11**: 347–355.

39. Haffner SM, Katz MS, Dunn JF. Increased upper body and overall adiposity is asociated with decreased sex hormone binding globulin in postmenopausal women. *Int J Obes* 1991; **15**: 471–478.

40. Ley CJ, Lees B, Stevenson JC. Sex-and menopause-associated changes in body-fat distribution. *Am J Clin Nutr* 1992; **55**: 950–954.

41. Haarbo J, Marslew U, Gotfredsen A, Christiansen C. Postmenopausal hormone replacement therapy prevents central distribution of body fat after menopause. *Metabolism* 1991; **40**: 1323–1326.

42. Espeland MA, Stefanick ML, Kritz-Silverstein D, Fineberg SE, Waclawiw MA, James MK, *et al.* Effect of postmenopausal hormone therapy on body weight and waist and hip girths. *J Clin Endocrinol Metab* 1997; **82**: 1549–1556.

43. Kritz-Silverstein D, Barrett-Connor E. Long-term postmenopausal hormone use, obesity and fat distribution in older women. *JAMA* 1996; **275**: 46–49.

44. Hassager C, Christiansen C. Estrogen/gestagen therapy changes soft tissue body composition in postmenopausal women. *Metabolism* 1989; **38**: 662–665.

45. Gambacciani M, Ciaponi M, Cappagli B, Piagggesi L, De Simone L, Orlandi R, Genazzani AR. Body weight, body fat distribution and hormonal replacement therapy in early postmenopausal women. *J Clin Endocrinol Metab* 1997; **82**: 414–417.

46. Jensen J, Christiansen C, Rødbro. Oestrogen–Progestogen replacement therapy changes body composition in early post-menopausal women. *Maturitas* 1986; **8**: 209–216.

47. Haffner SM, Stern MP, Hazuda HP, Mitchell BD, Patterson JK. Cardiovascular risk factors in confirmed prediabetic individuals. Does the clock for coronary heart disease start ticking before the onset of clinical diabetes? *JAMA* 1990; **263**: 2893–2898.

48. Dunaif A, Green G, Futerweit W, Dobrjansky A. Suppression of hyperandrogenism does not improve peripheral or hepatic insulin resistance in the polycystic ovary syndrome. *J Clin Endocrinol Metab* 1990; **70**: 699–704.

49. Moghetti P, Tosi F, Castello R, Magnani CM, Negri C, Brun E, *et al.* The insulin resistance in women with hyperandrogenism is partially reversed by antiandrogen treatment: evidence that androgens impair insulin action in women. *J Clin Endocrinol Metab* 1996; **81**: 952–960.

50. Shoupe D, Lobo RA. The influence of androgens on insulin resistance. *Fertil Steril* 1984; **41**: 385–388.

51. Diamanti-Kandarakis E, Mitrakou A, Raptis S, Tolis G, Duleba AJ. The effect of a pure antiandrogen receptor blocker, Flutamide, on the lipid profile in the polycystic ovary syndrome. *J Clin Endocrinol Metab* 1998; **83**: 2699–2705.

52. Falkeborn M, Persson I, Adami HO, Bergström R, Eaker E, Lithell H, *et al.* The risk of acute myocardial infarction after oestrogen and oestrogen-progestogen replacement. *Br J Obstet Gynaecol* 1992; **99**: 821–828.

53. Falkeborn M, Persson I, Terént A, Adami H-O, Lithell H, Bergström R. Hormone replacement therapy and the risk of stroke. *Arch Intern Med* 1993; **153**: 1201–1209.

54. Grodstein FG, Stampfer MJ, Colditz GA, Willett WC, Manson JAE, Joffe M, *et al.* Postmenopausal hormone therapy and mortality. *N Engl J Med* 1997; **336**: 1769–1775.

55. Heckbert SR, Weiss NS, Kepsell TD, Lemaitre RN, Smith NL, Siscovick DS, *et al.* Duration of estrogen replacement therapy in relation to the risk of incident myocardial infarction in postmenopausal women. *Arch Intern Med* 1997; **157**: 1330–1336.

56. Grodstein FG, Stampfer MJ, Manson JAE, Colditz GA, Willett WC, Rosner B, *et al.* Postmenopausal estrogen and progestin use and the risk of cardiovascular disease. *N Engl J Med* 1996; **335**: 453–461.

57. Hulley S, Grady D, Bush T, Furberg C, Herrington D, Riggs B, *et al.* Randomized trial of estrogen plus progestin for secondary prevention of coronary heart disease in postmenopausal women. *JAMA* 1998; **280**: 605–613.

58. Reis SE, Gloth ST, Blumenthal RS, Resar JR, Zacur HA, Gerstenblith G, *et al.* Ethinyl estradiol acutely attenuates abnormal coronary vasomotor response to acetycholine in postmenopausal women. *Circulation* 1994; **89**: 52–60.

59. The Writing Group for the Estradiol Clotting Factors Study. Effect on haemostasis of hormone replacement therapy with transdermal estradiol and oral sequential medroxyprogesterone acetate: a 1-year, double blind, placebo-controlled study. *Thromb Haemost* 1996; **75**: 476–480.

60. Kroon U-B, Silfverstolpe G, Tengborn L. The effects of transdermal estradiol and oral conjugated estrogens on haemostasis variables. *Thromb Haemost* 1994; **71**: 420–423.

61. Godsland IF. The influence of female sex steroids on glucose metabolism and insulin action. *J Intern Med* 1996; **240** (Suppl 738): 3–60.

62. Andersson B, Mattsson L-Å, Hahn L, Mårin P, Lapidus L, Holm G, *et al.* Estrogen replacement therapy decreases hyperandrogenicity and improves glucose homeostasis and plasma lipids in postmenopausal women with non-insulin-dependent diabetes mellitus. *J Clin Endocrinol Metab* 1997; **82**: 638–643.

63. Brussard HE, Leuven JA, Frölich M, Kluft C, Krans HMJ. Short-term estrogen replacement therapy improves insulin resistance, lipids and fibrinolysis in postmenopausal women with NIDDM. *Diabetologia* 1997; **40**: 843–849.

64. Andersson B, Mattsson L-Å. The effect of transfermal estrogen replacement therapy on hyperandrogenicity and glucose homeostasis in postmenopausal women with NIDDM. *Acta Obstet Gynecol Scand* 1999; **78**: 260–261.

65. Mosnier-Pudar H, Faguer B, Guyenne TT, Tchobroutsky G. Effects of deprivation and replacement by percutaneous 17 β-oestradiol and oral progesterone on blood pressure and metabolic parameters in menopause patients with non-insulin-dependent diabetes. *Arch Mal Coeur Vaiss* 1991; **84**: 1111–1115.

66. Kugami S, Holmäng A, Björntorp P. The effect of oestrogen and progesterone on insulin sensitivity in female rats. *Acta Physiol Scand* 1993; **149**: 91–97.

67. Rincon J, Homäng A, Wahlström EÖ, Lönnroth P, Gjörntorp P, Zierath JR, *et al.* Mechanisms behind insulin resistance in rat skeletal muscle following oophorectomy and additional testosterone treatment. *Diabetes* 1996; **45**: 615–621.

68. Matute M, Kalkhoff RK. Sex steroid influence on hepatic gluconeogenesis and glycogen formation. *Endocrinology* 1973; **92**: 762–768.

69. Veldhuis JD, Liem AY, South S, Weltman A, Weltman J, Clemmons DA, *et al.* Differential impact of age, sex steroid hormones, and obesity on basal versus pulsatile growth hormone secretion in men as assessed in an ultrasensitive chemiluminescence assay. *J Clin Endocrinol Metab* 1995; **80**: 3209.

70. Veldhuis JD, Iranmanesh A, Ho KKY, Waters MJ, Johnson ML, Lizarralde G. Dual effects in pulsatile growth hormone secretion and clearance subserve the hyposomatotropism of obesity in man. *J Clin Endocrinol Metab* 1991; **72**: 51–59.

71. Hartman ML, Clayton PE, Johnson ML, Celniker A, Perlman AJ, Alberti KGMM, Thorner MO. A low dose euglycemic infusion of recombinant human insulin-like growth factor I rapidly suppresses fasting-enhanced pulsatile growth hormone secretion in humans. *J Clin Invest* 1993; **91**: 2453–2462.

72. Mårin P, Kvist H, Lindstedt G, Sjöström L, Björntorp P. Low concentrations of insulin-like growth factor-I in abdominal obesity. *Int J Obes* 1993; **17**: 83–89.

73. Frystyk J, Vestbo E, Sklærbæk C, Morgensen CE, ¢rskov H. Free insulin-like growth factors in human obesity. *Metabolism* 1995; **44**: 37–44.

74. Iranmanesh A, Lizarralde G, Veldhuis JD. Age and relative adiposity are specific negative determinants of the frequency and amplitude of growth hormone (GH) secretory bursts and the half-life of endogenous GH in healthy men. *J Clin Endocrinol Metab* 1991; **73**: 1081–1088.

75. Vahl N, Jørgensen JOL, Skjærbæk C, Veldhuis JD, ¢rskov H, Christiansen JS. Abdominal adiposity rather than age and sex predicts mass and regularity of GH secretion in healthy adults. *Am J Physiol* 1997; **272**: E1108–1116.

76. Bengtsson B-Å. The consequences of growth hormone deficiency in adults. *Acta Endocrinol* 1993; **128**(Suppl 2): 2–5.

77. Rosén T, Bengtsson B-Å. Premature mortality due to cardiovascular diseases in hypopituitarism. *Lancet* 1900; **336**: 285–288.

78. Rasmussen MH, Hvidbeerg A, Juul A, Main KM, Gotfredsen A, Skakkebæ NE, Hilsted J. Massive weight loss restores 24-hour growth hormone release profiles and serum insulin-like growth factor-I levels in obese subjects. *J Clin Endocrinol Metab* 1995; **80**: 1407–1415.

79. Kopelman PG, Pilkington TRE, White N, Jeffcoate SL. Evidence for existence of two types of massive obesity. *BMJ* 1980; **281**: 82–83.

80. Jung RT, Campbell RG, James WPT, Callingham BA. Altered hypothalamic and sympathetic response to hypoglycaemia in familial obesity. *Lancet* 1982; **i**: 1043–1046.

81. Rosmond R, Björntorp P. The interactions between hypothelamic-pituitary-adrenal axis activity, testosterone, insulin-like growth factor I and abdominal obesity with metabolism and blood pressure in men. *Int J Obes* 1998; **22**: 1184–1196.

82. Bengtsson B-Å, Brummer R, Edén S, Bosaeus I, Lindstedt G. Body composition in acromegaly: the effect of treatment. *Clin Endocrinol* 1989; **31**: 481–490.

83. Bengtsson B-Å, Edén S, Lönn L, Kvist H, Stokland A, Lindstedt G, *et al.* Treatment of adults with growth hormone (GH) deficiency with recombinant human GH. *J Clin Endocrinol Metab* 1993; **76**: 309–317.

84. Lönn L, Johannsson G, Sjöström L, Kvist H, Odén A, Bengtsson B-Å. Body composition and tissue distributions in growth hormone deficient adults before and after growth hormone treatment. *Obes Res* 1996; **4**: 45–54.

85. Johansson J.-O, Fowelin J, Landin K, Lager I, Bengtsson B-Å. Growth hormone-deficient adults are insulin-resistant. *Metabolism* 1995; **44**: 1126–1129.

86. Hew FL, Koschmann M, Christopher M, Rantzau C, Vaag A, Ward G, Beck-Nielsen H, Alford F. Insulin resistance in growth hormone-deficient adults: defects in glucose utilization and glycogen synthase activity. *J Clin Endocrinol Metab* 1996; **81**: 555–564.

87. Kissebah AH, Peiris AN, Evans DJ. Mechanisms associating body fat distribution to glucose tolerance and diabetes mellitus: Window with a view. *Acta Med Scand* 1988; **723**: 79–89.

88. Peiris AN, Struve MF, Mueller RA, Lee MB, Kissebah AH. Glucose metabolism in obesity: influence of body fat distribution. *J Clin Endocrinol Metab* 1988; **67**: 760–767.

89. Bouchard C, Després J-P, Mauriége P. Genetic and nongenetic determinants of regional fat distribution. *Endocr Rev* 1993; **14**: 72–99.

90. Kissebah AH, Krakower GR. Regional adiposity and morbidity. *Physiol Rev* 1994; **74**: 761–811.

91. Cuneo RC, Salomon F, Watts GF, Hesp R, Sönksen PH. Growth hormone treatment improves serum lipids and lipoproteins in adults with growth hormone deficiency. *Metabolism* 1993; **42**: 1519–1523.

92. Johannsson G, Oscarsson J, Rosén T, Wiklund O, Olsson G, Wilhelmsen L, Bengtsson B-Å. Effects of 1 year of growth hormone therapy on serum lipoprotein levels in growth hormone-deficient adults: influence of gender and apo(a) and apoE phenotypes. *Arterioscler Thromb Vasc Biol* 1995; **15**: 2142–2150.

93. Rudling M, Norstedt G, Olivecrona H, Reihnér E, Gustafsson J-Å, Angelin B. Importance of growth hormone for the induction of hepatic low density lipoprotein receptors. *Proc Natl Acad Sci USA* 1992; **89**: 6983–6987.

94. Oscarsson J, Ottosson M, Johansson J-O, Wiklund O, Mårin P, Björntorp P, Bengtsson B-Å. Two weeks of daily injections and continuous infusion of recombinant human

growth hormone (GH) in GH-deficient adults: II. Effects on serum lipoproteins and lipoprotein and hepatic lipase activity. *Metabolism* 1996; **45**: 370–377.

95. Reaven GM. Pathophysiology of insulin resistance in human disease. *Physiol Rev* 1995; **75**: 473–486.

96. Reaven GH. Role of insulin resistance in human disease. *Diabetes* 1988; **37**: 1595–1607.

97. Rosmond R, Björntorp P. Blood pressure in relation to obesity, insulin and the hypothalamic-pituitary-adrenal axis in Swedish men. *J Hypertens* 1998; In press.

98. Julius S, Esler MD, Randall OS. Role of autonomic nervous system in mild human hypertension. *Clin Sci Mol Med* 1975; **48**: 243–252.

99. Sverrisdóttir YB, Elam M, Bengtsson B-Å, Johannsson G. Intense sympathetic nerve activity in adults with hypopituitarism and untreated growth hormone deficiency. *J Clin Endocrinol Metab* 1998; **83**: 1881–1885.

100. Böger RH, Skamira C, Bode-Böger SM, Brabant G, von zur Mühlen A, Frölich JC. Nitric oxide may mediate the hemodynamic effects of recombinant growth hormone in patients with acquired growth hormone deficiency. *J Clin Invest* 1996; **98**: 2706–2713.

101. Edén S, Widlund O, Oscarsson J, Rosén T, Bengtsson B-Å. Growth hormone treatment of growth hormone-deficient adults results in a marked increase in Lp(a) and HDL cholesterol concentrations. *Arterioscl Thromb Vasc Biol* 1993; **13**: 296–301.

102. Caidahl K, Edén S, Bengtsson B-Å. Cardiovascular and renal effects of growth hormone. *Clin Endocrinol* 1994; **40**: 393–400.

103. Fowelin J, Attvall S, Lager I, Bengtsson B-Å. Effects of treatment with recombinant human growth hormone on insulin sensitivity and glucose metabolism in adults with growth hormone deficiency. *Metabolism* 1993; **42**: 1443–1447.

104. Johannsson G, Mårin P, Lönn L, Ottosson M, Stenlöf K, Björntorp P, Sjöström L, Bengtsson B-Å. Growth hormone treatment of abdominally obese men reduces abdominal fat mass, improves glucose and lipoprotein metabolism, and reduces diastolic blood pressure. *J Clin Endocrinol Metab* 1997; **82**: 727–734.

33

Why Quality of Life Measures Should Be Used in the Treatment of Patients with Obesity

Marianne Sullivan, Jan Karlsson, Lars Sjöström and Charles Taft

Sahlgrenska University Hospital, Göteborg, Sweden

The aims of this chapter are

- To introduce a new discipline—quality of life assessment: its development, purposes, concepts, definitions, and basic tools
- To describe the current status of quality of life research in obesity
- To illustrate the usefulness of quality of life assessment in obesity

BACKGROUND AND RATIONALE

This section looks at health-related quality of life: its past, present and future status, what it is and the reasons for measuring it.

How the Need for Quality of Life Measures in Medicine Evolved

From Negative to Positive Health Concepts

The mission of health care services today is not only to cure disease, restore function, and alleviate ailment, but also to prevent disease and promote health. After World War II the 'academic world' tried to reorient the concept of health by broadening its definition. The net result of these efforts was that the patient perspective in medical care was emphasized by WHO in their 1948 definition of health, which included not only absence of disease or infirmity, but also a state of complete physical, mental and social well-being. The first attempts to quantify the new health definition began about a decade later. The principal focus in the 1960s on the physical aspects of health, primarily activities of daily living, later shifted to incorporate mental and social aspects, resulting in comprehensive health status questionnaires. During that decade the clinical trial (randomized or controlled) was proffered as the pre-eminent experimental model in clinical research. It was noteworthy that it took about two decades before this model was fully recognized by the medical profession (the Society of Clinical Trials was inaugurated in 1978), a fact that should be taken into account by those who complain that the integration of quality of life in medicine is moving slowly. The International Society for Quality of Life Research was created in 1994.

Classification of Medical Care by Level of Knowledge and Relation to Quality of Life

The need for quality of life assessment in medicine should be considered in relation to several key components of medical care: level of knowledge, efficiency, costs and evaluation. It may therefore be

International Textbook of Obesity. Edited by Per Björntorp.

helpful to view today's clinical medicine along a continuum from cure to supportive therapy.

1. Therapy with genuinely conclusive knowledge (top level),

i.e. treatment where the cause of the disease is known and can be influenced or eliminated. Long and intense basic research characterizes the scientific breakthroughs making causal therapy and prophylactic measures possible. Such therapy is very inexpensive compared with earlier treatments. Examples include a number of virogenic (e.g. polio, childhood viroses) and bacterial epidemics (e.g. tuberculosis, syphilis), now treated by immunization and antibiotics or chemotherapy, respectively. Another example is substitution therapy used when a certain substance is lacking or insufficient, e.g. in pernicious anaemia, hypothyroidism and diabetes. Apart from the last condition, the cost/benefit ratio at this level is very beneficial, the need for alternative therapies in principle is little, and the need for quality of life measures minimal. Diabetes is, however, not easily classified along the continuum despite the life-saving insulin therapy. Long-term features call for multimodal treatments to prevent negative sequelae and quality of life assessments are thus useful endpoints.

2. Therapy with a certain biological long-term effect (intermediate level),

i.e. treatment that reduces morbidity and mortality despite incomplete knowledge of the underlying disease mechanisms. Large and significant groups of diseases are represented here, e.g. non-generalized tumour diseases, kidney failure and coronary heart disease. Treatment at this level is often technically sophisticated and expensive but primitive from a biological perspective. Genuine cure for the disease is not the issue, rather the aim of treatment is to try to save a life at any cost. Treatment comprises a series of multimodal efforts with an increasing number of more and more specialized members of the treatment team at each rung up the treatment ladder, where surgical intervention is the precipitating first-order action available (e.g. tumour surgery, transplantation surgery). Today's treatment team is exemplified by the chain of care providers for patients with coronary heart disease from intensive care unit to outpatient rehabilitation and check-ups: ambulance staff, surgeons, cardiologists, nurses, psychologists, dieticians, physiotherapists, etc.

Outcome assessment is also multidisciplinary, often with improvements differing in various domains. The final common pathway from the multi-causal aetiology to the pathogenic mechanism is not yet available, i.e. the monocausal model exemplified at level 1 does not apply. The cost/benefit ratio is not beneficial, largely independent of the calculation method, e.g. cost/utility measures such as QALYs (quality-adjusted life years). A substantial and wide array of research attempts contribute to improved and safer therapy, e.g. improvement in transplantation outcome due to increasing knowledge about the immune system. The comprehensive evaluation of results often applied nowadays includes quality of life measures as secondary endpoints.

3. Therapy with no certain biological long-term effect (bottom level),

i.e. treatment of diseases where the cause is basically unknown and probably not possible to influence in the long run. This level comprises a great number of chronic diseases or conditions which place extreme demands on societal resources from an economic as well as humanitarian point of view. Among the many examples of such diseases are degenerative processes in the nervous system and supportive tissue, chronic pain conditions, many cancer diseases and mental diseases, degenerative diseases of ageing, and severe obesity. The goal of caretaking is effective symptom control and palliation, and the primary outcome is optimal quality of life. The health care system can offer a wide range of alternatives and combinations of treatments. Apart from providing transient symptom relief, traditional medical treatment is usually not applicable at this level; rather treatment is concerned with creating a psychologically positive therapeutic environment. Therapeutic teams provide functional training, compensation for functional impairments, physical conditioning, diet, supportive therapy to infuse hope, console, deal with psychosocial problems, etc.

Despite the availability of a vast number of therapeutic options, the benefits from treatments according to currently available clinical measures are more marginal than at level 2. The total effects of care are difficult to evaluate in all respects because there is no standardized way of weighing transient 'objective' and varying 'subjective' improvements in clinically applicable terms. The impact on quality of life typically needs to be measured by an extensive battery of generic and condition-specific measures to be satisfactorily understood. A cost/benefit ratio would probably be very high, i.e. disadvantageous, if such calculations were found to be feasible. Cost/ utility measures, sometimes supplementing the evaluation system of level 2, are also tested here. Although hard to validate, they offer new ways of thinking about resource allocation and ethics.

The need for quality of life assessment is naturally dependent on the relations between the key components of medical care, i.e. the lower the level of knowledge, the more complicated the evaluation will be. Treatment effects are dependent on the experienced change per se and people's expectations before, during and after therapy. It is thus necessary to include various patient-based measures in order to interpret treatment benefits versus placebo and adaptation effects.

How Quality of Life Measures Were Introduced in Clinical Trials

Early Milestones

Early studies (mid-1960s) in rehabilitation medicine used one social criterion (return to work) as central evidence of wisely spent resources. Later, evaluation of specialized medical care, e.g. coronary by-pass surgery, also defined treatment success in terms of return to work, often labelled quality of life. The health-related, or rather illness/sickness-related, quality of life assessment was introduced as an emerging research area in medicine in the 1970s, when today's methods were created and field-tested for the first time. During the 1980s a few large-scale clinical trials specified secondary quality-of-life aims. A well-known example of this trend was the COPD (chronic obstructive pulmonary disease) intervention study by McSweeney *et al.* (1), where different expectations of quality of life were linked to the alternative treatment options under examination. A frequently cited trial from oncology (limb-sparing vs. amputation in patients with soft tissue sarcoma) showed that inclusion of comprehensive quality of life measurements added new and valuable knowledge for subsequent clinical practice (2). Clinical cancer trials have recognized and incorporated quality of life measures increasingly ever since (3,4). Cardiology and rheumatology were also

among the early application areas. For example, the first recognized international demonstration of the need for quality of life research in clinical medicine took place in the cardiovascular field, i.e. the 1983 workshop under the auspices of the National Heart, Lung and Blood Institute (5) and the well-known multicentre study of antihypertensive therapy and quality of life (6). In rheumatology, the attempts to document patient-based effects of treatment in rheumatoid arthritis moved from mere registration of functional aspects of daily living to the use of the multidimensional self-report measures in the early 1980s (7).

Evidence-based Medicine and the Patient's Viewpoint

It was not until the WHO meeting in 1986, however, that health promotion objectives were made explicit and the health promotion hospital movement was launched to supplement disease orientation with health development. The importance of this goal was strongly emphasized and evaluation of health gains therefore expanded to include self-rated health/quality of life as an important endpoint. Methodological meta-analyses and evidence-based medicine were introduced to the medical establishment, all directed toward improving the arsenal of therapeutic measures. First, the traditional outcomes, readily understood by the medical profession, were evaluated; e.g. tumour response in cancer trials and walking distance in trials from rheumatology, pulmonary medicine and cardiology. Quite recently, this development has enabled us to approach outcome assessment from a different vantage point, the patient's (8,9). The validity and usefulness of assessing people's own perceptions of their health have now been documented in a multitude of studies (10). For example, self-rated global health has proved a more powerful predictor of mortality than traditional clinical measures, such as diagnostic criteria or laboratory measurements (11).

Current Status and Future

The Rationale of Quality of Life Outcomes: 'Why Measure It?'

The rationale behind measuring quality of life in health care concerns the 'paradox of health', i.e.

Table 33.1   Core dimensions of health-related quality of life in clinical research

Concepts	Definitions
Physical complaints/well-being	For example, disease- and treatment-related symptoms, general symptoms, fitness
Psychological distress/well-being	For example, anxiety and depressive symptoms, positive affect, cognitive disturbance
Functional status	For example, activities of daily living
Role functioning	For example, occupational and housework activities
Social functioning/well-being	For example, interpersonal relations, quantity and quality of social interaction, leisure
Health/quality of life perception	For example, global ratings

Reproduced from Sullivan (77) with permission.

better health state according to traditional indicators is not automatically accompanied by improved well-being or perceived health gain (12). Quality of life outcome evaluation is especially important in incurable conditions, when the self-evident and realistic goal of care is to make the patient's life as comfortable, functional, and satisfying as possible. Although traditional clinical outcome measures of signs and symptoms, together with data on survival, disease-free survival and time without symptoms of disease and toxicity of treatment, are certainly important in evaluating benefits of interventions, all this says little about people's overall health and the quality of their lives. Such information can be obtained only from the patient him/herself. It cannot be emphasized enough that quality of life studies should be conducted to get *new information of clinical value*, information that can be applied in further research and eventually in clinical practice.

Toward an Operational Definition of Health-related Quality of Life: 'What It Is'

Since the inception of quality of life research in medicine about 30 years ago, a controversy has existed concerning the potentials of quality of life questionnaires. Advocates have pointed to the centrality of these measures in all outcome assessments in chronic conditions. Others have thought of quality of life data as mainly qualitative, not amenable to meaningful statistical analysis and interpretation. So, when quality of life research first attracted attention in clinical studies it was met by a series of challenges: conceptual and methodological barriers to be overcome as well as attitudinal and practical hindrances due to lack of experience (3,13). It took several decades of conceptual analysis, pragmatic definitions and development and testing of basic tools before the current multidimensional,

psychometrically sound measures became available.

It is not possible to define all aspects of health or quality of life distinctly; these concepts are truly subjective and situational. If the concepts are considered solely unidimensionally and globally, they become practically undefined; e.g. 'how would you rate your quality of life?' Indicators like this are of questionable value because it is hard to interpret them; they do not provide the specific information needed to evaluate effects of treatment, to assist medical decisions, or to improve care. Problems in defining quality of life have paved the way for a joint behavioural/clinical effort to agree on operational definitions of a set of core dimensions that incorporates both broader and narrower elements, most often called *health-related quality of life* (Table 33.1) (14–16). The rationale behind this pragmatic solution may be readily understood through Figure 33.1. In the figure the dimensions are summarized in relation to obesity to reflect functional limitations and well-being along the continuum from condition-specific to general aspects of physical and mental health. Examples of specific and generic instruments currently used in obesity research are shown.

'Consensus' on concepts and definitions has led to the development of standardized questionnaires with well-established psychometric properties. Quality of life outcome measures in medicine are thus multidimensional, quantitative, and developed in accordance with psychometric theory to form multi-item scales, profiles and indexes. Most often clinical research questions require a combination of condition-specific and generic questionnaires. Condition-specific measures are often designed for clinical use and to be sensitive to changes after treatment. On the other hand, generic measures capture dimensions that are not specific to the condition and enable comparisons to be made between groups. Their central points concern health-related

Concepts: **condition-specific and generic**	Instruments: **obesity-related and generic**		
Condition-specific	IWQOL	TFEQ	OP
Complaints/consequences	• Health • Social/Interpersonal • Work • Mobility • Self-esteem • Sexual life • Activities of daily living • Comfort with food	• Restraint eating • Disinhibition • Hunger	• Obesity-related psychosocial problems
Functional health: generic Physical/mobility oriented consequences	SIP • Overall index • Physical dimension • Ambulation, mobility, body care and movement • Sleep and rest, eating, home management, work, recreation and pastimes		
	SF-36 • Physical component score • Physical functioning • Role–physical • Bodily pain • General health		
Social/emotional/cognitive consequences	SIP • Psychosocial dimension • Social interaction, emotional behaviour, alertness behaviour, communication		
Mental health: generic Distress/well-being	HAD • Depression • Anxiety		
	SF-36 • Mental component score • Mental health • Role–emotional • Social functioning • Vitality		
Overall quality of life	Global ratings		

Figure 33.1 Conceptual and measurement model of health-related quality of life assessment in obesity: a continuum of concepts and instruments. IWQOL: Impact of Weight on Quality of Life (40); TFEQ: Three-Factor Eating Questionnaire (54); OP: Obesity-related Problem scale from the SOS Quality of Life Survey (39); SIP: Sickness Impact Profile (69); SF-36: Short Form-36 Health Survey (34); HAD: Hospital Anxiety and Depression scale (72). Reproduced from Sullivan *et al.* (78) with permission

functioning and behaviour in everyday life. Thus, they usually include items related to aspects of physical functioning, e.g. mobility, but also to role and social functioning, and other common dimensions of health status such as pain, sleep, sexual functioning, general health perceptions and aspects of well-being, e.g. mood. It should be noted, however, that despite close points of similarity among generic instruments, they tend to vary widely in

their focus on core dimensions of health as well as in their capacity to detect relevant differences between study populations and within treatment groups over time.

Quality of life measures play an increasingly important role in evidence-based medicine since information from patients is not highly correlated with ratings of care professionals and significant others or with laboratory tests and other surrogate clinical

Table 33.2   Main psychometric features of health-related quality of life instruments

Concepts	Definitions
Reliability	For example, internal consistency (Cronbach's α), Reproducibility (test–retest correlation)
Validity	For example, content-related (acceptable to patients, relevant to clinicians or other focus groups), Construct-related (convergent and discriminant—multitrait or multitrait-multimethod analysis), Criterion-related (concurrent or predictive—known groups or events analysis)
Responsiveness	For example, sensitivity to clinically relevant changes (effect sizes—standardized response means)
Interpretability	For example, reference values (patient and general population databases)
Practicality	For example, respondent burden (self or proxy report), Administrative burden (alternative forms)
Cross-cultural applicability	For example, translation criteria (conceptual and linguistic equivalence), Psychometric evaluation (source instrument comparison)

Based on Instrument Review Criteria (22). Reproduced from Sullivan *et al.* (78) with permission.

outcomes. The inclusion of quality of life endpoints in intervention studies of obese persons is, however, a more recent phenomenon than in several other disciplines such as rheumatology, cardiology, and oncology, and has yet to gain wide acceptance among scientists and clinicians involved in the progress of obesity research (17–19). The most recent, comprehensive text on quality of life and pharmacoeconomics in clinical trials (20) addresses research activities from a wide variety of areas, but not obesity. In line with a general trend in health care, however, new standards proposed for evaluating the success of obesity interventions include quality of life assessments (21).

Authorized Measures: Psychometric Criteria

A summary of all the basic requirements of standardized quality of life questionnaires in medicine was formally established in the 1990s (22). By making the instrument criteria presented in Table 33.2 publicly available (23), the Medical Outcomes Trust contributes to quality assurance of outcome instruments, as the standards may be used: (a) to choose appropriate measures; (b) to assess the adequacy of findings, e.g. in the peer review of publications; and (c) to evaluate claims for new pharmaceutical agents where major focus is placed on quality of life.

Authorization of instruments today includes, beyond a clear conceptual and measurement model, evidence of reliability, validity, responsiveness, interpretability, practicality and cross-cultural applicability (Table 33.2). There are now well-established and feasible methods available to perform

careful construction of questionnaires and determine their psychometric properties to ensure interpretability of results (16,24–26). This methodology is also helpful for shortening instruments (27,28) and for cultural and language adaptations (29–31). The availability of computer services such as The On-Line Guide to Quality-of-Life Assessment, OLGA (32) helps today's selection and application of standardized instruments.

The process of instrument development thus implies many different steps of analysis to determine if the questionnaire measures the presumed constructs or dimensions of health status/quality of life (Table 33.2). Evidence of the construct validity of questionnaires is of particular importance when quality of life methods are being developed and incorporated in a new research field, as is now the case in obesity. It should be especially recognized that basic psychometric testing goes beyond the traditional calculation of Cronbach's alpha coefficients, which gives an estimate of the reproducibility of a measure. Modern testing is now more focused on the internal structure of an instrument, e.g. convergent and discriminant validity. A good example of this process is found in the Medical Outcomes Study approach, representing a broad range of self-reported functioning and well-being measures from which the Short Form 36-item Health Survey is derived (33–36). The increasing use of quality of life assessments as major endpoints in clinical trials places certain demands on instruments to demonstrate satisfactory responsiveness (37,38). The sensitivity of instruments to detect change in health over time has been studied far less than other aspects of validity (19).

Clinical Relevance

While the use of quality of life data in clinical trials is dictated by the research questions or hypotheses specified in the protocol, the clinical value may differ. In general, quality of life data may help care providers in: (a) evaluating the total burden of a disease; (b) estimating the effects of different treatment options; (c) detecting morbidity, psychosocial problems and special needs; (d) improving quality of care (communication, clinical decision-making and caretaking); and (e) educating staff, patients, families and others. With self-report questionnaires, patients have a better opportunity to selectively perceive and evaluate important symptoms and signs, impacts and side effects of therapy, and thus become responsible partners in the treatment process. Compliance rates may also improve. Outside the inner circle of medical care, health planners may find guidance in prioritizing and developing new care programmes.

In summary, quality of life measures today are

- Standardized, with cross-cultural applicability
- Established part of technology assessment in clinical research
- Newly introduced in treatment evaluation in obesity research

HEALTH-RELATED QUALITY OF LIFE (HRQL) AND OBESITY: WHAT DO WE KNOW?

Current 'State of the Art' in Obesity

As obesity is considered a chronic and incurable disease, the outcome of treatment can only be measured through changes in the degree of overweight and its consequences, not in terms of cure rate. The primary goal of treatment could be expressed in terms of controlling concomitant diseases, symptoms and complaints, and minimizing psychosocial adverse effects by reducing weight. Under these circumstances, the obvious outcome of therapy is the effect it has on the patients' everyday life and well-being. Health-related quality of life assessment in intervention studies of obesity, and the potential clinical value of such data, will thus be focused on below. Primary prevention of obesity will certainly

benefit from knowledge about the self-report methods discussed (Figure 33.1), although this issue is beyond the scope of this chapter.

An indication of the current state of HRQL in obesity research may be obtained by examining the published literature. Table 33.3 presents a list of publications obtained from a recent Medline search of quality of life methods used in obesity research. Studies were included if quality of life was approached in a multidimensional way, research questions were distinctly addressed and assessments accounted for in the methods section.

In a nutshell, this summary of main purposes and methods of the papers substantiates: (a) the newness of the field; (b) the scarcity of controlled studies; (c) the variety of selected instruments; and (d) the rapidly growing number of epidemiological and clinical studies using HRQL methods. It is also notable that most clinical studies have been conducted to evaluate the effects of weight-reduction surgery, while only two or three have been carried through to assess quality of life change during non-surgical weight loss treatment. To date, only a few attempts have been made to develop and validate HRQL methods in obese populations (39–43). Further careful evaluations of instrument properties are needed in longitudinal field studies, where the contribution of specific questionnaires vis-a-vis generic ones can be clarified. This process will take several years to complete. A number of recent publications have measured health status in the obese using the generic SF-36 Health Survey. Due to its well-documented high psychometric standards and multinational applicability, the SF-36 will undoubtedly be increasingly used, with or without other condition-specific measures (44).

HRQL and Obesity: Interpretation Strategies

Proposed strategies for interpreting quality of life data are multifaceted (37,45) and various illustrative examples related to obesity will be presented below. Statistical significance testing should not be used as the sole criterion for interpreting the clinical meaning of quality of life findings. For example, content-based interpretation strategies are a useful means to communicate the basic meaning of questionnaire scores. Elaborate examples of this approach can be

Table 33.3　Health-related quality of life (HRQL) studies in obesity: study design, main purpose and methods

	Main purpose	Study	HRQL assessment/method
Review article	HRQL assessment in obesity	Sullivan et al. (17) Kral et al. (18) Sarlio-Lähteenkorva et al. (79)	
Validation study	Development of obesity-specific HRQL instruments	Sullivan et al. (39) Kolotkin et al. (40) Kolotkin et al. (41) Mathias et al. (42) Le Pen et al. (43)	OP IWQOL IWQOL 'HRQL questionnaire' OSQOL
Cross-sectional study	Impact of obesity on HRQL	Sullivan et al. (39) Fontaine et al. (57) Fontaine et al. (58) Han et al. (51) Le Pen et al. (43) Brown et al. (52)	Battery: SOS Quality of Life Survey Generic: SF-36 Scales Generic: SF-36 Summary Scores Generic: SF-36 Scales Generic: SF-36 Scales Specific: OSQOL Generic: SF-36 Scales and Summary Scores
Retrospective study	Treatment effects of weight-reduction surgery	Carr et al. (80) Hafner et al. (81)	Interview Specific: Gastric Bypass Questionnaire
Controlled retrospective study	Treatment effects of weight-reduction surgery	Isacsson et al. (82) Van Gemert et al. (83)	Battery: Gothenburg Quality of Life Scale and others Generic: Nottingham Health Profile
Prospective study	Treatment effects of weight-reduction surgery Quality of life in obese patients after primary hip arthroplasty Effects of cardiac rehabilitation, exercise training and weight reduction in obese coronary patients	Larsen (84) Choban et al. (85) Chan and Villar (86) Lavie and Milan (87)	Battery: Quality of Life Index and others Generic: SF-36 Scales Generic: Rosser Index Specific: Harris hip score questionnaire Generic: SF-36 Kellner questionnaire
Controlled clinical trial	Effects of weight-reduction surgery vs. conventional treatment	Karlsson et al. (19)	Battery: SOS Quality of Life Survey
Randomized controlled trial	Prediction and effects of long-term dieting in moderately obese women randomized to a lacto-vegetarian vs. regular diet Effects of a combined 12-week weight loss programme in moderately obese women	Karlsson et al. (55) Rippe et al. (65)	Generic: Sickness Impact Profile (SIP), Mood Adjective Check List (MACL) Specific: Three-Factor Eating Questionnaire (TEFQ) Generic: SF-36 and others

found in the interpretation guidelines for the SF-36 Health Survey (35).

Since quality of life measurement scores have no direct commonly understood meaning, the clinical significance of different scale levels may be difficult to interpret for the inexperienced user. To be more user-friendly scores are sometimes transformed into a 0-to-100 scale, which facilitates the understanding of differences in scores and also enables scores of different measures within an instrument to be compared along a uniform scale (cf. SF-36 health profiles in Figures 33.2 and 33.3), A common way to evaluate the impact on quality of life is to relate patient scores to the scores of reference groups.

'Known group' comparisons may include norm-based interpretation linked to the analysis of score distributions in characterized clinical as well as general populations (cf. SIP category and index scores of severely obese vs. those of healthy subjects and cancer survivors in Figures 33.4 and 33.6, respectively). It is also useful to calculate the percentage of the study sample with no reported limitation on the different functional health scales, versus proportions with small-to-moderate and large dysfunction. Among other distribution-based interpretation methods to convey differences in quality of life scores, calculation of effect sizes should be mentioned. Effect size estimates allow direct comparisons across different measures regardless of scoring system and the clinical significance of differences between groups may be judged against standard criteria proposed by Cohen (46).

The clinical meaning of change in intervention studies is another important issue. To arrive at meaningful interpretations, quality of life change scores may be compared, or anchored to other established criteria for clinical change. Obviously, effects of obesity interventions on quality of life may be related to weight change and to reductions in morbidity. It should be noted, however, that initial weight loss or participation per se in weight management programmes is likely to produce unrealistic short-term changes, and repeated post-treatment assessments, including long-term follow-up of quality of life, are strongly recommended (19,47). The issue of clinically meaningful change could also be elucidated by calculating effect sizes of change (48). Standardized response means, SRM (49), is one of several methods used to estimate the responsiveness of measures in intervention studies (cf. SOS Quality of Life Survey change over time in Figure 33.8). Changes in score levels can also become meaningful by comparing them with 'normality' defined by population norms or with the impact of observed life events, such as being laid off from work.

Understanding individual scores sometimes requires thresholds indicating current or future morbidity, e.g. to estimate the prevalence of mood disorder in obese populations (cf. HAD scale and probabilities of depression in Figure 33.10). These well-established means of interpretation are all the more important in the field of obesity where the experience of quality of life measures is scanty.

HRQL and Obesity I: Obese Subjects vs. General Population Norms

The impact of obesity on quality of life has mainly been studied in clinical investigations where it is not known if samples are representative of the total obese population. It has been shown that obese subjects who seek treatment for their obesity report greater psychopathology than those who do not seek treatment (50). Both obese groups in that study, however, reported more distress than did normal weight controls. In the Swedish Obese Subjects (SOS) study, the severely obese who chose surgical treatment had generally lower levels of quality of life before treatment than their matched obese controls (19). Thus, it is crucial to perform population studies that include generic questionnaires in order to determine the extent and nature of the burden of obesity in relation to general population norms. Recently, three studies have used the SF-36 Health Survey to study the impact of obesity on quality of life in general population samples. The SF-36 is a widespread, generic short-form instrument, which comprises eight core domains of health-related quality of life: physical functioning, role functioning-physical, bodily pain, general health, vitality, social functioning, role functioning-emotional, and mental health (35,36,44).

Le Pen et al. (43) compared the SF-36 health profiles of subjects classified as non-obese (BMI < 27), overweight (BMI 27–30) or obese (BMI ≥ 30) in a French community sample. The overweight group did not differ from the non-obese except for a slight but significant decrease in physical functioning. The obese group, however, showed impaired quality of life compared to the non-obese on five of eight SF-36 scales: physical functioning, role functioning-physical and bodily pain (scales which mainly reflect physical health aspects) and in general health and vitality (scales reflecting both physical and mental health aspects). Unexpectedly, no differences between groups were observed on the mental health scales (social functioning, role functioning-emotional, and mental health).

Han et al. (51) used the SF-36 to evaluate the impact of abdominal fat (large waist circumferences) as well as generalized obesity (high BMI) on quality of life in a Dutch population sample. The total sample was divided by sex and tertiles of waist circumference and BMI. Odds ratios were cal-

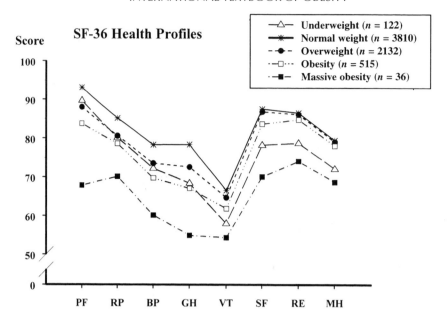

Figure 33.2   SF-36 health profiles in relation to body mass index (BMI) in a Swedish population study. A higher score (range 0–100) on the SF-36 scales represents better health status. Subjects are grouped in five categories of BMI: underweight (BMI < 18.5), normal weight (18.5 ≤ BMI < 25), overweight (25 ≤ BMI < 30), obesity (30 ≤ BMI < 40) and massive obesity (BMI ≥ 40). Calculations of BMI are based on self-reported height and weight. PF, physical functioning; RP, role-physical; BP, bodily pain; GH, general health; VT, vitality; SF, social functioning; RE, role-emotional; MH, mental health

culated (adjusted for age, socioeconomic and life-style factors) for poor health status, defined as a scale score below 66.7 (score range 0–100). Men and women in the upper tertiles of waist circumference (mean 104.3 cm) as well as BMI (mean 29.6) were more likely to have poor physical functioning. Subjects with generalized obesity were more likely to report bodily pain and women also reported poorer general health perceptions. No adverse effects of abdominal fat or generalized obesity were observed on role functioning-physical, vitality, social functioning, role functioning-emotional, and mental health.

Brown *et al.* (52) presented SF-36 data from a large (*n* = 14 431) population-based study of Australian women 45–49 years of age. Around half of the sample had a BMI > 25. The study corroborated earlier findings that the physical aspects of HRQL (physical functioning, bodily pain and general health) and vitality deteriorate with increasing BMI. Furthermore, even after adjusting for area of residence, education, smoking, exercise and menopausal status they found both high and low BMI to be associated with worse HRQL. The study pro-

vided additional support from the HRQL perspective for an optimal BMI range of 20–25.

We will use SF-36 data from two Swedish population studies to further illustrate this type of norm-based interpretation. In the first example, SF-36 health profiles from subjects with underweight and increasing degrees of overweight are compared with the normal weight persons in a 1997 population study in a Swedish county (Figure 33.2; Ulf Larsson *et al.*, unpublished data). The total postal survey comprised a random sample of the adult population (*n* = 8751, 72% response rate). We used a sub-sample of subjects between 16 and 65 years of age to avoid confounding physical health with increasing age.

As shown in Figure 33.2 the pattern of impact is quite clear; the more overweight the worse the health profile and more so for physical aspects of health (physical functioning, role-physical, bodily pain and general health) than mental. There is a dramatic negative impact on all aspects of health when obesity is massive (BMI ≥ 40). The difference, expressed in effect sizes, between the massively obese and normal weight subjects, was particularly

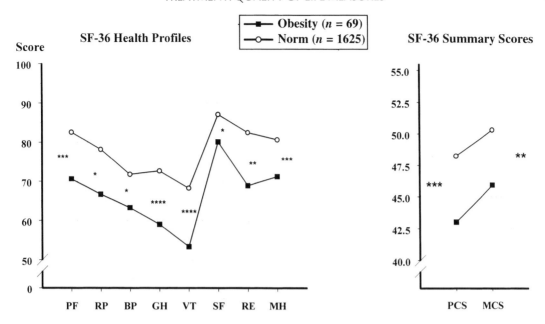

Figure 33.3   Comparison of SF-36 health profiles and summary scores between an obese (BMI ≥ 30) population sample and age- and sex-matched Swedish population norms. Calculations of BMI are based on self-reported height and weight. A higher score on the SF-36 scales (range 0–100) and summary components represents better health status. The physical (PCS) and mental (MCS) component summary scores are weighted indexes (mean 50, SD 10) of the eight scales. The physically oriented scales (PF, RP, BP and GH) have the highest impact on PCS, while the mentally oriented scales (MH, RE, SF and VT) have the highest impact on MCS. A score of 50 on PCS and MCS represents the mean of the general Swedish population. PF, physical functioning; RP, role-physical; BP, bodily pain; GH, general health; VT, vitality; SF, social functioning; RE, role-emotional; MH, mental health; PCS, physical component summary score; MCS, mental component summary score. Differences between groups were tested by Fisher's non-parametric permutation test: $*P < 0.05$, $**P < 0.01$, $***P < 0.001$, $****P < 0.0001$

large on physical functioning and general health, and moderate on social functioning, bodily pain, vitality and mental health (data not shown). A lower health profile compared with the normal weight group can also be seen in the physical areas for obese persons (BMI 30–39.9) and for those with overweight (BMI 25–29.9). Vitality and social functioning are affected in the obese group (BMI 30–39.9) but, unexpectedly, not mental health. It is also notable that underweight persons (BMI < 18.5) report worse mental health in all aspects compared with the obese and overweight groups and worse physical health than the normal weight group.

Mental health scores among the normal weight, overweight and obese in the French, Dutch, Australian and Swedish population samples were unexpectedly similar. This finding indicates that the prevalence of mood disorders in a random population sample of overweight and obese persons does

not, unlike the massively obese (BMI ≥ 40.0), differ from that of the general population. However, the sensitivity of the mental health scale of the SF-36 to detect mental disturbances in overweight and obese samples should be further investigated.

In Figure 33.3, an obese population group (BMI ≥ 30) is compared with a perfect age- and sex-matched Swedish SF-36 norm population (53), i.e. reference values representing the general population. The accuracy of comparisons with norm values requires that known systematic differences in self-rated health by demographics be taken into consideration. For example, physical health in particular decreases with age and women show generally lower health profiles than men. Thus, the advantage of a perfectly matched reference group is obvious. As shown in Figure 33.3, the health profile of the obese is clearly worse in all respects than the population norm. The SF-36 physical and mental summary scores are displayed to further emphasize the large differences between groups. It should be noted though that the health profile of the obese sample in Figure 33.3 is worse than that of the corresponding group (BMI 30–39) in Figure 33.2. The reasons for this are probably related to sample differences and thus more research is needed to clarify the impact of obesity on quality of life in general population samples.

There is no 'gold standard' quality of life instrument by which to assess the burden of obesity. On the contrary, since obesity is associated with a wide range of chronic conditions it would most likely be advantageous to compare results from different generic instruments. In the next example, the Sickness Impact Profile (SIP) is used to assess functional health in a sample of severely obese subjects. The SIP is a well-established self-report measure of health-related limitations in 12 defined areas of everyday life: body care and movement, mobility, ambulation, sleep and rest, eating, home management, work, recreation and pastimes, social interaction, communication, alertness behaviour and emotional behaviour. A physical, psychosocial, and overall index is also calculated.

In Figure 33.4, SIP dimension and index scores in a group of severely obese subjects from the SOS methods study (27) are compared with healthy reference subjects (39). The main features of the SOS registry and intervention studies can be seen in Figure 33.5.

The severely obese report more functional limitations in nearly all aspects of everyday life. Mobility-oriented areas are the most affected (body care and movement, mobility, and ambulation) together with home management, recreation and pastimes, and social interaction, all of which contain statements refering to mobility. SIP physical, psychosocial, and overall indexes show small to moderate effect sizes, i.e. the obese suffer from a wide variety of negative consequences in their ordinary lives compared with people in general. Also, more emotional behaviour dysfunction is reported by the obese. Behaviours not limited by obesity are: communication (primarily speech pathology), eating (mainly insufficient nutrition), and alertness behaviour (cognitive functioning). As shown in Figure 33.4b, effect size calculations are informative about both level and strength of the burden perceived by an obese sample compared with a reference group.

A disadvantage of the SIP is that eating problems of significance to obese people are not covered by the eating category. Rather SIP items comprise problems associated with poor nutrition due to lack of appetite, impairment, dexterity difficulties, etc. As an alternative to the SIP eating category, the Three-Factor Eating Questionnaire (TFEQ, Figure 33.1) is an appropriate and comprehensive measure of eating behaviour related to overweight and obese subjects (19,54–56).

Summary: How Obese Persons Differ From the General Population

- Poorer functioning and well-being, more in physical than mental aspects
- The more overweight, the worse HRQL
- Both physical and mental aspects affected in the massively obese
- Poorer HRQL in massive obesity than in underweight

HRQL and Obesity II: Obese Subjects Seeking Treatment vs. Other Groups of Chronically Ill and Disabled

In a US study, Fontaine et al. (57,58) used the SF-36 to assess quality of life in a consecutive sample of obese subjects seeking outpatient treatment. The obese scored significantly worse on all of the eight SF-36 scales compared with general US population norms. The largest differences were noted for the bodily pain and vitality scales. Further comparisons with reference values for other chronic medical conditions indicated that the impact of pain among obese subjects seeking treatment is considerable, equivalent to that of chronic migraine patients. This finding is of clinical importance and the effect of weight loss on chronic pain should be investigated.

In the next example, SIP category and index scores of the severely obese are compared with cancer survivors. As can be seen in Figure 33.6a, functional limitations in everyday life are in most areas worse in the severely obese than in an unselected group of cancer survivors 2–3 years after diagnosis (59). The differences are significant for several of the SIP categories and for all three summary indexes: physical, psychosocial, and overall. Restrictions are as common among the obese as in cancer survivors in areas representing mobility, sleep and rest, home

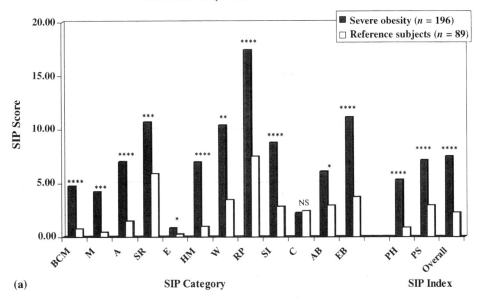

(a)   SIP Category   SIP Index

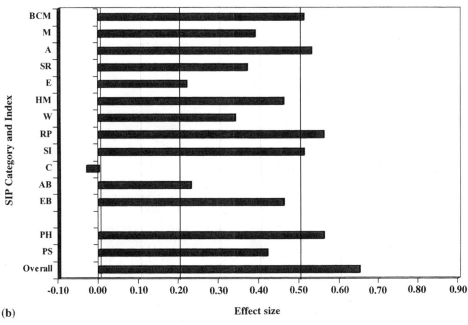

(b)   Effect size

Figure 33.4(a) Mean scores of SIP categories and indexes for severely obese subjects (SOS) vs. reference subjects from the general population. High scores on SIP categories and indexes represent dysfunction.
BCM, body care and movement; M, mobility; A, ambulation; SR, sleep and rest; E, eating; HM, home management; W, work; RP, recreation and pastimes; SI, social interaction; C, communication; AB, alertness behaviour; EB, emotional behaviour; PH, physical index (mean of BCM, M and A); PS, psychosocial index (mean of SI, C, AB and EB); Overall, total SIP index (mean of all 12 categories). Differences between groups were tested by Fisher's non-parametric permutation test. ****$P < 0.0001$, ***$P < 0.001$, **$P < 0.01$, *$P < 0.05$, NS, not significant.
(b) Effect sizes of SIP categories and indexes for severely obese subjects (SOS) vs. reference subjects from the general population. Effect size was calculated as the mean scale score difference between groups divided by the pooled standard deviation

> *The SOS study* is an ongoing nationwide, multicentre project which comprises a registry study and an intervention trial. Since its start in October 1987 about 7000 severely obese persons have been accepted in the registry study. Inclusion criteria are age at accrual (37–57 years) and BMI $\geq 34\,\mathrm{kg/m^2}$ for males and BMI $\geq 38\,\mathrm{kg/m^2}$ for females.
>
> *The intervention study* is a controlled clinical trial designed to test if the negative effects of severe obesity on mortality, morbidity and quality of life are reduced during long-term weight reduction. The outcomes of surgical vs. conventional weight reduction treatment will include 2000 surgical cases and their matched controls followed for 10 years.
>
> *Health-related quality of life, HRQL.* A battery of study-specific and generic questionnaires was designed to assess quality of life in the SOS study (see Appendix). Well-established HRQL measures, assumed to cover a broad range of health impacts of obesity, were supplemented by condition-specific parts, all suitable for large-scale mailout–mailback data collection.

Figure 33.5   The Swedish Obese Subjects (SOS) study

management, work, and communication. Effect size calculations (Figure 33.6b) further illustrate the relative strength of functional impacts in the obese versus cancer survivors. The recreation and pastimes and social interaction domains are most negatively affected by obesity, although effect sizes are small to moderate (interval 0.20–0.50). Additional comparisons showed that the impact of obesity was equal to that of a subgroup of cancer survivors with one or more known recurrences. Only limitations in mobility were significantly worse in the recurrence group (data not shown).

In contrast, the level of impact of obesity on functional health is modest compared with disabling conditions such as rheumatoid arthritis or chronic pain syndrome, where limitations according to SIP overall index are three to four times greater (60). However, the severely obese report worse mental well-being (Mood Adjective Check List; see Appendix) than a number of chronically ill or injured patient populations such as rheumatoid arthritis sufferers, cancer survivors with no recurrence 2–3 years after diagnosis, and people with spinal cord injuries several years after injury (39). The well-being of obese persons matches that of cancer survivors with recurrence and people with spinal cord injuries less than 2 years after injury. Only non-responders to treatment among patients with chronic pain syndrome score lower. Moreover, the severely obese report more symptoms of anxiety and depression (Hospital Anxiety and Depression scale; see Appendix) compared with spinal cord injured and disease groups such as generalized malignant melanoma and intermittent claudication.

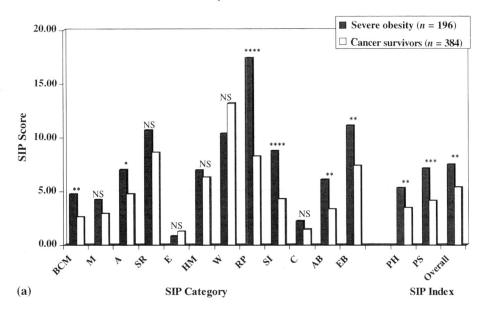

(a)

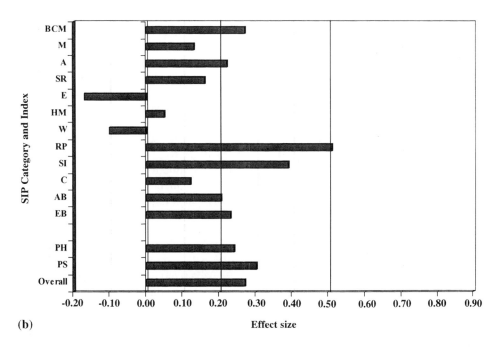

(b)

Figure 33.6(a) Mean scores of SIP categories and indexes for severely obese subjects (SOS) vs. unselected cancer survivors. High scores on SIP categories and indexes represent dysfunction. BCM, body care and movement; M, mobility; A, ambulation; SR, sleep and rest; E, eating; HM, home management; W, work; RP, recreation and pastimes; SI, social interaction; C, communication; AB, alertness behaviour; EB, emotional behaviour; PH, physical index (mean of BCM, M and A); PS, psychosocial index (mean of SI, C, AB and EB); Overall, total SIP index (mean of all 12 categories). Differences between groups were tested by Fisher's non-parametric permutation test. ****$P < 0.0001$; ***$P < 0.001$; **$P < 0.01$; *$P < 0.05$; NS, not significant.
(b) Effect sizes of SIP categories and indexes for severely obese subjects (SOS) vs. unselected cancer survivors. Effect size was calculated as the mean scale score difference between groups divided by the pooled standard deviation

Table 33.4 Obesity-related psychosocial problems (OP) in everyday life in severely obese men and women. Answers to the question: 'Are you bothered because of your obesity as regards the following activities?' (Scale range: definitely not bothered, not so bothered, mostly bothered, definitely bothered)

	Percentage mostly or definitely bothered							
	Body mass index (BMI; kg/m^2)						Total	
	30.0–34.9		35.0–39.9		40.0 +			
Items in OP scale	Men $n = 596$	Women $n = 87$	Men $n = 1112$	Women $n = 1375$	Men $n = 538$	Women $n = 1479$	Men $n = 2246$	Women $n = 2941$
Private gatherings in my own home	25.2	40.2	26.1	38.6	30.5	36.6	26.9	37.6
Private gatherings in a friend's or relative's home	31.0	47.1	34.5	48.4	42.2	46.5	35.4	47.4
Going to restaurants	30.5	57.5	36.7	61.8	44.1	62.4	36.8	62.0
Going to community activities, courses, etc.	27.2	51.7	34.6	55.0	41.6	56.0	34.3	55.4
Holidays away from home	28.3	62.1	34.8	55.6	41.5	56.7	34.7	56.3
Trying on and buying clothes	68.0	87.4	74.6	91.3	80.2	88.7	74.2	89.9
Bathing in public places (beach, public pool, etc.)	55.7	83.9	62.6	87.2	71.9	89.1	63.0	88.1
Intimate relations with partner	25.6	50.0	32.5	43.8	38.9	42.7	31.9	43.4
OP scale score[a] (mean and 95% CI[b])	37.0 34.9–39.1	56.9 51.2–62.5	41.7 40.1–43.3	57.8 56.4–59.2	48.0 45.6–50.4	57.9 56.6–59.3	42.0 40.9–43.1	57.8 56.9–58.8

[a]OP scores are transformed to a 0–100 scale. A higher score indicates greater problems.
[b]Confidence interval.

Summary: How Obese Patients Differ From other Chronic Populations

- Poorer functioning and mental well-being than unselected cancer survivors 2–3 years after diagnosis; comparable to those with recurrence
- The more overweight, the worse HRQL
- Better functioning than patients with disabling conditions, e.g. rheumatoid arthritis, chronic pain conditions
- Poorer mental well-being than the disabled, e.g. those with rheumatoid arthritis or with spinal cord injuries more than 2 years after injury

HRQL and Obesity III: Psychosocial Functioning

Impairment in psychosocial functioning among obese subjects has been documented in several reports during the last decades (18,61). Most studies, however, have been conducted in small samples of severely obese subjects before and after surgical treatment for obesity and generalizations are therefore uncertain. The validity of these studies is fur-

ther hampered by the high dropout rates and their failure to include control subjects, long-term follow-ups and standardized instruments, which greatly jeopardize the interpretability of the data.

Psychosocial dysfunction related to overweight is probably not well covered by generic instruments and an obesity-specific scale (Obesity-related Problem scale, OP; see Appendix) was developed in the SOS study to assess the impact of obesity on psychosocial functioning. The module comprises eight questions on how bothered patients are by their obesity in everyday life activities. Psychometric properties were shown to be satisfactory in the first 1743 subjects examined (39), later cross-validated in more than 2000 consecutive SOS subjects (62). The OP scale showed only moderate correlations ($r = 0.41$–0.54) with other HRQL measures and thus provides unique information on the quality of life of obese subjects. Table 33.4 illustrates that the psychosocial burden of obesity is substantial. Women perceived markedly more problems in every area regardless of degree of overweight, while men reported more problems the higher their BMI. As expected, the general trend for both men and women pointed to more concerns regarding activities in public places, such as trying on and buying clothes and bathing in public places. It has also been documented in the SOS intervention study that obese who choose surgical treatment report markedly more psychosocial dysfunction at baseline than do matched obese controls (19).

Summary: How Obesity-related Psychosocial Problems are Perceived

- Worst in public places, e.g. trying on and buying clothes, bathing
- Women much worse than men
- In men, the more overweight, the more psychosocial problems

HRQL and Obesity IV: Responsiveness to Weight Loss

Surprisingly little is known about the influence of weight reduction on psychosocial functioning and well-being in overweight or obese persons (63), and very few studies have measured the effects of weight loss on physical functioning, role functioning, vitality or other important aspects of health status. It is also unclear how weight gain which occurs after initial weight loss during the course of treatment affects the quality of life of the obese patients (64). Some recent studies that have used standardized self-report instruments for outcome assessment suggest that weight loss in obese subjects (e.g. after diet and lifestyle modification treatment) is mostly associated with improvements in mood (63). Positive long-term changes in functional health (Sickness Impact Profile) in moderately obese women were found after compliance in a 2-year weight loss programme (55). In a recent study, the SF-36 Health Survey was used to assess quality of life change in moderately obese women after a 12-week weight loss programme (65). Significant improvements in physical functioning, vitality and mental health were found in the intervention group, while no such improvements were noted in the control group.

Several studies on the outcome of weight-reduction surgery in severely obese subjects have reported very positive effects on psychosocial functioning and well-being (18). Responsiveness to weight loss after obesity surgery on the different

quality of life domains is, however, still unclear, especially in the long-term perspective. Obviously, it would be of great clinical value to clarify how the magnitude of weight loss affects quality of life, e.g. how much weight reduction is required to improve the general health perceptions of the patient. With regular use of well-established, standardized HRQL instruments in obesity research it would be possible to calculate a dose–response relation between weight loss and the various quality of life parameters.

HRQL Change in the SOS Intervention Study: the SOS Quality of Life Survey

The following examples are based on severely obese patients followed for 4 years in the SOS intervention study (Karlsson *et al.*, unpublished data). A battery approach was applied in the SOS study to assess quality of life. The SOS Quality of Life Survey (see Appendix) is intended to tap a broad range of health impacts of obesity, and generic instruments or subscales on functioning and well-being are supplemented by obesity-specific modules.

Poor HRQL at baseline was dramatically improved after obesity surgery, while stable ratings over time were observed in the control group. Powerful improvements after 6 and 12 months in the surgical group were followed by a slight to moderate decline at 2- 3- and 4-year follow-ups. It was demonstrated that improvements in HRQL after 6 months were weakly related to weight loss, while this association was strengthened at 2-year follow-up (19). Thus, short-term change on HRQL indicators in weight loss studies should be interpreted with caution. Long-term follow-up is most likely necessary to confirm the effects of obesity interventions on quality of life.

In Figure 37.7, the percentage bothered on each item of the Obesity-related Problem scale (OP) are shown at baseline and at 2- and 4-year follow-ups. Great improvements can be seen from baseline to intermediate (2-year) and long-term (4-year) follow-ups in all activities covered by the OP scale. The OP scale has proved the most responsive HRQL measure in relation to weight loss over 4 years in the SOS intervention study (19,66). The results are strengthened by the fact that the dropout rate in the surgery group was extremely low even after 4 years (about 17%).

To enable comparisons of the effect of obesity

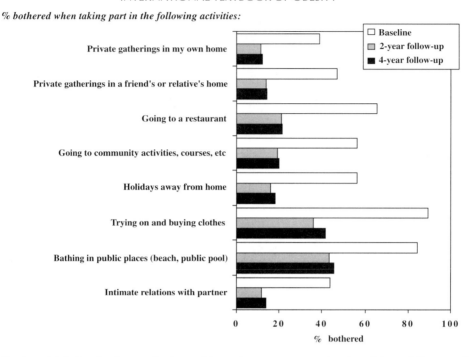

Figure 33.7 Psychosocial dysfunction in severely obese subjects prior to treatment and at 2- and 4-year follow-ups after surgical intervention in the SOS study ($n = 213$). The percentage bothered (mostly bothered and definitely bothered) is given for each item of the OP scale

surgery on the different quality of life domains, change scores from baseline to follow-ups were transformed to standardized response means (SRM; $Mean_{diff}/SD_{diff}$) (49). Effect sizes of HRQL change after 6, 24 and 48 months are displayed in Figure 37.8. SRMs for weight change were also calculated as a point of reference and, as expected, the effect size after gastric surgery was large (data not shown). SRM for weight loss was largest after 6 months (2.75) but declined after 2 years (1.95) and 4 years (1.60). A similar trend was noted for the HRQL measures. Great changes in eating behaviour (TFEQ) were observed after surgical intervention, i.e. patients reported more restrained eating (RE) and less disinhibition (DI) and hunger (HU). The early changes, however, declined slightly over time. Improvements in functional health (SIP) were largely in leisure activities (RP) and social interaction (SI). Relatively small improvements (SRMs around 0.20 to 0.50) were seen in the general health (GHRI-CH) and mental health (MACL, HAD, SE) domains as well as in global quality of life (QL).

HRQL Improvements in Relation to Weight Loss After Surgical Treatment

HRQL changes 4 years after obesity surgery were related to the magnitude of weight loss; improvements were stable over time in patients with substantial weight loss (> 30 kg; around 30%), while a regression was observed in patients with less weight reduction. If weight loss was minor (< 10 kg), patients tended to return to their baseline levels.

A dose–response relation was observed between weight loss and improvements in psychosocial functioning (OP). The surgically treated subjects were grouped by amount of weight loss (kg) 4 years after surgery and the mean OP-scale scores were calculated for each measurement time point. There were no significant differences between groups at baseline. After 6 months, levels of psychosocial problems were substantially reduced in all groups, with a more positive trend seen in subjects with major long-term weight reduction. A distinct pattern of change among groups was observed, namely, subjects with more favourable long-term weight

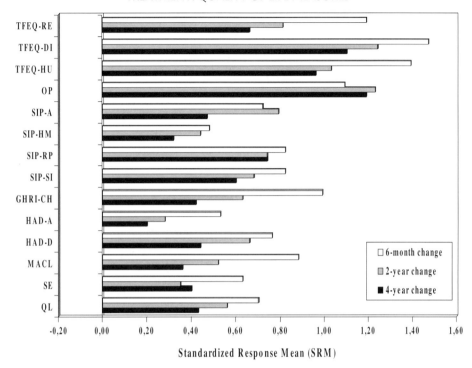

Figure 33.8 Effect of obesity surgery on health-related quality of life (HRQL) at short-term (6 months), intermediate (2 years) and long-term (4 years) follow-ups in the SOS intervention study. HRQL change scores from baseline to follow-up are transformed to standardized response means (SRM). SRM is calculated as the mean change score divided by the standard deviation of change ($Mean_{diff}/SD_{diff}$, Katz et al. (49)).
TFEQ, Three-Factor Eating Questionnaire; RE, restrained eating; DI, disinhibition; HU, hunger.
OP, Obesity-related Psychosocial Problems.
SIP, Sickness Impact Profile; A, ambulation; HM, home management; RP, recreation and pastimes; SI, social interaction.
GHRI, General Health Rating Index; CH, current health.
HAD, Hospital Anxiety and Depression scale; A, anxiety symptoms; D, depression symptoms.
MACL, Mood Adjective Check List. SE, Self-esteem. QL, Overall quality of life

reduction reported significantly lower levels of obesity-related psychosocial problems.

As shown in Figure 33.9, effect sizes of long-term change in quality of life were associated with the amount of weight loss at 4-year follow-up (66). Where there was substantial weight reduction ($\geq 25\%$ of preoperative body weight), large effects (> 0.8 SRM) were noted for obesity-related measures reflecting eating pattern and psychosocial problems but also for general health and functional health domains such as ambulation, recreation and pastimes, and social interaction. Interpretation of effect sizes proved that long-term effects of major weight loss on mental well-being were beneficial. Moderate effect sizes ($0.5 < SRM < 0.8$) were noted for depressive symptoms (HAD-D), self-esteem (SE), and overall mood (MACL), while the effect on anxiety symptoms was minor ($0.2 < SRM < 0.5$).

The matched control group, conventionally treated in primary health care, improved their eating pattern (decreased Disinhibition and Hunger scores) as well as their obesity-related psychosocial problems; however, the effects were small. Neither generic measures nor body weight changed beyond the trivial level in controls (Figure 33.8). They had gained 1.7 kg on average (SD 10.3) at 4 years.

Is poor HRQL reversible after substantial weight loss, i.e. to levels of a group of healthy subjects? Are improvements maintained over time? In most instances the answer seems to be yes and definitely so regarding psychosocial functioning and mental well-being. Whether impacts on physical functioning are permanently reversed needs more attention, particularly concerning how weight loss affects concomitant conditions. The SOS study will shed more light on this issue.

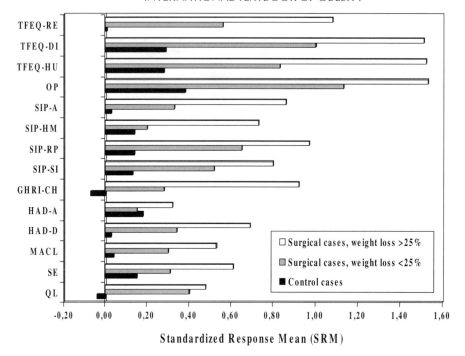

Standardized Response Mean (SRM)

Figure 33.9 Treatment effects on health-related quality of life (HRQL) in surgical cases and controls after 4 years in the SOS intervention study. The surgical cases are grouped by magnitude of weight loss after 4 years. HRQL change scores from baseline to 4-year follow-up are transformed to standardized response means (SRM). SRM is calculated as the mean change score divided by the standard deviation of change (Katz *et al.* (49)).
TFEQ, Three-Factor Eating Questionnaire; RE, restrained eating; DI, disinhibition; HU, hunger.
OP, Obesity-Related Psychosocial Problems.
SIP, Sickness Impact Profile; A, ambulation; HM, home management; RP, recreation and pastimes; SI, social interaction.
GHRI, General Health Rating Index; CH, current health.
HAD, Hospital Anxiety and Depression scale; A, anxiety symptoms; D, depression symptoms.
MACL, Mood Adjective Check List. SE, Self-esteem. QL, Overall quality of life

Summary: How Improvements are Evaluated and Related to Weight Loss

- Key to success: need for both condition-specific and generic measures, long-term follow-up, large samples, matched controls
- Poor quality of life is mostly reversible if weight loss is substantial
- Obesity-specific measures most responsive to weight reduction

HRQL and Obesity V: Detecting Mood Disorders

Studies of the prevalence of psychopathology in obese persons have yielded inconsistent results (61). The reasons for this are probably related to dif-

ferences in study populations as well as assessment methods. Obese men and women in the SOS registry study showed significantly more self-assessed psychiatric morbidity than reference subjects and other patient groups (39), emphasizing the high distress level associated with severe obesity. Self-assessment measures are of potential use in clinical practice for detecting mood disorders. For example, the Hospital Anxiety and Depression scale (HAD; see Appendix) could be used in the assessment of HRQL to increase attention to mental health aspects. The instrument was designed to detect mood disorders, particularly in the somatically ill. Therefore, the HAD does not involve any somatic items frequently found in similar instruments assessing psychiatric morbidity, e.g. Beck's Depression Inventory (67). The latter measure includes questions about appetite loss and weight change, which may be accurate indicators of depression in normal

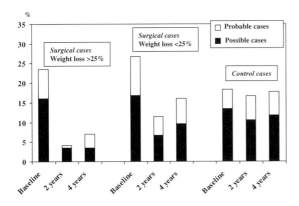

Figure 33.10 Prevalence (%) of clinical depression according to HAD classifications in surgical cases and controls prior to treatment and at 2- and 4-year follow-ups in the SOS intervention study. The surgical cases are grouped by magnitude of weight loss after 4 years

weight individuals but are likely to confound the occurrence of depression in obese populations.

The two cut-offs of the HAD scale for possible and probable clinical cases of anxiety or depression have proved clinically valid in a number of studies within our research programme. Figure 33.10 illustrates the prevalence figures for depression in the SOS surgery group by amount of weight loss after 4 years compared with corresponding data in the control group. Baseline, 2- and 4-year values are given. The conclusion is clear: patients who choose surgery more frequently showed distress levels indicating depression than those who served in the control group. Degree of improvement neatly followed amount of weight loss. Controls showed slight weight gain on average after both 2 and 4 years but prevalence figures indicating possible disorder were somewhat lower regarding the lower cut-off.

Questionnaires with validated thresholds like the HAD scale are well suited for the clinical setting and can thus aid specialists, GPs, dieticians and other allied health professionals in detecting mood disorders among the obese. Further, other condition-specific measures such as the OP scale and the TFEQ (see Appendix) should be of value to care providers once the relevant threshold values have been established. Progress in this area is foreseen within the SOS study.

Summary: Detecting Psychiatric Morbidity

- HAD scale thresholds effective in the obese
- High prevalence of depression reversible if weight loss is substantial

CONCLUSIONS

Resource allocations for the management of obesity and other so-called lifestyle disorders demonstrating small or uncertain treatment effects have diminished concurrently with increasing health care service costs. At the same time obesity is growing to pandemic proportions and costs for treating diseases associated with obesity are consuming more and more of health care budgets. Obesity has become 'a time bomb to be defused' (68). If attention is paid to the total burden of overweight, both in terms of personal suffering and healthcare expenditures, there is probably enough strong evidence to demand allocation of resources for serious clinical action to fight obesity.

The introduction of health-related quality of life (HRQL) to obesity research, prevention and clinical management may further strengthen the evidence. First, since the goals of weight reduction interventions are not only to normalize metabolic risk factors, reduce morbidity, prolong life, but also to restore or enhance functioning and well-being, HRQL endpoints must be included when evaluating treatments. Second, it has become increasingly recognized in clinical epidemiology and evidence-based medicine that systematic and comprehensive documentation of treatment efficacy should incorporate HRQL outcome measures. Third, pharmaceutical regulatory agencies, such as the FDA in the USA and EMEA in Europe, are currently integrating HRQL assessment into their clinical development plan. Fourth, new guidelines and recommendations will move pharmaceutical claims, also for severe obesity, towards a more 'fair balance' between clinical findings/ surrogate measures and the patient's viewpoint, i.e. HRQL.

Summary: Quality of Life and Obesity—What Do We Know?

- Health-related quality of life—a useful concept in research, prevention and clinical medicine
- Methodological 'know how' readily available

- Health-related quality of life—a new endpoint for industry
- Health-related quality of life—a new tool to identify patients suitable for different interventions

APPENDIX: SWEDISH OBESE SUBJECTS (SOS) QUALITY OF LIFE SURVEY

Conceptual and measurement model of health-related quality of life in obesity

Concepts: condition-specific and generic	Instruments: obesity-related and generic
Condition-specific	TFEQ OP

Complaints/ consequences	• Restraint eating • Obesity-related
	    • Disinhibition psychosocial
	    • Hunger problems

Generic
 Functional health
    Physical/ mobility oriented
    consequences
	SIP
	    • Ambulation
	    • Home management
	    • Work
	    • Recreation and pastimes

Social/ emotional/ cognitive
    consequences
	SIP
	    • Social interaction

General health perceptions	GHRI • Current health

Mental health
    Distress/ well-being
	HAD
	    • Depression
	    • Anxiety

	MACL
	    • Overall mood score
	    • Pleasantness
	    • Activation
	    • Calmness

	SE • Self-esteem
Overall quality of life	Global rating

TFEQ: Three-Factor Eating Questionnaire(54, 55)
OP: Obesity-related Problem scale from the SOS Quality of Life Survey(39)
SIP: Sickness Impact Profile(69, 70)
GHRI: General Health Rating Index(39, 71)
HAD: Hospital Anxiety and Depression scale(39, 72)
MACL: Mood Adjective Check List(39, 73)
SE: Self-Esteem scale(74) (75)
Global rating: Overall quality of life(76)

TFEQ: Three-Factor Eating Questionnaire (54,55); OP: Obesity-related Problem scale from the SOS Quality of Life Survey (39); SIP: Sickness Impact Profile (69,70); GHRI: General Health Rating Index (39,71); HAD: Hospital Anxiety and Depression scale (39,72); MACL: Mood Adjective Check List (39,73); SE: Self-Esteem scale (74,75); Global rating: Overall quality of life (76).

Brief description of the SOS Quality of Life Survey

Self-assessment of eating behaviour. The three-factor eating questionnaire (TFEQ) includes 36 statements with an agree/disagree response format, 14 questions on a four-point response scale, and one rating on a 0–10-point scale. Responses are dichotomized and summed into three factors: restrained eating, disinhibition, and hunger. A short-form version is developed within the SOS Study.

Obesity-related psychosocial problems. A study-specific module was created (OP) to assess how bothered obese persons are in everyday life because of their obesity. It contains eight items on a four-point response scale to cover the perceived impact of obesity on selected activities known central to obese persons. Responses are summed into one score.

Physical and role functioning. Ambulation (A), home management (HM), work (W), and recreation and pastimes (RP), four categories from the Sickness Impact Profile (SIP), were selected to cover limitations in daily life activities. They contain 12, 10, 9 and 8 statements, respectively. Respondents simply agree to those statements that describe a limitation related to their health. Items agreed to are summed according to predetermined weights, divided by the sum of all weights in each category and multiplied by 100.

Psychosocial functioning. Social interaction (SI), the main psychosocial category from the SIP, was chosen to assess health-related dysfunction in social life; quality and quantity of social contacts within the family, among friends, and in the community. It has 20 statements with the same format as described above.

General health perceptions. Overall health was measured by the current health scale (CH) selected from the General Health Rating Index (GHRI). The scale aggregates nine statements on a four-point response format.

Mood disorders/distress. The Hospital Anxiety and Depression scale (HAD) was used to describe levels of psychological distress, screening for possible or probable mood disorder in the somatically ill. The instrument has 14 questions on a four-point response scale, summed to anxiety and depression scores with cut-offs for clinical cases.

Mental well-being. Mental well-being was measured by the short version of the Mood Adjective Check List (MACL) comprising 38 adjectives on a four-point response scale, summed into pleasantness, activation and calmness dimension scores and an overall index. A self-esteem scale (SE) comprising 10 questions on a four-point response scale was added to include the psychological self-image.

Overall quality of life. A global question was posed in accordance with a standardized wording using a seven-point response scale with anchors 'very poor' and 'excellent'.

ACKNOWLEDGEMENTS

This contribution was made possible through support by the Swedish Council for Social Research (grant no. 97-0355: 1b), the Swedish Foundation for Health Care Sciences and Allergy Research (grant no. V96 065), the Swedish Medical Research Council (grant no. 05239) and the Faculty of Medicine, University of Göteborg.

REFERENCES

1. McSweeney AJ, Grant I, Heaton RK, Adams KM, Timms RM. Life quality of patients with chronic obstructive pulmonary disease. *Arch Intern Med* 1982; **142**(3): 473–478.
2. Sugarbaker PH, Barofsky I, Rosenberg SA, Gianola FJ. Quality of life assessment of patients in extremity sarcoma clinical trials. *Surgery* 1982; **91**(1): 17–23.
3. Osoba D (ed.) *Effect of Cancer on Quality of Life*. Boca Raton, FL: CRC Press, 1991.
4. Godyear MDE, Fraumeni MA. Incorporating quality of life assessment into clinical cancer trials. In: Spilker B (ed.) *Quality of Life and Pharmacoeconomics in Clinical Trials*, 2nd edn. Philadelphia: Lippincott-Raven, 1996: 1003–1013.
5. Wenger NK, Mattsson ME, Furberg CD, Elinson J (eds.) *Assessment of Quality of Life in Clinical Trials aof Cardiovascular Therapies*. New York: Le Jacq, 1984.

6. Croog SH, Levine S, Testa MA, *et al.*. The effects of anti-hypertensive therapy on the quality of life. *N Engl J Med* 1986; **314**(26): 1657–1664.

7. Bombardier C, Ware J, Russell IJ, Larson M, Chalmers A, Read JL. Auranofin therapy and quality of life in patients with rheumatoid arthritis. Results of a multicenter trial. *Am J Med 1986;* **81**(4): 565–578.

8. Ellwood PM. Shattuck lecture—outcomes management. A technology of patient experience. *N Engl J Med* 1988; **318**(23): 1549–1556.

9. Ware JE Jr. Measuring patients' views: the optimum outcome measure. SF-36: a valid, reliable assessment of health from the patient's point of view. *BMJ* 1993; **306**: 1429.

10. Ware JE Jr. The status of health assessment 1994. *Annu Rev Public Health* 1995; **16**: 327–354.

11. Björner JB, Kristensen TS, Orth-Gomér K, Tibblin G, Sullivan M, Westerholm P. *Self-Rated Health—a useful concept in research, prevention and clinical medicine.* Stockholm: Swedish council for planning and coordination of research, 1996.

12. Barsky AJ. The paradox of health. *N Engl J Med* 1988; **318**(7): 414–418.

13. Patrick DL, Deyo RA. Generic and disease-specific measures in assessing health status and quality of life. *Med Care* 1989; **27**(3 Suppl): S217–232.

14. Patrick DL, Erickson P. Assessing health-related quality of life for clinical decision-making. In: Walker SR, Rosser RM (eds) *Quality of Life Assessment. Key Issues in the 1990s.* Dordrecht: Kluwer Academic Publishers, 1993: 11–63.

15. McSweeny AJ, Creer TL. Health-related quality-of-life assessment in medical care. *Dis Mon* 1995; **41**(1): 1–71.

16. Shumaker SA, Berzon R (eds). *The International Assessment of Health-Related Quality of Life: Theory, Translation, Measurement and Analysis.* Oxford: Rapid Communications, 1995.

17. Sullivan MB, Sullivan LG, Kral JG. Quality of life assessment in obesity: physical, psychological, and social function. *Gastroenterol Clin North Am* 1987; **16**(3): 433–442.

18. Kral JG, Sjöström LV, Sullivan MB. Assessment of quality of life before and after surgery for severe obesity. *Am J Clin Nutr* 1992; **55**(2 Suppl): 611S–614S.

19. Karlsson J, Sjöström L, Sullivan M. Swedish obese subjects (SOS)—an intervention study of obesity. Two-year follow-up of health-related quality of life (HRQL) and eating behavior after gastric surgery for severe obesity. *Int J Obes Relat Metab Disord* 1998; **22**(2): 113–126.

20. Spilker B (ed.) *Quality of Life and Pharmacoeconomics in Clinical Trials,* 2nd edn. Philadelphia: Lippincott-Raven, 1996.

21. Atkinson RL. Proposed standards for judging the success of the treatment of obesity. *Ann Intern Med* 1993; **119**(7 Pt 2): 677–680.

22. Committee MOT. Instrument review criteria. *Medical Outcomes Trust Bulletin* 1995; **3**(4 (Suppl)): I-IV.

23. Lohr KN, Aaronson NK, Alonso J, *et al.* Evaluating quality-of-life and health status instruments: development of scientific review criteria. *Clin Ther* 1996; **18**(5): 979–992.

24. Streiner DL, Norman GR. *Health Measurement Scales. A Practical Guide to their Development and Use.* Oxford: Oxford University Press, 1989.

25. Nunnally JC, Bernstein IH. *Psychometric Theory,* 3rd edn.

New York: McGraw-Hill, 1994.

26. McDowell I, Newell C. *Measuring Health: a Guide to Rating Scales and Questionnaires,* 2nd edn. New York: Oxford University Press, 1996.

27. Karlsson J, Sjöström L, Sullivan M. Swedish Obese Subjects (SOS)—an intervention study of obesity. Measuring psychosocial factors and health by means of short-form questionnaires. Results from a method study. *J Clin Epidemiol* 1995; **48**(6): 817–823.

28. Ware JE Jr, Kosinski M, Keller SD. *How to score the SF-12 Physical and Mental Summary Scales.* Boston: New England Medical Center: The Health Institute, 1995.

29. Salek S (ed.) *Compendium of Quality of Life Instruments.* Chichester: Wiley, 1998.

30. Gandek B, Ware JE Jr, Aaronson NK, *et al.* Tests of data quality, scaling assumptions, and reliability of the SF-36 in eleven countries: results from the IQOLA Project. (International Quality of Life Assessment). *J Clin Epidemiol* 1998; **51**(11): 1149–1158.

31. Conway K, Méar I. Cultural adaptation of quality of life instruments by MAPI Research Institute. *Quality of Life Newsletter* 1998; (20): 4–5.

32. Hendrick SC, Taeuber RC, Erickson P. On learning and understanding quality of life: a guide to information sources. In: Spilker B (ed.) *Quality of Life and Pharmacoeconomics in Clinical Trials,* 2nd edn. Philadelphia: Lippincott-Raven, 1996: 59–64.

33. Stewart AL, Ware Jr JE (eds) *Measuring Functioning and Well-Being: The Medical Outcomes Study Approach.* Durham: Duke University Press, 1992.

34. Ware JE Jr, Sherbourne CD. The MOS 36-item short-form health survey (SF-36). I. Conceptual framework and item selection. *Med Care* 1992; **30**(6): 473–483.

35. Ware JE Jr, Snow KK, Kosinski M, Gandek B. *SF-36 Health Survey Manual and Interpretation Guide.* Boston: New England Medical Center: The Health Institute, 1993.

36. Ware JE Jr, Kosinski M, Keller SD. *SF-36 Physical and Mental Health Summary Scales—A User's Manual.* Boston: New England Medical Center: The Health Institute, 1994.

37. Lydick EG, Epstein RS. Clinical significance of quality of life data. In: Spilker B (ed.) *Quality of Life and Pharmacoeconomics in Clinical Trials,* 2nd edn. Philadelphia: Lippincott-raven, 1996: 461–465.

38. Staquet MJ, Hays RD, Fayers PM (eds) *Quality of Life Assessment in Clinical Trials. Methods and Practice.* Oxford: Oxford University Press, 1998.

39. Sullivan M, Karlsson J, Sjöström L, *et al.* Swedish obese subjects (SOS)—an intervention study of obesity. Baseline evaluation of health and psychosocial functioning in the first 1743 subjects examined. *Int J Obes Relat Metab Disord* 1993; **17**(9): 503–512.

40. Kolotkin RL, Head S, Hamilton M, Tse CK. Assessing impact of weight on quality of life. *Obes Res* 1995; **3**(1): 49–56.

41. Kolotkin RL, Head S, Brookhart A. Construct validity of the impact of weight on quality of life questionnaire. *Obes Res* 1997; **5**(5): 434–441.

42. Mathias SD, Williamson CL, Colwell HH, *et al.* Assessing health-related quality-of-life and health state preference in persons with obesity: a validation study. *Qual Life Res* 1997; **6**(4): 311–322.

43. Le Pen C, Levy E, Loos F, Banzet MN, Basdevant A. 'Speci-

fic' scale compared with 'generic' scale: a double measurement of the quality of life in a French community sample of obese subjects. *J Epidemiol Community Health* 1998; **52**(7): 445–450.

44. Ware JE Jr, Gandek BL, for the IQOLA Project. Overview of the SF-36 Health Survey and the International Quality of Life Assessment (IQOLA) Project. *J Clin Epidemiol* 1998; **51**(11): 903–912.

45. Ware JE Jr, Gandek BL, Keller SD, IQOLA Project Group. Evaluating instruments used cross-nationally: methods from the IQOLA Project. In: Spilker B (ed.) *Quality of Life and Pharmacoeconomics in Clinical Trials*, 2nd edn. Philadelphia: Lippincott-Raven, 1996: 681–692.

46. Cohen J. *Statistical Power Analysis for the Behavioral Sciences*. New York: Acedemic Press, 1978.

47. Wing RR, Epstein LH, Marcus MD, Kupfer DJ. Mood changes in behavioral weight loss programs. *J Psychosom Res* 1984; **28**(3): 189–196.

48. Hays RD, Anderson R, Revicki D. Psychometric considerations in evaluating health-related quality of life measures. *Qual Life Res* 1993; **2**(6): 441–449.

49. Katz JN, Larson MG, Phillips CB, Fossel AH, Liang MH. Comparative measurement sensitivity of short and longer health status instruments. *Med Care* 1992; **30**(10): 917–925.

50. Fitzgibbon ML, Stolley MR, Kirschenbaum DS. Obese people who seek treatment have different characteristics than those who do not seek treatment. *Health Psychol* 1993; **12**(5): 342–345.

51. Han TS, Tijhuis MA, Lean ME, Seidell JC. Quality of life in relation to overweight and body fat distribution. *Am J Public Health* 1998; **88**(12): 1814–1820.

52. Brown WJ, Dobson AJ, Mishra G. What is a healthy weight for middle aged women? *Int J Obes Relat Metab Disord* 1998; **22**(6): 520–528.

53. Sullivan M, Karlsson J, Ware JE, Jr. *SF-36 Hälsoenkät: svensk manual och tolkningsguide (Swedish Manual and Interpretation Guide)*. Göteborg: Sahlgrenska University Hospital, 1994.

54. Stunkard AJ, Messick S. The three-factor eating questionnaire to measure dietary restraint, disinhibition and hunger. *J Psychosom Res* 1985; **29**(1): 71–83.

55. Karlsson J, Hallgren P, Kral J, Lindroos AK, Sjöström L, Sullivan M. Predictors and effects of long-term dieting on mental well-being and weight loss in obese women. *Appetite* 1994; **23**(1): 15–26.

56. Lindroos AK, Lissner L, Mathiassen ME, *et al.* Dietary intake in relation to restrained eating, disinhibition, and hunger in obese and nonobese Swedish women. *Obes Res* 1997; **5**(3): 175–182.

57. Fontaine KR, Cheskin LJ, Barofsky I. Health-related quality of life in obese persons seeking treatment. *J Fam Pract* 1996; **43**(3): 265–270.

58. Fontaine KR, Barofsky I, Cheskin LJ. Predictors of quality of life for obese persons. *J Nerv Ment Dis* 1997; **185**(2): 120–122.

59. Sullivan M, Cohen J, Branehög I. *A Psychosocial Study of Surviving Cancer Patients in California, USA and the Western Region of Sweden. Part II: Response Patterns and Determinants of Adjustment to Cancer in Sweden*. Göteborg: Sahlgrenska University Hospital, 1988.

60. Augustinsson LE, Sullivan L, Sullivan M. Chronic pain in functional neurosurgery: function and mood in various diagnostic groups with reference to epidural spinal electrical stimulation. *Schmertz, Pain, Douleur* 1989; **10**: 30–40.

61. Stunkard AJ, Wadden TA. Psychological aspects of severe obesity. *Am J Clin Nutr* 1992; **55**(2 Suppl): 524S–532S.

62. Karlsson J, Sjöström L, Sullivan M. Construct validity and responsiveness of the obesity-related problem scale (OP). *Qual Life Res* 1999; **8**(7): 603.

63. Wadden TA, Steen SN, Wingate BJ, Foster GD. Psychosocial consequences of weight reduction: how much weight loss is enough? *Am J Clin Nutr* 1996; **63**(3 Suppl): 461S–465S.

64. Foster GD, Wadden TA, Kendall PC, Stunkard AJ, Vogt RA. Psychological effects of weight loss and regain: a prospective evaluation. *J Consult Clin Psychol* 1996; **64**(4): 752–757.

65. Rippe JM, Price JM, Hess SA, *et al.* Improved psychological well-being, quality of life, and health practices in moderately overweight women participating in a 12-week structured weight loss program. *Obes Res* 1998; **6**(3): 208–218.

66. Karlsson J, Sjöström L, Sullivan M. Swedish obese subjects (SOS)—an intervention study of obesity. Measuring effects of weight loss on quality of life in the severely obese. *Qual Life Res* 1997; **6**(7/8): 667.

67. Steer RA, Beck AT. Modifying the Beck Depression Inventory: reply to Vredenburg, Krames, and Flett. *Psychol Rep* 1985; **57**(2): 625–626.

68. Bray GA. Obesity: a time bomb to be defused. *Lancet* 1998; **352**(9123) 160–161.

69. Bergner M, Bobbitt RA, Carter WB, Gilson BS. The Sickness Impact Profile: development and final revision of a health status measure. *Med Care* 1981; **19**(8): 787–805.

70. Sullivan M, Ahlmén M, Archenholtz B, Svensson G. Measuring health in rheumatic disorders by means of a Swedish version of the Sickness Impact Profile. Results from a population study. *Scand J Rheumatol* 1986; **15**(2): 193–200.

71. Davies AR, Sherbourne CR, Peterson JR, Ware Jr LE. *Scoring Manual: Adult Health Status and Patient Satisfaction Measures Used in RAND's Health Insurance Experiment*. Santa Monica, CA: The RAND Corporation, 1988.

72. Zigmond AS, Snaith RP. The Hospital Anxiety and Depression scale. *Acta Psychiatr Scand 1983;* **67**(6): 361–370.

73. Sjöberg L, Svensson E, Persson LO. The measurement of mood. *Scand J Psychol* 1979; **20**(1): 1–18.

74. Rosenberg M. *Society and the Adolescent Self-Image*. Princeton: Princeton University Press, 1965.

75. Rydén A, Karlsson J. Persson LO, Sjöström L, Sullivan M. Mental health, personality and severe obesity—before and after surgery. *Int J Obes* 1998; **22**(Suppl 3): 284.

76. Aaronson NK, Ahmedzai S, Bergman B, *et al.* The European Organization for Research and Treatment of Cancer QLQ-C30: a quality-of-life instrument for use in international clinical trials in oncology. *J Natl Cancer Inst* 1993; **85**(5): 365–376.

77. Sullivan M. Quality of life assessment in medicine. Concepts, definitions, purposes, and basic tools. *Nord J Psychiatr* 1992; **46**: 79–83.

78. Sullivan M, Karlsson J, Taft C. How to assess quality of life in medicine: rationale and methods. In: Guy-Grand B, Ailhaud G (eds) *Progress in Obesity Research: 8*, London: Libbey, 1999: 749–755.

79. Sarlio-Lähteenkorva S, Stunkard AJ, Rissanen A. Psychoso-

cial factors and quality of life in obesity. *Int J Obes* 1995; **19**(Suppl 6): S1–S5.

80. Carr ND, Harrison RA, Tomkins A, *et al.* Vertical banded gastroplasty in the treatment of morbid obesity: results of three year follow up. *Gut* 1989; **30**(8): 1048–1053.

81. Hafner RJ, Watts JM, Rogers J. Quality of life after gastric bypass for morbid obesity. *Int J Obes* 1991; **15**(8): 555–560.

82. Isacsson A, Frederiksen SG, Nilsson P, Hedenbro JL. Quality of life after gastroplasty is normal: a controlled study. *Eur J Surg* 1997; **163**(3): 181–186.

83. van Gemert WG, Severeijns RM, Greve JWM, Groenman N, Soeters PD. Psychological functioning of morbidly obese patients after surgical treatment. *Int J Obes* 1998; **22**: 393–398.

84. Larsen F. Psychosocial function before and after gastric banding surgery for morbid obesity. A prospective psychiatric study. *Acta Psychiatr Scand Suppl* 1990; **359**: 1–57.

85. Choban PS, Onyejekwe J, Burge JC, Flancbaum L. A health status assessments of the impact of weight loss following Roux-en-Y gastric bypass for clinically severe obesity. *J Am Coll Surg* 1999; **188**(5): 491–497.

86. Chan CL, Villar RN. Obesity and quality of life after primary hip arthroplasty [see comments]. *J Bone Joint Surg Br* 1996; **78**(1): 78–81.

87. Lavie CJ, Milani RV. Effects of cardiac rehabilitation, exercise training, and weight reduction on exercise capacity, coronary risk factors, behavioral characteristics, and quality of life in obese coronary patients. *Am J Cardiol* 1997; **79**(4): 397–401.

34

Surgical Treatment of Obesity

John G. Kral

SUNY Downstate Medical Center, New York, USA

Those who cannot remember the past
are condemned to repeat it.
(G. Santayana)

Surgical treatment of obesity ('bariatric surgery'; anti-obesity surgery) passes the pragmatic test: it works, most of the time. It is also cost-effective and on a cost per-kg-lost basis is superior to any other method of weight loss for class II and III obesity. Most important: the results are durable, defined as providing maintenance of medical significant weight loss for more than 5 years.

Why, then, is surgical treatment not more widely appreciated or performed? A recent survey of attendees of a weight-loss clinic showed that most of the obese patients were willing to take a 6% risk of immediate death if they were guaranteed to reach their desired weight and 25% of the patients were willing to take a 21% risk of dying (1). Yet only a small fraction of eligible patients undergo anti-obesity surgery, this most effective treatment with a mortality rate below 1%. Men in particular do not have such surgery though their relative risk of dying from obesity is substantially higher than the risk of women of equal body mass index (BMI) (2) and also higher than their risk of dying from anti-obesity surgery. There are many causes for a relative under-utilization of anti-obesity surgery, some of which are frankly irrational.

Developments during the past decade effectively address earlier concerns over safety and reliability. This text will describe the fundamental principles of the three most common surgical techniques, will discuss safety and will attempt to define crucial problems influencing the outcome of anti-obesity surgery. Recent trends in this field threaten to repeat mistakes from the 1960s and 1970s.

METHODS

Operations systematically performed to achieve weight loss first appeared in the early 1950s, initially as removal of long segments of small bowel, subsequently as bypass of even longer intestinal segments excluded from the nutrient stream but available for reattachment should the need arise (*intestinal bypass*; jejuno-ileal bypass). Stomach operations, pioneered by Edward E. Mason of Iowa in the 1960s, similarly evolved from gastric resection into *gastric bypass*, excluding a large portion of the stomach, attaching the remnant to a loop of small bowel (Figure 34.1). Mason was convinced that the mechanism of weight loss was mechanical restriction of intake through the small gastric remnant ('pouch'). Thus, he went on to develop a purely restrictive operation, *gastroplasty*, consisting of a stapled pouch with an externally banded conduit into the stomach proper. The small size of the pouch (< 15 ml) and the small diameter of the outlet (9 mm) physically limit the amount of food that can be consumed during a single meal.

Gastric bypass provides greater weight loss, sustained for longer periods of time in a larger proportion of patients than does gastroplasty. This implies that gastric bypass functions through other mechanisms than restriction alone. Undigested nutrients

International Textbook of Obesity. Edited by Per Björntorp.
© 2001 John Wiley & Sons, Ltd.

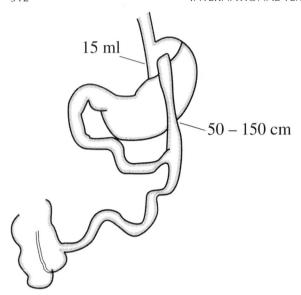

Figure 34.1   Gastric bypass. Roux-en-Y gastric bypass with a Roux limb measuring 50–150 cm in length

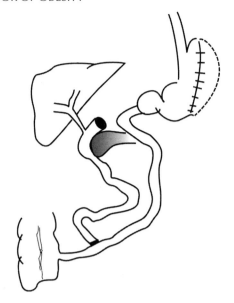

Figure 34.2   Biliopancreatic bypass with duodenal switch. Sleeve gastrectomy (hatched) and duodeno-ileostomy with 150 cm common limb

emptying from the small stomach pouch into the segment of small bowel (jejunum) evoke satiety signals via mechanoreceptors. Calorically dense liquid or soft food rapidly emptying into the small bowel causes weight loss through 'dumping', an aversive physiological response associated with release of vasoactive gastrointestinal peptides elicited by chemoreceptors, portal chemoreceptors and possibly potentiated by peptide receptors in the brain. Regardless of mechanism, gastric bypass achieves greater weight loss than purely restrictive gastric operations.

Variants of gastric bypass use longer limbs of bypassed small bowel (Figure 34.1) causing more maldigestion and adding malabsorption leading to greater weight loss, appropriate in heavier patients (those with BMI ≥ 50). Predictably, these operations have greater potential for causing deficiencies. The first of these more aggressive gastrointestinal bypass operations, *biliopancreatic diversion* (BPD), was introduced in 1976 by Nicola Scopinaro of Genoa. In its original form it included resection of the stomach with diversion of digestive bile and pancreatic secretions to the terminal 50 cm of ileum. These more malabsorptive operations have been performed in a few centers worldwide, though the series have been fairly large. A recent modification of biliopancreatic bypass, maintaining the pylorus and a portion of the duodenum, called 'duodenal

switch' (Figure 34.2) seems to improve protein absorption and cause fewer side effects than the biliopancreatic bypass of Scopinaro (3,4). This improved side-effect profile, replicated in several centers, is leading to wider adoption of these types of operations, such that they can be considered to be a legitimate alternative in selected patients.

Laparoscopic Surgery

All types of surgery have been dramatically transformed during the last decade owing to the technical advances making possible the development of laparoscopic techniques. Insertion of tiny fiberoptic light sources and cameras into inflated body cavities for transmission of images to video screens allows insertion and operation of instruments through smaller incisions with less surgical trauma—aptly called 'minimally invasive' surgery.

These techniques are especially appropriate in obese patients who generally require large incisions for exposure. Because of their reduced hemodynamic and respiratory reserves, obese patients withstand trauma less well than their lean counterparts, which is why they are considered to be higher operative risks. This is one of many

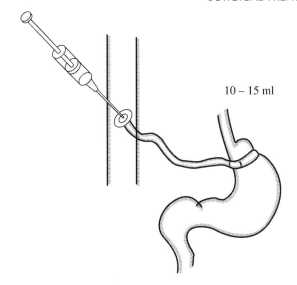

10 – 15 ml

Figure 34.3 Laparoscopic adjustable gastric band. The inflatable band is attached to an intramuscularly placed injectable port

factors that traditionally has led to underutilization of surgical services among the obese. Minimally invasive techniques, with their shorter recovery times and shorter periods of postoperative rehabilitation, have made operations safer for obese patients, thus expanding their access to surgery.

The first bariatric surgical procedure to capitalize on the minimally invasive approach was circumgastric adjustable banding. This is a truly restrictive procedure, originally developed for open surgery by Lubomyr Kuzmak of New Jersey around 1985. An inflatable Silastic ring is placed just below the esophagogastric junction and is attached via tubing to a subcutaneous injectable port (Figure 34.3). As the patient's eating behaviour changes and the gastric wall adapts, the functional inner diameter of the conduit may change. The adjustable band allows titration of the desirable degree of restriction.

Vertical banded gastroplasty and gastric bypass became feasible laparoscopically with the development of laparoscopic stapling instruments. As with all surgery, laparoscopic or open, there is a learning curve until technical mastery can be achieved, with its attendant reduced complication rate. As of the end of 2000, there are reports of series of patients who have undergone these laparoscopic stapling operations. None have the appropriate 5-or-more year period of observation in sufficient numbers of patients necessary to evaluate the efficacy of these

approaches. However, it does appear as if the safety of performance of these operations via laparoscopy is at least equivalent to that of the open procedures.

Staged Surgery

Because of the high degree of safety of performance of laparoscopic adjustable gastric banding, with very quick postoperative return to full function, and the relative ease of completely reversing the operation because of the non-reactive nature of the Silastic implant (band + tubing), it is reasonable to expand the availability of this very effective method for achieving weight loss. Patients developing complications and *unmanageable* side effects of the gastric restriction would be candidates for reversal of the operation as would be patients with inadequate weight loss. Given the > 95% recidivism of obesity and its comorbities after reversal of any bariatric operation, such patients should be offered a malabsorptive type of operation such as gastric bypass at the time of the reversal. Staged surgery appears to be a logical strategy in the overall management of severely obese patients (5).

RESULTS

The simplest outcome measure, *weight reduction*, can be expressed in absolute or relative terms, with the latter based on percentage of preoperative body weight or reduction of 'excess' body weight determined from life insurance tables of desirable weight for height. As a 'rule of thumb' weight loss is approximately one-third of initial (maximum) weight after gastric bypass compared to 20–25% after gastric restriction and 40% after biliopancreatic diversion or duodenal switch. In terms of reduction of excess weight (% excess weight loss, % EWL), gastric restriction achieves 50–55%, gastric bypass 60–65% and BPD around 75%. Variations in these weight losses are related to initial body weight and to differences in setting, location and patient selection between different series.

The majority of severely obese patients undergoing anti-obesity operations (women, aged 35–40 years with BMI around 42 kg/m^2) want sufficient weight loss to become 'lean' or at least not visibly obese regardless of health implications. Most sur-

Table 34.1 Response of comorbidity to surgically induced weight loss

	% cured[a]	% improved[b]
Asthma	95	100
Diabetes	90–95	100
Dyslipidemia	70	85
Heart failure	60	90
Hypertension	60–65	90
Sleep apnea	100	100

[a]No need for further treatment.
[b]Reduced medication dosage.

Table 34.2 Complications of open gastric bypass

Complication	%	Complication	%
Mortality	1	Wound infection	
		severe	3.5
		minor	10
Thromboembolism	2	Marginal ulcers	6
Leaks	1.5	Bowel obstruction	2
Pneumonia	1.9	Abscess	2.5
Splenectomy	2.7	Arrhythmia	1.5
Hemorrhage	1		

geons, wishing to please their patients, comply with defining 'success' in terms of weight loss. Indeed, the whole concept of % EWL is predicated on reducing excess weight to bring the patient to an 'ideal' or 'desirable' non-obese weight. However, the weight-for-height standards are derived from large populations of individuals who have not lost weight, particularly not large amounts of weight. There are no actuarial standards for people who have lost significant amounts of weight after being severely obese (BMI ≥ 35) because people at these weight levels are undersampled in population studies.

Since severely obese patients generally have increased body cell mass, reflected in large organ sizes, elevated cell numbers and increased bone mass, it is neither realistic, nor necessarily 'healthy' to reduce 100% of excess weight. It is obvious from the post-surgical weight loss figures cited above that loss of 100% of excess is rarely attained and thus should be of little concern. However, both surgeons and patients need to understand the physiological limitations on weight loss in order to avoid unrealistic, potentially unhealthy expectations.

Reduction of comorbidity with attendant increases in longevity and improved quality of life should be the appropriate goal of anti-obesity surgery. Solely for the purpose of amelioration of comorbidity, it seems that sustained reductions of 10% of body weight are sufficient and a large population study of women showed a 25% reduction in mortality with intentional loss of $\geq 9\,\mathrm{kg}$ (6). There is very little evidence that non-surgical methods are able to maintain this degree of weight loss for periods of 5 years or more, especially in patients with BMI greater than $33\,\mathrm{kg/m^2}$.

Table 34.1 lists obesity comorbidities in surgical patients and their response to surgically induced weight loss. These impressive results, particularly with respect to type 2 diabetes, beg the question whether it is ethical to withhold surgical treatment from obese patients with insulin-resistant diabetes. Before answering the question, it is necessary to scrutinize the side effects, complications and costs of anti-obesity surgery.

Complications

Since reviewing this topic in 1994 including a presentation of definitions and analysis of the quality of the data (7), more information has become available, particularly regarding laparoscopic approaches. Table 34.2 lists early complications of open gastric bypass operations in three centers performing large numbers of gastric bypasses yearly. The early mortality rate of 1% is based on the total experience from the mid-1980s. Subsequently mortality seems to have dropped well below 1%. In general, complication rates are similar in gastric restrictive procedures though gastroplasty operations are less complex. This is because gastroplasty is performed more widely in hospitals less familiar with bariatric surgery than the highly specialized centers performing gastric bypass.

As mentioned earlier, the laparoscopic approaches have not been available sufficiently long to provide adequate assessment of safety or efficacy. The surgeons who have pioneered the laparoscopic bariatric operations are naturally especially dedicated during the development phase. Early results from laparoscopic bypass in centres reporting between 35 and 700 patients over the last 4 years have not demonstrated any mortality, though reoperations have been required for various technical reasons. One series has been plagued by anastomotic strictures, requiring endoscopic dilatation and in

Table 34.3 Rules of eating after gastric restriction

Eat slowly in a quiet setting—no stress
Advance your diet from liquids to purees to solids
Chew properly before swallowing
Stop eating immediately when your pouch is full
Never drink with your food
Wait at least 1 hour before drinking after food

If you vomit or regurgitate:
Identify the reason(s)
Wait 4 hours before drinking
Advance your diet, only if tolerated
If not tolerated: contact your surgeon

some cases reoperation.

The best documented series of laparoscopic adjustable banding revealed only one early complication in 273 patients, an infected reservoir site (8). Among late postoperative complications the authors encountered obstructing prolapse of the stomach through the band in 22% of their first 100 patients. After small technical changes, they have not had any such complication in their last 100 cases (8).

Side Effects

It seems intuitively obvious that vomiting might be an effect or side effect of gastric restriction, while diarrhea would follow malabsorptive operations bypassing large segments of small bowel. Although it is true that vomiting and diarrhea might be mechanisms of weight loss in these procedures, it is a common misconception that they are obligate (and thus acceptable) sequelae.

Vomiting, with the rare exception of organic or band-related stricture or stenosis, is a behavioral failure preventable by proper education in the majority of patients. If patients have learned and adhere to the 'rules of eating' (Table 34.3; Kral (9)), vomiting is a rare (< 10%) event (7).

Diarrhea, similarly, can be controlled by cognitive means—at least after an initial (approximately 3 months) postoperative phase of intestinal adaptation. The amount and the timing of liquid intake determines the number and consistency of stools, especially when combined with reduced intake of fat. Otherwise there is a medical problem which needs to be addressed (10). The most important cause of adverse outcomes after intestinal bypass operations, which led to their virtual abandonment,

was the failure of the medical profession to respond to diarhea as an unacceptable symptom caused by bacterial overgrowth and/or some other hazardous inflammatory condition when it did not respond to dietary manipulation.

The same type of mistake is now being repeated by the profession by accepting vomiting as an obligate effect of gastric anti-obesity operations. Over the long term vomiting gives rise to deficiencies and acid–base disturbances as well as esophagitis (potentially carcinogenic) and the risk of aspiration leading to acute or chronic lung disease. If vomiting does not respond to behavior modification, an organic cause must be sought. Furthermore, it is necessary to be vigilant for development of bulimic behavior (11), though this does not appear to be a risk after gastric bypass (12).

Deficiencies

The purpose of all bariatric surgery is to reduce the intake and/or absorption of nutrients. Ideally this 'programmed undernutrition' should preferentially shunt non-essential lipid calories, while maintaining essential macro- and micronutrients. Clearly this is not feasible without routine supplementation of nutrients predictably at risk for depletion. Most bariatric procedures have the potential to create deficiencies of hemic precursors (iron and vitamin B_{12}), while gastric bypass also affects calcium and biliopancreatic diversion in addition causes malabsorption of protein (reviewed in Cannizzo and Kral (13)). By routinely prescribing at-risk supplements and regularly monitoring blood levels it is possible to prevent all types of deficiencies. There is, however, no method for guaranteeing that patients, in spite of being fully informed of the adverse consequences, cooperate with treatment plans. This, of course, is perceived as a weakness of the surgery.

CRITIQUE

Cost–benefit analyses of treatments for obesity are lacking (14). For non-surgical treatments this is expected since such treatments are unable to provide durable, truly long-term weight loss allowing such analyses. A few studies have attempted to perform econometric analyses of anti-obesity surgery focusing on employment status, consumption of medical services and sick-leave, while others have attempted to assess global changes in quality of life (15). In general, the outcomes are extremely favorable for surgical treatment of severe obesity, but there are some serious limitations in the representativity of the populations and the scope of the studies.

The short-term success brought about by the relative safety and ease of performing anti-obesity operations laparoscopically and the lure of the burgeoning market of candidates for such surgery pose serious threats to this field. Just as was the case with intestinal bypass operations in the 1960s and 1970s, when any reasonably technically competent, enterprising surgeon performed them without any knowledge of or desire for managing the sequelae of the operation, there is now a recruitment of 'handymen' willing to demonstrate their technical proficiency in the belief that others will step in to take care of the specific needs of such patients. Unfortunately, there are no such 'others'. Internists, whether endocrinologists, nutritionists, gastroenterologists or generalists, have no interest in taking care of these 'surgical' cases. Indeed, many view the surgeons as (well-paid) competitors in this market, and would rather see them fail than recognize this as an opportunity to improve the quality of care for these patients.

It is tragic that the internists' focus on the development of new drugs (16), and the surgeons' lack of understanding of the importance of behavioral modification, patient selection, and psychodynamics for the outcome of gastric restrictive operations stand in the way of progress in this field. Entrenched, often adversarial positions encumber the necessary interdisciplinary collaborations that might otherwise improve the treatment of severely obese patients.

Most surgeons performing bariatric surgery, whether newcomers to the field or seasoned veterans, are committed to one type of procedure: gastric restriction for the newcomers and gastrointestinal bypass for the veterans. The arguments over 'gold standard', procedure-of-choice or even standard of care embody an anti-intellectual and hazardous failure to recognize the complexity of the disease of obesity and the need to individualize. The complexity goes beyond the advances in molecular genetics and cell biology, which as yet have not translated into clinical practice or improved patient satisfaction. Unfortunately many surgeons engaged in treating obesity do not seem to have realized that this surgery is not simply a technical exercise but rather a behavioral intervention requiring *patient education* (9), not just 'informed consent'. Furthermore, patient selection requires more refinement than has been brought to bear by practitioners of the behavioral sciences (17).

SUMMARY

Anti-obesity surgery has increasingly become safer and its efficacy is indisputably superior to any other existing treatment. However, there are numerous problems impeding wider use of surgery, some political and some conceptual. Surgeons fail to recognize the contribution of behavioral factors to side effects and complications, possibly because they are usually less severe than obesity and its comorbidities. Internists, behaviorists and nutritionists seem unwilling, if not unable to be involved in the care of these 'surgical' patients. There is a lack of outcome predictors to aid in the selective assignment of patients to appropriate treatment modalities and much remains to be done to improve pre- and postoperative patient education.

In the final analysis, before the prevalence of obesity is drastically reduced by prevention, surgical treatment should be further refined, not as a technical exercise, but as an integrated component of broad-based treatment requiring education of patients as well as the interdisciplinary team of professionals necessary to treat this complex disease on an individualized basis.

REFERENCES

1. Weiss B, Klein S, Nease R. What risks will obese patients take to lose weight? 2000; submitted for publication.
2. Calle EE, Thun MJ, Petrelli JM, Rodriguez C, Heath Jr CW. Body-mass index and mortality in a prospective cohort of US adults. *N Engl J Med* 1999; **341**: 1097–1105.
3. Scopinaro N, Adami GF, Marinari GM, *et al*. Biliopancreatic diversion. *World J Surg* 1998; **22**: 936–946.
4. Marceau P, Hould FS, Simard S, *et al*. Biliopancreatic diversion with duodenal switch. *World J Surg* 1998; **22**: 947–954.
5. Kral JG. Overview of surgical techniques for treating obesity. *Am J Clin Nutr* 1992; **55**: 552S–555S.
6. Williamson DF, Pamuk E, Thun M, Flanders D, Byers T, Clark H. Prospective study of intentional weight loss and mortality in never-smoking overweight US white women aged 40–64 years. *Am J Epidemiol* 1995; **141**: 1128–1141.
7. Kral JG. Side effects, complications and problems in anti-

obesity surgery: Introduction of the obesity severity index. In: Angel A, Anderson H, Bouchard C, Lau D, Leiter L, Mendelson R (eds) *Progress in Obesity Research: 7*. London: John Libbey, 1996: 655–661.

8. O'Brien PE, Brown WA, Smith A, McMurrick PJ, Stephens M. Prospective study of a laparoscopically placed, adjustable gastric band in the treatment of morbid obesity. *Br J Surg* 1999; **85**: 113–118.

9. Kral JG. The role of surgery in obesity management. *Int J Risk Safety Med* 1995; **7**: 111–120.

10. Kral JG. Current procedures in bariatric surgery. In: Haubrich W, Schaffner F, Berk JE (eds) *Bockus Gastroenterology*, 5th edn. Philadelphia: WB Saunders. 1994: 3231–3239.

11. Hsu LKG, Betancourt S, Sullivan SP. Eating disturbance before and after vertical banded gastroplasty: A pilot study. *Int J Eat Disord* 1996; **19**: 23–34.

12. Rand CSW, Macgregor AMC, Hankins GC. Eating behav-

ior after gastric bypass surgery for obesity. *South Med J* 1987; **80**: 961–964.

13. Cannizzo Jr F, Kral JG. Obesity surgery: A model of programmed undernutrition. *Curr Opin Clin Nutr Metab Care* 1998; **1**: 363–368.

14. Martin LF, White S, Lindstrom Jr W. Cost-benefit analysis for the treatment of severe obesity. *World J Surg* 1998; **22**: 1009–1017.

15. Kral JG, Sjöström LV, Sullivan MBE. Assessment of quality of life before and after surgery for surgical obesity. *Am J Clin Nutr* 1992; **55**: 611S–614S.

16. Heymsfield SB, Greenberg AS, Fujioka K, *et al*. Recombinant leptin for weight loss in obese and lean adults. *JAMA* 1999; **282**: 1568–1575.

17. Kral JG. Surgical treatment of obesity. In: Kopelman PG, Stock MJ (eds) *Clinical Obesity* London: Blackwell Science, 1998: 545–563.

35

Swedish Obese Subjects, SOS

Lars Sjöström

Sahlgrenska University Hospital, Göteborg, Sweden

Swedish Obese Subjects (SOS) is an ongoing inter-vention study of obesity that was started in 1987. At that time it was not known if long-term intentional weight loss would decrease the elevated morbidity and mortality of obesity. Thirteen years later we still do not know, and SOS is so far the only study that has been designed to answer this question. SOS results on hard endpoints such as myocardial in-farction and total mortality cannot be expected un-til 2004 to 2008, but several reports on changes in risk factors, cardiovascular function, health econ-omy and quality of life induced by intentional weight loss have been published. In this review, reference is given to the number of patients in the published reports rather than to currently (Febru-ary 2000) available patients (if not stated otherwise).

Some parts of this chapter overlap with a similar review in Swedish to be written for The Swedish Council on Technology Assessment in Health Care and with a review on obesity surgery printed in *Endocrine* (1).

SOS AIMS

The main goal of SOS is to examine if large and long-term intentional weight loss will reduce the elevated morbidity and mortality of obese subjects. Several secondary aims, related to the genetics of obesity, quality of life and health economics, have also been defined (2).

STUDY DESIGN

SOS originally consisted of one registry study and one intervention study (2). Later one randomized reference study and one genetic sib pair study were added.

In the registry study 6000–7000 obese men (BMI ≥ 34) and women (BMI ≥ 38) in the age range 37–60 years are examined by GPs at 480 of the 700 existing primary health care centres in Sweden. From the registry, patients are recruited into the intervention study consisting of one surgically treated group (goal $n = 2000$, February 2000, $n = 1870$) and one matched control group (same numbers) treated conventionally at the 480 primary health care centres. The surgically treated patients obtain (variable) banding, vertical banded gastrop-lasty (VBG) or gastric bypass (3) (Figures 35.1–35.3).

SOS is a matched and not a randomized study since, in 1987, ethical approval for randomization was not obtained due to the high operative mortal-ity (1–5%) observed in most surgical study groups from the 1970s and 1980s. Thus, partients choose for themselves if they want surgical or conventional treatment. When a surgical patient has been accep-ted according to a number of inclusion and exclu-sion criteria, a matching programme taking 18 dif-ferent matching variables into account selects the optimal control among eligible individuals in the registry study (2). The selection is based on an algo-rithm moving the mean values of the matching

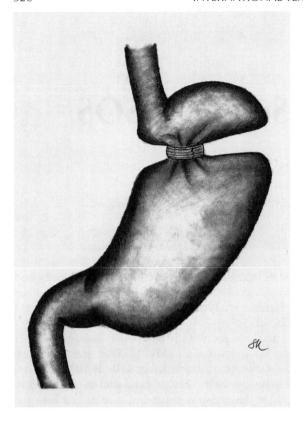

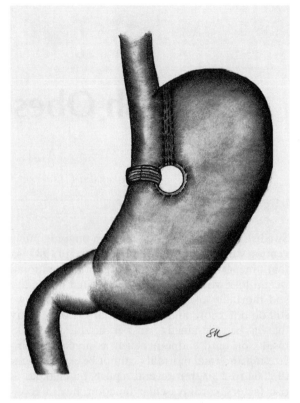

Figure 35.1 Gastric banding as originally described by Bö (59) and Solhaug (60). Later adjustable gastric banding was introduced (61–63). Copyright Sofia Karlsson and Lars Sjöström

Figure 35.2 Vertical banded gastroplasty as described by Mason (64, 65). Copyright Sophia Karlsson and Lars Sjöström

variables of the control group towards the current mean values of the surgically treated patients. Thus a group match rather than an individual match is undertaken. The participating centres cannot influence the matching programme.

The surgically treated patient and the control start the intervention on the operation day of the former. Both patients are examined just before inclusion and then after 0.5, 1, 2, 3, 4, 6, 8 and 10 years. According to the original protocol the follow-up was planned to be 10 years for both groups, but recently, it was decided to add one 15- and one 20-year examination. Centralized biochemistry is obtained at 0, 2, 10, 15 and 20 years. All visits are automatically booked by a computer at the SOS secretariat and all centres obtain the necessary forms, test tubes etc. for a given visit some weeks before the booked appointment. If information is not coming back as expected from patients or centres, the programme is automatically sending out reminders or asks the staff of the secretariat to solve the problem by phone.

WEIGHT LOSS

In one 2-year report on 767 surgically treated patients and 712 obese controls, the weight loss was 28 ± 15 kg (means $\pm$ SD) and 0.5 ± 8.9 kg, respectively (4). The percentage reductions after gastric bypass, VBG and banding were 33 ± 10, 23 ± 10 and $21 \pm 12\%$, respectively. Similar 2-year changes in body weight were recently reported for 1210 surgically treated and 1099 control subjects of SOS (5).

The energy intake before and during weight loss was studied by means of a validated dietary questionnaire (6,7) in 365 patient operated with VBG or banding and in 34 patients operated with gastric

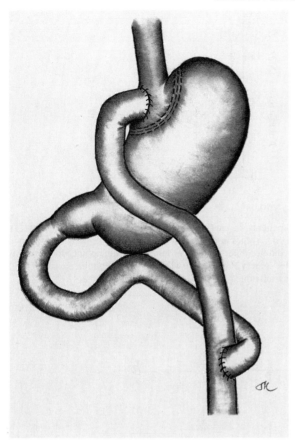

Figure 35.3   Gastric bypass as originally described by Mason (66,67) and later modified by several investigators (53,70–72). Copyright Sofia Karlsson and Lars Sjöström

bypass (8). Although the weight loss was 38.6 kg in the gastric bypass group but only 26.7 kg in the combined VBG and banding group, the energy intake before and after surgery did not differ between the groups (Figure 35.4). It has been shown that gastric bypass is associated with increased energy expenditure (9), perhaps due to an increased secretion of glucagon-like peptide 1 (GLP-1) (10,11).

In another report, 346 surgically treated patients and 346 controls were followed for 8 years (12). At 8 years, 251 surgically treated patients (73%) and 232 controls (67%) had completed the study. All dead individuals are included among non-completers since mortality figures are not yet released from the safety monitoring committee of SOS. Weight changes of completers in the four groups are shown in Figure 35.5. As in the 2-year report, there was no significant weight change in the control group while the surgically treated groups reached minimum

weights after one year. As expected, gastric bypass was more efficient than VBG and banding. Between the end of year 1 and the end of year 8, a slow relapse was seen in all of the surgically treated groups. However, as compared to inclusion, the surgically induced weight loss was still 20.1 ± 15.7 kg (16.5%) after 8 years, while the controls had increased their body weight 0.7 ± 12.0 kg. The difference in the 8-year body weight change between the two groups was highly significant ($P <$ 0.001).

Figure 35.5 illustrates also that conventional, non-pharmacological treatment of severe obesity is of little benefit when undertaken by non-specialized treatment units. This implies personal tragedies for millions of obese persons not having access to specialized treatment and immense consequences from a public health point of view.

SURGICAL COMPLICATIONS

Four postoperative deaths in 1870 operated patients have occurred in the SOS study (0.21%, February 2000). Three of these fatal cases were due to leakage that was detected too late. One death was caused by a technical mistake during a laparoscopic operation.

Peri- and postoperative complications have been calculated on 1164 patients followed for 4 years (13, and unpublished observations). During the primary stay at the hospital the following complications occurred: bleeding 0.5%, embolus and/or thrombosis 0.8%, wound complications 1.8%, deep infections (leakage, abscess) 2.1%, pulmonary 6.1%, other complications 4.8%. The number of complications was 193 and the number of patients with complications 151 (13%). In 26 patients (2.2%) the postoperative complications were serious enough to cause a reoperation.

Over 4 years 12% of the 1164 patients were reoperated, usually due to poor weight loss, but in some cases due to vomiting or other side effects. Usually banding and VBG were converted to gastric bypass but in some cases the original operation was repaired.

Over the 4 years a number of other operations were undertaken in both groups. In the control group 10.1 operations per 100 person-years were undertaken while the corresponding figures in the

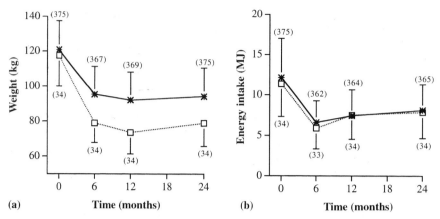

Figure 35.4 Weight loss (a) and energy intake (b) over 2 years in SOS patients who underwent gastropalsty (★) or gastric bypass (□). The gastroplasty operations were banding and VBG pooled. Mean ± SD. Values in parentheses indicate number of patients at each examination. Energy intake, estimated with validated technique (6,7), did not differ between groups at any time point. Body weights were significantly lower in gastric bypass patients at all time points after surgery P < 0.0001), whereas body weight before surgery did not differ significantly between groups. From Lindroos *et al.* (8) with permission

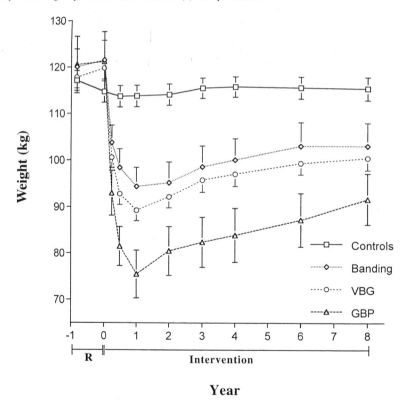

Figure 35.5 Weight change (95% CI) in 232 obese controls and 251 surgically treated patients from matching until end of year 8 in the SOS intervention study. Analysis based on completer population. R, registry study with collection of matching variables. Banding, *n* = 63. Vertical banded gastroplasty, VBG, *n* = 164, gastric bypass, GBP, *n* = 24. Each one of the surgical groups had a significantly (*P* < 0.01) larger weight reduction than the controls. From C.D. Sjöström *et al.* (12), with permission

Table 35.1 BMI and risk factors in 50-year-old men and women from SOS and in 50-year-old randomly selected reference subjects. Risk factor levels for other age groups, see Sjöström *et al.* (2)

	SOS males	Ref. males	*P* <	SOS females	Ref. females	*P* <
No.	102	220		121	398	
Age (years)	48–52	50		48–52	50	
BMI	37.3 ± 3.9	24.0		41.4 ± 4.4	24.8	
Systolic (mmHg)	146 ± 16	137 ± 22	0.001	147 ± 18	140 ± 22	0.01
Diastolic (mmHg)	94 ± 9	90 ± 14	0.01	89 ± 9	85 ± 11	0.001
Blood glucose (mmol/L)	5.9 ± 2.0	4.7 ± 1.3	0.001	5.5 ± 1.6	4.2 ± 0.9	0.001
Insulin (mU/L)	31 ± 25	9.6 ± 8.0	0.001	22 ± 12	14 ± 5	0.001
Triglycerides (mmol/L)	2.7 ± 2.0	1.3 ± 0.8	0.001	2.0 ± 1.0	1.3 ± 0.6	0.001
HDL cholesterol (mmol/L)	1.2 ± 0.4	1.6 ± 0.4	0.001	1.4 ± 0.4	—	
Total cholesterol (mmol/L)	6.2 ± 1.2	6.4 ± 1.3	NS	6.1 ± 1.1	7.2 ± 1.1	0.001

From L. Sjöström *et al.* (2), with permission.

surgical groups was 15.2. Operations due to ventral hernia, gallbladder disease, intestinal obstruction and surplus of skin were more common in the surgical group while, on average, operations due to malignancy, gynaecological disorders and all other reasons taken together were more common in the control group.

RISK FACTORS AT BASELINE

In an early cross-sectional analysis of 450 men and 556 women from the registry study of SOS it was shown that as compared to randomly selected controls most cardiovascular risk factors were elevated in the obese (Table 35.1) (2). The exception was total cholesterol, which was similar in obese and non-obese males and lower in obese women as compared to reference women.

Later, risk factors have also been analysed in relation to body composition in 1083 men and 1367 women from the SOS registry study (14). This analysis revealed one body compartment–risk factor pattern and one subcutaneous adipose tissue distribution–risk factor pattern. Within the first pattern risk factors were positively and strongly related to the visceral adipose tissue mass and, somewhat more weakly, also to the subcutaneous adipose tissue mass. Some risk factors, such as glucose and triglycerides in men and insulin in women, were negatively related to lean body mass. In addition, the subcutaneous adipose tissue distribution was related to risk factors both when and when not taking the body compartments into account statis-

tically. A preponderance of subcutaneous adipose tissue in the upper part of the trunk, as indicated by the neck circumference, was positively related to risk factors while the thigh circumference was negatively related to risk factors. These two risk factor patterns have also been observed longitudinally, i.e. changes in risk factors and changes in body composition and adipose tissue distribution are related (15) in the same way as in the cross-sectional observations (14).

RISK FACTOR CHANGES

In a 2-year report of 282 men and 560 women, pooled from the surgically treated group and the control group, risk factor changes were examined as a function of weight change (15). Ten kilogram weight loss was enough to introduce clinically significant reductions in all traditional risk factors except total cholesterol (Figure 35.6). Although it is known that total cholesterol is reduced short term (1–6 months) by moderate weight losses (16,17), Figure 35.6 illustrates that 30 to 40 kg maintained weight loss is required to achieve a preserved reduction in total serum cholesterol after 2 years.

In another 2-year report on 767 surgically treated patients and 712 controls, the weight loss of the surgical group resulted in dramatic reductions in the incidence of hypertension, diabetes, hyperinsulinaemia, hypertriglyceridaemia and low HDL cholesterol (4) (Figure 35.7). In the case of diabetes a 32-fold risk reduction was observed while the incidence of other risk conditions was reduced 2.6- to

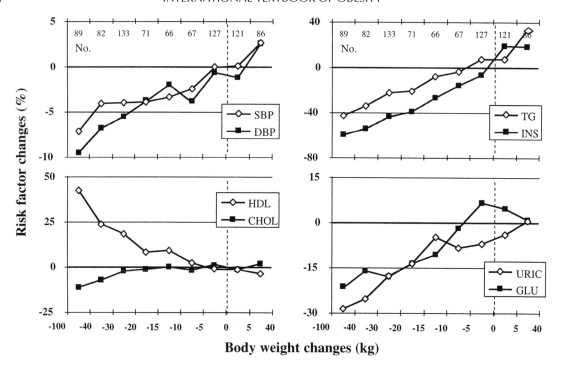

Figure 35.6 Adjusted risk factor changes (%) in relation to body weight changes (kg) over 2 years in 842 obese men and women pooled from the surgically treated group and the obese control group of the SOS Intervention study. The percentage change in each risk factor was adjusted for the basal value of that risk factor, initial body weight, sex, age and height. The number of subjects in each weight-changing class is shown at the top of the figure (as No). SBP and DBP, systolic and diastolic blood pressure; HDL, serum HDL cholesterol; CHOL, serum total cholesterol; TG, serum triglycerides; INS, serum insulin; URIC, serum uric acid; GLU, blood glucose. All serum samples collected after overnight fast. From C.D. Sjöström *et al.* (14), with permission

10-fold. In analogy with Figure 35.6, weight loss had no effect on the incidence of hypercholesterolaemia (figure 35.7). To give a visual impression of the weight loss necessary to prevent development of diabetes, the surgically treated group and the control group were pooled and the diabetes incidence plotted by decentiles of weight change (18). As can be seen in Figure 35.8, weight changes close to zero were associated with a 2-year diabetes incidence of 7–9%. A Mean weight loss of 7% was still associated with a 2-year diabetes incidence of 3% while no new cases of diabetes were seen for mean weight losses 12% or larger.

In the 8-year follow up (12) the incidence of diabetes was still five times lower in the surgical group than in the control group (figure 35.9). However, there was no difference between the two groups with respect to the 8-year incidence of hypertension (Figure 35.9). This was the case with or without multiple adjustments in the completer population as well as in the intention-to-treat population (12).

In a follow-up study, the final blood pressure has been shown to be closely related to recent weight changes and the length of the follow-up but more weakly associated with initial weight and the initial weight loss (19).

Unpublished 10-year data from SOS show that insulin, glucose, triglycerides and HDL cholesterol are improved by surgical treatment while blood pressure and total cholesterol are not.

While short-term weight losses improve all cardiovascular risk factors (see Figure 35.6 and (16,17)), several observational epidemiological studies have shown an association between weight loss and increased total as well as cardiovascular mortality, even in those who were obese at baseline (20). This discrepancy has usually been explained by the inability of observational studies to separate intentional from unintentional weight loss. Williamson has provided some evidence for this in women (21) but not in men (22). The 8-year study discussed above (12) suggests another possibility: long term,

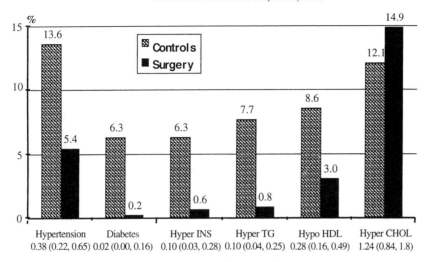

Figure 35.7   Two-year unadjusted incidence of indicated conditions in 712 obese controls (striped bars) and in 767 surgically treated completers (filled bars) from the SOS intervention study. Below bars, Odds Ratios (95% CI) adjusted for baseline values of age, sex, weight smoking and matching value of perceived health. $P < 0.001$ for all differences between groups except for hypercholesterolemia. Abbreviations as in Figure 35.6. From C.D. Sjöström *et al.* (4), with permission

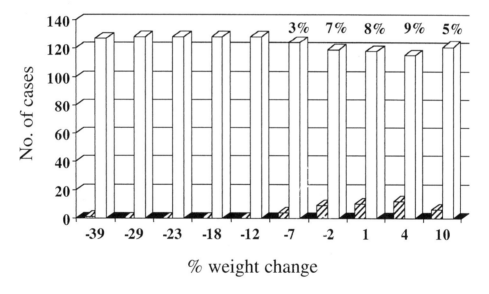

Figure 35.8.   Two-year incidence of diabetes by decentile of percentage weight change in the SOS intervention study. Pooled data from 1281 obese controls and surgically treated subjects not having diabetes at baseline. Striped bars indicate new cases of diabetes. At bottom, the average percentage weight change within each decentile. At top, the 2-year incidence of diabetes within each weight change decentile. Data based on ref. (4) and figure reproduced from C.D. Sjöström (18), with permission

some risk factors, such as blood pressure, may relapse in spite of maintained weight loss.

A third explanation may be that non-traditional risk factors deteriorate during weight loss. Recently, 10-year data from SOS have demonstrated that homocysteine increases with increasing weight loss, independent of method of weight loss (surgery or conventional), also when adjusting for changes in folate and B_{12} (23). Homocysteine levels have been shown to be related to cardiovascular mortality (24). Since homocysteine and folate are negatively related and since folate intake is reduced during

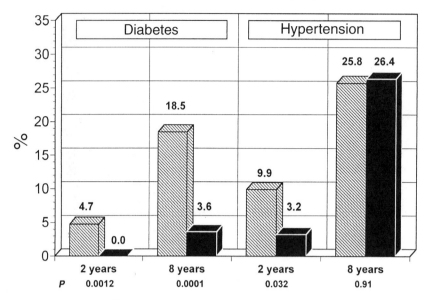

Figure 35.9 Two- and 8-year unadjusted incidence of diabetes and hypertension in 232 obese controls (striped bars) and 251 surgically treated patients (filled bars) from the SOS intervention study. Calculations based on completer population. Almost identical odds ratios were obtained with and without adjustments in completer and intention-to-treat populations (now shown). From C.D. Sjöström *et al.* (12), with permission

caloric restriction, our observations suggest that all weight-reducing treatments, whether surgical or not, should be accompanied by substitution with multivamin pills, folic acid and possibly B_{12} in order to counteract an increased incidence of cardiovascular disease due to hyperhomocystein-aemia.

EFFECTS ON THE CARDIOVASCULAR SYSTEM

In subsamples of the SOS study, cardiac function was examined at baseline and after 1 to 4 years of follow-up.

At baseline a surgically treated group ($n = 41$) and an obese control group ($n = 31$) were compared with a lean refrence group ($n = 43$) (25,26). As compared to lean subjects, the systolic and diastolic blood pressure, left ventricular mass and relative wall thickness were increased in the obese while the left ventricular ejection fraction (systolic function) and the E/A ratio (diastolic function) were decreased at baseline. After 1 year, all these variables had improved in the surgically treated group but not in the obese control group. When pooling the two obese groups and plotting left ventricular mass

or E/A ratio as a function of quintiles of weight change, a 'dose' dependency was revealed, i.e. the larger the weight reduction, the larger the reduction in left ventricular mass (Figure 35.10) and the more pronounced the improvement in diastolic function (Figure 35.11). Unchanged weight was in fact associated with a measurable deterioration in diastolic function over 1 year.

In other small subgroups from SOS, heart rate variability from 24-hour Holter ECG recordings and 24-hour catecholamine secretion were examined (27). As compared to lean subjects, our examinations indicated an increased sympathetic activity and a withdrawal of vagal activity at baseline. Both these disturbances were normalized in the surgically treated group but not in the obese control group after 1 year of treatment.

Furthermore, questionnaire data from 1210 surgically treated patients and 1099 obese SOS controls examined at baseline and after 2 years were analysed with respect to various cardiovascular symptoms (5). At baseline the two groups were comparable in most respects. After 2 years, dyspnoea and chest discomfort were reduced in a much larger fraction of surgically treated as compared to controls. For instance, 87% of the surgically treated reported baseline dyspnoea when climbing two flights of stairs while only 19% experienced such

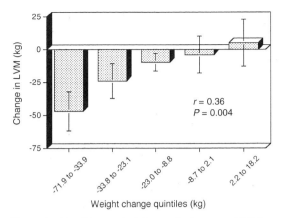

Figure 35.10 Changes in left ventricular mass (LVM) as a function of 1-year weight change quintiles (kg) in the SOS intervention study. Mean ± SEM. Pooled echocardiographic data of 38 surgically treated patients and 25 obese controls. Correlation for trend based on individual observations ($n = 63$). From Karason *et al.* (25), with permission

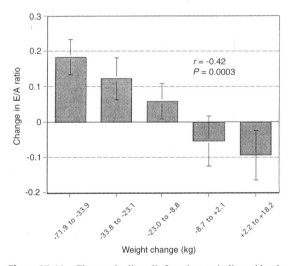

Figure 35.11 Changes in diastolic function, as indicated by the E/A ratio, in relation to 1-year weight change quintiles (kg) in the SOS intervention study. Mean ± SEM. Pooled transmitral Doppler data of 41 surgically treated patients and 30 obese controls. Correlation for trend based on individual observations ($n = 71$). From Karason *et al.* (26), with permission

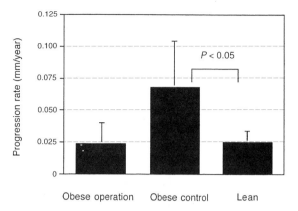

Figure 35.12 Annual progression rate of intima-media thickness in the carotid artery bulb in surgically treated obese patients ($n = 14$), obese controls ($n = 9$) and lean controls ($n = 27$) matched for gender, age and height. Mean ± SEM. Progression rate measured ultrasonographically over 4 years in the two obese groups and over 3 years in the lean reference group. The weight change was -22 ± 10 kg in the operated group and 0 ± 13 kg in the obese control group. From Karason *et al.* (28), with permission

Physical inactivity was observed in 46% of the surgically treated group before weight reduction but only in 17% after 2 years. Corresponding figures in the obese control group were 33 and 29%, respectively ($P < 0.001$) (5). Thus physical inactivity not only contributes to the development of obesity but obesity prevents physical activity. This vicious circle is broken by surgical treatment.

Finally, the intima-media thickness of the carotid bulb was examined by means of ultrasonography at baseline and after 4 years in the SOS intervention study (28). A randomly selected lean reference group matched for gender, age and height was examined at baseline and after 3 years. As shown in Figure 35.12 the annual progression rate was almost three times higher in the obese control group ($n = 9$) as compared to lean reference subjects ($P < 0.05$). In the surgically treated group, the progression rate was normalized. Although resuls from this small study group need to be confirmed in larger trials, this study nevertheless offers the first data on hard endpoints after intentional weight loss.

We have also shown that the pulse pressure increases more slowly in the surgically treated group than in the obese control group after a mean follow-up of 5.5 years (19). In gastric bypass individuals the pulse pressure is in fact decreasing. These observa-

dyspnoea at the 2-year follow-up. In the obese control group the corresponding figures were 69 and 57%, respectively ($P < 0.001$ for difference in change between groups).

Similarly, a high likelihood for sleep apnoea was observed in 23% of the surgically treated patients at baseline but only in 8% after 2 years of treatment. In the control group the corresponding figures were 22 and 20%, respectively ($P < 0.001$).

tions are of interest since it has been shown that, at a given systolic blood pressure, a high pulse pressure is associated with increased arterial stiffness (29), increased intima-media thickness (30) and increased cardiovascular mortality (31). Thus pulse pressure changes (19) as well as ultrasonographic measurements (28) indicate that surgical treatment is slowing down the increased atherosclerotic process in the obese.

ECONOMIC CONSEQUENCES OF OBESITY AND WEIGHT LOSS IN SOS

In cross-sectional studies of SOS patients it was shown that independent of age and gender, sick leave was twice as high and disability pensions twice as frequent as in the general Swedish population (32–34). The annual extra indirect costs (sick leave plus disability pension) attributable to obesity were estimated to be 6 billion SEK, or 1 million US dollars per 10 000 inhabitants per year.

The number of lost days due to sick leave and disability pension the year before inclusion into the SOS intervention was almost identical in the surgically treated group and the obese control group (104 and 107 days, respectively, Figure 35.13) (35). The year after inclusion the number of lost days were higher in the surgically treated group but over years 2 to 4 after inclusion the lost days were lower in the surgically treated group (figure 35.13). This was particularly evident in those individuals above median age (46.7 years) (not shown) (35).

The direct costs attributable to obesity and their changes after weight loss are currently being examined in the SOS study. So far we know that weight loss is associated with decreased costs for medication for diabetes and cardiovascular disease (36).

QUALITY OF LIFE BEFORE AND AFTER WEIGHT LOSS

Cross-sectional information from 800 obese men and 943 women of the SOS Registry study demonstrated that obese patients have a health-related quality of life (HRQL) that is much worse than in the age-matched reference groups (37). In fact, HRQL in the obese was as bad as, or even worse than, in patients with severe rheumatoid arthritis,

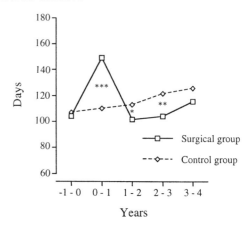

Figure 35.13 Days of sick leave plus disability pension per year in 369 surgically treated and 371 obese controls the year before inclusion and over 4 years after inclusion into the SOS intervention study. All data adjusted for age, gender, and several predictive variables. During years 1–4, the number of days are also adjusted for days of sick leave plus disability pension the year beforre inclusion. Significant differences between groups indicated as $*P < 0.05$, $**P < 0.01$, $***P < 0.001$. From Narbro *et al.* (35), with permission

generalized malignant melanoma or spinal cord injuries. The measurements were performed with general scales such as General Health Rating Index, Hospital Anciety and Depression scale, Mood Adjective Check List and Sickness Impact Profile in original or short form (37,38) and with an obesity-specific psychosocial scale (37). All scales have been validated during Swedish measuring conditions.

In 2- (39) and 4-year (see Chapter 33) reports, results from all measurement instruments are improving dose dependently, i.e. the larger the weight loss, the larger the improvement in HRQL, and in particular in the obesity-specific psychosocial scale (Figure 35.14).

OTHER STUDIES COMPARING NON-SURGICAL AND SURGICAL TREATMENT

While SOS has compared surgical treatment with treatment delivered by general practitioners at 480 primary heath care centres in Sweden (2), three other studies have compared surgical treatment with dietary treatment undertaken by more or less specialized obesity clinics (40–45).

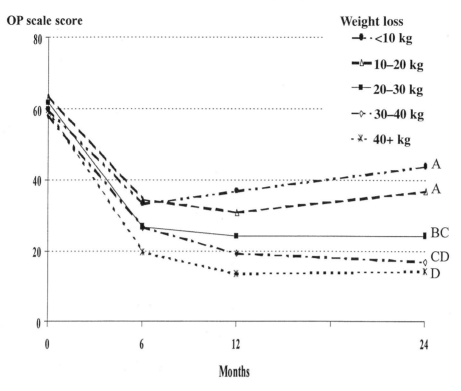

Figure 35.14 Obesity-related psychosocial problems in everyday life by weight reduction during 2 years intervention in the SOS study. Indicated weight change classes obtained after pooling of 487 surgically treated patients and 487 obese controls followed for 2 years. The psychosocial problems were estimated with the validated OP instrument. High scores represent dysfunction. Groups with different letters are significantly different at 2-year follow-up ($P < 0.05$, Turkey's range test). From Karlsson *et al.* (39), with permission

Jejuno-ileal Bypass vs. Diet

In 'The Danish Obesity Project' (40,41) 202 patients were randomized in the proportions 2:1 to jejuno-ileal bypass or diet treatment. Six patients never came to treatment. The remaining 130 surgically treated and 66 diet treated patients were followed for 2 to 3 years. After 2 years, the weight loss was 42.9 kg in the surgically treated group and 5.9 kg in the diet group. Quality of life as well as blood pressure were markedly improved in the surgical group. However, the surgical group had a large number of complications some of which were serious. As discussed below, jejuno-ileal bypass is no longer recommended due to serious side effects.

Horizontal Gasroplasty vs. VLCD Followed by Diet

In another early Danish study 60 patients were

randomized to horizontal gastroplasty or very low calorie diet (VLCD) followed by traditional dieting. A 2-year (42) and 5-year (43) report appeared in the mid-1980s. Unfortunately, less than 50% of the patients had in fact been followed for 2 and 5 years, respectively, when the reports were written. At 2 years the weight loss was 30.6 kg in the gastroplasty group and 8.2 kg in the VLCD/diet group. Weight losses are not reported at 5 years. Instead, a 'cumulated success rate' defined as more than 10 kg maintained weight loss was given. This success rate was 16% in the patients operated with horizontal gastroplasty and 3% in the VLCD/diet group. Horizontal gastroplasties are no longer in use due to poor long-term results (1,44,45).

Gastric Bypass vs. VLCD and Diet

In a prospective, non-randomized, non-matched study Martin *et al.* compared gastric bypass (GBP)

($n = 201$) with VLCD followed by diet ($n = 161$) 46). After VLCD, the diet group was offered one counselling session per week for 18 months and then annual follow-ups. The follow-up ranged from 2 to 6 years. At 6 years the follow-up rate was 34.5% in the GBP group and 19.7% in the VLCD/diet group. In the GBP group BMI dropped from 49.3 kg/m^2 to a minimum of 31.8 after 2 years. At 6 years BMI was 33.7 kg/m^2. In the VLCD/diet group the corresponding figures were 41.2, 32.1 and 38.5. As compared to VLCD/diet treatment, GBP thus resulted in twice as large a BMI drop and in a much smaller relapse.

BMI CUT-OFFS

At the consensus conference 1991, the National Institutes of Health (NIH) recommended that obesity surgery should be restricted to individuals with BMI ≥ 40 kg/m^2 although a somewhat lower cut-off could be accepted in subjects with pronounced metabolic complications (47). At that time the SOS project had already used the BMI cut-off 38 kg/m^2 for women and 34 kg/m^2 for men for 4 years. Our preliminary impression in the early 1990s did not make us change our cut-off and today it is obvious that a cut-off of 40 kg/m^2 leaves a larger fraction of the obese population virtually without efficient treatment and often in very bad shape in spite of the fact that new anti-obesity drugs have been added to the therapeutic arsenal.

In a preliminary report, Näslund (13) has analysed effects and complications in surgically treated SOS patients with BMI < 40 and BMI ≥ 40 kg/m^2. In absolute terms, weight loss was larger in the heavier group while this was not the case in relative terms. The frequency of complications was similar in both groups and from a risk factor point of view both groups benefited similarly from surgical treatment.

SURGICAL METHODS OF CHOICE

GBP results in larger weight loss than vertical banded gastroplasty (VBG) and gastric banding. The two latter techniques give similar weight reductions. Banding is associated with more reoperations than GBP and VBG. GBP is technically more de-

manding than VBG and banding and it results in iron and B$_{12}$ insufficiency that must be treated. It is not known whether GBP will cause negative calcium balance or other malabsorptive problems in a 10- to 30-year perspective. Such hypothetical problems are less likely with VBG and banding since these methods do not change the normal passage of food through the gastrointestinal tract. Finally, patients subjected to GBP cannot easily have their stomach examined endoscopically, which makes examinations of sucpect malignancy more complicated.

Taken together these circumstances suggest that GBP should be reserved for individuals with a considerable degree of obesity (BMI ≥ 40 kg/m^2) while VBG according to SOS experience can be used in the BMI interval 34–45 kg/m^2. Banding in its original form (SOS data) as well as all forms of horizontal gasroplasties (48) should not be used due to the increased need for revisions. Variable banding has not been evaluated in randomized studies but seems to have a place in the obesity therapy, particularly when used with laparoscopic techniques (49,50).

Several efficient techniques that have not been included in the SOS study have been developed. Jejuno-ileal bypass (JIB) is as effective as gasric bypass (51). However, JIB is associated with a large number of serious side effects and therefore not recommended any longer (52). The biliopancreatic diversion (53) is outstanding in achieving weight reduction but it is also associated with malabsorption of protein, fat-soluble vitamins and calcium (53,54). Treatment with this technique should be reserved for the heaviest (BMI > 45) and should only be undertaken by surgical departments (rather than individual surgeons) that are prepared to take a lifelong responsibility for the patients. The experience with biliopancratic diversion with duodenal switch (55) is still limited. It seems as if this technique is at least as efficient as the original biliopancreatic diversion and associated with less frequent and milder side effects (56,57).

Randomized studies comparing gastric bypass, biliopancreatic diversion and biliopancreatic diversion with duodenal switch are urgently needed. While randomized studies were fairly common in the early days of bariatric surgery no such studies seem to have been published since 1993 (1).

OVERALL CONCLUSIONS

The prevalence of obesity is high and rapidly increasing (58) and obesity is associated with a dramatically increased morbidity and mortality.

Surgery is the only obesity treatment resulting in more than 15% average weight loss over 10 years. This treatment has dramatic positive effects on most but not on all risk factors over a 10-year period. Large weight reductions achieved by surgery improve the cardiovascular system in several respects. Long-term direct and indirect costs seem to be reduced after surgical obesity treatment and quality of life is markedly improved.

Conventional treatment at specialized obesity units may achieve 5% weight loss over 2 to 5 years of follow-up. This is not enough to keep risk factors down long term. Non-pharmacological, conventional obesity treatment at primary health care centres is not associated with weight loss, short or long term (4,12), and unfortunately most obese patients worldwide have no access to specialized obesity treatment.

Treatment with currently available anti-obesity drugs results in 8–12% weight reduction over 2 years as compared to 4–6% in the placebo groups (16). This is encouraging even if more efficient drugs are needed in the future. So far no randomized drug trials with a longer duration than 2 years have been published.

Primary health care centres will constitute the worldwide basis for obesity treatment in the future. Within the next 5–10 years, treatment given by these centres will hopefully improve with better programmes and more efficient anti-obesity drugs.

There is an urgent need for one specialized obesity centre per approximately 500 000 inhabitants. At these centres, internists, nurses and dietitians need to work full-time with obese subjects referred to them from GPs. The demand for such treatment is almost unlimited. In a region with 500 000 inhabitants, obese patients overall will be in need of at least 20 000–30 000 visits annually.

While waiting for more efficient anti-obesity drugs, the surgical treatment of obesity must increase dramatically. The real need is 500–1000 operations annually per 500 000 inhabitants in most Western countries, even if the current demand for operations is smaller. All obese patients with BMI $\geq 40\,\mathrm{kg/m^2}$ need detailed information on surgical treatment options and a very large number of individuals with BMI above as well as below $40\,\mathrm{kg/m^2}$ will benefit from surgical treatment. Surgical treatment is particularly important in obese patients with associated cardiovascular risk factors.

REFERENCES

1. Sjöström L. Surgical intervention as a strategy for treatment of obesity. *Endocrine* (Suppl): 2000; in press.
2. Sjöström L, Larsson B, Backman L, Bengtsson C, Bouchard C, Dahlgren S, *et al.* Swedish Obese Subjects (SOS). Recruitment for an intervention study and a selected description of the obese state. *Int J Obes Relat Metab Disord* 1992; **16**: 465–479.
3. Deitel M. *Surgery for the Morbidity Obese Patient.* Philadelphia: Lea & Febiger, 1989.
4. Sjöström CD, Lissner L, Wedel H, Sjöström L. Reduction in incidence of diabetes, hypertension and lipid disturbances after intentional weight loss induced by bariatric surgery: the SOS Intervention Study. *Obes Res* 1999; **7**: 477–484.
5. Karason K, Lindroos AK, Stenlöf K, Sjöström L. Relief of cardiorespiratory symptoms and increased physical activity after surgically induced weight loss. Results from the SOS study. *Arch Intern Med* 2000; **160**: 1797–1802.
6. Lindroos AK, Lissner L, Sjöström L. Validity and reproducibility of a self-administered dietary questionnaire in obese and non-obese subjects. *Eur J Clin Nutr* 1993; **47**: 461–481.
7. Lindroos AK, Lissner L, Sjöström L. Does degree of obesity influence the validity of reported energy and protein intake? Resultws from the SOS dietary questionnaire. *Eur J Clin Nutr* 1999; **53**: 375–378.
8. Lindroos Ak, Lissner L, Sjöström L. Weight change in relation to intake of sugar and sweet foods before and after weight reducing gastric surgery. *Int J Obes Relat Metab Disord* 1996; **20**: 634–643.
9. Flancbaum L, Choban PS, Bradley LR, Burge JC. Changes in measured resting energy expenditure after Roux-en-Y gastric bypass for clinically severe obesity. *Surgery* 1997; **122**: 943–994.
10. Mason EE. Ileal [correction of ilial] transposition and enteroglucagon/GLP-1 in obesity (and diabetic?) surgery. *Obes Surg* 1999; **9**: 223–228.
11. Orskov C, Poulsen SS, Moller M, Holst JJ. Glucagon-like peptide I receptors in the subfornical organ and the area postrema are accessible to circulating glucagon-like peptide I. *Diabetes* 1996; **45**: 832–835.
12. Sjöström CD, Peltonen M, Wedel H, Sjöström L. Differentiated long-term effects of intentional weight loss on diabetes and hypertension. *Hypertension* 2000; **36**: 20–21.
13. Näslund I. Effects and side-effects of obesity surgery in patients with BMI below and above 40 in the SOS study. *Int J Obes* 1998; **22** (Suppl 3): S52.
14. Sjöström CD, Håkangård AC, Lissner L, Sjöström L. Body compartment and subcutaneous adipose tissue distribution—risk factor patterns in obese subjects. *Obes Res* 1995; **3**: 9–22.

15. Sjöström CD, Lissner L, Sjöström L. Relationships between changes in body composition and changes in cardiovascular risk factors: the SOS Intervention Study. Swedish Obese Subjects. *Obes Res* 1997; **5**: 519–530.

16. Sjöström L, Rissanen A, Andersen T, Boldrin M, Golay A, Koppeschaar HP, *et al.* Randomised placebo-controlled trial of orlistat for weight loss and prevention of weight regain in obese patients. European Multicentre Orlistat Study Group [see also editorial]. *Lancet* 1998; **352**: 167–172.

17. Wadden TA, Anderson DA, Foster GD. Two-year changes in lipids and lipoproteins associated with the maintenance of a 5% to 10% reduction in initial weight: some findings and some questions. *Obes Res* 1999; **7**: 170–178.

18. Sjöström CD. Effects of surgically induced weight loss on cardiovascular risk factors (PhD thesis). Göteborg: Göteborg University, 2000: 1–87.

19. Sjöström CD, Peltonen M, Sjöström L. Blood and blood pressure during long-term weight-loss in the obese: the SOS intervention study.

20. Pamuk ER, Williamson DF, Serdula MK, Madans J, Byers TE. Weight loss and subsequent death in a cohort of US adults. *Ann Intern Med* 1993; **119**: 744–748.

21. Williamson DF, Pamuk E, Thun M, Flanders D, Byers T, Heath C. Prospective study of intentional weight loss and mortality in never-smoking overweight US white women aged 40–64 years [published erratum appears in *Am J Epidemiol* 1995 Aug 1; **142**: 369]. *Am J Epidemiol* 1995; **141**: 1128–1141.

22. Williamson DF, Pamuk E, Thun M, Flanders D, Heath C, Byers T. Prospective study of intentional weight loss and mortality in overweight men aged 40–64 years (Abstract). *Obes Res* 1997; **5**(Suppl): 94.

23. Jacobson P, Lindroos AK, Sjöström CD, Sjöström L. Long-term changes in serum homocystein following weight loss in the SOS study (Abstract). *Int J Obes* 2000; in press.

24. Moghadasian MH, McManus BM, Frohlich JJ. Homocyst(e)ine and coronary artery disease. Clinical evidence and genetic and metabolic background [published erratum appears in *Arch Intern Med* 1998 Mar 23; 158: 662]. *Arch Intern Med* 1997; **157**: 2299–2308.

25. Karason K, Wallentin I, Larsson B, Sjöström L. Effects of obesity and weight loss on left ventricular mass and relative wall thickness: survey and intervention study. *BMJ* 1997; **315**: 912–916.

26. Karason K, Wallentin I, Larsson B, Sjöström L. Effects of obesity and weight loss on cardiac function and valvular performance. *Obes Res* 1998; **6**: 422–429.

27. Karason K, Molgaard H, Wikstrand J, Sjöström L. Heart rate variability in obesity and the effect of weight loss. *Am J Cardiol* 1999; **83**: 1242–1247.

28. Karason K, Wikstrand J, Sjöström L, Wendelhag I. Weight loss and progresion of early atherosclerosis in the carotid artery: a four-year controlled study of obese subjects. *Int J Obes Relat Metab Disord* 1999; **23**: 948–956.

29. Nichols WW, O'Rourke MF. *McDonald's Blood Flow in Arteris.* Philadelphia: Lea & Febiger, 1998.

30. Boutouyrie P, Bussy C, Lacolley P, Girerd X, Laloux B, Laurent S. Association between local pulse pressure mean blood pressure, and large-artery remodeling. *Circulation* 1999; **100**: 1387–1393.

31. Franklin SS, Khan SA, Wong ND, Larson MG, Levy D. Is pulse pressure useful in predicting risk for coronary heart disease? The Framingham heart study. *Circulation* 1999; **100**: 354–360.

32. Narbro K, Jonsson E, Waaler H, Wedel H, Sjöström L. Economic consequences of sick leave and disability pension in obese Swedes (Abstract). *Int J Obes* 1994; **18**(Suppl 2): 14.

33. Sjöström L, Narbro K, Sjöström D. Costs and benefits when treating obesity. *Int J Obes Relat Metab Disord* 1995; **19** (Suppl 6): S9–12.

34. Narbro K, Jonsson E, Larsson B, Waaler H, Wedel H, Sjöström L. Economic consequences of sick-leave and early retirement in obese Swedish women. *Int J Obes Relat Metab Disord* 1996; **20**: 895–903.

35. Narbro K, Ågren G, Jonsson E, Larsson B, Näslund I, Wedel H, *et al.* Sick leave and disability pension before and after treatment for obesity: a report from the Swedish Obese Subjects (SOS) study. *Int J Obes* 1999; **23**: 619–624.

36. Narbro K, Ågren G, Näslund I, Sjöström L, Peltonen M. Decreased medication for diabetes and cardiovascular disease after weight loss (Abstract). *Int J Obes* 2000; in press.

37. Sullivan M, Karlsson J, Sjöström L, Backman L, Bengtsson C, Bouchard C, *et al.* Swedish Obese Subjects (SOS)—an intervention study of obesity. Baseline evaluation of health and psychosocial functioning in the first 1743 subjects examined. *Int J Obes Relat Metab Disord* 1993; **17**: 503–512.

38. Karlsson J, Sjöström L, Sullivan M. Swedish Obese Subjects (SOS)—an intervention study of obesity. Measuring psychosocial factors and health by means of short-form questionnaires. Results from a method study. *J Clin Epidemiol* 1995; **48**: 817–823.

39. Karlsson J, Sjöström L, Sullivan M. Swedish Obese Subjects (SOS)—an intervention study of obesity. Two-year follow-up of health-related quality of life (HRQL) and eating behavior after gastric surgery for severe obesity. *Int J Obes Relat Metab Disord* 1998; **22**: 113–126.

40. The Danish Obesity Project: Randomised trial of jejunoileal bypass versus medical treatment in morbid obesity. *Lancet* 1979; **ii**: 1255–1258.

41. Stokholm KH, Nielsen PE, Quaade F. Correlation between initial blood pressure and blood pressure decrease after weight loss: A study in patients with jejunoileal bypass versus medical treatment for morbid obesity. *Int J Obes* 1982; **6**: 307–312.

42. Andersen T, Backer OG, Stokholm KH, Quaade F. Randomized trial of diet and gastroplasty compared with diet alone in morbid obesity. *N Engl J Med* 1984; **310**: 352–356.

43. Andersen T, Stokholm KH, Backer OG, Quaade F. Long-term (5-year) results after either horizontal gastroplasty or very-low-calorie diet for morbid obesity. *Int J Obes* 1988; **12**: 277–284.

44. Lechner GW, Elliott DW. Comparison of weight loss after gastric exclusion and partitioning. *Arch Surg* 1983; **118**: 685–692.

45. Pories WJ, Flickinger EG, Meelheim D, Van Rij AM, Thomas FT. The effectiveness of gastric bypass over gastric partition in morbid obesity: consequence of distal gastric and duodenal exclusion. *Ann Surg* 1982; **196**: 389–399.

46. Martin LF, Tan Tl, Horn JR, Bixler EO, Kauffman GL, Becker DA, *et al.* Comparison of the costs associated with medical and surgical treatment of obesity. *Surgery* 1995; **118**: 599–606.

47. NIH. Gastrointestinal surgery for severe obesity: National Institutes of Health Consensus Development Conference Statement, March 25–27, 1991. *Am J Clin Nutr* 1992; **55**(suppl): 615S–619S.

48. Sugerman HJ, Wolper JL. Failed gastroplasty for morbid obesity. Revised gastroplasty versus Roux-Y gastric bypass. *Am J Surg* 1984; **148**: 331–336.

49. Belachew M, Legrand M, Vincent V, Lismonde M, Le Docte N, Deschamps V. Laparoscopic adjustable gastric banding. *World J Surg* 1998; **22**: 955–963.

50. Fried M, Peskova M, Kasalicky M. Assessment of the outcome of laparoscopic nonadjustable gastric banding and stoma adjustable gastric banding: surgeon's and patient's view. *Obes Surg* 1998; **8**: 45–48.

51. Griffen WO, Jr, Young VL, Stevenson CC. A prospective comparison of gastric and jejunoileal bypass procedures for morbid obesity. *Ann Surg* 1977; **186**: 500–509.

52. O'Leary JP. Gastrointestinal malabsorptive procedures. *Am J Clin Nutr* 1992; **55**(2 Suppl): 567S–570S.

53. Scopinaro N, Gianette E, Adami GF, Friedman D, Traverso E, Marinari GM, *et al.* Biliopancreatic diversion for obesity at eighteen years. *Surgery* 1996; **119**: 261–268.

54. Chapin BL, LeMar HJ, Jr, Knodel DH, Carter PL. Secondary hyperparathyroidism following biliopancrteatic diversion. *Arch Surg* 1996; **131**: 1048–1052; discussion 53.

55. Hess DS.Biliopancreatic diversion with duodenal switch procedure (Abstract). *Obes Surg* 1994; **4**: 105.

56. Marceau P, Hould FS, Simard S, Lebel S, Bourque RA, Potvin M, *et al.* Biliopancreatic diversion with duodenal switch. *World J Surg* 1998; **22**: 947–954.

57. Rabkin RA. Distal gastric bypass/duodenal switch procedure, Roux-en-Y gastric bypass and biliopancreatic diversion in a community practice. *Obes Surg* 1998; **8**: 53–59.

58. World Health Organization. *Obesity. Preventing and Managing the Global Epidemic.* WHO/NUT/NCD/98.1 ed. Geneva: WHO, 1998.

Index